CABINET
181 Wyckoff Street
Brooklyn, NY 11217 USA
phone + 1 718 222-8434
fax + 1 718 222-3700
info@cabinetmagazine.org
www.cabinetmagazine.org

Issue 61, Spring–Summer 2016

Cover: Detail from a Lakota "winter count" calendar. Pictographic histories typically inscribed on animal hide, winter counts were maintained by "the calendar keeper," an individual charged with selecting, often in consultation with tribal elders, one particularly memorable event from the past year to represent the entire year. Each year's pictograph was added to those of previous years, producing a sequential chronicle that could be used to remember and recount the collective history of the particular band, or *tiošpaye*, comprising some 150 to 300 individuals. These calendars were known to the Lakota as *waniyetu wowapi*: *waniyetu* meaning "year," which they measured from first snowfall to first snowfall, and is therefore often translated as "a winter," and *wowapi*, meaning anything that is marked on a flat surface and can be read or counted.

The winter count depicted here is a copy of one kept on cloth by Battiste Good, a Brulé Lakota who was the calendar keeper for his band. Good, whose Indian name Wapóštangi translates as Brown Hat, made the copy on nineteen pages in a sketchbook in 1880 at the request of Army surgeon William H. Corbusier. The numbers, which would not have been used in the original, are in Good's hand and list the years, as well as certain clarifying details. Before dying, the calendar keeper would usually designate a successor, often a son or a nephew; after the death of Good, who lived on the Rosebud Reservation in present-day South Dakota, his son High Hawk took over his duties as keeper of the band's winter count.

The detail reproduced here depicts years from the mid-eighteenth century, including 1742 ("attacked-them-while-gathering-turnips winter"), the drawing for which depicts an attack on a group of women from the band, and 1764 ("many-sticks-for-drying-beef winter"), whose pictograph commemorates a year in which the band had so much meat to dry that the entire village was crowded with drying racks.

POSTMASTER
Please send address changes to Cabinet, 181 Wyckoff Street, Brooklyn, NY 11217.

Cabinet (USPS # 020-348, ISSN 1531-1430) is a quarterly magazine published by Immaterial Incorporated, 181 Wyckoff Street, Brooklyn, NY 11217. Periodicals Postage paid at Brooklyn, NY, and additional mailing offices.

Printed in Belgium by Die Keure, a printer for all seasons.

ADVERTISING
phone + 1 718 222-8434
advertising@cabinetmagazine.org

DISTRIBUTION
Cabinet is available in the US and Canada through Disticor, which distributes both using its own network and through Ingram, Ubiquity, Small Changes, Cowley Distribution, Kent News, MSolutions, the News Group, Chris Stadler, and Don Olson Distribution.

To carry Cabinet through one of these distributors, contact Melanie Raucci at Disticor: phone + 1 631 587-1160, mraucci@disticor.com

Cabinet is available in Europe and elsewhere through Central Books, London: orders@centralbooks.com

Cabinet is available worldwide as a book, with an ISBN, through DAP: phone + 1 212 627-1999, dap@dapinc.com

For further information, contact: circulation@cabinetmagazine.org

INDIVIDUAL SUBSCRIPTIONS

1 year (4 issues):	2 years (8 issues):
US $32	US $60
Canada $38	Canada $72
Western Europe $40	Western Europe $76
Elsewhere $50	Elsewhere $96

Please send a check in US dollars made out to "Cabinet," or mail, fax, or email us your Visa/MC/AmEx/Discover info to:

181 Wyckoff Street
Brooklyn, NY 11217 USA
phone + 1 718 222-8434
fax + 1 718 222-3700
subscriptions@cabinetmagazine.org
www.cabinetmagazine.org/subscribe

INSTITUTIONAL SUBSCRIPTIONS
Institutional subscriptions are available through library agencies such as EBSCO, or directly from Cabinet:
www.cabinetmagazine.org/subscribe

SUBMISSIONS
We only accept submissions via email. Guidelines available at:
www.cabinetmagazine.org/information/submissions.php

Editor-in-chief
Sina Najafi

Senior editor
Jeffrey Kastner

Editors
D. Graham Burnett, Christopher Turner

UK editor
Brian Dillon

Associate director
Kelley Deane McKinney

Art director
Everything Studio

Associate editor
Julian Lucas

Editorial assistant
Evdoxia Ragkou

Website directors
Ryan O'Toole, Luke Murphy

Editors-at-large
Saul Anton, Sasha Archibald, Mats Bigert, Brian Conley,
Christoph Cox, Jeff Dolven, Leland de la Durantaye, Jesse Lerner,
Jennifer Liese, Ryo Manabe, Alexander Nagel, Sally O'Reilly, George
Prochnik, Frances Richard, Daniel Rosenberg, Aaron Schuster, David
Serlin, Debra Singer, Justin E. H. Smith, Margaret Sundell, Allen S.
Weiss, Eyal Weizman, Margaret Wertheim, Gregory Williams,
Jay Worthington, Tirdad Zolghadr

Contributing editors
Molly Blieden, Eric Bunge, Pip Day, Charles Green, Adam Jasper,
Srdjan Jovanovic Weiss, Lytle Shaw, Cecilia Sjöholm, Carl Michael
von Hausswolff, Sven-Olov Wallenstein

Digital Artist-in-Residence
Ryota Sato

Events
Bryony Quinn (London)

Cabinet national librarian
Matthew Passmore

Erratum:
Charlie Fox's "A Mind of Winter" (Cabinet no. 59) mistakenly
stated that the photographs of Robert Walser's body lying in the
snow after his death were taken by Walser's friend Carl Seelig.
They were in fact taken by a medical examiner.

Cabinet is a non-profit 501(c)(3) magazine published by Immaterial
Incorporated. Our survival depends on support from generous
foundations and individuals. Please consider supporting us at whatever
level you can. Donations are tax-deductible for those who deal with
Uncle Sam. All gifts are acknowledged online. Contributions of $25
or more will be acknowledged in the next possible issue; those above
$100 will be noted in four issues. Checks to "Cabinet" can be sent to
our office; please write "This will make winter feel like autumn" on the
envelope.

Cabinet wishes to thank the following visionary foundations and
individuals for their support of our activities during 2016–2017.
Additionally, we will forever be indebted to the extraordinary
contribution of the Flora Family Foundation from 1999 to 2004;
without their support, this publication would not exist. We would
also like to extend our enormous gratitude to the Orphiflamme
Foundation and the Opaline Fund for their generous support.

$100,000
The Lambent Foundation

$50,000
The Warhol Foundation for Visual Arts

$15,000
The New York City Department of Cultural Affairs

$10,000
The National Endowment for the Arts

$8,000
The New York State Council on the Arts

$6,000
Margaret Sundell & Reinaldo Laddaga

$3,000
The Danielson Foundation

$1,500–$2,500
Stina & Herant Katchadourian, Terry Winters

$501–$1,000
Anonymous, Martha & Thomas G. Armstrong, Sara Clugage,
Spencer Finch, Steven Rand & Nancy Wender, Christian
Scheidemann, Sandy Tait & Hal Foster

$500 or under
Pamela Cederquist, Steven Igou, Deborah Lovely, Meredith Martin
& Joshua Siegel & Maisie Martin Siegel, Lenore & Richard Niles

$250 or under
Tauba Auerbach, Jeff Beall, Freya Cooper Kiddie, Mia Enell &
Nicholas Fries, George Ganat, Jair Gonzalez, Alex Goodfriend,
Cynthia Hansen, Peter Hapstak, Peter Jaszi, Craig Kalpakjian,
James Katzenberger, Carin Kuoni & John Oakes, Scott LeBouef,
Tod Lippy, Deborah Lovely, Paul McConnell, Elizabeth Merena,
Helen Mirra, Jason Olin, Andrew Pederson, John Sargent, Eric
Schmid, Pooja Shah & Rebecca Ward, John Sherburne, James Siena,
Debra Singer & Jay Worthington, Jude Tallichet & Matt Freedman,
Volker Welter, Margaret Wertheim

$100 or under
James Baker, Mark Bartlett, Zachary Cowan, Jeffrey Cunard,
Loic Darques. Joseph Fratesi, Cynthia Hansen, Fredrika Jacobs,
Paul Kehoe, Jim Martin, Marina McDougall, Jan Peuker, Catherine
Rogers, Gregory Shelnutt, Amanda Taylor, Pamela Tibbetts

CONTRIBUTORS

Saïda Bloom is a graduate student based in New York and Beirut. She is currently writing on fictitious calendrical systems in Middle Eastern literature.

D. Graham Burnett is an editor of *Cabinet* and teaches at Princeton University. Recent collaborative work includes "The Ketchem Screen" at Manifesta 11 in Zurich, and "Presenting and Representing the W-Cache" at the Museum of Jurassic Technology in Los Angeles. He is affiliated with the collective ESTAR(SER). For more information, visit <estarser.net>.

Brian Dillon is UK editor of *Cabinet*, and teaches critical writing at the Royal College of Art, London. His books include *The Great Explosion* (Penguin Books, 2015), *Objects in This Mirror: Essays* (Sternberg Press, 2014), *I Am Sitting in a Room* (Cabinet Books, 2012), and *The Hypochondriacs* (Faber & Faber, 2010). He writes regularly for *Artforum*, *frieze*, the *Guardian*, and the *London Review of Books*. He is working on a book about essays and essayists.

Nicholas Gaskill is an assistant professor in the Department of English at Rutgers University, New Brunswick, where he teaches nineteenth- and twentieth-century US literature, visual culture, and philosophy. He is currently writing a book on theories of color experience in the era of aniline dyes.

Byron Ellsworth Hamann teaches art history at Ohio State University. He is an editor of *Grey Room*; codirector (with Liza Bakewell) of "Mesolore: Exploring Mesoamerican Culture"; project manager (for Dana Leibsohn and Barbara Mundy) of "Vistas: Visual Culture in Spanish America, 1520–1820"; and author of *The Translations of Nebrija: Language, Culture, and Circulation in the Early Modern World* (University of Massachusetts Press, 2015).

Adam Herring teaches art history at Southern Methodist University in Dallas. He is the author of *Art and Writing in the Maya Cities, AD 600–800: A Poetics of Line* (Cambridge University Press, 2005) and *Art and Vision in the Inca Empire: Andeans and Europeans at Cajamarca* (Cambridge University Press, 2015).

Adam Jasper is a postdoctoral researcher at Eikones NCCR Iconic Criticism, located in Basel. He is an editor of the *Architectural Theory Review*, and was recently guest coeditor of an issue of *Future Anterior*.

Agnieszka Kurant, a Polish artist based in New York, is currently a visiting artist at MIT's Center for Art, Science & Technology. Recent projects include a commission for the Guggenheim Museum, New York, and a solo exhibition at the Sculpture Center, New York. Her work has been exhibited at the Palais de Tokyo, Paris; Tate Modern, London; Moderna Museet, Stockholm; Witte de With, Rotterdam; Musée d'art moderne et contemporain, Geneva; and the Performa Biennial, New York, among others. In 2017, her work will be presented at the Guggenheim Bilbao and at the Kitchen, New York.

Justine Kurland is a New York–based photographer. Her debut monograph *Highway Kind*, published by Aperture, was released in the fall of 2016. She is represented by Mitchell-Innes & Nash gallery, New York.

Oliver Preston is a writer and designer living in Brooklyn.

Justin E. H. Smith writes from Paris. He is the author, most recently, of *The Philosopher: A History in Six Types* (Princeton University Press, 2016).

Christopher Turner is an editor of *Cabinet* and director of the London Design Biennale.

Allen S. Weiss has most recently published *The Grain of the Clay: Reflections on Ceramics and the Art of Collecting* (Reaktion Books, 2016). In 2016, he produced and directed, with Tom Rasky, *Poupées des ténèbres* (Dolls of Darkness), a documentary film on the art of Michel Nedjar in relation to the Holocaust.

Lawrence Weschler is the author of over a dozen books, including *Seeing Is Forgetting the Name of the Thing One Sees* (University of California Press, 1982; updated and expanded edition, 2008); *Mr. Wilson's Cabinet of Wonder* (Pantheon, 1995); *Vermeer in Bosnia* (Pantheon, 2004); and, most recently, *Waves Passing in the Night: Walter Murch in the Land of the Astrophysicists* (Bloomsbury USA, 2017). For more information, visit <lawrenceweschler.com>.

Tony Wood studies history at New York University. A member of the editorial board of *New Left Review*, he is the author of *Chechnya: The Case for Independence* (Verso Books, 2007) and is completing a book on Putin's Russia.

COLUMNS

INGESTION / THE HUNGER ARTISTS
Oliver Preston

"Ingestion" is a column that explores its topic within a framework informed by history, aesthetics, and philosophy.

———

A shrunken man, wearing only tights, sits on a bed of straw, in the middle of a cage. A throng of faces encircles the cage. They show mild amusement; they look up at the man for a few minutes before drawing back, satisfied. The children in the crowd stare more earnestly and for longer. A few faces are familiar to the man, though he rarely looks at them. They reappear beside the cage each day and, unlike the others, remain stiff with something—an expectation they themselves seem not to understand. The man is always being watched, if not by the passing spectators then by paid wardens, who are meant to enforce his pledge to live for forty days without food. When the wardens are not on their shifts authenticating the man's claim, they work in the town, we are told, as butchers.

This is the basic situation of Franz Kafka's "A Hunger Artist," a short story first published in a 1922 issue of the Berlin literary magazine *Die neue Rundschau* and later included in a 1924 collection, which took the story's name.[1] Like all of Kafka's stories, "A Hunger Artist" seems to visit us from another world. It is hermetic, to borrow Theodor Adorno's word. If it is a joke, its punch line is written in Morse code. If it is an allegory, its referents are irretrievable. Adorno offers that, reading Kafka, one might feel overcome by perpetual and unanswerable *déjà vu*. Apparently agreeing, Walter Benjamin insists that Kafka's writing belongs to a pre-mythical epoch.[2]

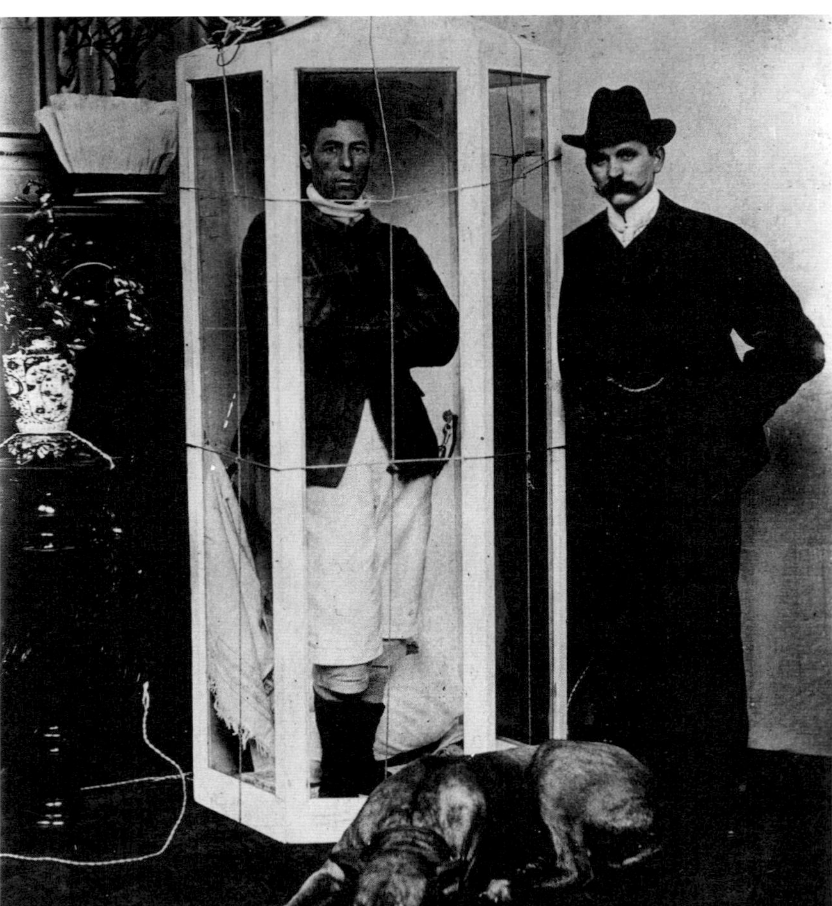

Hunger artist Papus, who was active around the turn of the twentieth century, is here pictured in his sealed glass box at the Passage-Panoptikum in Berlin. Courtesy bpk Bildagentur / Art Resource.

None of which is to say, however, that the figure of the hunger artist hails from the same cosmic no-place as the Odradek.[3] The first sentence of "A Hunger Artist," "During these last decades the interest in professional fasting has markedly diminished," might as well have been lifted from a newspaper article.[4] Beginning more or less precisely in 1880, hunger performances surged in popularity across Europe and the United States; by 1930, the fad was in decline. Kafka thus lived and died alongside the hunger artists. In the final years of the nineteenth century, the Italian Giovanni Succi toured Milan, Vienna, London, and New York, fasting for up to forty-five days at a time under the watch of journalists, medical examiners, and paying fans. Beginning in 1906, Clare de Serval, the "Apostle of Hunger" from Berlin, repeatedly shut herself inside a specially made glass box for weeks at a time in an attempt to prove the health benefits of self-starvation, telling one reporter that she was always reluctant to break her fasts.[5] Another Berliner, Siegfried Hertz, faced prosecution when it was discovered that a wire connected to his radio—one of the few furnishings in his fasting box—was in fact a straw through which the performer had been furtively sipping hot chocolate. Kafka likely saw a 1916 report on a hunger artist in the *Prager Tagblatt*, a newspaper in Prague that he read often. That he himself saw a hunger

performance is not entirely out of the question.[6]

Though in one sense it is. Nobody, after all, can see a hunger performance. To witness more than an excerpt would require an endurance outmatching the faster's. One would have to stay awake while the faster slept, eyes never relinquishing their hold on the body before them, tracking all the countless movements—accidental or gestural, brief or sustained—that make up the material of its slow, staged diminution. "No one could possibly watch the hunger artist continuously, day and night," Kafka writes, "and so no one could produce first-hand evidence that the fast had really been rigorous and continuous; only the artist himself could know that, he was therefore bound to be the sole completely satisfied spectator of his own fast."[7]

But then it seems that the appeal of the hunger artist resides only in his authenticity—satisfaction, here, is critical. The spectators face a paradox. In order to determine that the hunger artist is worthy of being watched in the first place, they must commit him to constant, seamless watching. Unless they can resign themselves to faith, in which case they won't need to lay eyes on the faster, the spectators will watch the act with only its authentication in mind. An attempt to authenticate is also always an attempt to thwart. Those who come closest to witnessing the whole performance—I mean "witness" both in the phenomenological sense of "seeing" and in the legal sense of "legitimating"—will be sustained not by their benign interest but by their doubt. Doubt which they, pricked by rage, continually renew against a backdrop of boredom.

This problem of witnessing—of how to see a hunger performance— especially vexed those medical regimes whose authority the extraordinary claims of fasters threatened. To understand this we must widen the frame of our inquiry. In fact, the

hunger artists of Kafka's day represent just a minor, carnivalesque outcropping of a broad tradition. Self-starvation as spiritual practice has, of course, a history in Europe. For Christian—especially Catholic—mystics, fasting for short spells has long constituted an important expression of piety. Cases of extreme, apparently miraculous abstemiousness among the devout have garnered attention and skepticism at regular intervals since at least the thirteenth century: famously, the saints Angela of Foligno and Catherine of Siena were said to subsist on the Eucharist alone. Young women were involved in most of these cases, and the nineteenth century saw a remarkable proliferation of "fasting girls," reports of which were appearing by midcentury in newspapers across Britain and the United States.[8]

Sarah Jacob was born in 1857. The daughter of Welsh farmers, she grew up in a stone cottage with dirt floors. She was a precocious student, writing poetry and reading the Bible assiduously. When she was eight, she and her five family members fell ill with scarlet fever. They all recovered, but Sarah retained certain baffling symptoms: she complained of unbearable stomach pain and often fell into seizures. She became bedridden. Over the course of a year, her diet dwindled to virtually nothing; for a time, her daily meal consisted of "nothing but a little apple, about the size of a pill, in a teaspoon."[9] After visiting her, a local vicar wrote a letter to the *Welshman*, an English-language newspaper, in which he claimed Jacob "had not partaken of a single grain of any kind of food whatever for over sixteen months."[10] The news spread; soon, people from across Eng and were appearing by her bedside. They found her dressed in white, her hair crowned with ribbons and flowers, her apparently paralyzed body surrounded by open books.

On 24 April 1869, a report on Sarah Jacob appeared in the *British*

Medical Journal, in which a Welsh doctor recounted his visit to the fasting girl and offered a litany of measurements he had collected—her pulse, her temperature, the length and girth of her arms. In the final paragraph, he called on "those who have the leisure and scientific ardour to visit the case, and investigate and judge for themselves."[11] Robert Fowler, a physician from London, had both leisure and ardor. While vacationing in Cardigan, Wales, that August, he paid a visit to Jacob, and became fixated on exposing the now-twelve-year-old girl as a fraud: she was, in his mind, a run-of-the-mill, deceitful hysteric who was being goaded on by her criminal parents and a superstitious public.

He made these accusations public in a long letter to the London *Times*, which further excited the zeal of the English medical establishment. Encouraged at least in part by Fowler's tirade, several Welsh doctors arranged for a watch that December. They were unsatisfied by the findings of an earlier committee of locals, who had committed Jacob to a two-week period of surveillance— seven volunteers, all male, had taken turns watching her every move—and found no foul play. (One volunteer had dozed off during his watch; another was blind-drunk on gin.) The doctors enlisted three trained nurses as wardens and specified a more rigorous, invasive protocol: Sarah was to be frequently removed from her bed, stripped, her person searched. Her temperature and pulse would be recorded often, her waste examined.

After six days, Jacob was *in extremis*. Another four days and she was dead. Her parents, who had refused to call off the watch, were tried for manslaughter and imprisoned. Fowler, triumphant, immediately compiled and published a history of the case, in which he punctuates long excerpts from newspaper reports, eyewitness accounts, and legal transcripts with his own eager rebukes

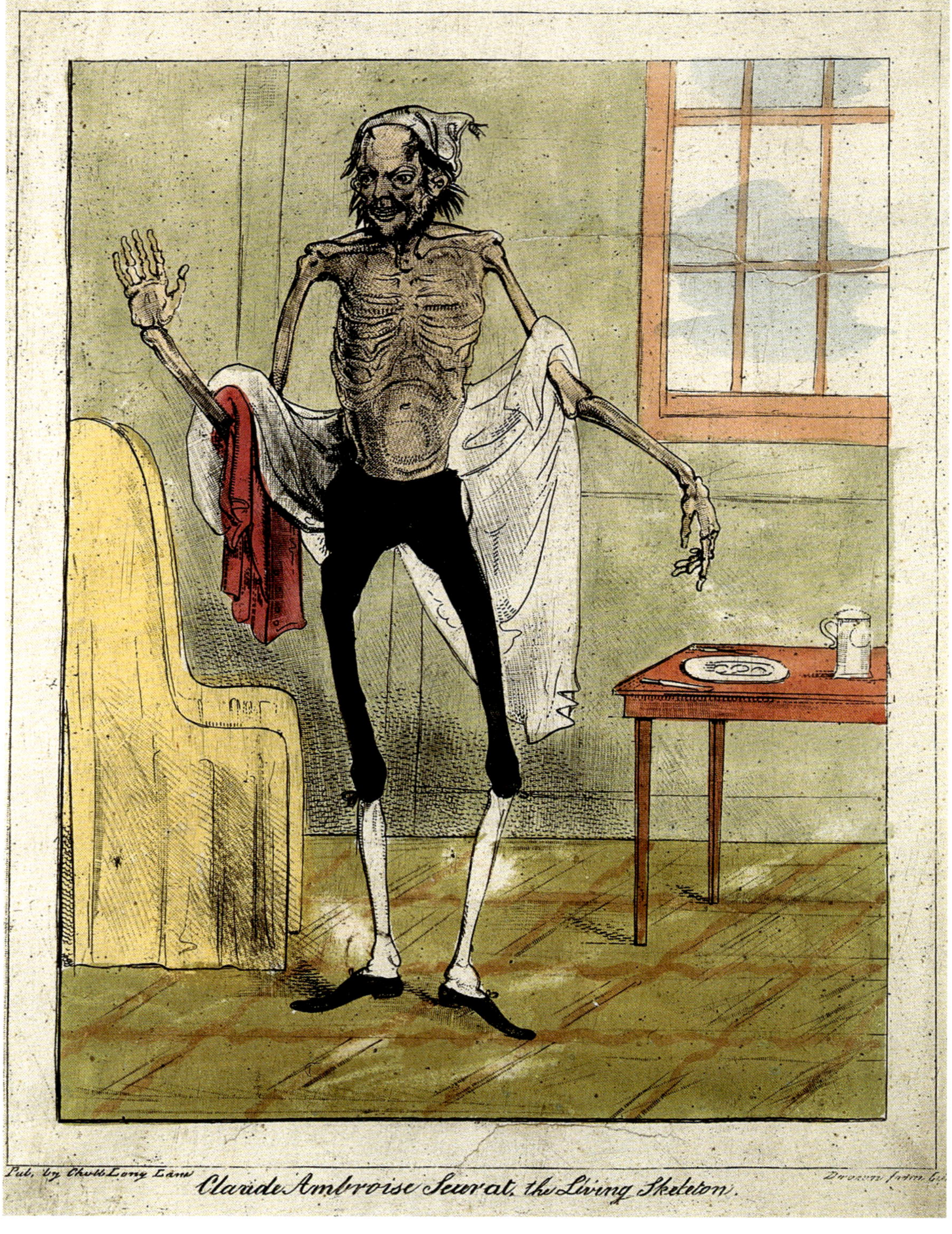

Although the hunger artist first emerged in the late nineteenth century, the public display of "living skeletons" goes back to at least the eighteenth century. What distinguished these individuals from hunger artists was that the former did not claim to abstain from food, while thinness was not necessarily part of the hunger artist's appeal. This etching depicts Claude Ambroise Seurat, a well-known "living skeleton" who was on display in France and Britain in the early nineteenth century. Courtesy Wellcome Images.

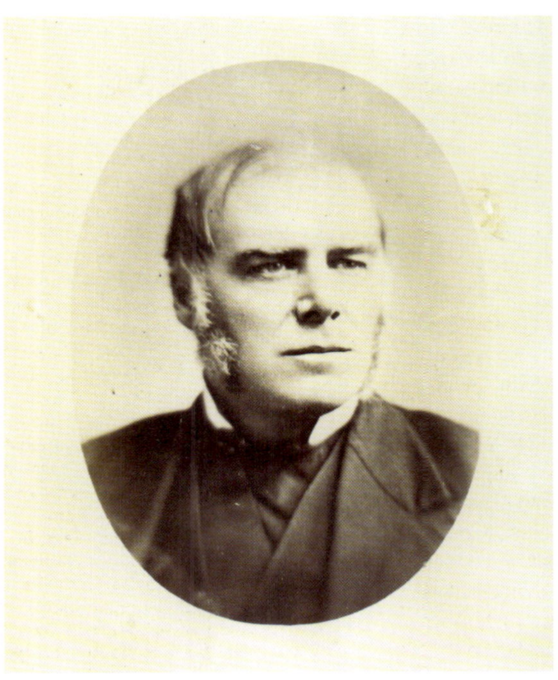 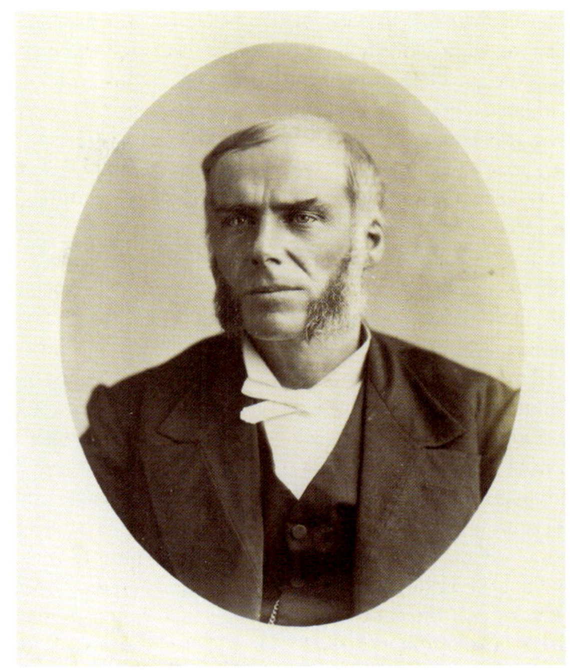

of the Jacob family. The book's centerpiece is an exhaustive, brutally minute account of the watch. Here, Sarah Jacob's body—its surface, its dark interior movements, even its sounds—is pulled sharply into cold light, held by a steady and indifferent gaze.

The watch was a strange kind of trial. The judicial body, consisting of Fowler, the Welsh doctors, and the relay of nurses, exacted punishment even as it was collecting evidence of Jacob's so-called guilt. The two activities were in fact indistinguishable. Fowler concludes his history with this sentence, astonishing for its rage: "For a morbid persistence in a perverse determination, the girl (when surrounded by an impregnable cordon) of a necessity paid the last penalty demanded by the unerring Laws of outraged Nature!"[12] The penalty included the indignities and humiliations attendant on surveillance—she was stripped naked before strangers, her bowel movements were subjected to intense scrutiny—but amounted ultimately to death.

Nine years later, Mollie Fancher,

a woman living in Brooklyn, gained notoriety for her miraculous abstemiousness. As in the Jacob case, a skeptical doctor took immediate interest. In 1879, William Hammond, a leading neurologist and former Surgeon General of the United States army, published *Fasting Girls: Their Physiology and Pathology*, which sought to debunk a great number of historical cases of sustained fasting and, in so doing, impugn Fancher and her followers. The book devotes nearly an entire chapter to Sarah Jacob, whose case Hammond calls "one of the most remarkable histories of folly, credulity, and criminality which the present day has produced."[13] He was apparently enamored of the methods used in the Jacobs case, and, in the appendix of his book formally challenged Fancher to fast for a month under surveillance. If she succeeded, he would pay her $1,000. Fancher refused.

Enter Henry S. Tanner, a grave, portly man from Minnesota. Tanner was an "eclectic" physician, a member of a then-sizeable minority of medical practitioners invested

in herbal alternatives and generally skeptical of neurologists such as Hammond, with their pretensions of objectivity and their growing monopoly over medical truth. It was his understanding that humans could, by simple force of will, enter long periods of trance-like abstention—in this regard, humans were no different from bears. He came to this conclusion after the breakup of his marriage, when, despondent and dyspeptic, he tried to starve himself to death. After thirty days of not dying, he found himself cured of his depression and his gastric troubles. Invigorated and intent on spreading the news, Tanner wrote a letter to the *New York Times* on 9 January 1880, in which he offered to accept Hammond's challenge in Fancher's place. Hammond, interviewed the following day by the newspaper, agreed, but doubted that Tanner was a real person: "I am inclined to think that the whole thing is a huge Western

———

Above: Photographs of Henry S. Tanner taken prior to his fasting performance in 1880 at New York's Clarendon Hall, and at its conclusion.

joke," he surmised.[14] When, four months later, a decidedly embodied Tanner appeared in Hammond's office in New York, Hammond turned him away, and evaded all of Tanner's ensuing solicitations.

Tanner was undeterred. He planned to spend forty days in an auditorium in Clarendon Hall, a building owned by the United States Medical College, an "eclectic" institution. He would be under the constant watch of members of the college, and the hall would be left open to the public during the day. The *New York Times* described the scene on the eve of the fast: "A bed, two chairs, a table, and a pint of water daily are all that he will be allowed during the six weeks, and as he is not likely to eat the furniture, the result is looked forward to with some interest."[15]

Indeed, Tanner attracted hundreds of visitors. After he survived the first six days, the newspaper published at least one dispatch from Clarendon Hall every day for the remaining thirty-four days of his fast. The reports follow Tanner's movements and attitudes with unsettling and, ultimately, boring precision. Every one of his actions is raised to a single plane of significance, a uniformity that estranges rather than clarifies his being.[16] He appears by turns chummy and utterly irascible, inconsolably depressed and merely blank. Though it seems the *New York Times* reporters wrote a sentence every time he turned over in his sleep, the many gestures recorded in print never resolve into an identity. This may be because Tanner was insane. It may also be that the insistent formlessness of surveillance, which treats every accident of the body with equal suspicion, can never fully recognize the subject it hopes to expose.

The drama of "A Hunger Artist"—if the story can be said to have anything so conventional—inheres in just such a problem of recognition. Kafka's hunger artist wants to be watched. He prefers the skeptical wardens, who keep a floodlight trained on him through the night, over those who turn their backs. But because fasting requires only abstention, inaction, it offers no clear, soliciting ensign around which attention and meaning can gather. The gesture in which the fast consists, rather than meet the spectator's experience at a right angle, moves alongside it, in real time. The temporality of the performance, a homogenous nonevent, is indistinguishable from life itself, and so is incapable of impressing itself upon it. The life of the faster and the life of the spectator are aligned in perfect separation. This is why a public fast is always hopelessly diffuse. Even those who remain are waiting for a revelation that never arrives.

Tanner survived the forty days without much incident. Despite this, the feat failed to convince Hammond and the medical establishment, as he had hoped. Instead, Tanner unwittingly inaugurated a fad. Giovanni Succi took after Tanner, and many took after Succi. By the time Kafka was writing his story, there was a café in Berlin that boasted an in-house faster. Bedraggled and gaunt, he sat inside a human-sized bell jar, silently smoking while the surrounding patrons ate forkfuls of Wiener schnitzel and chatted.[17]

---

1 Released posthumously, the book was the last Kafka prepared for publication, thus narrowly escaping its author's final disavowal: in 1924, dying of tuberculosis, Kafka ordered Max Brod, his friend and literary executor, to incinerate his remaining manuscripts and papers. Brod never carried out his friend's request.

2 See Walter Benjamin, *Illuminations*, ed. Hannah Arendt, trans. Harry Zohn (New York: Schocken Books, 1968), p. 117, and Theodor Adorno, *Prisms* (Cambridge, MA: The MIT Press, 1981), p. 246.

3 The central figure of Kafka's parable "The Cares of a Family Man," the Odradek is a mysterious creature with a star-shaped spool for its head and a kind of wooden crowbar for its body. Though apparently ancient, it strikes the narrator as childlike. It speaks only in clipped sentences.

4 Franz Kafka, "A Hunger Artist," in Franz Kafka, *The Complete Stories*, ed. Nahum N. Glatzer, trans. Edwin and Willa Muir (New York: Schocken Books, 1971), p. 268.

5 Alfred Gradenwitz, "An Apostle of Hunger," *The Technical World Magazine*, vol. 13, no. 3 (May 1910).

6 I have gleaned most of this information from the fifth chapter of Walter Vandereycken and Ron van Deth's *From Fasting Saints to Anorexic Girls: The History of Self-Starvation* (New York: New York University Press, 1990), which contains the most comprehensive overview of hunger artists I have encountered. American newspapers reported on Giovanni Succi often (for starters, see "Succi's Long Fast," *The New York Times*, 6 November 1890), and in 1890, *The British Medical Journal* published detailed findings from his London fast—see "The Fasting Man," *The British Medical Journal*, 21 June 1890.

7 Franz Kafka, "A Hunger Artist," in Franz Kafka, *The Complete Stories*, p. 270.

8 There was a great deal of scholarly interest in fasting women in the 1980s, especially among historians trying to understand the historical precursors of anorexia nervosa. Of the books written on the subject, Caroline Walker Bynum's *Holy Feast and Holy Fast: The Religious Significance of Food to Medieval Women* (Berkeley: University of California Press, 1987) and Joan Jacobs Brumberg's *Fasting Girls: The History of Anorexia Nervosa* (New York: Vintage, 2000) provide the most comprehensive and nuanced accounts. Rudolph Bell's *Holy Anorexia* (Chicago: University of Chicago Press, 1985) offers an impressive catalogue of fasting women in medieval Italy, but shoulders the bizarre project of diagnosing every one of them—even those whose historicity is uncertain—with anorexia nervosa. For a more recent history of self-starvation and its political dimensions, see Patrick Anderson's fascinating book *So Much Wasted: Hunger, Performance, and the Morbidity of Resistance* (Durham, NC: Duke University Press, 2010).

9 Henry Harries Davies (the Jacobs family doctor), cited in Robert Fowler, *The Complete History of the Case of the Welsh Fasting Girl* (London: Henry Renshaw, 1871), p. 7.

10 Frederic Rowland Young, "A Strange Case," cited in Robert Fowler, *The Complete History*, p. 15.

11 J. Lewis, "The Case of a Young Girl Who Is Said to Have Fasted for the Last Seventeen Months," *The British Medical Journal*, 24 April 1869, cited in Robert Fowler, *The Complete History*, p. 25.

12 Robert Fowler, *The Complete History*, p. 259.

13 William A. Hammond, *Fasting Girls: Their Physiology and Pathology* (New York: G. P. Putnam's Sons, 1879), p. 30.

14 Robert A. Gunn, *Forty Days without Food!: A Biography of Henry S. Tanner, M.D.*, (New York: Albert Metz & Co., 1880), p. 34.

15 "Dr. Tanner's Fast," *The New York Times*, 24 June 1880. The fast was originally scheduled to begin on 24 June but was postponed until 28 June. It ended on 7 August.

16 See the *New York Times* from 6 July to 12 August 1880.

17 Walter Vandereycken and Ron van Deth, *From Fasting Saints to Anorexic Girls*, p. 89.

LEFTOVERS /
VAPOR TRAILS
D. Graham Burnett

"Leftovers" investigates the cultural significance of detritus.

———

In early October 1918, a young American army captain named Ward Wells found himself bivouacking with his unit in a patch of forest a little northwest of Verdun, just as a tremendous bombardment up ahead shattered the bright autumn morning. He described what he saw in a from-the-trench letter to his brother back in Iowa:

Our attention was first drawn to the sky by the sudden appearance of several strange and startling clouds— long, graceful, looping ribbons of white. These were tapering to a point at one end, and at the other, where they dissolved into nothingness, 60 degrees across the sky, were about as broad as the width of a finger held arm's distance from the eye.

He and his fellow doughboys had never seen anything quite like it, and they scrutinized the celestial calligraphy with squinting faces:

On close observation we noticed some distance ahead of each cloud point the tiny speck of a chasse plane. Apparently the churning of the air was all that was needed to upset the delicately balanced meteorological conditions and precipitate this strange cloud formation.

It was an astute interpretation of an as-yet untheorized bit of aerodynamics and atmospheric chemistry. Young Captain Wells, who had some scientific training, closed his letter with a poetic flourish:

I had seen ships leave their tracks in the clouds, similar to those of little sea animals in the wet sands at the shore, but never before had I seen a plane writing in white upon the blue slate of the sky.[1]

This was not, of course, "skywriting"—at least not in the conventional sense of an airplane making smoke intentionally for the purpose of inscribing messages in the air. Such skywriting did not yet really exist in its conventional form, and anyway the aces dueling for position over the battlefield had no time for playful tracery. What Ward Wells and his comrades witnessed on that otherwise cloudless morning was in fact one of the very earliest documented occurrences of a meteorological phenomenon now familiar to all of us—what have come to be called *contrails*, the streak-like white wisps that (sometimes) lace the sky where planes have passed.[2]

I turn my head right now and look out the window, and there are two of them overhead: one a loose and tufted relic, only distinguishable from the cirrus ribs with which it lies on account of a slight skew; the other presently streaming in fresh billows from a silver jet raking the cerulean vault.

What are contrails? Why do they form? To whom do they matter?

Bracketing a powerful strain of paranoia-spectrum analysis that has vexed these questions in the last decade (to which I will return), the physics of contrail formation is helpfully disclosed in the etymology of the term itself, a portmanteau contraction of *condensation* and *trail*. Contrails are visible ribbons of water vapor suspended in the atmosphere, which is to say, they really are clouds—linear, anthropogenic clouds. They happen under two quite different scenarios.

Let's do the less important (and less common) one first. Most powered flight works by creating (via a precisely shaped wing or propeller slicing through the air) local regions of low pressure. Depending on just how low that pressure gets, and how fast it gets low (and some other factors that have to do with the mechanics of vortices), you can actually get a substantial sudden drop in temperature in these low-pressure regions. This is not totally unrelated to the phenomenon that causes your canister of compressed gas to get very cold when you vent its contents. If these low-pressure zones get cold enough in relation to the humidity of the air in question, you hit the "dew point"—that sweet spot of pressure and temperature at which a gaseous substance (in this case H_2O in its gaseous state in the atmosphere) becomes a liquid (in this case liquid H_2O, suspended in droplets in the air), i.e, *condensation*.[3] A stream of that finely particulate condensation flowing out behind the wing or propeller tip will be a whitish streak of contrail. It's even possible that the temperature drops so low that the tiny water drops *freeze*, which actually looks about the same, as far as the contrail is concerned—if perhaps a little whiter and often slightly more durable as the indicative mist hangs in the empty air.

Contrails of this first type (sometimes called "visible wing-tip vortices" or "aerodynamic contrails") tend to be short-lived, and mostly appear during high-strain and/or high-speed maneuvers. Fighter jets generate them as they bank hard or climb fast. But passenger planes can produce them too, generally speaking only at takeoff and landing, and only if the weather conditions are just right.

Usually when people talk about contrails, however, they are talking about the other kind—like the high, straight, persistent ones outside my window right now. These are the product of the same basic "event" (the airborne condensation/freezing of gaseous water) but the key water in question in this second type of contrail is not water just "there" in the air as the plane passes. It is, rather,

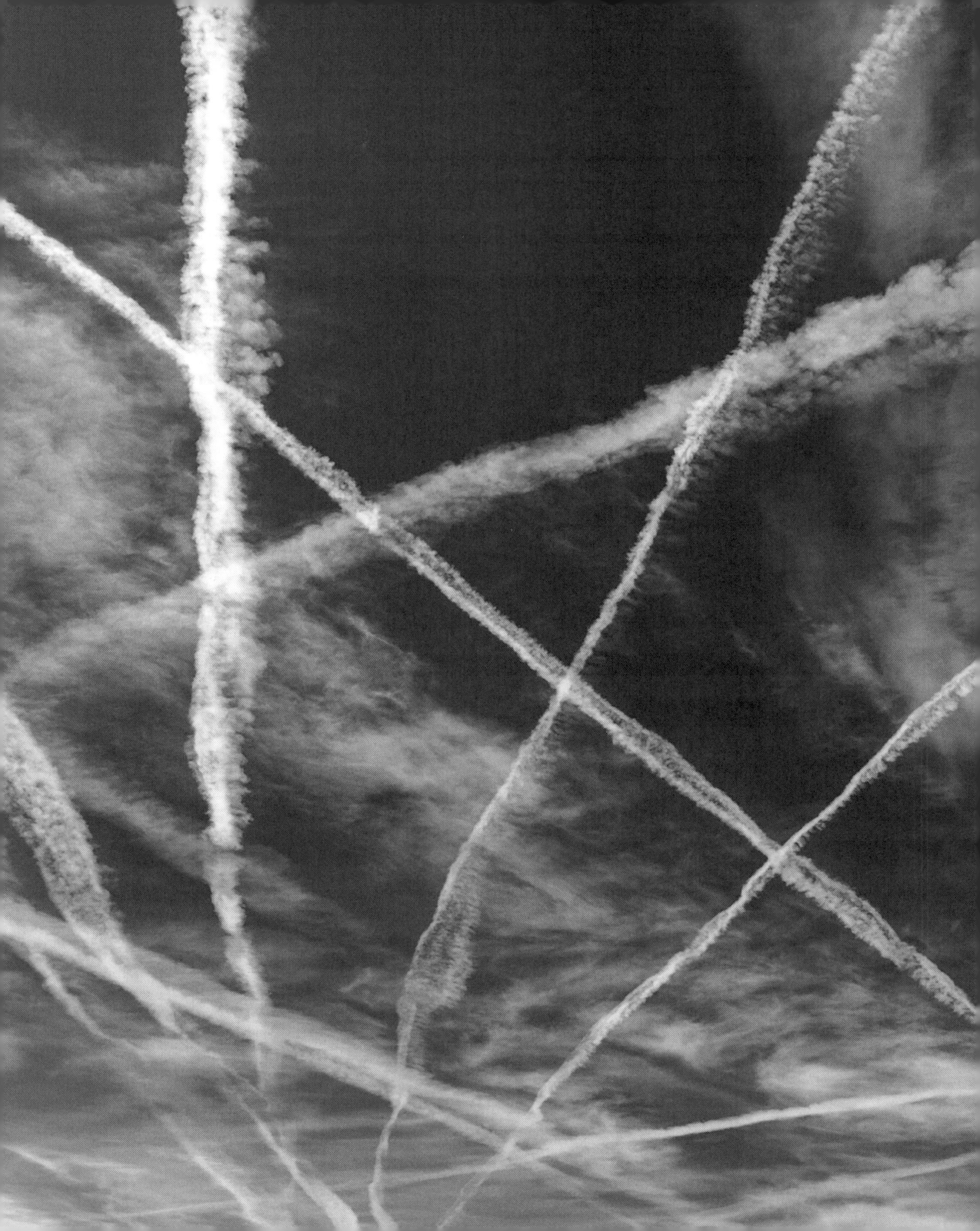

the water that results from the combustion of fossil fuels—water, that is, in the exhaust of the plane's engines.

When you "burn" a hydrocarbon (methane, butane, gasoline, jet fuel, etc.), what you are doing is ripping up some bonds between atoms of hydrogen and carbon by means of a rapid chemical reaction (i.e., *combustion*) with molecules of oxygen. The main products of this violent recombination, besides a lot of energy, are carbon dioxide and water. So airplane engines, like basically all engines (whether jet or internal combustion), release a lot of gaseous water into the atmosphere. If you do that at thirty-five thousand feet or so, where it is, say, minus sixty-five degrees Fahrenheit, that water vapor is very likely to condense and instantly turn into ice crystals—leaving a wake of white cirrus trailing behind your engines. These are the contrails of the high sky—the cold darts and long tracks that tail the metal birds.[4]

The history of contrails is difficult to separate from the history of aviation. As Ward Wells's letter makes clear, streamer clouds trailing airplanes were a novelty in 1918—novel enough that his correspondence eventually found its way to publication in *Scientific American* the following year, as evidence for a hitherto unseen phenomenon, a phenomenon in need of an explanation. While heavier-than-air aviation was by then already more than a decade old, it took the exigencies of war (together with the derring-do of stunt pilots) to push the early flying machines to the extremes of force and altitude that generate vapor trails. For instance, another of the earliest published accounts of the phenomenon accompanied a breathless report on Major Rudolph W. Schroeder's near-fatal attempt on the world altitude record in September of 1919. Running out of oxygen around thirty-six thousand feet, Schroder apparently lost consciousness, and dropped some

thirty-three thousand feet in less than three minutes, as the ice in his goggles froze over his eyelids:

For a brief time residents of Dayton [Ohio] were sure a comet had appeared in the sky. They had mistaken the trail of vapor escaping from the machine as it sped downward for a "stranger in the heavens."

The exhaust gas from the airplane, freezing in the frigid temperature, caused a cloud-like formation, resembling the tail of a comet, to hang below the clouds. Inasmuch as the airplane was not visible, speculation varied as to what it was. Some witnesses were inclined to the belief that a strange body was coming with a message from Mars. Professor William Beck, the astronomer at St. Mary's College, making observations through a telescope, discerned the airplane.[5]

Schroeder lived (though he did not recover his sight for some time), and his vapor trail streaked the upper limits of powered flight in those years.

More high-altitude flights in the decades ahead made the phenomenon less exotic, but it would take the rise of reliable jet aviation in the period immediately following World War II to make the avionic vapor trail sufficiently commonplace as to demand a new word. The term *contrail* was coined in the mid-1940s. By that time, long, thin, pointer-clouds pricking out high-flying bombers (and their fighter escorts) had become all too familiar to civilians and military personnel alike across much of Europe and the Pacific, causing considerable concern to those engaged in the sneak-attack game of strategic air warfare.[6]

And it was in this context that a US Air Force–trained meteorologist named Herbert Appleman set to work on the problem, with an eye toward developing a quantitative model for the conditions under which exhaust contrails could be expected to occur.

The result, published in 1953, can be thought of as a rule-of-thumb guide for high-flying pilots trying to avoid divulging their daytime location.[7] If you plotted the relevant variables (altitude, humidity, temperature), you ought to be able to find a flight path that kept you out of vapor-trail zones. The Appleman chart and its descendants duly became standard tools in contrail avoidance, but they were never foolproof—there being enough wonky factors in the weather and the behavior of air around fast-moving bodies to make for plenty of undesirable contrail surprises.[8] The problem was sufficiently serious (there being no obvious way to eliminate engine exhaust) that a pinnacle technology of secret Cold War surveillance, the U2 spy plane, was forced to rely on an ultra-low-tech hack to minimize contrail disasters: a little rearview mirror on the side of the plane. If the pilot saw a contrail behind his craft, he was supposed to change altitude in a hurry. Down on the ground, sky-watching civilian Cold Warriors, like members of Britain's Aircraft Recognition Society, read up on how to identify specific airplanes by their contrails, and later sentinels scoped out other details of celestial tracking: "distrails," for instance ("negative" contrails—clear streaks made through cloudy skies by the passage of aircraft), and contrail *shadows* (sometimes visible on the underside of light clouds), which could disclose the passage of a high-flying airplane above the cloud ceiling.[9]

· · ·

This 1950s nexus of military-industrial paranoia, anthropogenic cloud monitoring, and civilian sky gazers has proven strangely durable—if also unsettlingly plastic. For about a decade now, a vast conspiracy-theory subculture out there in the interwebs has promoted, with stupefying energy and commitment, the notion that some, many, or even all visible contrails are in fact properly

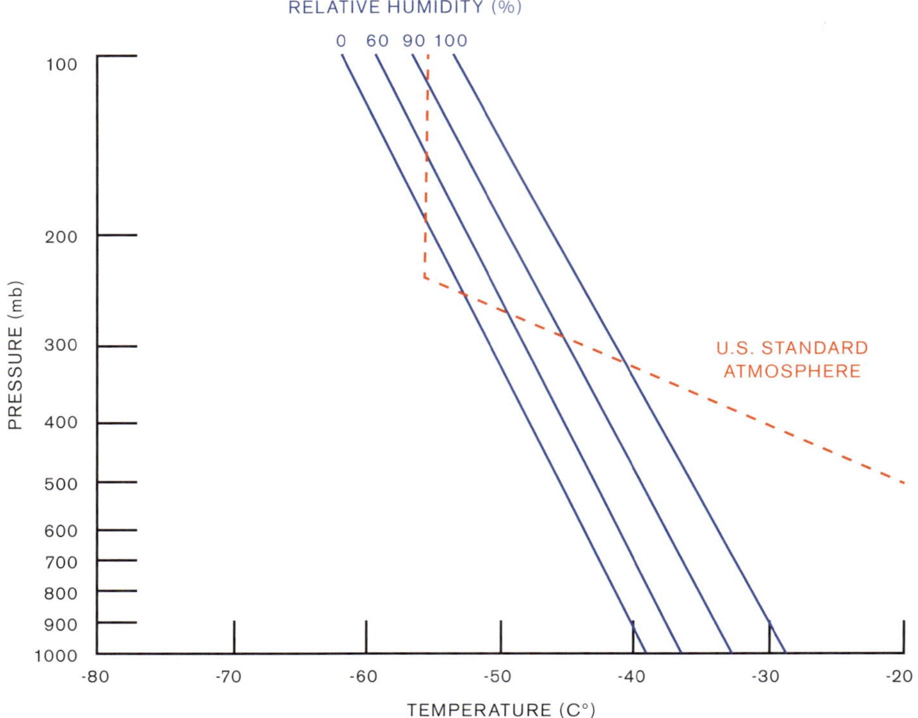

understood as *chemtrails*: miasmatic evidence of a sweeping government plot to deploy aerosol spraying across the country (and perhaps the world). Many argue that this has something to do with climate change geo-engineering, but others allege large-scale human experimentation, genetic manipulation of populations, and possible military objectives. It is a passionate community, if somewhat shadowy, and at times genuinely enraged. For all that, its partisans have had some success in forcing their issue to the edges of respectable investigative reporting and non-fringe documentary filmmaking.

I could be wrong, of course, but I spent some time with the available material, and it seems that there is nothing to it at all. Contrails are contrails. They have been around for a long time. They are not new, and the things that are streaming out of the airplanes outside my window are contrails. There is a lot of good evidence for all this. While from time to time

people do spray stuff from airplanes, and while this has surely been, on a number of notable occasions, a very bad idea, commercial airlines are not being deployed in a secret, large-scale plot to defeat our enemies, willfully transform the earth and its inhabitants, or poison us by nefarious means. While contrails themselves, it turns out, may indeed be slightly altering the weather (because they actually slightly add to the earth's total cloud cover), this has absolutely nothing to so with so-called chemtrails, which, in a basic sense, do not exist.[10]

When I first turned to the topic of contrails, I was motivated by what seemed to me the poetry (and poignancy) of these ephemeral indications of human movements through the upper atmosphere. If on earth, we leave expressive threads of footprints, and in the water we open the self-closing sea-wound of a wake, then the air-equivalent of these marks of passage would be the contrail, a kind of

comet tail to our celestial ambitions. I thought I would sift some forgotten sources in an effort to recover the records of the early encounters with the phenomenon, in the hopes of finding a freshness of perspective on a sky effect that has long since become a commonplace—but that I suspected would once have been met with surprise, and even wonder.

But the surprise, in the end, was entirely my own: there is, in fact, really no such thing as a "forgotten source" bearing on contrails. As a direct result of more than a decade of hot Internet conflict between

---

Above: Herbert Appleman's nomogram, 1953. Temperature and pressure measurements falling in the region to the left of the 0 percent humidity line could be assumed to constitute contrail-forming conditions, according to the Appleman model, while the region to the right of the 100 percent line could be assumed to be contrail-free. For the intervening zone, contrails would be assumed to form behind a passing jet at a given pressure (altitude) if the temperature fell to the left of the relevant line indicating the observed ambient relative humidity.

chemtrail advocates and their equally impassioned opponents/debunkers, *essentially every single historical instance of the observation of a vapor trail in the sky* has not only been tugged up from the archives of oblivion, it has also likely been subject to layers of critical scrutiny and trenchant commentary. We basically have crucible-tested knowledge of the full universe of contrail appearances of any and all imaginable forms across the twentieth century. Thousands and thousands of photographs of contrails dating back to the interwar period have been posted to websites dedicated to this purpose in the belief that the long and well-documented existence of contrails refutes the conspiracists' arguments concerning the ostensibly nefarious innovation of chemtrailing.[11] You can quickly find, for instance, that a shockingly anachronistic contrail streaks the backdrop sky thirty-four seconds after the title credits in John Ford's elegiac 1964 western, *Cheyenne Autumn*—set in 1878. Interested in the history of contrails being seen as meteors or even UFOs? There are extensive and well-documented online discussions of both matters.

For the historian, it is an incredible thing: crowd-sourced, paranoia-driven, globally aggregated research of a sort heretofore entirely beyond the dreams of the most dogged student of the dusty shelves. The resulting archive of contrails may be the best-documented collection of sources on anything that I have ever encountered.

I have, of course, written this piece out of that archive, and as I now push away from the desk, I am struck, looking out the window, by the strange weather and the weird vortices that sometimes cause the passage of time, winging by, to leave dense trails of visible condensation hanging before the eye.

Dichten = Condensare.

1 These extracts from Wells's communication survive because his brother conveyed the observations to *Scientific American*, which published them on 7 June 1919 (vol. 120, no. 23, pp. 600–601).

2 For an impressively detailed account of the early sightings and their interpretations, see Donald R. Baucom, "Wakes of War: Contrails and the Rise of Air Power, 1918–1945—Part I: Early Sightings and Preliminary Explanations, 1918–1938," *Air Power History*, vol. 54, no. 2 (Summer 2007).

3 It should be said that a significant factor in this process, as in any process of atmospheric condensation (rain, snow, fog), is the availability of "condensation nuclei," e.g., little particles of dust, etc., that facilitate the transition of gaseous water to its liquid form. In the case of exhaust contrails, particles of various exhaust products provide these nuclei in abundance.

4 As it happens (this is nuance, but worth getting right), with big, persistent contrails the majority of the visible water you are seeing actually *is* atmospheric water—it is atmospheric water the condensation of which has been catalyzed by the initial condensation of the water of combustion streaming out of the airplane engines.

5 "Major Schroeder in New Altitude Flight," *Aircraft Journal*, vol. 6, no. 12 (20 March 1920), p. 14. This account of the formation of the contrail is surprisingly precise, given the many theories that circulated around these apparitions in the early years. As it happens, a brief scientific account of the phenomenon did appear in 1920, authored by the great German polar researcher and geophysicist Alfred Wegener, but it was not abstracted in the English-language literature until 1921: Alfred Wegener, "Frostübersättigung und Cirren," *Meteorologische Zeitschrift*, vol. 37 (1920).

6 A valuable index of the general understanding of vapor trails among English-language aviators and aviation professionals at the outbreak of the war is afforded by *Flight* magazine's pair of publications in 1940: "Visible Vortices?" (18 July 1940) and "Visible Vortices" (5 September 1940). The former served as a call for correspondence from those who had seen vapor trails and "who have any additional facts to add or any alternative explanations to give." The latter summarized the results of the query.

7 Herbert Appleman, "The Formation of Exhaust Condensation Trails by Jet Aircraft," *Bulletin of the American Meteorological Society*, vol. 34, no. 1 (January 1953). For a sense of similar (non-classified) work through the war, consider A. M. Descamps, "Les traînées blanches d'avions," *Ciel et Terre*, vol. 61, nos. 7–8 (July–August 1945).

8 For a detailed treatment, see Frank G. Noppel, "Contrail and Cirrus Cloud Avoidance Technologies" (PhD thesis, Cranfield University, 2007).

9 "Identification by Contrails," *Flight*, vol. 70, no. 2480 (3 August 1956). See also "Contrails and the GOC [Ground Observer Corps]," *The Aircraft Flash* (published by the US Air Defense Command), vol. 2 (1953).

10 The idea that aviation-induced clouds might have a measurable effect on weather patterns appears to have been first mooted in 1970 by the American geophysicist Wallace B. Murcray in his "On the Possibility of Weather Modification by Aircraft Contrails," *Monthly Weather Review*, vol. 98, no. 10 (October 1970). He ends his meditation on the question with a solid invocation of Dr. Strangelove-esque anxiety: "In conclusion, it should be stated that if contrails are affecting the weather it is not necessarily for the worse, although if there is any considerable change it is sure to make someone unhappy. The Russians might well be pleased with an ice-free Arctic Ocean; but if it leads to major glaciation in central Canada, it is unlikely that the Canadians and Americans would regard it as favorable." For a useful recent review essay on the question, see Ulrich Schumann, "Formation, Properties and Climatic Effects of Contrails," *Comptes Rendus Physique*, vol. 6, nos. 4–5 (May–June 2005). Perhaps the most striking recent work in this area has been that of Rob MacKenzie, now at the University of Birmingham. He and his colleagues used historical records of World War II bombing raids, which produced dense contrail cover, to assess local climate variation. See A. C. Ryan, A. R. MacKenzie, S. Watkins, and R. Timmis: "World War II Contrails: A Case of Aviation-Induced Cloudiness," *International Journal of Climatology*, vol. 32, no. 11 (September 2012).

11 See, for example, <contrailscience.com/about>.

INVENTORY / THE SAVOY FILES
Christopher Turner

"Inventory" examines or presents a list, catalogue, or register.

———

In the famously elegant Savoy Hotel on the Strand in London, there used to be a secret room in the lobby, situated on a mezzanine above the revolving doors. It was made almost invisible by mirrors that reflected the columns and Grecian frieze of the spacious entrance hall. Only the staff would have known the room was there. Inside, in a library filing cabinet, thousands of yellow four-by-six-inch index cards were stored, dating back to 1918—there are a few blue and red cards from even earlier—with carefully collected data on each of the guests that passed through the portals below.

The lobby has since been restored, and the card index room removed (it was replaced in 1982 by computerized records), but its contents have been preserved in the Savoy's basement archive. Susan Scott, who has administered this collection for the past two decades, showed me several boxes of these alphabetically arranged, yellowing records: they include well-thumbed cards, sometimes with newspaper clippings attached, on earls and counts, prime ministers and business-men, conductors and army captains, maharajahs and movie stars.

As well as recording names and addresses, the arrival date and length of stay, and the amount charged for each suite, the cards have a sec-tion to document the number of V(isitors), C(hildren) and S(ervants). When the luxury hotel opened in 1890, built by the theatrical producer Richard D'Oyly Carte with profits from his Gilbert and Sullivan operas, it was the first British institution to boast elevators, electric lights, en suite bathrooms, and twenty-four-hour service; its seventh floor was earmarked for guests' maids and valets. (The hotel took its name from the Savoy Palace that used to occupy the site but was burned down in the Peasants' Revolt of 1381.) The cards sometimes also have a box in which the number of pieces of a visitor's luggage is marked. In 1961, Dorothy McGuire, a cabaret singer, arrived with forty-five valises. A clip-ping attached to her card from the *Evening News* refers in the headline to her "mountain of luggage."

The cards of more famous visitors are distinguished with red metal tags, and the Savoy has hosted an impres-sive constellation of stars—past guests include Oscar Wilde (who carried out his affair with Lord Alfred Douglas at the hotel), Noël Coward, Fred Astaire, Zeppo Marx, Maria Callas, Frank Sinatra, Ava Gardner, Coco Chanel, and Bianca Jagger (then married to Mick), who appar-ently sometimes checked in under the pseudonym Mrs. B. Fitzgerald or Miss Barry. Alongside practical information, and brief descriptions of the subject's profession ("famous dancer"), the cards carry records of recent achievements, such as appearances in new films or plays—trivia that enabled a slick concierge to compliment clients with flattering familiarity.

Many of the cards include a sec-tion labeled "Special Requirements," documenting the tastes and prefer-ences of significant guests in neat, handwritten notes: "Always wants large bed," "Please Note: Give special attention to floor service in future," "River view," "Do not give rubber mat in bath." Marlene Dietrich's card says that she wished to be greeted on arrival with twelve pink roses and a refrigerated bottle of Dom Pérignon. The actor Richard Harris's card notes the exact tem-perature he liked his porridge. He spent the last few years of his life living in the hotel, and when he was carried out from the Savoy Grill on a stretcher, famously warned fellow diners, "It was the food!"

Some cards are bookmarked with black clips, forming a list of undesir-ables: "No cheques to be accepted or credit allowed," "Cheque returned marked signature unknown," "Unpaid account written off as bad debt." On the card of one gentleman, a company director who had recently lost his job and was no longer the beneficiary of an expense account, is written, "Please treat with caution" and security were instructed to keep an eye on him. Most on this blacklist were to be refused future reserva-tions. Some are dismissed on their cards with the damning note, written in scarlet ink, "Not Savoy class."

Others are singled out for special treatment: "Very good people—per Mr. Ward." Anyone who aroused the remotest suspicion was investigated by the Savoy's house detectives, men who were all ex-Scotland Yard. They checked names against addresses, and marginalia confirmed if the per-son on the card was a "Householder" or "Appears correctly in social regis-ter." "Cannot trace at above address," reads one pencil note. During the war, army officers were given a ten percent discount, and questions are raised over the status of numerous "majors" and "captains," their cards marked, "Not on army list."

Some cards, such as that of a Mrs. Despina del Maestres, include descriptions of their subjects. "Dresses in expensive clothes. Well spoken. Bills not paid. per Security Officer 4.9.63." Another for a Mr. E. M. Ling, dated 1954, reads like a police identification of a potential suspect. "5'6"; hair black; high fore-head; clean shaven; red complexion. Very well spoken. Ex-Guards officer type." He was an inspector, working

———

Overleaf: Samples of cards from the Savoy hotel's secret guest catalogue. Courtesy Savoy Archive.

Name RUSTAD (PETER WARWICK) CAPT.
Res. Address GLEN BRAE, CLAYGATE, SURREY.
Business Address
Information BRITISH. Last in Army Rgt. Cannot trace at above address.
16.3.44 Furze Hill, Claygate. Surrey

Booked by
wife's add. Spring Cottage, Robinhare, Clevedon Som.

Arrived	Departed	Length of Stay	Room No.	No. of Party V. C. S.	Amount per Diem for Apartments
19.3.43	20.3.43	1.	633. 6%	1	1 10 —
16.3.44	17.3.44	1	285 (W. mrs Mary Joyce Rustad) 10%	2	2 7 6

Name HITCHCOCK (ALFRED J.   SIR
Res. Address 10957 BELLAGIO ROAD, BELAIR, W. LOS ANGELES, 24. CALIF. USA
Business Address
Deceased 29 4 80
Per Times 30. 4. 80
Information BRITISH. Film director. Shown in Motion Picture Almanac. Married 1926 Alma Reville. Films include The Lady Vanishes. Lifeboat. Spellbound, Rope etc.

Created Knight Commander Order of British Empire NEW YEARS HONS
SEE ALSO WIFES CARD MRS ALMA LUCY HITCHCOCK LIST 1980
Booked by   Wife is American. SAN. FRAN. 25995.

K5576

Name LOEWENSTEIN. (Alfred) Capt.   I.
Res. Address Pinfold, Thorpe Satchville, Melton Mowbray.
Business Address 35. rue de la Science, Brussels.
Information Belgian. Dir. of Cos. (The well known millionaire)

DECEASED. Fell out of an aeroplane crossing the Channel.

Booked by Claridge's Hotel, London.

Arrived	Departed	Length of Stay	Room No.	No. of Party V. C. S.	Amount per Diem for Apartments
10.11.26	18.11.26.	8.	241/2 : 234/7 : 274 : 280 : 275/255/287 : 786/161 : W. Raoul Dufresne de la Chevalrie; C.L. Fisher; Julian Dupont: Mr Archinard; Julie C.A. Chiraussel (Eng.); Miss E.M. Frisby; Arthur E. Hodgson;	10 3	24 14 6.
note a/c my					
all this own acct					
Capt. L. himself					
Diff	11.11.26	1			see over

Name CHANEL. (Gabrielle) Mme
Res. Address 29. rue du Fbg. St. Honoré, Paris.
Business Address
Information (Famous dressmaker & fashion designer)
Special Requirements No booking

Arrived	Departed	Length of Stay	Room No.	No. of Party V. C. S.	Amount per Diem for Apartments
9.5.24	10.5.24	1	434/7/8 & 804. (w. Vera A. Bate & Elise Zehren maid)	2 1	11 11 . 10 6
16.5.24.	19.5.24	3.	441/42/822. w. Elise Zehren. maid	1	7 7 .

LING E.M. Age - 32/35; height 5'6"; hair black;

high forehead; clean shaven; red complexion. Very

well spoken. Ex-Guards officer type.

The British Hotels and Restaurants Association.
1st February, 1952.

Name MARX. (Zeppo)
Res. Address 169, East 78th St., N.Y.C.
Business Address U.S.A.
Information Actor. (one of the Marx Bros. — vaudeville artistes — of Cocoanuts fame) (correct in Tel. Dir. at res. add. — full name Zeppo Herbert Marx. Married Barbara Blakeley fashion model
Booked by
Bankers See also
Deceased 28.11.79 per D. Telegraph 1.12.79
see attached cutting 21/9/59. S.S. Paris.

Arrived	Departed	Length of Stay	Room No.	No. of Party V. C. S.	Amount per Diem for Apartments
30.12.30	1.2.31	33.	435. (w. Mrs. M.) 31.12.30 to 329: charge £12 per week since arr.	2	12 . - per week

for the British Hotels and Restaurant Association, and alert staff had to be sure to recognize him so as to be able to discreetly give him preferential treatment.

The files were kept up to date by cross-checking against newspapers' death notices, and some cards are written over in red ink with "Deceased," the date of death, and the source of this information (for example, *The Times*). Case closed. One for Captain Alfred Loewenstein, who is described in a parenthesis as "The well known millionaire," includes the intriguing detail: "Fell out of an aeroplane whilst crossing the Channel." Loewenstein had only stayed in the Savoy once, for eight days, but managed to fill three cards as reception struggled to keep track of his sizeable entourage as they kept changing rooms.

Loewenstein, it turns out, was a financier, once known as the third-richest man in the world, but later pursued by investors, and his death in July 1928 remains a mystery. He was flying back to his native Belgium from England when he went to the lavatory—his Fokker plane was the first to include such a facility—but, absent-mindedly, he supposedly opened the exit door directly opposite, plunging to his death. Tests revealed that the exit door, clearly signed as such, was incredibly hard to open in midflight even for two men and, though no one was ever prosecuted, murder was suspected, or even a faked death.

Sometimes the hotel's manager sent letters of condolence to surviving relatives. In the archive is a handwritten response on headed paper from Oona Chaplin, fourth wife of Charlie, then living in Switzerland. In 1952, the year *Limelight* came out, they had been photographed together on the roof of the Savoy, with Charlie Chaplin shown pointing out to her his birthplace south of the river. It was his first visit to England in twenty-one years, and he would be refused reentry into the United States, accused of being a communist. "Your letter touched me very much," she replied. "Just thinking about the Savoy brings back happy memories—he loved it so."

The Savoy's scrupulously maintained index offers a snapshot of British class and privilege, and the Jeevesian discretion of the hotel staff. During World War II, at the same time as the Savoy's staff were filling in these cards, other secret information was being collated in other parts of the hotel. Lieutenant Colonel Claude Dansey, the deputy chief of the secret intelligence services who was known as Colonel Z, took lunch every day in the restaurant, where he interviewed potential recruits. Winston Churchill liked to bring his entire cabinet there for lunch, taking advantage of the restaurant's exemption from the restrictions of wartime rationing. (In 1940, the Italian restaurant manager, suspected of leading a Fascist cell, was interned, along with many of his waiters.) Guy Liddell, MI5's director of counterespionage, held meetings over midday cocktails in the American Bar. And, upstairs, intelligence officers—using aliases now buried in the Savoy archive—conducted interrogations and debriefings in hired rooms.

SENTENCES /
FAIR HOPES OF
ENDING ALL
Brian Dillon

"Sentences" is a column by Brian Dillon each installment of which examines the mechanics and style of a single sentence chosen by the author.

———

"Wee have a *winding sheete* in our Mothers wombe, which growes with us from our conception, and wee come into the world, wound up in that winding sheet, for wee come to *seeke a grave*; And as prisoners discharg'd of actions may lye for fees; so when the *wombe* hath discharg'd us, yet we are bound to it by *cordes* of flesh, by such a *string* as that wee cannot goe thence, nor stay there."
—John Donne

The poet and preacher John Donne died from stomach cancer in the spring of 1631. He had likely been sick for a year, but continued in his office of dean at St. Paul's cathedral, where his weekly sermons were admired for their erudition, piety, and extremes of metaphorical invention. When illness made him quit the capital for his daughter's house in Essex, rumors arose that Donne was already dead, or was feigning his distemper. Gathering his strength, he returned to London in March, quite sensible of his hourly decline but resolved to deliver a last sermon, at the palace of Whitehall before King Charles I and his court. As Donne's first biographer Izaak Walton tells us, the poet's friends were appalled at his appearance—he had left about him "but so much flesh as did only cover his bones"—and they tried to dissuade him from his homiletic duty. When he rose as appointed on the first day of

Lent and in a hollow voice began to speak of dissolution, decay, and the life to come, it seemed to them that he had composed his own funeral oration.

Such was Donne's devout insouciance in the face of death that in the days before he spoke this sermon—and in it the astonishing sentence that is today's lesson—he contrived its visual counterpart, his own ghastly monument. He summoned a painter to his sickroom, who found the learned dean shrouded head to foot, his eyes closed and limbs arranged as if already in the grave. Donne had the resulting portrait set by his bedside so he could look upon it in his last days—as the critic Frank Kermode put it, the dying man seemed possessed of an "almost histrionic composure." It was on this picture (now lost) that the sculptor Nicholas Stone based the monument to Donne that still stands in St. Paul's. An engraving from the same source formed the frontispiece to the final sermon when it was published in 1632: here is the ailing divine embarked on his ultimate spiritual migration, oblivious to the world of flesh even as he makes us stare at its grisly remnant.

In print, the sermon is called "Deaths Duell," though Donne never titled his sermons: nothing came before the biblical quotation that gave each one its subject and its structure. In this case the lesson is from Psalm 68, verse 20: "And unto God the Lord belong the issues of death." As was sermonic convention, Donne approaches this ambiguous line via an explicit tripartite plan. His task as preacher is, first, closely to read this text for its diverse meanings; second, to set it in the context of biblical and theological authority; third, to lay out nakedly, in a kind of moral anatomy, the lessons and models that may be taken away. "Deaths Duell" begins with another triad: a somewhat distracting architectural conceit by which Donne thinks of the psalmic

text as a building, with foundations, buttresses, and joints or "contignations." But we are soon amid the fundamental truths of the text, of which there are also three. "And unto God the Lord belong the issues of death" means: He will deliver us *from* death, to eternal life; *in* death, because he will save us from undue suffering; and *by* death, for this trial is necessary to attain our reward.

So far so schematic, so theologically and rhetorically conventional. But "Deaths Duell" is also a cabinet of baroque horrors, a repository of gruesome images cast in sentences that are themselves errant or deformed. In spite of Donne's insistence on our deliverance, and his own, into eternal life, it seems at the same time that death never ends, that it reigns either side of the actual event of our leave-taking. The world, writes Donne, "is but an *universal church-yard*, but our *common grave*; and the life and motion that the greatest persons have in it, is but as the shaking of buried bodies in their graves, by an *earth-quake*." So too, one might say, the text of his sermon itself, which is planted everywhere with corpses, some of which are in disguise as living persons. There is, of course, the noisome reality of the grave, and our being gnawed away by worms. But the most pristine picture of health is shadowed by death: even in youth, even in our infancy, even in the wombe, we are already dying.

The deliciously dismal effect of all this unceasing decease is partly a matter of Donne's prose style. He wrote at a time when—better to say, he quickened the process whereby—in English the orotund Ciceronian period, a balanced type of sentence made of hierarchical clauses, complexly deferring its dying fall (or alternatively: its *o altitudo!*), was being shaken loose by a less formal, Senecan, model—a sentence onto the end of which one could dash new clauses, carelessly. Donne could do Ciceronian, for sure: in his

160 surviving sermons, there are many exquisitely ordered examples. In "Deaths Duell," he even deploys a neatly balanced sentence to tell us that life and death conspire to produce, precisely, a circular Ciceronian period: "As the first part of a sentence peeces wel with the last, and never respects, never hearkens after the *parenthesis* that comes betweene, so doth a *good life* here flow into an *eternall life*, without any consideration, what manner of *death* wee dye."

More frequently in Donne, however, we encounter the loose sentence, which is paratactic, episodic, serial, and seems in "Deaths Duell" the aptest form to describe the unending triumph of death. And the sentence that does this best in the sermon is this one: "Wee have a *winding sheete* in our Mothers wombe, which growes with us from our conception, and we come into the world, wound up in that winding sheet, for wee come to *seeke a grave*; And as prisoners discharg'd of actions may lye for fees; so when the *wombe* hath discharg'd us, yet we are bound to it by *cordes* of flesh, by such a *string*, as that wee cannot goe thence, nor stay there." At this point, Donne has already invited us, his congregation, to imagine the infant in the womb, sightless and without sound, being "*fed with blood*" and "fitted for *workes of darkenes*." Why so monstrous, vampiric even? Because the child is like a worm that feeds on the body of its mother; but also resembles a corpse in the grave, that breeds then kills worms when the body is spent. A grotesque chain of associations is forged here, of which our sentence is the last rotten link, with its suggestion that the caul or amniotic membrane is itself a shroud, and the umbilical cord a chain by which at birth we are imprisoned. At the end of the sentence, it's clear not only that death rules in the midst of life—a predictable enough idea—but that life is exactly a state of

being-between, almost undead.

Thrilled on its way by the already complete metaphor in the first clause, the logic of the sentence is inexorable, delirious. "Which," "and," "for": a hideous plausibility is being built here, soon to be mirrored in the "and," "so," "yet" of the second half of the sentence. It's possible to admire—that is, to fear and love—this sentence solely for the sleek, dire phrase at its center: "for wee come to seeke a grave." It might almost have served on its own, given how forcibly Donne has already insisted that death is present from conception. Instead, either side of this phrase, there hang more unwieldy images, barely contained by the syntax of argument. The legal metaphor—the discharged prisoner still has costs to pay, so remains in prison—is straight out of Donne the poet and student of law. But the remainder is more curious, even awkward, with its odd shift from plural to singular ("cordes" to "string") and its weak, stringy phrasing: "as that wee cannot go thence." In spite of various symmetries—the strong metaphors, the prepositions and conjunctions—I do not think the two halves of the sentence are equal. The first, ending at the grave, sounds all of a piece, held together by the newborn wail of all those *w*'s. The second part seems fractured by that extra semicolon, even if we know that it's perfectly conventional for the time—the rhetorical punctuation (like Donne's frequent *italics*) pointing more to sound than grammatical sense.

In fact, in certain editions of "Deaths Duell," the sentence is cloven after "*seeke a grave*" and becomes two sentences; the first, I suppose, is "better" than the second, sufficient and entire unto itself. In another version published not long after Donne's death, our sentence is conjoined with the previous one, which already tells of "the death of the wombe" and "the manifold deaths of this *worlde*." And in still another

text—the rendering favored by the editors of the Oxford University Press edition of all the sermons—fully four (or is it five?) shorter sentences are gathered into one long one: a paratactic heap of language that makes a funeral of birth, a mother's labor of life itself, and a swelling graveside mound of dirt out of such thoughts and their expression.

I remain attached to the version above, which happens to be the first I read. Its morbid extravagance, its botched symmetry, its alliteration, its repetitions—womb and winding sheet, the doubled discharge—all seem to dramatize thought itself. (It's this "peculiar convolution," wrote Mario Praz, that keeps us coming back to Donne.) Perhaps the insight is swifter and more wittily expressed in the first half, but no matter. Or perhaps that is the point, because by the end of the sentence we are left hanging—or *depending*, as Donne liked to say. (Unable to advance or return, dangling or buried, doesn't he sound now like one of those fretful, stilled narrators out of late Beckett?) At the end of the sermon, Donne asked his listeners to *depend* upon the image of Christ crucified, just as he *depended* from the Cross. "There wee leave you in that *blessed dependency*," he said, knowing very soon his own cord would be cut.

Opposite: In 1631, an ailing John Donne commissioned a portrait of himself as a corpse. This engraving, based on that portrait, was used as the frontispiece for the 1632 edition of *Deaths Duell*. Courtesy British Museum.

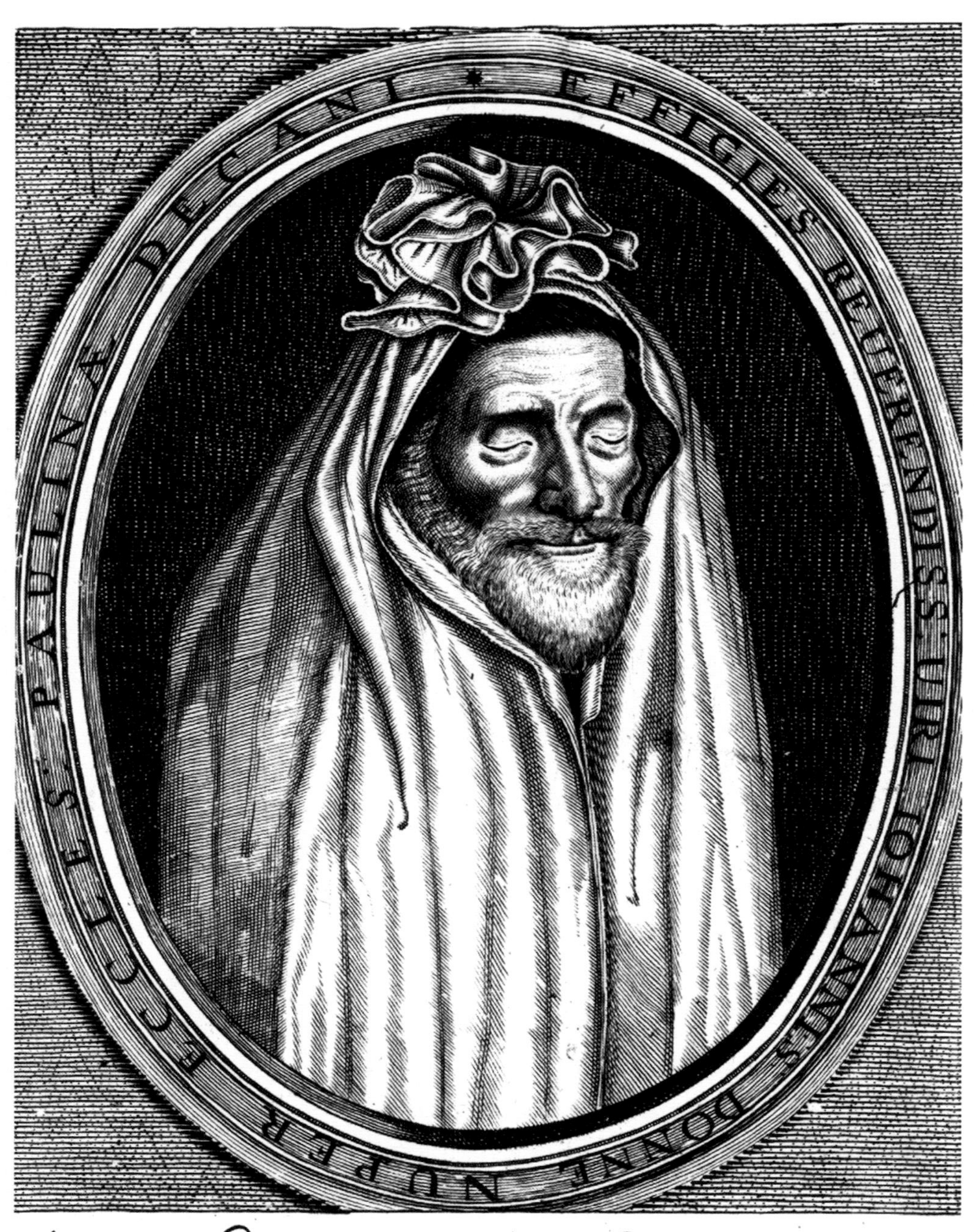

Corporis hæc Animæ sit Syndon, Syndon Jesu
Amen.

Martin ℗ scup. And are to be sould by R R and Ben: ffisher

F-HOLE
Justine Kurland

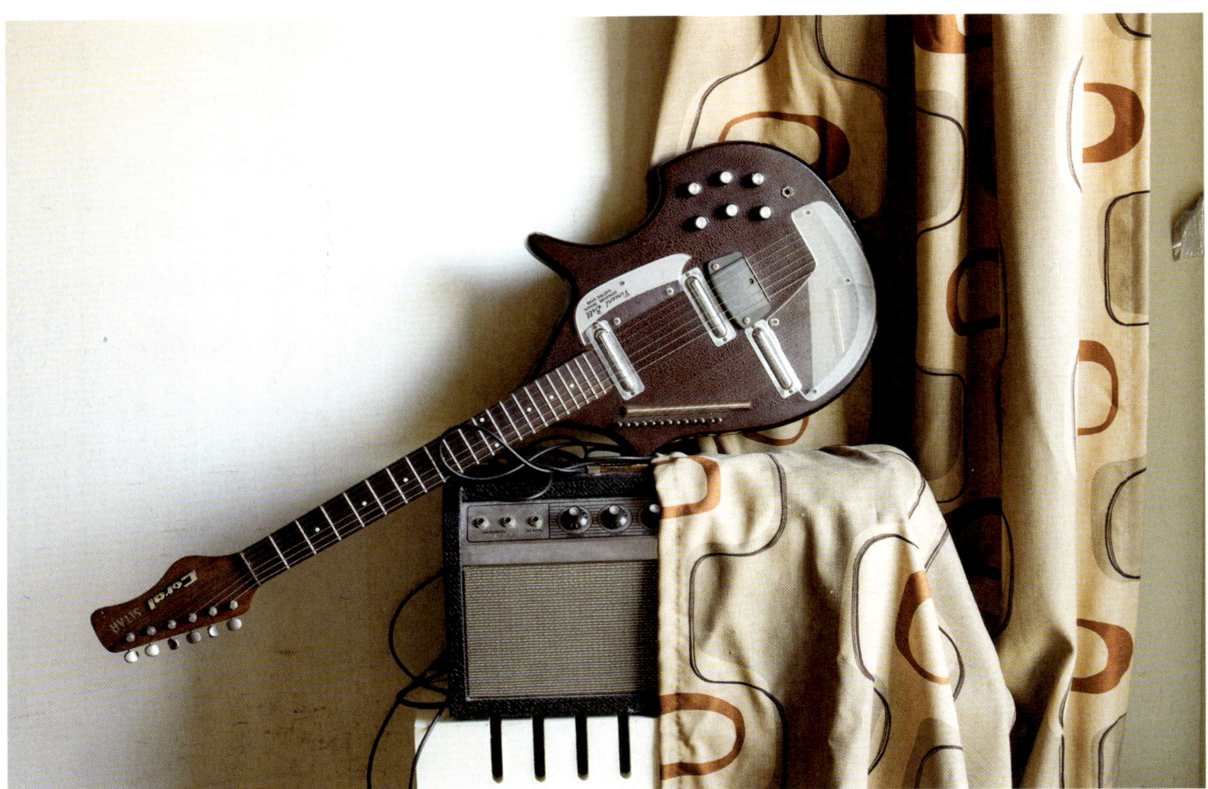

I want to tell you why I sold my van. It's not the first van I've left behind but it might be the last. I would like to publicly renounce a belief system that once seemed useful and true to me; I've outgrown the romantic escapism of this mode of travel. The boy who bought my van was excited to have it. He had just graduated from Bard and was planning to use it to drive to Marfa, where he had an internship. I felt like I was passing a baton. But exactly what kind of baton was it? Few things in the popular imagination are as symbolically loaded as cars. Or as guitars, for that matter. But let me start with vans.

The first one was our family car, by which I mean to say, my mother's van. She named it Ruby Blue. The exterior was tomato-soup-colored and the inside was pink. My older sister was fifteen at the time, which would make it 1980, and had kissed a man twice her age on a bed in the back. He owned the local bar. I remember my mother pulling him out of the van by his hair and my sister scampering away in embarrassment.

Sometimes when I remember it, I'm the one on the bed with the bar owner; perhaps he touches my face and tells me how beautiful I'll be when I grow up, the kind of woman who will make men fall off their bicycles. He did say that to me once. What I see clearly now is the cartoonish way he was expelled from the van—headfirst—by my mother's clenched fist. I don't think it's a stretch to say that the van was a feminist space.

The enclosure of a van is security to some and a threat to others. It's a space that seems to exist outside law and convention. I took pride in its wildness, in how feral I became when I traveled in my van. I didn't need anybody or anything; in my van, I was self-sufficient. If I stayed with a friend, my van was my bed. I could leave at any time of the night without waking anybody up.

When I drive, I'm simultaneously inside and outside. The interior driver is safely strapped into an

---

Above and throughout: Photos Justine Kurland.

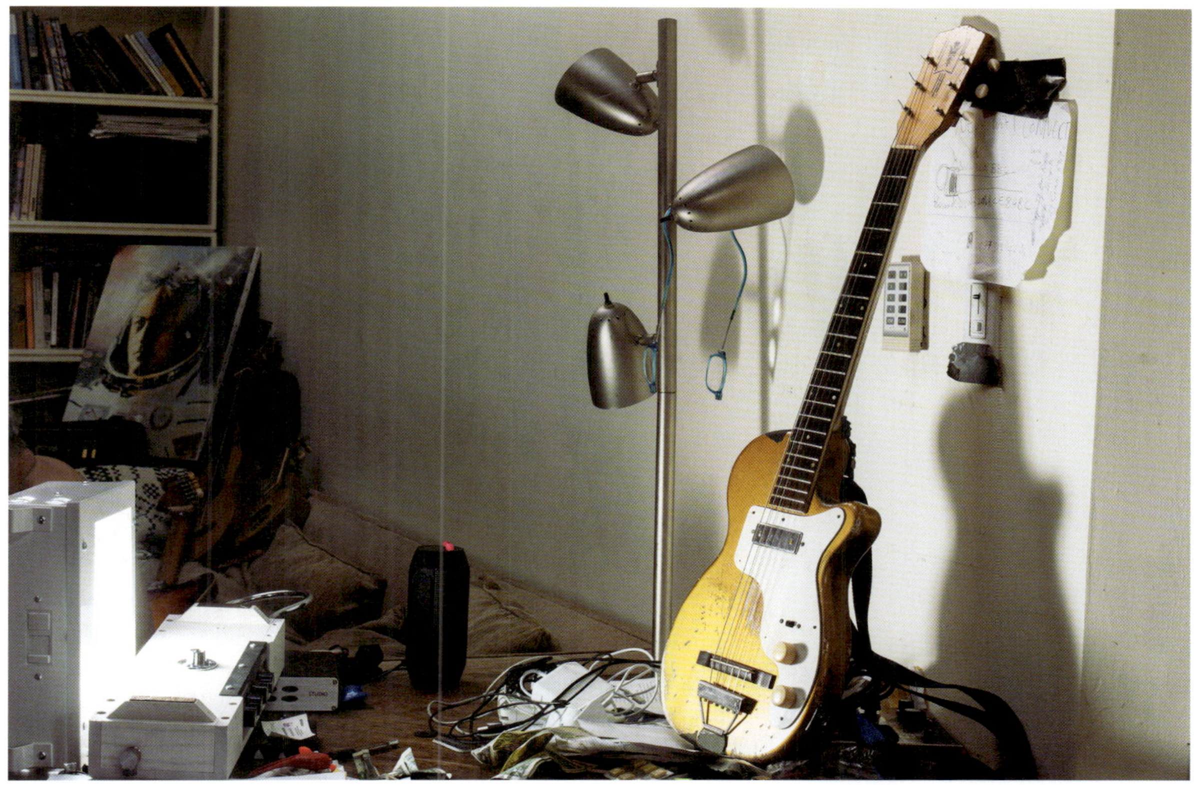

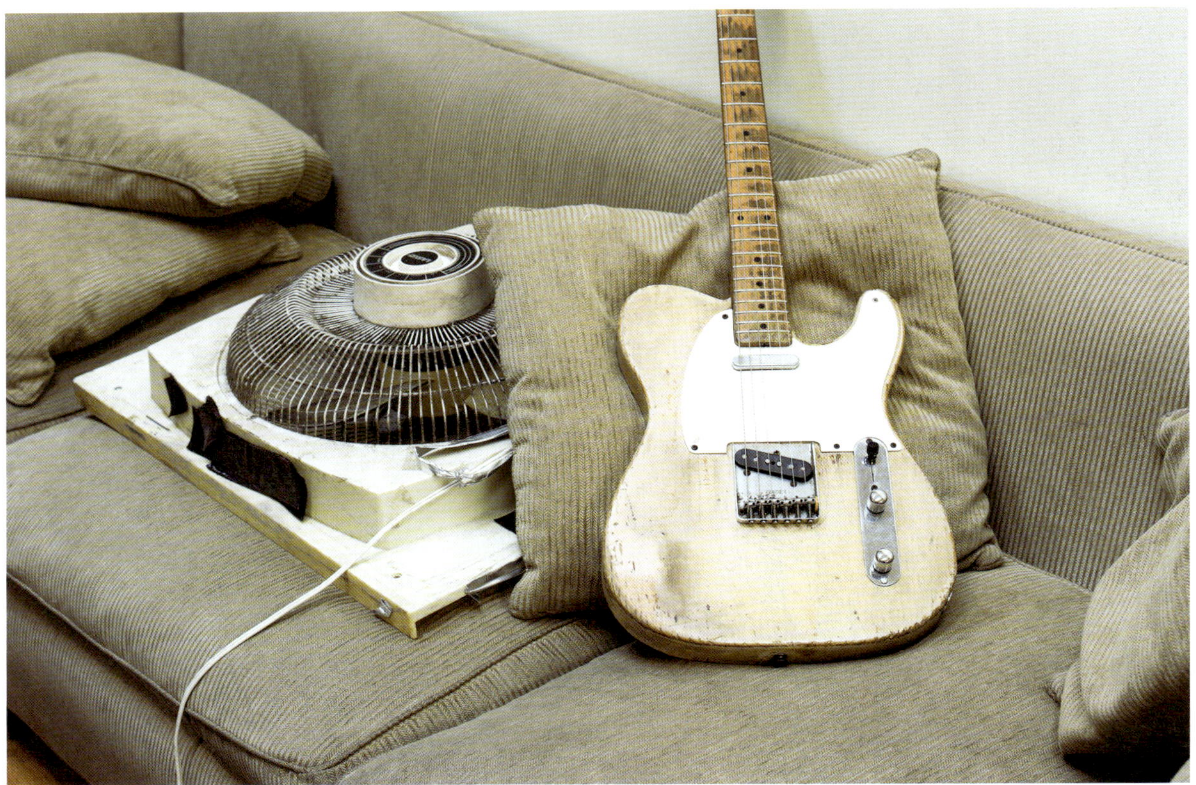

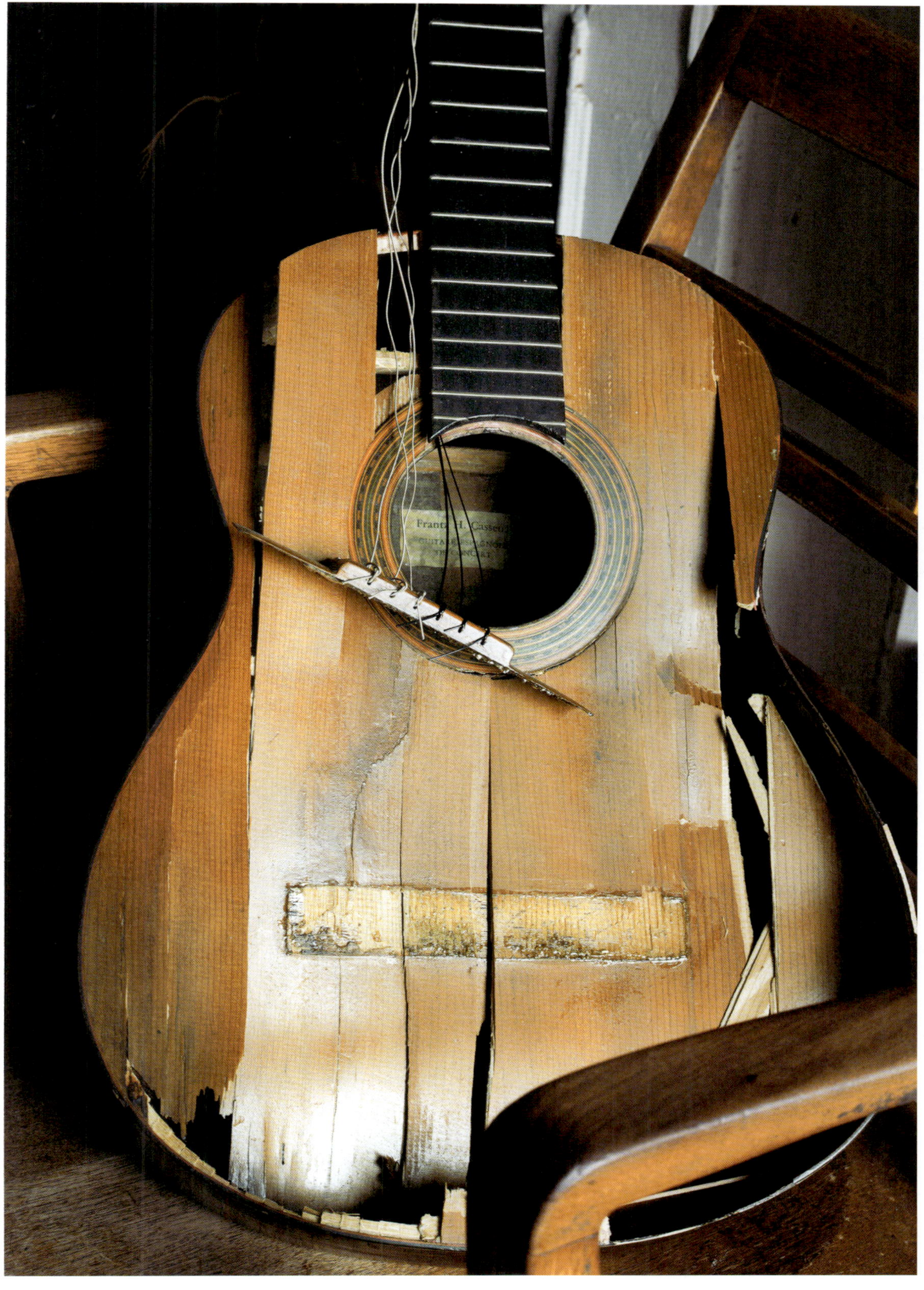

impenetrable private bubble, while the exterior driver navigates freely through the world and covers long distances. If I've been driving for a long time, I turn off the radio so I can hear the engine. What I'm listening for are problems, a misfiring piston or a metallic scrape. When I stop to pump some gas, I like smelling the exhaust fumes and how my ass vibrates for a while after the motor's been cut.

I'll probably die one day in an automobile accident. It will be raining and dark with low visibility. Construction on the road forces the four lanes of traffic to converge into two, and each oncoming car splashes another wave of dirty water against my windshield. Their headlights blind me and we scream with our horns. I'm hit head-on but I don't try to swerve— instead, I use my hands to protect my face.

My father died in 2013, the week before my winter break from teaching, which is when I usually go on a road trip to take photographs. I decided to go anyway that year, leaving the preparations for my father's memorial to my sister. I stopped the car only to sleep or to pee or to write emails inviting people to his service. I don't think I took a single usable photograph.

The van was a way to navigate through my grief. I imagined I was driving away from pain but in fact it filled the four corners of my vehicle. I drove the long way to LA, through the South and along the Mexican border. I listened to the same CD the whole way, on repeat for the entire month. It was in the stereo when I started the van and I never bothered to take it out. The CD was by a guitarist, someone I've had infrequent but periodic hookups with over the past twenty years; he'd given it to me four years earlier, the last time I'd seen him.

He's something of a genius improviser in the way he builds a melody and shatters it open. His music feels interior since it registers emotionally, but also exterior because, in order to structurally pull apart a song, there must be distance. A tune might turn itself inside out, negate itself, and devolve into atonality. Listening, I tumble into the lacuna that had once been a song. Later, I learned to recognize particular strains in his songs from the music of his teacher, a Haitian classical composer who, among other things, mimicked the sounds of voodoo drums with his guitar. You can hear it in the rumble of low chords oscillating back and forth, like jumping from your left foot to your right, the strings loose and dirty, slurring as if toothless and

drunk. He plays on his own on this CD, and the sound of solo guitar was especially affecting in my state of mind. His guitar became my soundtrack as I drove west and by the end of the trip, I was in love with him. We've been involved ever since. Until last month, when he broke up with me. Again.

I never felt comfortable photographing him, so I made pictures of his guitars. A guitar can stand in for a woman's curved form, or it can be phallic—increasingly so the lower it hangs on a torso. I wanted to unravel the myths surrounding guitars, even if I only cared about the ones that belonged to my Guitarist. I photographed his guitars in order to fix them in my own fantasy.

It's necessary to traverse a fantasy rather than go around it, if you want to unfasten its hold on reality. By moving through it, you have the possibility of understanding what it's made of. This isn't my idea; it's Žižek's, or Lacan's, or somebody's. Anyway, if you can bear to go the whole distance, you'll discover there's a void at the center, a huge abyss of nothingness, and that the journey is compelled by nothing more than cheap, everyday props and disposable promises. It's a little like driving a car, or soloing on guitar—once it's over, it's hard to know why you bothered. Vans are hollow inside and so are a lot of guitars, volumes of empty space designed to amplify sound or capacity.

I've had a few vans, but by the time I got this last one, I knew exactly how I wanted it. I designed the interior especially for road trips. The bed doubled as a shelving unit for camera gear; it had a bookcase, cupboards, and hardwood floors. The man who built it built houses and used fancy scrap lumber, birch and cherry. He also played the guitar.

Thoreau's transcendental philosophy underlies much of my motivation for driving, even if I often find his writings annoyingly self-righteous. Nevertheless, it's all there: my attraction to natural settings, as though going deep enough into a forest means I can walk into a time before I existed; my sense that isolation and self-reliance can solve the messy problem of other people. The part that most deeply resonates with me is his cabin. When I drew up the plans for my van and outfitted it with the things I would need, I felt complete in a way that's hard to quantify. Yes, I do happen to have a Phillips-head screwdriver, a pee jar, a cast-iron pan, a copy of *Let Us Now Praise Famous Men*, tampons, the Rand McNally road atlas, peanut butter,

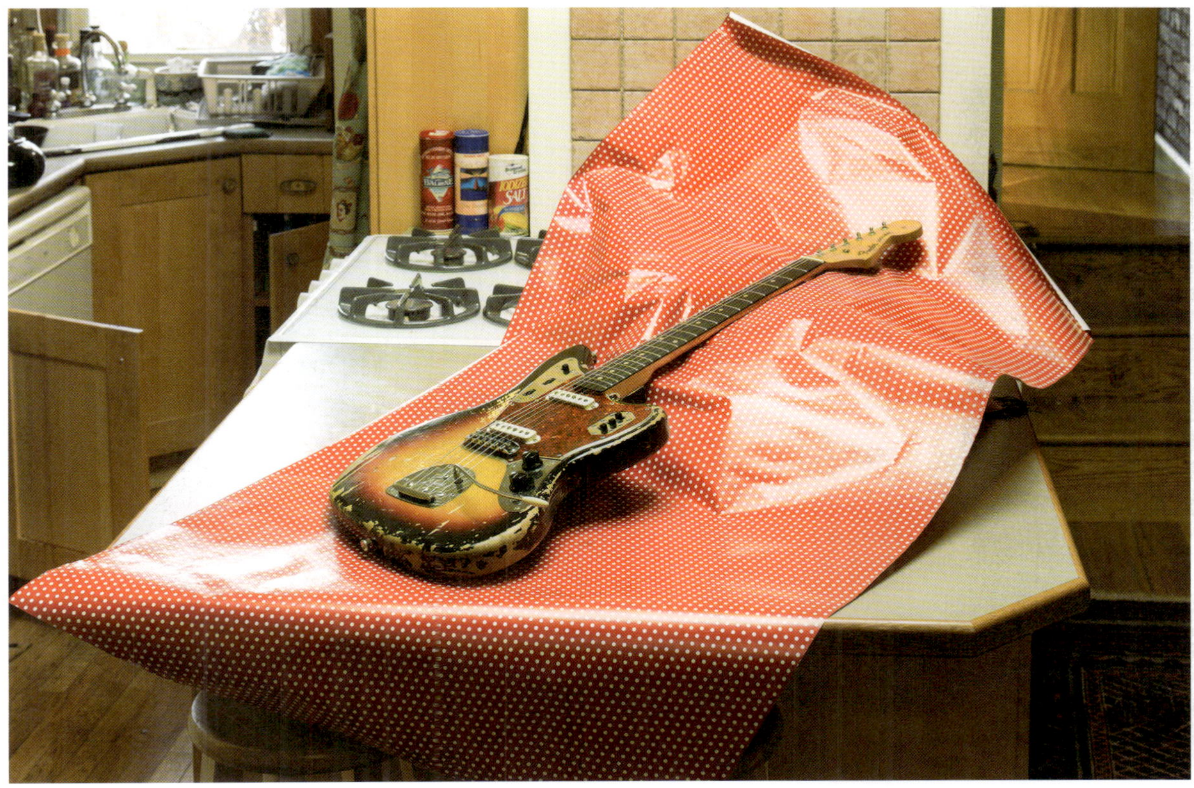

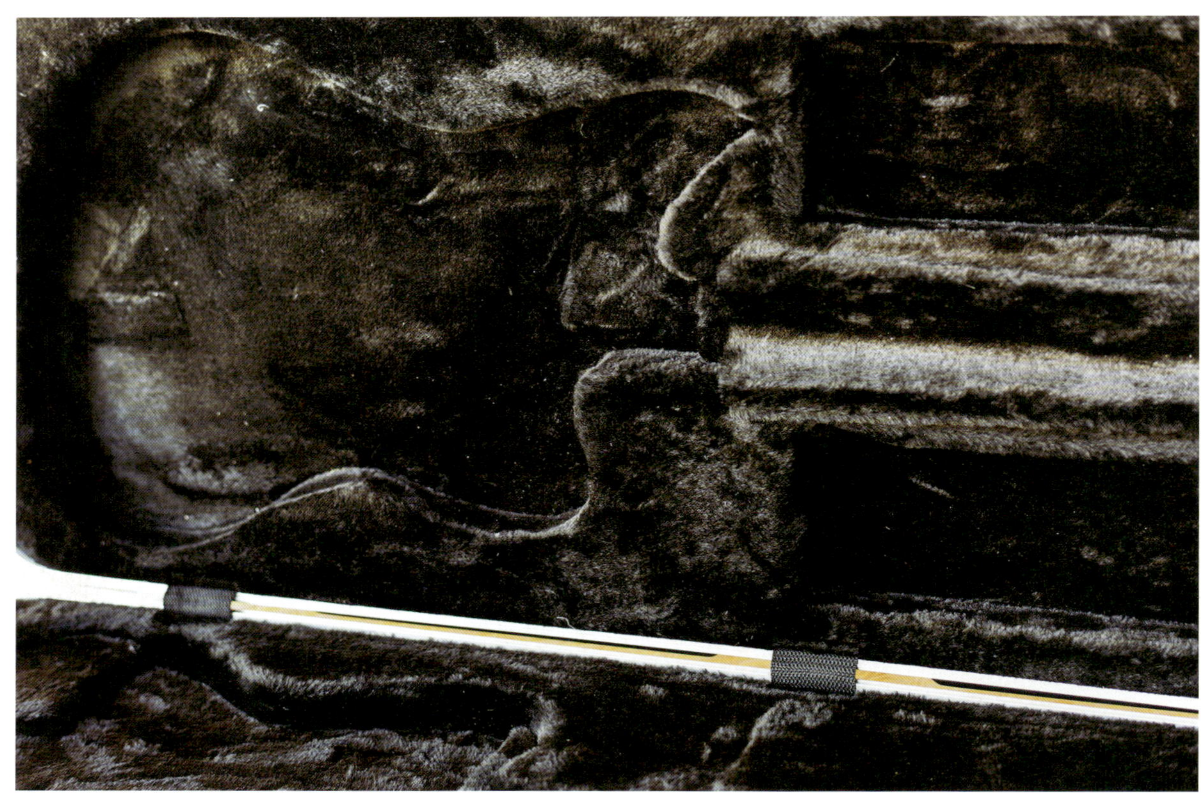

and a memory-foam mattress pad. But it's more than that, more like the love a turtle has for the color, rather than the usefulness, of her shell.

Maybe Thoreau is only a libertarian, claiming a freedom within the margins of his privilege. Haven't we all heard the story of how, during his two years at Walden, he would walk the four miles home every day for his mother's fresh-baked cookies? Think about how Virginia Woolf's "room of one's own" differs from Thoreau's cabin. If a woman's role in society tradition-ally demands her subjugation, then it might be wise for her to withdraw. Woolf writes of the necessity of "killing the angel of the house," which splits me in two when I see my eleven-year-old's body, damp and limp, innocently tangled in his sheets. What about my own responsibility to stick around? After all, someone has to bake the cookies.

After my father died, I walked through his house and photographed his things with my iPhone. I felt creepy doing it—not that he would have minded, but sometimes what a photograph shows isn't nice. He lived in deprivation and poverty. An angry stoicism marked his house, from his duct-taped orthopedic shoes to the DO NOT RESUSCITATE order taped over my son's drawing of a train on his refrigerator, aged by speckles of food. The walls were yellowed from nico-tine and furry from dust stuck on grease. There were carefully crafted models of Mussolini-era bombers and a table for tying flies: fighting and fishing. I never used the photographs for anything or even showed them to my sisters. But I think taking them changed how I photograph.

The Guitarist left a guitar at my house so he would have something to play on the rare occasions he came over. It was a beater—the wood had lost its tension and the bridge kept popping off—but he couldn't bear to throw it away because it had been a gift from his teacher. I didn't break the guitar out of anger alone. My aggression was tentative, even self-conscious. I only cracked the face at first, careful to keep the body intact. As the weeks went by, I took more liberties. But destroying the guitar was not some easy metaphor. I broke it into pieces because of a trajectory I had set in motion with the first photograph I took of it. I had been photographing his guitars to know what they were made of, to understand them as physical objects in the world, with a finite capacity for distress, and a fixed point of dissolution.

By the time I was done with it, the guitar was small enough to fit inside a tote bag. I brought it to a vacant lot to burn and remembered a story the Guitarist had told me about his teacher. I'll call him George. In the late forties, George left Haiti with his wife and moved to New York in order to pursue a career as a composer. He told her that he wouldn't have children with her, also because of his career. The story goes that, while he slept, she crept into his room and tried to cut off his fingers with a pair of scissors. George managed to keep all his digits and later became the father of Haitian classical guitar. But I'm not thinking about him now, I'm thinking about her. I wonder if she was enraged when she held his hand in hers, or merely being practical.

I'm shopping for another car now—a used economy compact, nothing to call home, just a car like any other car. My van had become a container that shaped not only what was inside it, but also what lay beyond. I sold it because it felt like a played-out story, in which freedom had become synonymous with isolation. I need to travel, but there are a lot of different ways to go. Even though I've shed my cabin, I'm keeping the wheels.

In William Faulkner's *Light in August*, Lena Grove travels in pursuit of her baby's father. She continues her journey long after it's clear that no father will materialize. He's not the reason she goes on, just her excuse for living on the road. "My, my. A body does get around," she sighs over and over again.

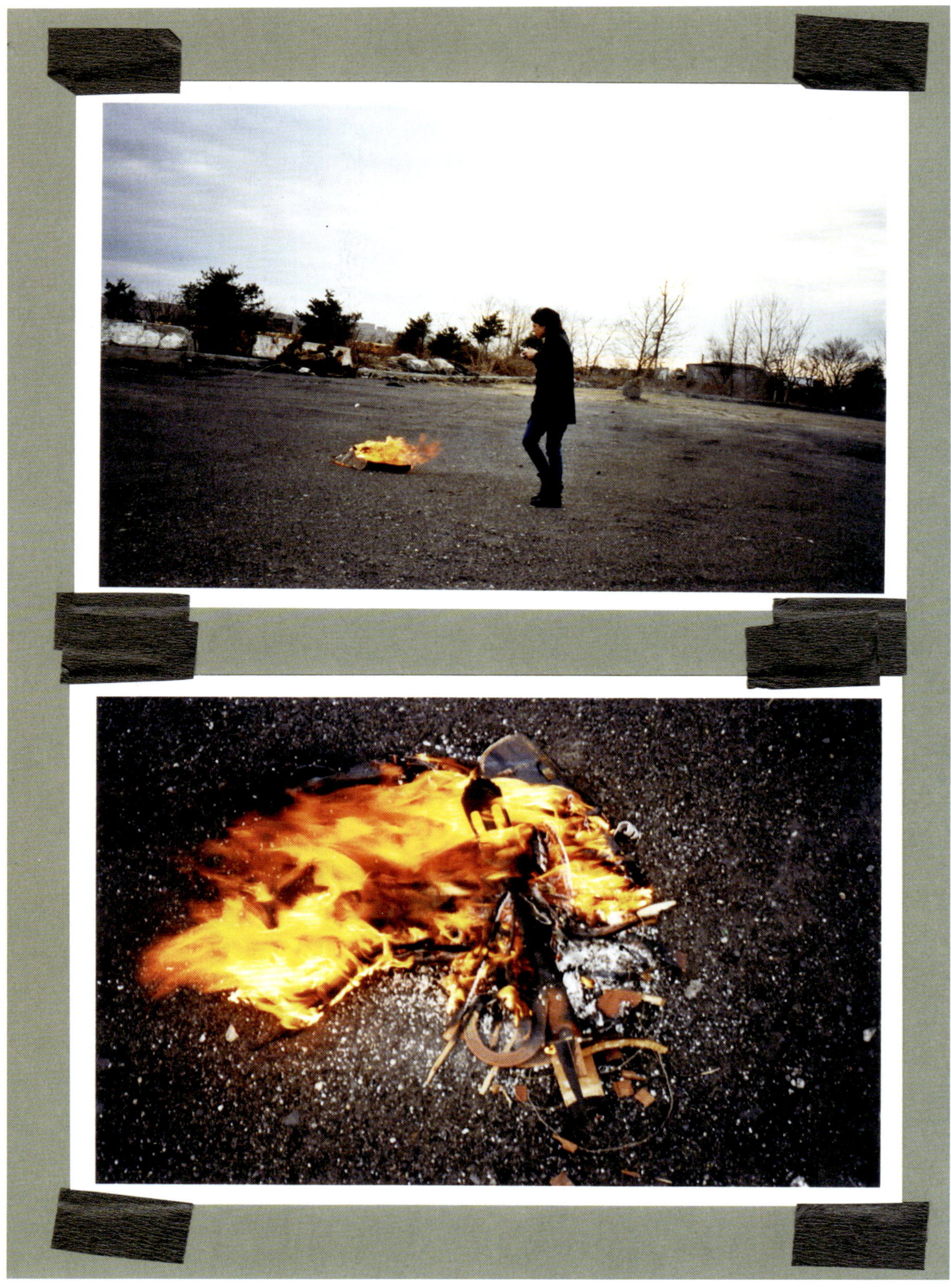

OF PRIMITIVES AND PRIMARIES
Nicholas Gaskill

Art education in the United States began as a colorless affair. Walter Smith, the spokesperson for the industrial drawing campaign that first put art instruction on the public school curriculum in the 1870s, advised teachers to avoid color work until high school, and even then to use it only sparingly.[1] Color, he reasoned, was ancillary both to industrial drawing's practical aims—its attempt to improve the quality of domestic goods by training the hands and eyes of future laborers—and to its metaphysical commitment to "form" as the "language of nature," as opposed to the mere "transient circumstance" of color.[2] Yet by the 1890s, these gray-scale lessons had given way to activities incorporating colored chalk, watercolors, bright parquetry blocks, crayons, and other colorful materials made newly available by advances in dying and color printing techniques. Far from being put off until high school, such chromatic exercises were now recommended particularly for young children, and were accompanied by dozens of books and articles advocating a range of competing approaches to color instruction. Everyone believed that color deserved a prominent place in the modern curriculum, but there was profound disagreement over which colors should be taught, and why.

The three most prominent color instruction systems at the turn of the century—those of game designer Milton Bradley, chromolithographer Louis Prang, and painter-turned-color-theorist Albert Munsell—offered divergent programs for training the vision of the next generation, rooted in conflicting beliefs about both color and childhood. They nonetheless shared a common goal that distinguishes them from the direction color education took after the 1920s. Using exercises in both looking and making, these pedagogues sought to enhance a distinct faculty of color perception known as the "color sense." And they claimed that this training, in turn, would give students the cognitive and social abilities befitting modern citizens, even as they disagreed about what these abilities were. More than a synonym for color perception, the color sense denoted a cultivated talent for seeing and feeling colors, both singly and in combination. It was thought to be trainable, possibly historical, and to vary across human populations.[3] Because it was a psychological rather than a physiological faculty—located in

the mind more than the eye—the work of training the color sense involved providing students with a clear "mental image" of color. Such a mental image, educators argued, would set color instruction on a "solid" or "objective" or "logical" foundation (the terms varied only slightly) and the practical work of installing it in the child's mind required that educators first agree on a set of color *standards*. What these standards were and how to derive them were the questions that most divided Bradley, Prang, and Munsell. The answers they generated reveal the historical concerns that brought color into the classroom and, in the process, made color perception a matter of pedagogical—at times even national—interest.

Perhaps the first point to make about the search for color standards at the end of the nineteenth century is that very few people, and none with any educational clout, advocated the familiar system of primary, secondary, and tertiary colors. In fact, what Milton Bradley mocked as the "red, yellow, and blue theory" was by 1890 considered positively outdated and unscientific, a relic of David Brewster's discredited optics that ignored the advances made by Hermann von Helmholtz and Thomas Young in the mid-nineteenth century.[4] And to be sure, all of the major color education systems aspired to be scientific; color instruction, in its early stages, was a clear outgrowth of the nineteenth-century quest to discover a "logic" or "grammar" of color harmonies. But there were practical considerations as well: as Bradley and Prang both noted, it was impossible to create a pure green by mixing the blue and yellow pigments available to schoolteachers. If not in the three primaries, then, where were the standards to be found?

Bradley proposed the six distinct colors of the solar spectrum: red, orange, yellow, green, blue, and violet. Note that it's six (plus intermediary steps) and not seven—because who sees indigo in the rainbow anyway? (Newton added it to get enough colors to

---

Opposite: Parquetry blocks produced by Milton Bradley, ca. 1890. The phrase "7th Gift" on the packaging refers to the blocks' position in the succession of pedagogical activities designed for young children by educator Friedrich Fröbel. Courtesy Norman Brosterman.

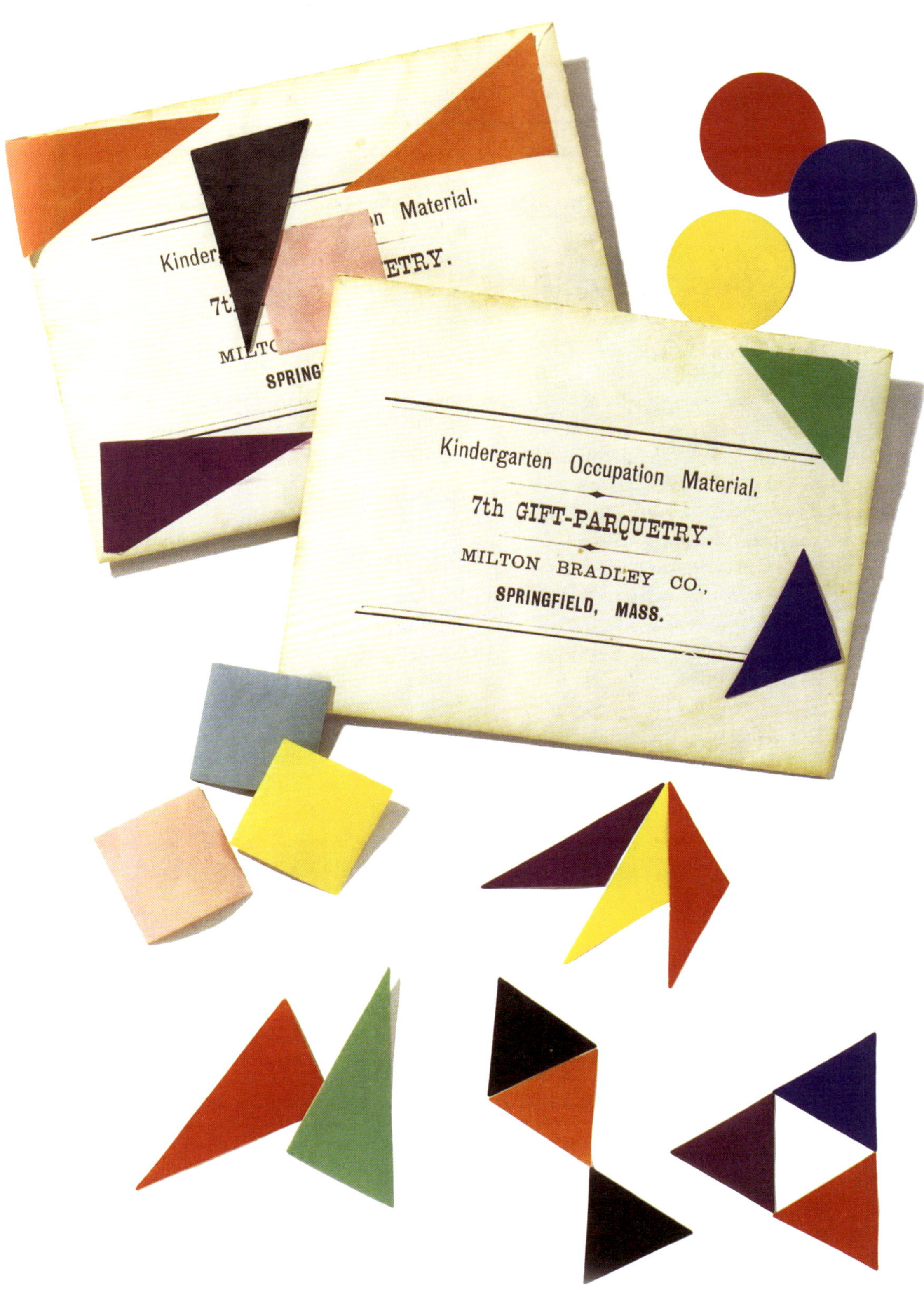
Kindergarten Occupation Material.
7th GIFT-PARQUETRY.
MILTON BRADLEY CO.,
SPRINGFIELD, MASS.

match the seven notes of the musical scale.) But before discussing the justifications for the spectrum standards, we should first explain why Bradley, a man most known as the printer and toy manufacturer who made a mint off *The Checkered Game of Life* (1860), cared about color education in the first place. Because he did indeed care: he published several books on color instruction in the 1890s, including the much-cited *Elementary Color* (1895), which built on his decades of experience manufacturing a full line of colored materials designed for school use. His interest in the topic had begun in the late 1860s after he attended a lecture by Elizabeth Peabody on the educational theories of Friedrich Fröbel, the inventor of kindergarten. Fröbel's system involved a series of "gifts"—including six worsted balls of different colors, sets of wooden cubes, spheres, and cylinders—and of activities he called "occupations," such as weaving, paper folding, and clay modeling. Peabody remarked that if the kindergarten movement were to take hold in America, these materials would need to be manufactured domestically. Bradley jumped at the opportunity. The lecture had made a convert of him, and he wanted to do his part to facilitate the kindergarten movement. Yet as a manufacturer, he immediately ran into trouble: many of the occupations called for colored paper, but Bradley's suppliers couldn't agree on what any particular hue should look like. Even worse, the same paper mill often failed to provide steady hues, and so Bradley "found it impossible to … insure his customers that any color he had furnished them could be duplicated."[5]

In the process of solving this problem for manufacturing, Bradley formulated his educational program. He established a system of color standards designed to communicate colors between his factory and the mill, and then used this system to shape students' engagements with the chromatic world. It's not surprising, then, that Bradley's course of study reflects the habits of thought well-suited to a factory owner: namely, an approach to the visible world that treated it as an

---

Below: The Prang Color Chart, showing the colors of an "ideal color unit." Published in Louis Prang, Mary Dana Hicks, and John S. Clark, *Color Instruction: Suggestions for a Course of Instruction in Color for Public Schools*, 1893.

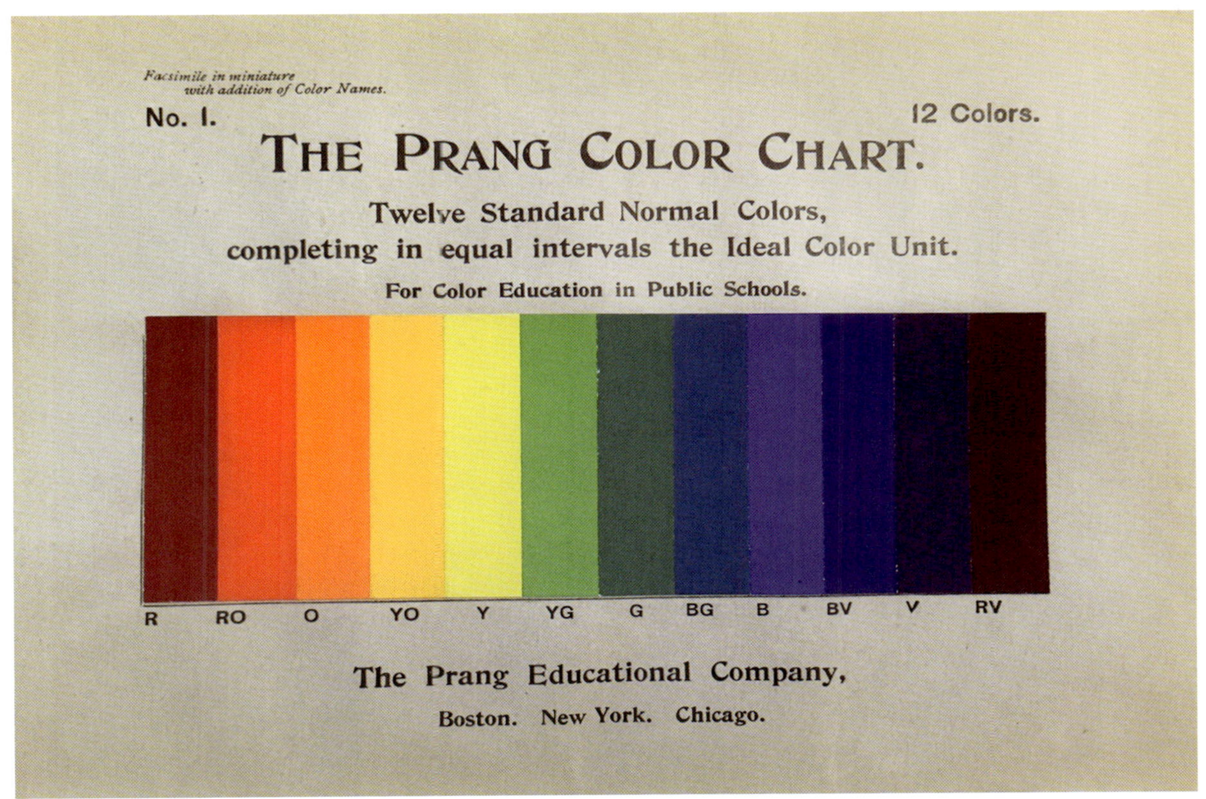

assortment of decomposable colors able to be reconstructed and mass-produced on demand. He chose the six hues of the prismatic spectrum as his standards because, he explained, they are the fundamental colors of light and therefore the fundamental colors of nature. The central conceit of the Bradley method is that these standard colors are somehow the world's realest colors and that the secret to developing the color sense is to create a "mental image of each of the six colors" as vividly present to the student "as that of the cube after it has been handled and modeled."[6] To this end, the students began their course by moving, hue by hue, through the standards, then studying the increments between them, then their mixtures with white, black, and gray, before finally—finally!—turning to the colors of the landscape, of household objects, and of flowers.

But even once they'd re-entered the realm of everyday color experience, their task was to treat it as a conglomeration of the abstract standards: the characteristic assignment in the Bradley system, detailed in Bradley's own books and in those of his followers, was the *color analysis*, in which children broke down the component parts of natural objects. On the one hand, the assignment aimed to "lead the pupil to closer observation, to see color where he has never thought of looking for it, to discover harmonies where he never knew before they could be found"—lofty goals that extended Fröbel's pedagogy further into the realm of color. On the other, it transformed the underlying principles of unity that Fröbel hoped kindergarten activities would reveal into stacks of colored material waiting to be called up from the warehouse and arranged in ever more spectacular chromatic goods. Indeed, Bradley completed his list of the benefits of color education by specifying that the more abstract attainments "should ultimately lead him [the pupil] to the practical application of what he has learned in the arts and manufactures."[7] This mixture of Romantic education and modern industry lies behind Bradley's boast that "the graduate from a two year's course in the kindergarten may have a better color sense than is at present enjoyed by the average business or professional man."[8] To be sure, all systems of color education emphasized the commercial benefits of training the color sense—this business-oriented brand of pedagogy was the legacy of the industrial drawing campaign—but Bradley's system built the assumptions of the manufacturer's world into its exercises most vividly, weaving

them into the framework he inherited from Fröbel and Peabody.

Where Bradley appealed to nature's standards as the basis for education, the authors of *Color Instruction* (1893)—Louis Prang, Mary Dana Hicks, and John Clark—argued that the only sound starting point for color training was in the preferences and discriminating powers of children. The idea, current in the psychological field of child study, was that children experienced colors differently than adults, that their eyes only responded to bright, saturated hues, leaving some colors barely distinguished at all. As the authors announce in their preface, "Hitherto color instruction has been based upon theory only, and colors have been arbitrarily given without any consideration of the power of color perception in the child. In this course an appeal to the color perception of the child is for the first time presented in the course of the exercises, leading to a knowledge of color through the development of the color sense."[9] Hicks—the real voice behind *Color Instruction*, despite the fact that Prang gets most of the credit—conducted her own experiments on "the child's power of color perception" in 1891. She concluded that children perceive light hues better than dark ones, and that they have a decided preference for yellow. Based on these findings, she suggested that color education begin with yellow and move through orange, red, violet, and blue before ending with green, though she also encouraged teachers to test their students early on and to tailor the course to their abilities.

This caveat, it turns out, is important. For just as surely as the Prang system expresses the basic tenet of both child study and progressive education—namely, that the child has its own interests and cognitive capacities that are distinct from those of the adult, and therefore that instruction must be tailored to the mind of the child—so too does it align itself with a contemporaneous line of anthropological inquiry into the correlation between color perception and civilization, one that posited variation in the color sense across racial groups. Hicks references this work explicitly in her essay "Color in Public Schools" (1894), citing figures who supposed that "the color-sense is the result of the development of the race" and that "the eyes of infants go through stages corresponding to race experience."[10] Even more, Hicks contributed to these studies by collecting data from the Carlisle Industrial Indian School, the Hampton Normal and Agricultural

Munsell's "color tree," his representation of color space. Illustration from Albert Munsell, *A Color Notation: A Measured Color System, Based on the Three Qualities Hue, Value, and Chroma*, 1907.

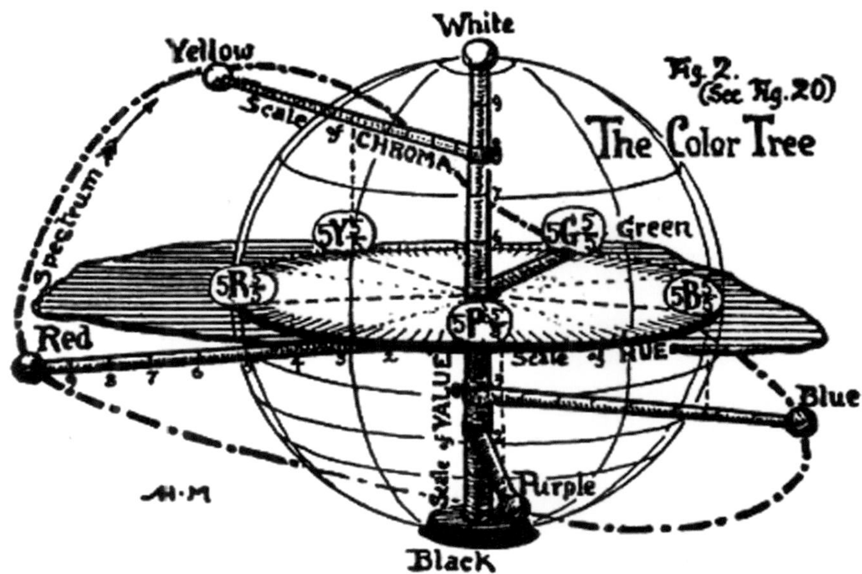

Institute, and—thanks to the help of Earl Barnes, the first director of Stanford University's education department—the "Chinese children of Oakland."[1] Unlike the white children, the Native Americans preferred blue, the "colored students" liked blue and violet, and the Chinese kids showed an inclination towards red-orange and yellow-green. But the particular preferences here are not as important as the fact that they were looked for and appealed to as part of a program of perceptual training. In the end, Hicks's insistence that "the color sense varies greatly in different individuals, because of heredity and because of the greater or less degree of cultivation" situates the Prang color system squarely within the racialization of color perception more explicitly invoked in late nineteenth-century anthropology.[12]

In *Color Instruction*, however, the focus is on cultivation, not heredity. In particular, the book provides a set of exercises designed to lead students from the rudimentary color perceptions available to them in the first grade to the nuanced and delicate harmonies enjoyed by civilized adults. As in Bradley's initiative to train the eyes of future manufacturers, this program required establishing a set of standards. But unlike Bradley's, Prang's standards were not given as natural, nor were they used to explain the colors of the world; rather, they were components of an "ideal color unit" that comprised twelve basic intervals: red, orange, yellow, green, blue, and violet, with half-steps between each. As befits a system that treats color perception as an

acquired skill related to mental development, the ideal color unit was presented strictly as a learning tool, not as nature's paint box; that is, it was a useful abstraction meant to get the child in closer working touch with her environment. "In early education," Prang and company write, "the essential aim is, or should be, to make the child acquainted with his environment," and "the study of color" makes this environment "more and more real to him."[13] Such contact is facilitated by a color unit constructed to sensitize the child to finer and finer distinctions in the visual world—distinctions of hue, distinctions of tone and complementarity, and even, toward the end of the course, distinctions of historical and cultural context provided through lessons in the history of ornamentation. This effort to teach the child to feel the *meaning* of color as well as its bare sensory force explains the most distinctive feature of the Prang system: its reliance on nineteenth-century poetry, specifically lyric poems in which the speaker describes a color experience, as models of a well-developed color sense. In short, Prang's course of study, in its movement from color preference tests in the first grade through poetry recitals at the advanced levels, sought to effect the movement from primitivism to civilization, enacted in the life of the child.

Bradley and Prang offered two distinct explanations for why young children should play with bright colors: either because these hues are nature's primaries (Bradley) or because the students are little

primitives whose color sense responds only to vivid stimuli (Prang). Our final pedagogue opposed both of these fundamental assumptions and launched his educational program to intervene in what he saw as the violent assault on the child's eye occurring in public schools. Citing those, like Hicks and Prang, who suggested that children need bright colors to excite their interest, Albert Munsell asked, "Does [the child] not also crave candy, matches, the bass drum and the carving knife?" We keep the child protected from other sensational extremes—loud noises, spicy flavors, frigid temperatures—why expose them to "loud" and "riotous" pigments? Munsell continues:

It is true that he dearly loves to play Indian in the back yard, to scalp his sister, shoot the cat, paint horrid hieroglyphs upon the stable door and make the cook shudder with his yells, but I have yet to visit a school where such exercises form the introduction to singing or dancing. Only in color does such savagery exist.[14]

Needless to say, Munsell did not think that teachers should encourage the child's savage instincts—there's none of Hicks's emphasis on meeting the child where she's at. Instead, Munsell insisted that "education aims at control of the body and the mind" and that it was "high time to apply logical methods in training the eye."[15] As such, his students were taught to curb their primitive impulses, a skill all the more necessary due to the discordant hues daily thrown up on billboards and tomato cans (Munsell's favorite examples) as the world of commerce increasingly became a world of enticing color.

Munsell referred to his program as "a measured training of the color sense."[16] The mental image he sought to install in his students was not a collection of fundamentals or an ideal color unit designed to better acquaint the child with her environment; rather, it was a kind of governor or regulator, something to calibrate the child's unbalanced responses to its chromatic environment. He called his collection of standards the "five middle hues": low-key versions of red, yellow, green, blue, and purple. (But not orange. He demoted orange from a basic color to an intermediary between yellow and red to correct what he saw as a brightness bias in other color systems.)[17] He arrived at these standards, he assured his readers, in the most scientific way. First, he mapped the whole of color space in three dimensions:

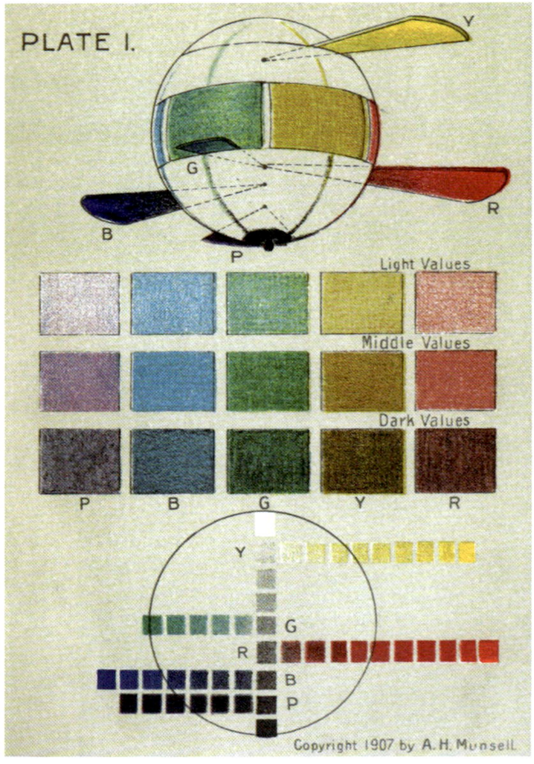

Albert Munsell's "five middle hues," shown relative to their position within the whole of color space. Illustration from Albert Munsell, *The Munsell Color System: Children's Studies in Measured Colors*, 1907.

hue (red, yellow, blue, etc.), value (lightness or darkness), and chroma (saturation or purity). His favorite image is that of a tree, where the trunk represents the scale from white to black, and the branches are the colors, each gaining in purity or "chroma" as it distances itself from the grayscale base. Some branches extend further than others. Red and yellow, for instance, reach greater intensities of chroma than green or purple. For Munsell, this disparity showed that the so-called spectrum standards, presented as equal in all but hue, were actually very different sorts of colors when described in terms of all three qualities of chromatic space. To arrive at his middle colors, his standards for education, Munsell carved a balanced color sphere from this uneven color tree. "The regular color sphere," he explained, "is contained within the irregular color solid, for if the latter be placed, as it were, in a lathe, and excess chroma cut away, there will remain the balanced color sphere, every hue of which is symmetrically disposed to the neutral center."[18]

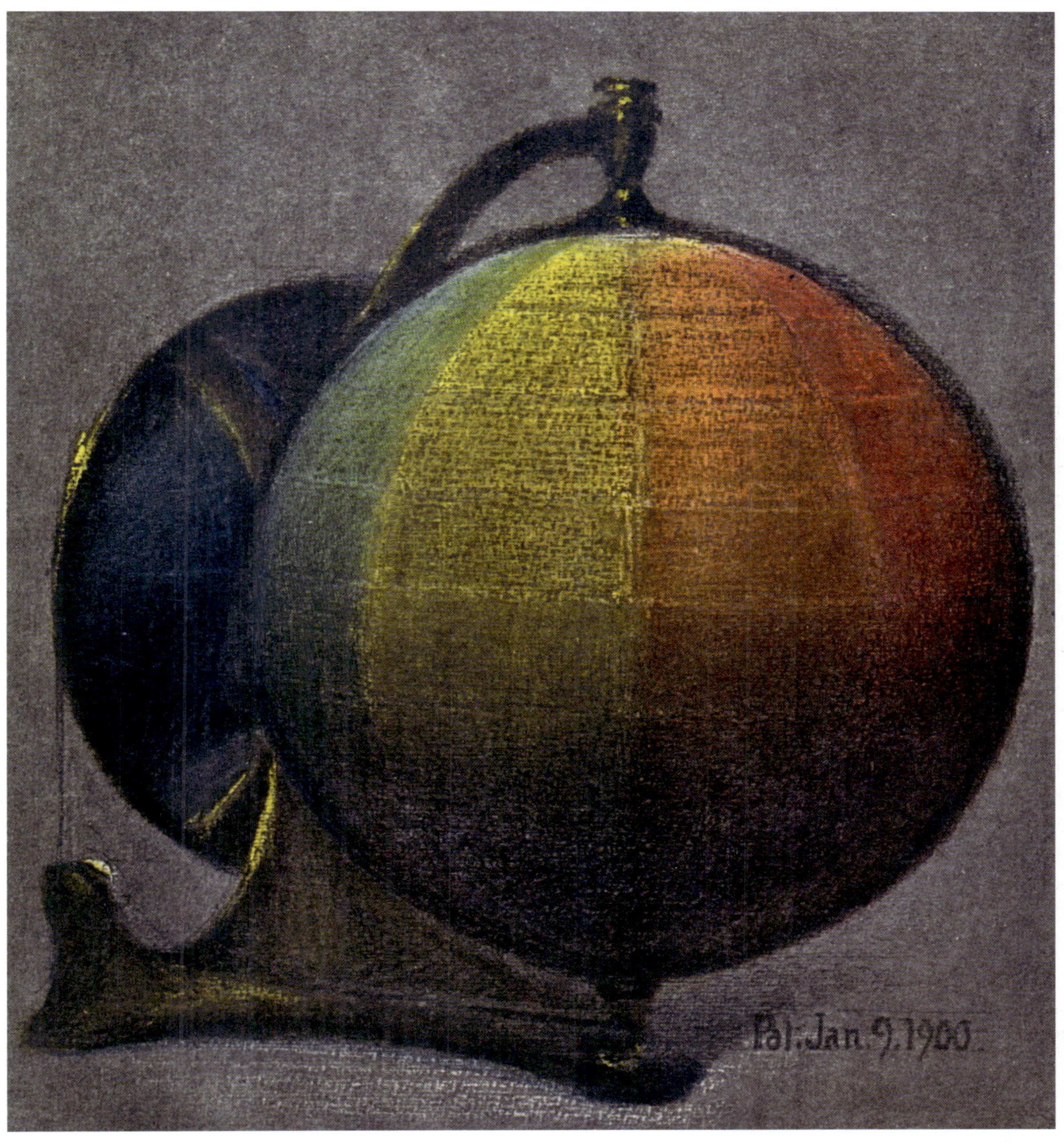

Munsell's "balanced color sphere," with the "excess" hues removed. Illustration from Albert Munsell, *A Color Notation: A Measured Color System, Based on the Three Qualities Hue, Value, and Chroma*, 1907.

The five distinct hues that make up the equator of this sphere were equidistant from the black and white poles (and so equal in value) and equally extended from the grayscale base (and thus poised between "the extremes of neutrality and maximum chroma").[19] These middle hues served as Munsell's standards—the colors of the crayons, watercolors, and other materials used by beginners in the Munsell system. They were, Munsell wrote, the "starting-points for training the eye"; and "only with such a trained judgment," he concluded, "is it safe to undertake the use of strong colors."[20]

Starting with these colors, and then working up to stronger combinations, all the while attending to the relations among colors mapped out in three dimensions, proponents of the Munsell system hoped to produce students with impeccable taste, children who, far from thrilling at bright reds and yellows, would shun them as discordant and take delight only in subdued palettes, with high color thrown in for spice. Public school teachers, however, rushed to protest. Some, like Hicks, argued that children simply couldn't see the middle colors very distinctly, and thus that using them as a basis was misguided. Others complained that children couldn't draw nice things like poppies and buttercups with these muted hues. Indeed, anyone who's been in a Toys"R"Us store or had children bring them artwork from kindergarten knows that Munsell lost this battle decisively, even as his three-dimensional color solid (the tree, not the sphere) became the standard for color nomenclature in American industry.[21]

But if that's the case, who won? Not exactly Bradley or Prang, even though their emphasis on bright hues certainly set the tone for the century that followed. Instead, by the 1920s, the fundamental premise of these three pedagogues—that the color sense required systematic training—had given way to a looser mode of instruction, one based on "free expression" and exemplified in the rise of finger painting in the 1930s. For teachers after World War I, the problem wasn't which system to adopt; the problem was with the very notion that systematic, top-down instruction could improve, rather than dampen, the child's enjoyment of color. But between 1890 and 1915, the linguistic and conceptual abstractions of color education were understood not as impediments to the immediacy of color but rather as the mediations required to intensify and enrich that immediacy, bringing within its range the social concerns and historical assumptions that marked the United States at the turn of the century. Bradley's students came to see the world as manufacturers; Prang's were treated as primitive perceivers working their way toward civilization; Munsell's were meant to embody the genteel reaction against the rise of consumer culture: and in all of these cases, color perception became imbued with specific cultural significance. This, finally, is the lesson of color pedagogy: it shows so clearly what is often so hard to see, the social meanings not just of colors but of our ways of seeing and feeling them.

1 Foster Wygant, *School Art in American Culture*, *1820–1970* (Cincinnati, OH: Interwood Press, 1993), p. 6.

2 Walter Smith, *Art Education, Scholastic and Industrial* (Boston: James R. Osgood & Co., 1872), p. 63.

3 For more on the color sense, see Guy Deutscher, *Through the Language Glass: Why the World Looks Different in Other Languages* (New York: Picador, 2010).

4 Milton Bradley, *Color in the Kindergarten: A Manual of the Theory of Color and the Practical Use of Color Material in the Kindergarten* (Springfield, MA: Milton Bradley Co., 1893), p. 6.

5 Ibid., p. 4. See also Bradley's account in his 1902 text "Early Days of the Kindergarten," reprinted in *Milton Bradley, A Successful Man: A Brief Sketch of His Career and the Growth of the Institution which He Founded* (Springfield, MA: Milton Bradley Co., 1910).

6 Milton Bradley, *Elementary Color* (Springfield, MA: Milton Bradley Co., 1895), p. 79.

7 Milton Bradley, *Color in the Kindergarten*, p. 32.

8 Ibid., p. 6.

9 Louis Prang, Mary Dana Hicks, and John S. Clark, *Color Instruction: Suggestions for a Course of Instruction in Color for Public Schools* (New York: Prang Educational Company, 1893), pp. iii-iv.

10 Mary Dana Hicks, "Color in Public Schools," *Proceedings of the National Education Association Convention, Asbury Park, N.J., 1894* (St. Paul, MN: National Education Association, 1895), p. 914.

11 Ibid., p. 913.

12 Josh Berson shows how the stadial theory of civilization that characterized nineteenth-century ethnographic inquiries into the color sense was revived—in a modified form—through the search for basic color terms in mid-twentieth-century linguistic anthropology. See Josh Berson, "Color Primitive," *Cabinet*, no. 52 (Winter 2013–2014).

13 Louis Prang, Mary Dana Hicks, and John S. Clark, *Color Instruction*, p. 13.

14 Albert Munsell, *Color and an Eye to Discern It* (Boston: printed by author, 1907), p. 14.

15 Ibid.

16 Albert Munsell, "A Measured Training of the Color Sense," *Education*, vol. 29, no. 6 (February 1909).

17 See Michael Rossi, "Orange," *Cabinet*, no. 41 (Spring 2011).

18 Albert Munsell, "A Measured Training of the Color Sense," p. 374.

19 Ibid., p. 365.

20 Ibid., p. 1.

21 Edward R. Landa and Mark D. Fairchild, "Charting Color from the Eye of the Beholder," *American Scientist*, vol. 93, no. 5 (September–October 2005).

BETWEEN THE MINE AND THE STREAM
Justin E. H. Smith

Gwalia, Western Australia, 1897. A young man, an American man, rides with his entourage into town, on camelback. He is covered with blackflies. He has the air of an arrogant yet honorable man. The ragged miners assembled there know that the man has recently earned a degree in geology from a university on the other side of the ocean. He has come to apply the most advanced knowledge of modern mine engineering to extract, with their labor, the metal riches from this continent of red dust.

The man succeeds. He cuts costs by employing desperate Italian immigrants, ready to work for lower wages, for any wages. They are scabs, as the English and Irish union militants see it, but they get the job done.

The man's employers, the London-based Bewick, Moreing & Co., are impressed, and send him to China to continue his work. He is now accompanied by his former Stanford sweetheart and new wife, Lou, née Henry. They will live through the Boxer Rebellion together, in Tianjin in 1900. Both, it is reported, show courage under siege and agility with firearms.

The man is made a partner in his company, and the couple will enjoy long sojourns in London, he directing mining operations around the world from an abstract distance, she continuing in her study of languages and literatures, notably Latin and Chinese. In 1905, she comes across a copy of Georgius Agricola's (or Georg Bauer's) 1556 work, *De re metallica*, on the subject of metals, mining, and metallurgy. It has never been translated into English. The couple decides to undertake this project together.

The resulting edition is published in London in 1912. It is the very model of what historians of science today call "Whiggish" scholarship. It is solid and rigorous as far as facts go, and precise in matters of translation (going so far as to include a thorough study of the sixteenth-century German mining vocabulary that Agricola had rendered, for the first time, into learned Latin). Yet it is also triumphalist, presentist, and hermeneutically blind, setting out from the premise that we, today, in 1912, know better than they did in the past, and that history has been a long, slow march out of foolishness, from a world of dark superstition to one of no-bullshit problem-solving: Agricola is

an impressive thinker "for his era." The translators do not seem to be worried that their own thought too is of an era, of which it may one day be taken as typical. (Curiously, Whiggism in science can coexist with the staunchest classicism in philology. Thus, in the translators' preface, we are told that Agricola's Latin is mostly free of "medieval corruption," yet regrettably "tainted with German construction."[1])

Leaving aside our translators' Whiggish bent, the British political party known as the Whigs do have a complicated historical relationship to the American party of our mining-engineer-turned-Latinist. In 1929, he will be elected, as a Republican, to the office of president of the United States.

When we speak of a "presidential philosophy," we do not ordinarily have in mind the intellectual debt a president may have had to Renaissance natural philosophy. But Herbert Hoover's intellectual development seems to require that we widen our ordinary scope. Hooverism may in fact be the last echo of a sort of statesmanly engagement with philosophy that probes somewhat deeper into the order of things, and into humanity's place in that order, than does the recent genre of campaign-minded, policy-focused, ghost-written memoirs.

Hoover's philosophy is continuous with a long American tradition, born in England, of engaging with nature, both for the wonder of the thing itself and for the more practical empiricist aim, typified already in the seventeenth century by Francis Bacon, of discovering better ways to dominate it and to put it to use for us. The idea that philosophy might be practical in this way has been almost completely erased from our consciousness today, above all in the professionalized

---

Opposite: In this engraving from Georgius Agricola's *De re metallica* (1556), two miners use forked divining rods to locate subterranean deposits of metal. According to Hoover, Agricola's is the first published description of such instruments, which were believed (barring any "impeding peculiarities" on the part of those using them) to begin rotating near veins of ore. Rods of different materials were paired with different minerals: hazel with silver, pitch pine with lead, iron (or steel) with gold. Agricola denounced their use as a superstition, which passed to miners "from its impure origin with the magicians."

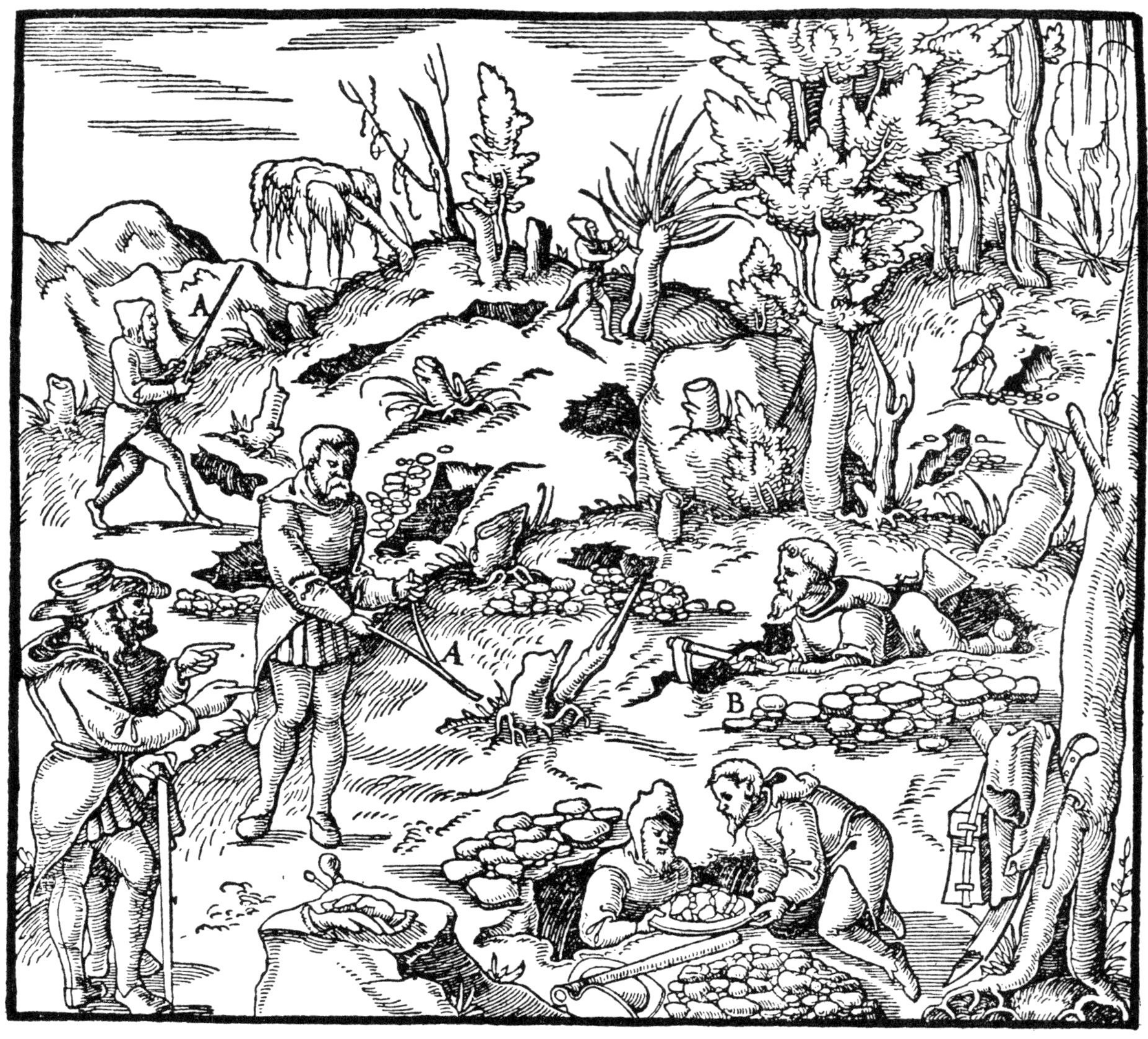
A
A
B

bubble of academic philosophy. Yet, from the sixteenth to the eighteenth centuries, the period from which Hoover drew the most, common usage of the term makes perfectly clear that what a "philosopher" does primarily is to inquire—as Socrates was, wrongly, accused of doing—into what goes on in the heavens above and the earth below (and everywhere between as well). In a characteristic usage of the term, John Evelyn, in his 1661 work *Fumifugium; Or, The Inconveniencie of the Aer and Smoak of London Dissipated*, speaks of "these unwholsome vapours, that distempered the Aer, to the very raising of Storms and tempests; upon which a Philosopher might amply discourse."[2] Or, as Agricola himself explains, "there are many arts and sciences of which a miner should not be ignorant. First there is Philosophy, that he may discern the origin, cause, and nature of subterranean things."[3]

Thomas Jefferson would amply discourse on the floral and faunal diversity of the New World, not least with his contemporary, the French natural historian Buffon, and also participate in ethnolinguistic surveys of the Native American groups of the Northeast. This sort of practical undertaking was one of the principal tasks of philosophy as commonly understood into the eighteenth century, and particularly so in the United States, where it was the only conception of philosophy that seemed appropriate for the nascent nation. Even those Americans who drew on supremely abstract continental systems, such as the one Hegel had lately produced, nonetheless understood that a philosophy that did not directly engage the hard resistant bodies of the physical world and their strange properties—metals and mines, electricity, hydraulics, and magnetism—had no place on a continent and on a frontier that had only just begun to be subjugated.[4]

Knowledge is power, Francis Bacon said, long before Michel Foucault would transform this evident truth to mean something different: that knowledge is *nothing but* the expression of power. The removal of supernatural beings and other products of ignorance from our imagination enabled the removal of precious metals from underground veins. Agricola cleared the mineshafts of gnomes and helped along the appropriation of all that lay hidden under the earth. Jefferson surveyed the natural diversity of a new continent, and the new knowledge of it fed the dream of the full conquest of it. Even the recording of Native languages was a prelude to the elimination of those who spoke

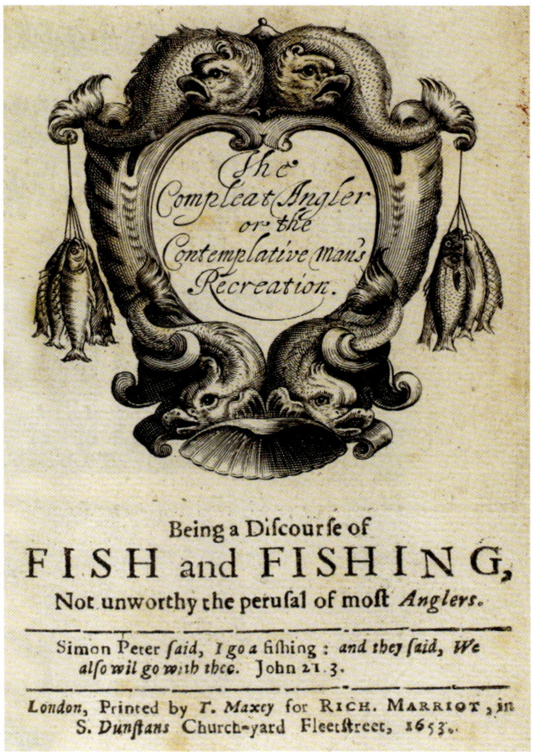

Frontispiece to Izaak Walton's *The Compleat Angler*, 1653.

them. And Hoover carried this project even further. Born in Iowa in 1874, while the so-called "Indian Wars" were raging, the first president from west of the Mississippi would continue westward still, to California, and from there he would cross the ocean, to new continents, to old new continents. The year after Hoover crossed the Pacific, the United States would annex Hawai'i as a territory and set up a military government in the Philippines. Knowledge is power, the young Stanford graduate must have thought to himself as he set out from California across the ocean. So powerful in fact that it cannot be stopped at the edge of a continent, but, manifestly, is destined to take over the world.

In *De re metallica*, Agricola felt compelled to neutralize a certain deep-seated and ancient anxiety about mining. It is one that Pliny the Elder expresses in his *Natural History* when he bemoans the absurd lengths to which men will go to rape the earth out of greed for gold. "We penetrate into her entrails ... as though each spot we tread upon were not sufficiently bounteous and fertile for us."[5] But in the new, modern

spirit, of which Agricola is an early harbinger, the earth does not have entrails, only resources. He no longer believes that minerals are born of a sort of seed in the earth's *matrix*: a Latin term that was common in geology into the eighteenth century, and that translates as "womb." As the Hoovers will later remark, it is interesting that Agricola preserves the term "vein" (*vena*), which, like *matrix*, is borrowed from the realm of biology.[6] But for him, this is the mere lexical fossil of an outdated concept, for the earth is no longer living, no longer to be comprehended in the same terms as the vital, pullulating creatures that move on its surface.

And so the ironically named Agricola defends mining against those who "glorify agriculture beyond measure."[7] The earth we tread on may be bounteous, and it is good that the farmers know to extract its fruits. "But let them leave to miners the gloomy valleys and sterile mountains, that they may draw forth from these, gems and metals which can buy, not only the crops, but all things that are sold."[8] Mining trumps farming because its "fruits" are exchangeable for any and all others. But the work of getting these fruits, as the ancients had warned, is dirty. Poisonous air hangs down there, as if to warn us away. A philosopher-miner might amply discourse on it, if he is not yet dead of asphyxiation.

Among Agricola's preferred methods of mineral extraction is fire setting, a technique that induces thermal shock in subterranean shafts and causes the ore to break away more easily. This method would become antiquated with the use of explosives and, later, of chemical processes such as cyanidation. A century or so after Agricola, the German philosopher Leibniz would propose using water pressure to extract silver from the Harz mountains.

By the time of Hoover's presidency, Pliny's admonitions against digging into the earth out of greed for gold would be entirely forgotten. In the nineteenth century, gold had itself become a significant motor in the westward motion of America, and by the late 1920s, the earth would be spotted with open mining pits—though these were still sparse and no one had yet thought of simply removing the tops of mountains in search of valuable metals, as they began to do in Appalachia in the 1970s. Union Carbide's Hawk's Nest Tunnel project in West Virginia, begun in 1927, resulted a few years later, during Hoover's presidency, in the death by silicosis of 476 miners tasked with pulling silica out of the earth for use in electroprocessing steel.

The subterranean world had been depopulated of its gnomes and ogres and mysterious powers; the spirit of rational Agricola had won out over the hallucinations of the seventeenth-century Jesuit Athanasius Kircher, who in his *Mundus subterraneus* of 1665 would give a rather detailed account of the malevolent beings one will encounter if one descends into the crater of a volcano.[9] The triumphalism of Herbert Hoover, had he thought about it, might have been tempered by the awareness that something down there, underneath the earth, deep in its veins, still wants to kill those who are compelled to go down there. Or, rather, it kills us without even wanting to, which is perhaps more terrifying still. And it is Pliny's forgotten warning that the ultimate cause of all this death is greed—that if the earth is killing us, this is only because we are probing into it without warrant or invitation—that points the way to a *tertium quid* that is neither ignorant superstition nor the triumphalism of the engineer, neither fear of nature nor domination of it, but rather the search after some sort of harmony with it.

This brings us to the second phase of Hoover's philosophical *Bildung*. If Agricola had been the guiding thinker of our president's early engagement with philosophy (conceived broadly, again, to include what was once called natural philosophy and is now called science), the inspiration for his later thought would be Izaak Walton, the author of the 1653 book *The Compleat Angler*. This is a work of natural history and practical philosophy at once, both describing and taxonomizing various species of fishes, but also, much more importantly, reflecting on the importance of devotion to a particular practice in one's life, such as fishing, as conducive to the attainment of true happiness.

In one conception, as we have already seen, philosophy is the activity of which Socrates was falsely accused: looking into what goes on in the heavens above and the earth below. In a parallel conception, one which way may indeed justly be attributed to the same Greek philosopher, it is nothing other than the cultivation, through practice, of virtue. For many schools of post-Socratic Greek philosophy, moreover, notably the Stoics, virtue and happiness are one and the same, or, perhaps better, they are coextensive: one cannot truly attain the one without attaining the other. It is such an understanding of philosophy that has caused some

scholars, notably Pierre Hadot, to describe ancient philosophy as a "way of life." Nor had this conception of philosophy gone extinct by the early modern period. In fact, philosophy as a way of life continued to coexist into the seventeenth century with the alternative model—philosophy as looking into things—sometimes in tension with it, sometimes in harmony.

Walton himself plainly understands philosophy in both senses. Thus he speaks of the "commendations which some philosophical brains have bestowed upon the freshwater Perch," as, for example, that they "have in their brain a stone, which is, in foreign parts, sold by apothecaries, being there noted to be very medicinable against the stone in the reins."[10] But he also concludes his treatise with an admission from the Hunter (one of three characters in the work, alongside the Fisherman and the Falconer) that "I will not forget the doctrine which you told me Socrates taught his scholars, that they should not think to be honoured so much for being philosophers, as to honour philosophy by their virtuous lives."[11] The Hunter, who the fisherman has urged to try his pastime, then promises: "You advised me to the like concerning Angling, and I will endeavour to do so."[12] He will endeavor, that is, to manifest virtue in his life by excelling at fishing, an activity that Walton conceives as salutary not in view of its outcomes, but rather in view of the contemplative nature of the process itself. "Virtue," here, is meant in the double sense of the Greek *arete*, which is to say, both goodness, with the moral valences that word carries today, and excellence, in the sense of perfecting a particular skill. Here, angling will do just as well as practicing dialectic or yoga in pursuit of the virtuous life. It is, to draw on Aristotle's distinction between the sorts of activities belonging variously to perfective and imperfective verbs, more like taking a walk than building a house: at any moment in the taking of a walk, it is the case that the walker has taken a walk, while it is only after completing the building of a house ("perfecting" the house) that a builder has built a house. One need not catch a fish in order to have fished, just as one need not come away from dialectical philosophy with some positive answer to a question. Whether angling really differs from hunting is a matter of debate—whether, that is, one can be said to have hunted even if one comes home empty-handed. But Walton's own view is clear: angling is an "imperfective" activity, and as such it belongs among those other

activities that are good not for how they finish, but for how they are before they've finished.

In 1927, Herbert Hoover, then secretary of commerce, gave a speech in Chicago at a meeting of the Izaak Walton League of America.[13] The arrogant young man who rode into Gwalia can still be made out, and yet there is at the same time a certain solicitude, a worry about preserving the harmony of nature. Fish are, in the end, ours for the taking, but we must still be careful not to take them all.

It may be that the difference of object—fish rather than metal—is in part responsible for the difference of temperament, but, whatever the reason, in contrast with the case of mining, Hoover is supremely skeptical of the presumption of progress in fishing. "Some millions of fishermen have invented thousands of new lures of seductive order," he observes, "and devised many new and fearful incantations with a host of new kinds of clothes and labor-saving devices to carry them about."[14]

This progress is in part a result of the global industry and trade that he himself has helped to drive: "We have arrived at the high state of a tackle, assembled from the steel of Damascus, the bamboos of Siam, the silk of Japan, the lacquer of China, the tin of Bangkok, the nickel of Canada, the feathers of Brazil, and the silver of Colorado—all compounded by mass production at Chicago, Ill., and Akron, Ohio."[15] And yet all this progress has not advanced the art of fishing in the least: "But I ask you if, in the face of all this over-whelming efficiency and progress, there is less time between bites?"[16]

As in philosophy understood as the cultivation of a virtuous life, in fishing there can be individual progress that comes through long attunement to the nature of the creature one seeks; but there can be no historical progress through advances in the associated technology, the "tackle." For the same reason, fishing also levels out class differences, as attunement to nature cannot be bought: "Nor do I need to repeat that fishing is not the rich man's sport," Hoover repeats, "though his incantations are more expensive. I have said elsewhere that all men are equal before fishes."[17]

As had been the case for Walton, fishing is particularly conducive to the good of the soul, particularly in

____

Opposite: Postpresidential fishing. Herbert Hoover tries his luck, 1936. Photo Harris & Ewing. Courtesy Library of Congress.

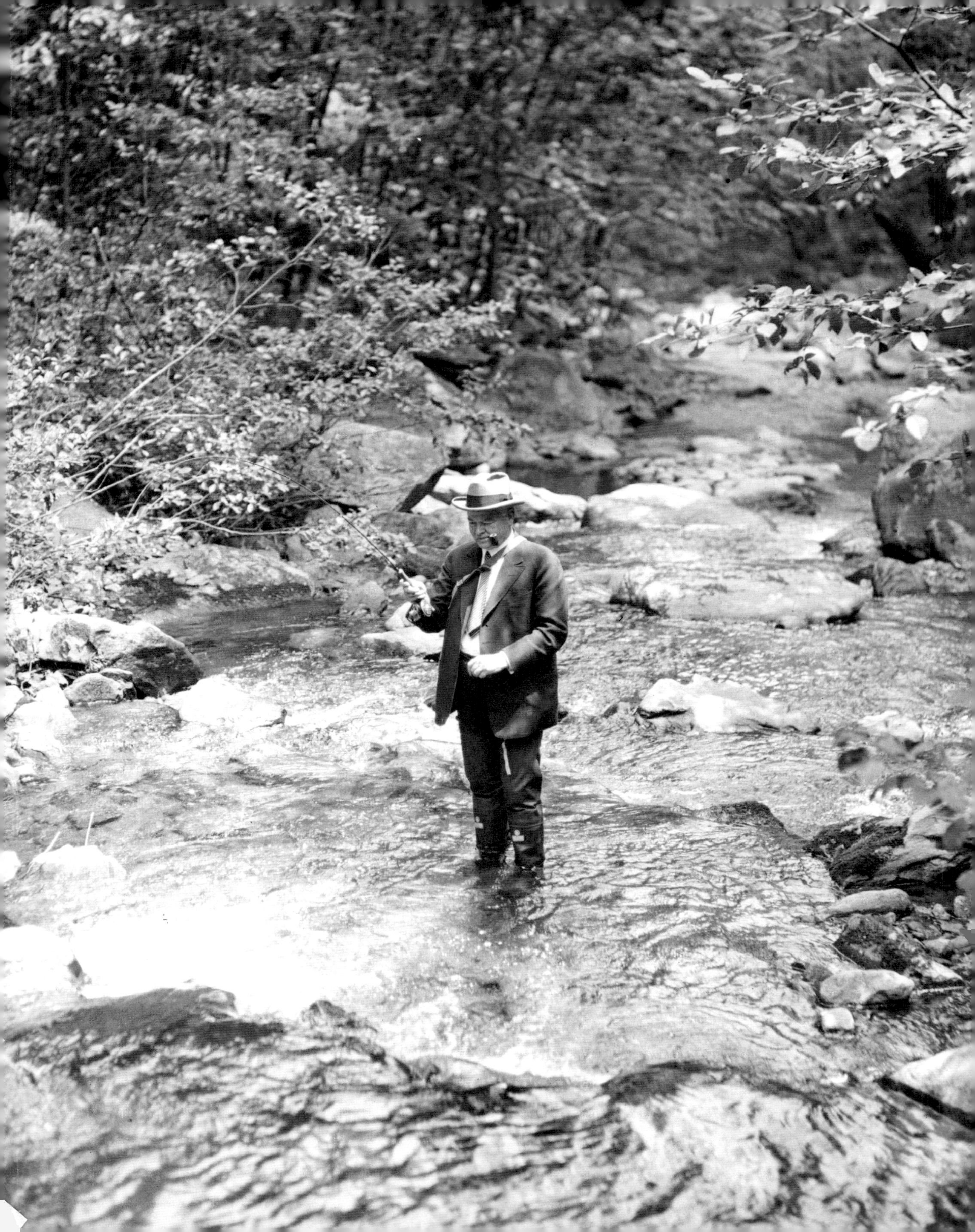

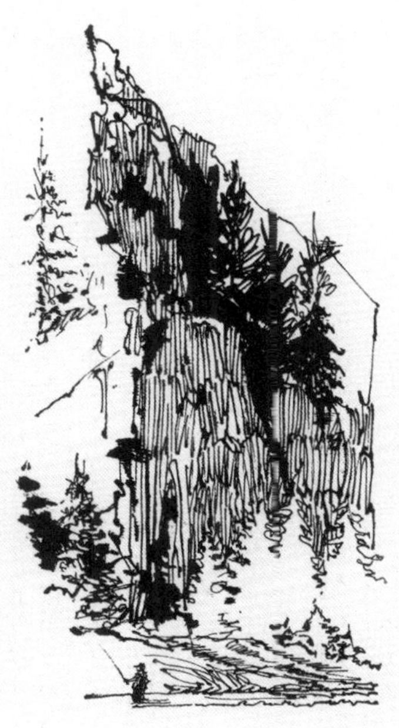

FISHING FOR FUN–

*And
To Wash Your Soul*

HERBERT HOOVER

Edited by William Nichols

RANDOM HOUSE
New York

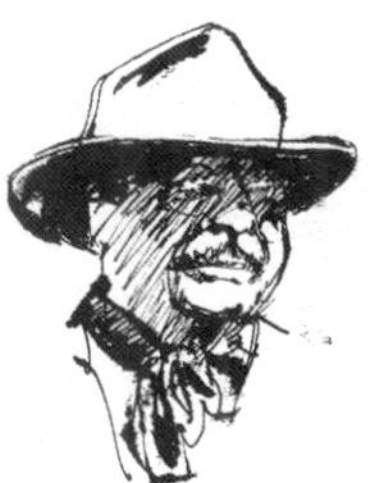

Everyone knows of the first Roosevelt that he was a valiant hunter of big animals, and generally an evangel of the strenuous life—which included fishing. He relates an adventure with an Adirondack stream when he was twelve years old:

"After dinner all of us began to 'whip' the rapids. At first I sat on a rock by the water but the black flies drove me from there, so I attempted to cross the rapids. But I had miscalculated my strength for before I was half way across the force of the current had

[72]

swept me into water which was above my head. Leaving the pole to take [care] of itself I struck out for a rock. My pole soon stuck and so I recovered it. I then went half wading, half swimming down stream, fishing all the time but unsuccessful."

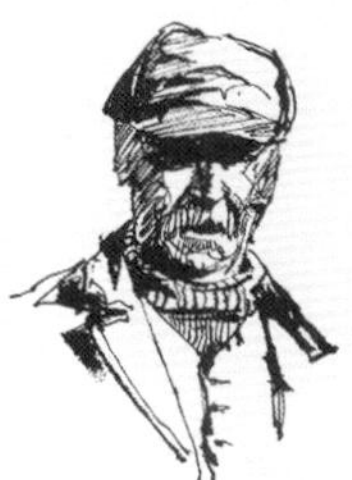

President Cleveland is author of a delightful little volume called *Fishing and Hunting Sketches*, in which he sets forth his ideas on the beatitudes of those sports. As a fisherman, he preferred small-mouthed black bass to trout,

[73]

contrast with hunting, because its sought-after object is in truth only an occasion for the exercise of pleasurable attention to, and within, nature. To induce people to take joy in nature, they "need some stimulant from the hunt, the fish, or the climb."[18] But for Hoover, the second of these options is not a stimulant like the others because it's not excitative, but rather pacifying. And this is the reason for his love of it: "I am for fish. Fishing is not so much getting fish as it is a state of mind and a lure to the human soul into refreshment."[19]

Hoover contrasts at some length the world of the 1650s with that of the 1920s. Walton, he says, "never got the jumps from traffic signals or the price of wheat."[20] His spiritual predecessor could also have had no idea of pollution, "the poison cup which we give to eggs, fry, fingerlings, adolescents, and adult fish alike."[21] If we want fish, he reasons with intentional obviousness, "we have to reserve for them some place to live."[22]

How do we do this? A sort of moderate conservationism would endure in Hoover's thinking until the end of his long life. His final work, published in 1963, the year before his death, bears the anodyne title *Fishing for Fun—And to Wash Your Soul*.[23] He explains in the preface that a publisher had approached him concerning his many public addresses and magazine articles on fishing over the decades and suggested that "these meditations would make a little book of good cheer." He found it hard to refuse: "In the daily grind of trying to find out why the Communists get that way, it would be an expedition into relief. So here they are."[24]

Hoover now openly acknowledges that water pollution comes from "ships, factories, coal mines, chemical works in cities and towns—to mention only a few of them. Many of these things damage public health, destroy the outdoor appeal of the streams, and all of them damage the fish."[25] And yet, "after all we are an industrial people. We have to work eight hours a day and all but a few weeks in the year, and we cannot abolish our industries and still pay for fishing tackle."[26] Fishing inculcates virtues that mining never could, but no lesson learned from fishing could ever refute or overturn the philosophical disposition that Hoover had developed, inherited from Agricola and Bacon, in his labors as a mining engineer.

____

Opposite: Pages from Herbert Hoover's *Fishing for Fun*, 1963.

Extracting the tin of Bangkok and the nickel of Canada may not help fishing to advance, but if our extractive activities prove harmful to the fish and threaten the very activity of the fisherman, then it is not by retreat, but by further advancement of the first sort of philosophical project Hoover knew, the project of science, that we might hope to eliminate the harm. Philosophy as figuring things out and thereby coming to master and appropriate them must act as the faithful guardian of that humbler, purer, and vastly more ancient articulation of philosophy, as cultivation of a life of virtue, through, for example, "contemplation of the eternal flow of the stream, the stretch of forest and mountain," which "all reduce our egotism, soothe our troubles, and shame our wickedness."[27]

Philosophy as cultivation of virtue is thus contained within philosophy as what Foucault might call "power/knowledge." National parks, first set up by Theodore Roosevelt at the encouragement of the wandering transcendentalist John Muir, are such worlds within a world. And old Herbert Hoover in retirement, down at the fishing hole—dreaming of his Iowa childhood, when spitting on the bait worm was the preferred incantation, and a hickory stick did as well as the finest store-bought pole; dreaming of that lost past, just as the Cold War was reaching its darkest hour, and the Americans and the Soviets who had "got that way" were targeting their intercontinental missiles—this too was a world within a world. But as we are reminded by "Gone Fishin'," the song made famous in 1951 by Bing Crosby and Louis Armstrong, when someone engages in an activity conducive to happiness without having first put in their time, they are likely to invite reproach from those who have stayed behind under the reign of "responsibility." In truth, the reproach to those who have not earned their right to "go fishin'" is this: You have escaped our world of power and disappeared into a world of happiness; how dare you.

Philosophy as the cultivation of virtue, I have said, has existed since antiquity alongside philosophy as inquiry into, and harnessing of, the forces of nature. Sometimes these two have been in harmony; sometimes they have not. Looking into the workings of nature—what goes on in the heavens above and in the earth below—has often been seen as a crucial component of the project of coming to understand our place in the cosmos, an understanding that is in turn

necessary to avoid being disappointed by mortality, by unanticipated turns for the worse, by the fates. Thus, no true happiness without knowledge of the workings of nature. But pursuit of this knowledge was always a charged affair, and could easily cross over from virtue to vice, as wonder gave way to curiosity gave way to greed. Pliny drew the boundary at the surface of the earth: explore and come to know what comes out of the earth, but do not try to find where it comes from, let alone to extract it yourself. Bacon sought to scrap this limit and pushed for a new spirit of inquiry into nature in which no domain of it is best left alone by us, and no amount of intervention or exploitation pushes nature beyond what it, in itself, is suited for. This is the spirit that Hoover himself would inherit, one that sees knowledge as desirable principally to the extent that it aids in the accumulation of power, not in the cultivation of happiness.

And yet, as his late work shows, Hoover, like Walton, remained committed to happiness as the end of a certain kind of philosophical practice. He continues to embody two fundamentally different, and sometimes opposed, conceptions of philosophy: the one that takes it as a probing into nature, which after

Bacon also becomes a violation of nature, and the other which takes it as the project of serenity, of ataraxia, of happiness. Of course, when Hoover is out fishing, he is not doing so in the same spirit as Bing or Satch. He is not shirking his responsibilities but rather basking in the certainty of having fulfilled them. In the manner of Cincinnatus, he acts the noble statesmen who, having made his contribution, then withdraws—not to the field, but to the pond.

He is also, perhaps, the last American president to embody, if mostly unconsciously, a connection to the two strands of philosophy we have identified, the one that accumulates knowledge as a means to power, and the other that cultivates virtue as equivalent to happiness. In him, they come together, while today, in the absence of any connection whatsoever between philosophy and the practice of politics, they appear opposed. Power tolerates happiness, until it gets in the way; and happiness ignores power, as long as it can. And American presidents come and go, each generally more violent than the last, and each generally more forgetful than the last of what "virtue" had once meant.

1 Herbert Clark Hoover and Lou Henry Hoover, "Translators' Preface," in Georgius Agricola, *De re metallica, Translated from the First Latin Edition of 1556, with Biographical Introduction, Annotations and Appendices upon the Development of Mining Methods, Metallurgical Processes, Geology, Mineralogy & Mining Law from the Earliest Times to the 16th Century*, trans. Herbert Clark Hoover and Lou Henry Hoover (London: The Mining Magazine, 1912), p. i.

2 John Evelyn, *Fumifugium; Or, The Inconveniencie of the Aer and Smoak of London Dissipated* (London: Godbid, Bedel, & Collins), 1772, p. 41ff.

3 Georgius Agricola, *De re metallica*, p. 3.

4 One group that modified Hegel to make him suitable for the United States were the St. Louis Hegelians. For more on the group, see John Kaag, "America's Hands-On Hegelian," in *Chronicle of Higher Education*, vol. 62, no. 28 (25 March 2016), and Matt Erlin, "Absolute Speculation: The St. Louis Hegelians and the Question of American National Identity," in

German Culture in Nineteenth-Century America: Reception, Adaptation, Transformation, ed. Lynn Tatlock and Matt Erlin (Rochester, NY: Camden House, 2005).

5 Pliny the Elder, Natural History, Book XXXII, ch. 1.1, "Metals." The translation I am using here is from *The Natural History of Pliny*, vol. 6, ed. and trans. John Bostock and H. T. Riley (London: Henry G. Bohn, 1857), p. 69.

6 As the translators note, *vena* is among the mining terms that Agricola inherits from Latin antiquity, though much of his vocabulary is also an attempt to render in Latin what had previously only been treated in writing in Ulrich Rülein von Calw's *Nutzlich Bergbüchlein*, (Useful little book of mining), published in Erfurt in 1527. A crucial distinction for Agricola is that between *venae profundae* and *venae dilatatae*, which had been earlier rendered in German as, respectively, *Gänge* and *schwebende Gänge*, or, in the equivalent terms the Hoovers identify in contemporary geology, "fissure veins" and "bedded deposits." See Georgius Agricola,

De re metallica, p. 43, footnote 1.

7 Ibid., p. 5.

8 Ibid., p. 6.

9 Athanasius Kircher, *Mundus subterraneus, quo universae denique naturae divitiae* (Amsterdam: Joannem Janssonium and Elizeum Weyerstraten, 1665).

10 Izaak Walton and Charles Cotton, *The Compleat Angler; or, The Contemplative Man's Recreation. Being a Discourse of Fish and Fishing, Not Unworthy of the Perusal of Most Anglers* (London: Thomas Nelson and Sons, 1900), pp. 153–154. The word 'reins' here indicates the kidneys. Walton continued to add to the book in subsequent editions; for the fifth edition, which was published in 1676, Cotton provided a second part. Walton is the sole author of all passages cited here.

11 Ibid., p. 206.

12 Ibid.

13 Herbert Hoover, *A Remedy for Disappearing Game Fishes: An Address by Herbert Hoover, Secretary of Commerce, Delivered Before the Izaak Walton League of America* (Washington, DC: US Government Printing

Office, 1927). The speech was delivered on 9 April 1927.

14 Ibid., p. 2.

15 Ibid.

16 Ibid.

17 Ibid.

18 Ibid., p. 12.

19 Ibid.

20 Ibid., p. 2.

21 Ibid., p. 9.

22 Ibid.

23 Herbert Hoover, *Fishing for Fun—And to Wash Your Soul* (New York: Random House, 1963). Hoover had described fishing as a "wash of the soul" already in his 1927 speech, and attributed this expression to the poet Edgar Guest. To impart some idea of the poet's stature, it is enough to cite a couplet by Dorothy Parker, referring to a certain examination for diagnosing syphilis: "I'd rather flunk my Wassermann test / Than read a poem by Edgar Guest."

24 Ibid., unpaginated preface.

25 Ibid., p. 51.

26 Ibid.

27 Herbert Hoover, *A Remedy for Disappearing Game Fishes*, p. 12.

UNCOMPUTABLES
Agnieszka Kurant

In his 1969 book *Calculating Space*, the German engineer Konrad Zuse, a pioneer of modern programming languages, was the first to suggest that the universe is a giant information processor or calculator, and that the entire cosmos could be described as the computational output of a "cellular automaton." Bacteria, fungi, whales, forests, crystals, rocks, seas, planets, stars, galaxies, cities, nations—today we know of no life form, nor any inert thing, that does not emit, receive, store, and process information. Everything computes.

In the twenty-first century, mass computation has become a new form of power. From cultural taste to global happiness, from climate change to high-frequency trading, everything is calculated using algorithms. At a time when global corporations use behavioral forecasting to capitalize on their ability to predict, and valorize, our future decisions, feelings, movements, habits, and interests, one wonders if anything remains uncomputable.

One phenomenon that does seem resistant to computation and prediction is that of emergence. The complex systems within which emergence occurs—from termite colonies to social movements and cities, from the human brain to the Internet—manifest nonlinear, unpredictable behaviors that nevertheless produce novel and coherent structures and patterns. These emergent structures, arising from the self-organizing processes of collective intelligence, are more than the sum of their components' behaviors. Recent discoveries in complexity science have drawn attention to the fact that the same principles and patterns underlie the processes of emergence and collective intelligence observed in both nature and culture. Modeling these phenomena through computer simulations has opened new fields of science, which range from growing artificial societies and artificial life to exploring new models of political conflict resolution to evolving so-called artificial artificial intelligence.

One of the most mysterious creatures displaying signs of intelligence is the slime mold *Physarum polycephalum*, an organism found on most forest floors. Despite the apparent lack of a nervous system, *Physarum* has shown in experiments that it can navigate obstacles in its search for food, even to the extent of passing through a labyrinth. Somewhere between

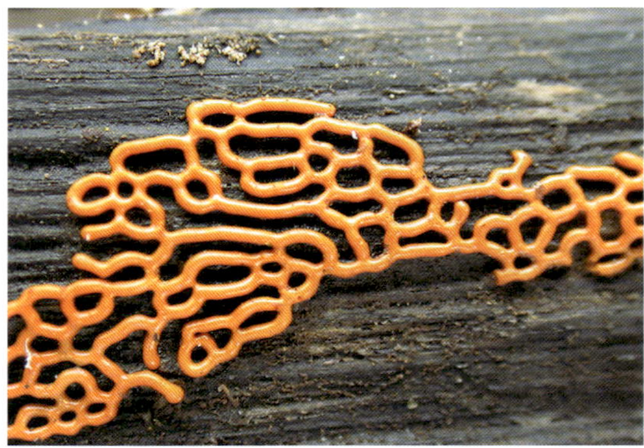

Hemitrichia serpula, the so-called pretzel slime mold. Photo Randy Darrah.

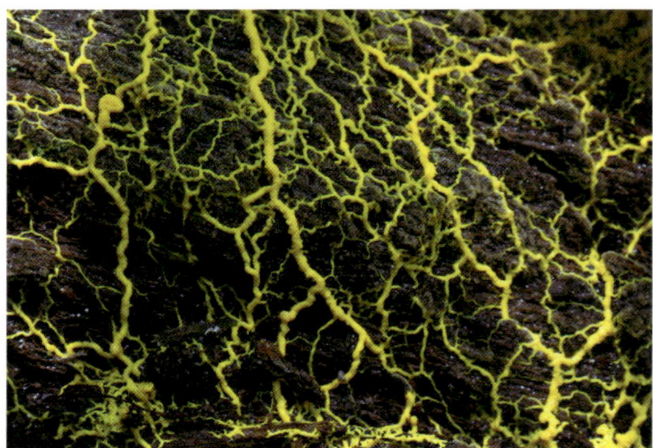

Physarum polycephalum on a decaying log. This slime mold is moving as a collective body and sending out branches to look for nutrients. Photo IamTK via Shutterstock.

an individual and a swarm, *Physarum* spends part of its life in the form of diffuse individual cells, each of which travels on its own. But under certain conditions, these single-celled amoebae fuse into a giant cell with multiple nuclei called a plasmodium and begin to move as a single body, sending out tubes that continue to branch out to search for food. Once a source of nutrition has been located, the unsuccessful branches it has sent out shrink, leaving only the most efficient route between it and the food source. This process allows the slime mold to survive even in adverse environments by adapting to fluctuating conditions. The intelligence of the slime mold is defined by its ability to change its morphology by removing the unproductive pathways so as to optimize the transfer of nutrients from food

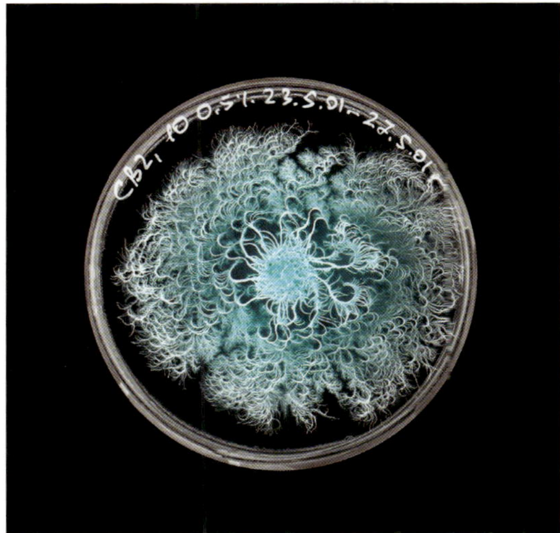

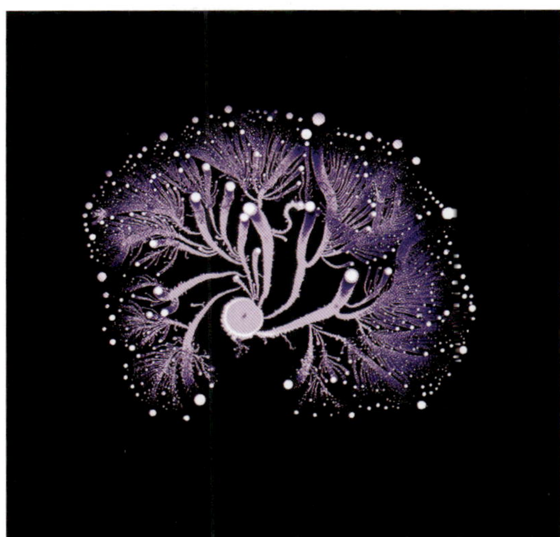

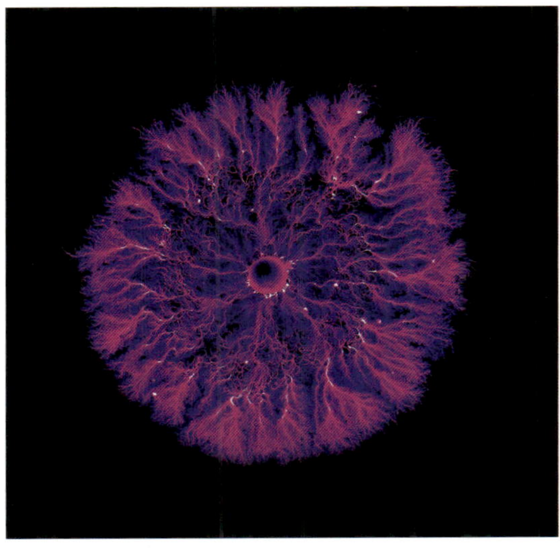

sources while maintaining its status as an aggregated organism.

Slime mold has recently been co-opted for computation. Because the mold is sensitive to light and certain chemicals, it can be used to find the optimal pathways between a number of points given certain constraints. Andrew Adamatzky and his fellow researchers at the International Center of Unconventional Computing at the University of the West of England are developing methods to harness the behavior of these organisms in order to perform computational tasks. They created a *Physarum* machine—an amorphous, programmable, living computer. This "plasmobot" is capable of solving, for instance, the classic, computationally intractable mathematical puzzle known as the Traveling Salesman Problem, for which no exact algorithm has been found, by using the physical movement of its body. It optimizes its foraging pattern—finding the shortest route to any food source using the protoplasmic tubes it sends out and then propagating the nutrients efficiently. The pathways of these nutrient networks represent a solution to the mathematical problem.

Slime mold is an example of an emergent structure, a behavior also found in other animal groups, including ants, termites, bees, fish, and birds. Emergent processes can be seen in many other contexts, such as cities, and in organizational phenomena discernible in computer simulations and cellular automata. Left to regulate themselves, groups of human beings also tend to produce spontaneous order out of which something new emerges: a pattern, a decision, a structure, or a change in direction. A classic traffic roundabout is a good example, with cars moving in and out with such effective organization that some modern cities have begun replacing stoplights at problem intersections with traffic circles. Open-source software and Wikipedia form an even more compelling illustration. Other examples of emergence include the stock market, the brain, the Internet, political parties, social movements, and the phenomenon of life.

Left: Colonies of *Paenibacillus dendritiformis* and *Paenibacillus vortex*, photographed by Eshel Ben-Jacob, the biological physicist who discovered them. The bacterial colonies exhibit collective decision-making processes, functioning like what the scientist calls "a super brain that receives signals and processes information." For these images, Ben-Jacob dyed the naturally colorless bacteria.

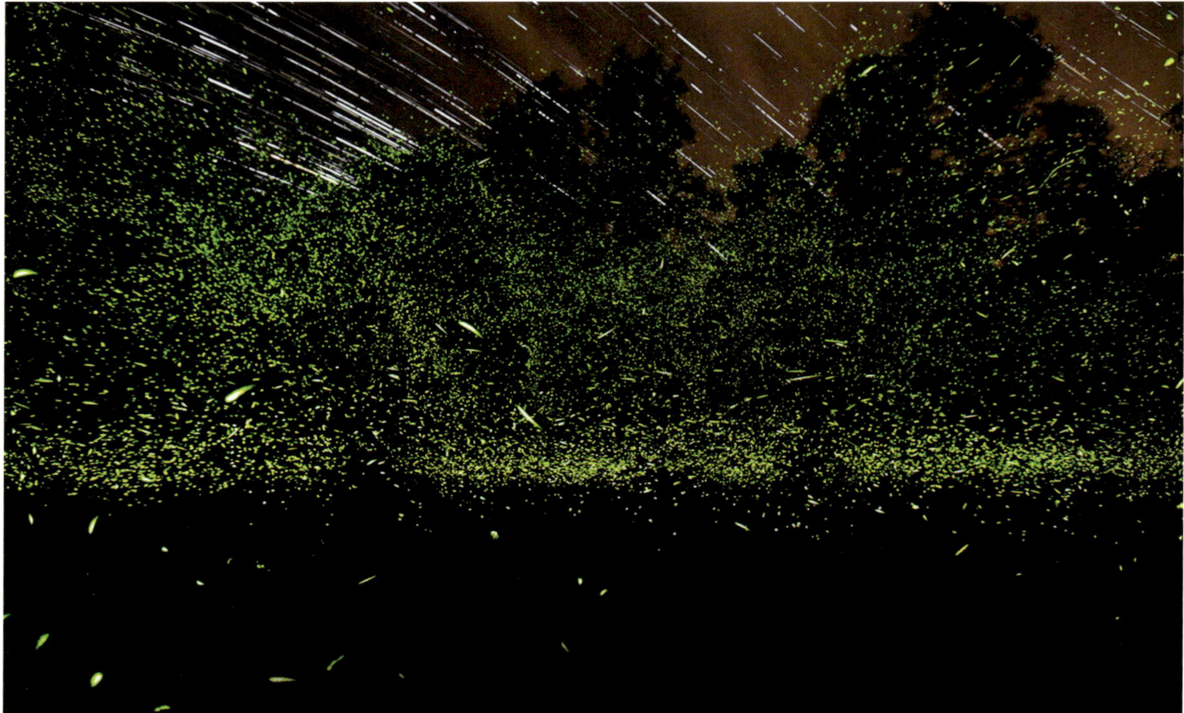

Under environmental stress, strains of the bacterium *Paenibacillus dendritiformis*, discovered in the early 1990s by a group led by physicist Eshel Ben-Jacob, form evolving, intricate, complex colonies through collective behavior. Ben-Jacob, who put forward the idea of bacterial decision-making, has demonstrated that bacteria are smart organisms with social intelligence and that they have genes specific to cannibalism and communication. When they are starved or exposed to other stressors, they release a chemical that kills off some of the colony so that the rest can survive. The decision circuits of the individual bacteria are integrated through the exchange of chemical messages, guaranteeing collective decision making for the group's benefit. *Paenibacillus dendritiformis* respond to extreme stress, such as starvation or poisoning, by creating spores, which are highly resistant to the outside environment as a result of their dormant states. The response involves more than five hundred genes and takes about ten hours. Each bacterium performs a sophisticated decision-making process. In addition to gauging its own internal stress, it also adjusts to the stress of its peers. Modeling this complex interplay enabled the scientists to assess the pros and cons of different choices in game theory, which attempts to model decision making by humans in scenarios where an individual's success in making choices depends on the choices of others. The bacteria's decision-making process is far more advanced than the game theory problem known as the Prisoner's Dilemma because the number of participants in a bacterial colony can be up to a hundred times the number of people on Earth, and this has provided crucial insights for economists and political scientists applying mathematical models to describe complex human decision making.

Termites, just like humans, belong to the few species in nature that have evolved to form complex worker societies (divided into farmers, nurses, soldiers, foragers, etc.). The by-product of their labor produces mounds with architectural qualities, often resembling the ruins of civilizations, pyramids, or cathedrals. The collective intelligence of the entire society is pooled to build one structure. It has been observed that various termite colonies display disparate collective behavior as varied as human personalities. Some colonies are more dynamic and adventurous while others are more sluggish and slow. Complexity scientists make similar

Above: Fireflies flashing in synchronicity, Great Smoky Mountains National Park, United States. Photo Cheng Niu.

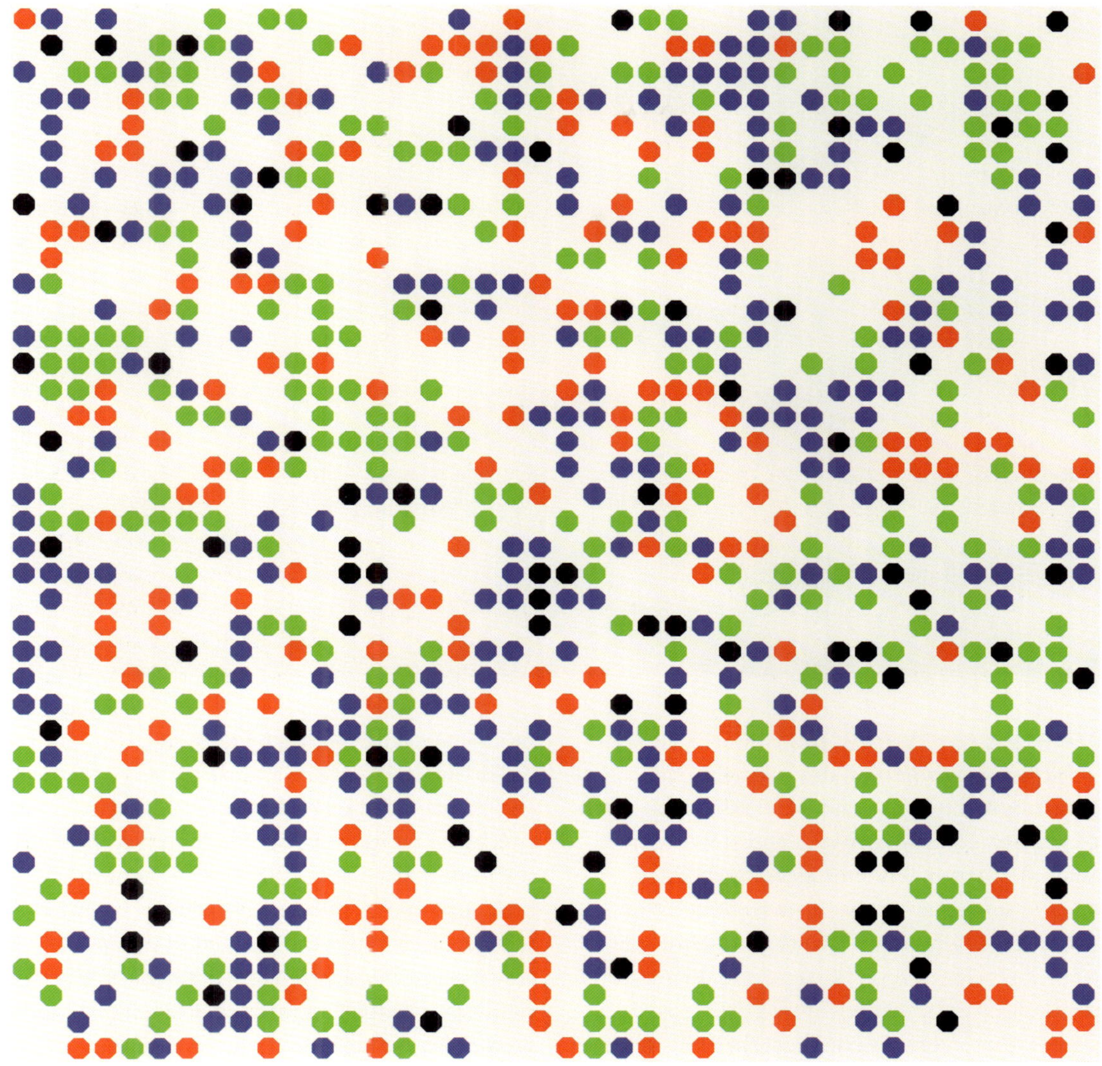

Joshua Epstein's artificial society model of ethnic tension and genocide, first outlined in a paper in 2002, presents an ethnically mixed zone in which violence can flare between two kinds of agents, represented by blue and green dots, who are safeguarded by police officers, represented by black dots. The blue and green agents can only "see" in their immediate vicinity. Each individual agent has its own personality—its own degree of privation or discontent, its level of ethnic hostility, and its willingness to risk arrest.

The higher the ethnic tension, the more likely it is that an agent will loot a neighbor's store, seize its house, or kill it; doing so turns the hostile agent red. Police officers look for red agents in order to put them in jail. A less belligerent agent might behave peaceably when a police officer is nearby, but as in real life, the violence, once begun, will spread rapidly because cops are overwhelmed in one neighborhood after another, thus reducing the risk of arrest.

observations about other systems of collective intelligence such as revolutionary movements, which display diversified personality traits as super organisms or "collective persons."

The mathematical biologist Steven Strogatz looks at emergence through synchronization. He shows how flocks of creatures (like birds, fireflies, and fish) manage to synchronize and act as a unit when no one is giving orders. The prototypical example that he offers is that of fireflies in East Asia blinking after dark. Along the tidal rivers of Malaysia, thousands of male fireflies congregate and flash in perfect unison at a rate of about three times every two seconds, a behavior intended to attract females. A similar phenomenon can be observed with thousands of crickets that chirp in unison. Strogatz explains how enormous systems can synchronize themselves, from the electrons in a superconductor to the pacemaker cells in our hearts, and shows that although these phenomena might seem unrelated on the surface, at a deeper level there is a connection, forged by the unifying power of mathematics. His research also investigates the ways in which humans sync in a social sense. He theorizes that the synchrony of networks may be fundamental in synced human phenomena as diverse as fads, traffic, the World Wide Web, the spread of disease, and even clapping. The outburst of clapping at the start of a round of applause often suddenly becomes synchronized, and this synchronization can disappear and reappear several times during the applause. The phenomenon is an expression of social self-organization.

Complexity scientists have noticed that the processes of rock sedimentation, or the ways in which crystals, glass, or ice are formed, are comparable to the crystallization and stratification of civilizations, societies, or social movements. This position derives from Artur Iberall's "homeokinetics" and was further analyzed by Manuel de Landa and, more recently, as the concept of "social physics" by Alex Pentland. Crystallizations of civilizations began with extensive trade and flows of goods among dispersed populations of hunter-gatherers, turning these loose structures into more dense forms. Subsequently three kinds of fictions that emerged—money, gods, and laws—allowed the self-organizing systems of human species to create overarching narratives in order to form larger societies of people who never met. The interplay of individual choices of citizens is a complex system with collective results that bear no close relation to the individual intent.

The new science of artificial societies suggests that real ones are both more predictable and more surprising than we thought. Since the late 1960s, economists and social scientists have used computer simulations of societies or groups of people to analyze socioeconomic phenomena and observe agent-based complex system behavior. This allows for testing social theories on a large scale. In the 1990s, Robert Axtell and Joshua Epstein decided to use emergent processes seen in coral reefs and flocks of birds to grow a simple artificial world in which little hunter-gatherer creatures would move around a landscape, finding, storing, and consuming the only resource—sugar. When they brought Sugarscape, as they called it, to life with the computer, they were startled to see that almost immediately their rudimentary artificial society produced a skewed distribution of sugar that looked very much like the skewed distribution of wealth in human societies, even though nothing about the agents' simple behavioral rules pointed to any such outcome. For several years, they built up and elaborated Sugarscape, and discovered that simple rules could produce complex social phenomena that mimicked migrations, epidemics, trade. Epstein and Axtell then began applying their technique, which they called agent-based modeling, to a variety of problems and questions. In Sugarscape, and in the other artificial societies that followed, they made their agents heterogeneous. This means that the artificial people, like real people, were different from one another. Each Sugarscape agent has its own "genetic code": a distinctive combination of metabolic rate (how much sugar each agent needs in order to stay alive), vision (how far the agent can "see" as it hunts for sugar), and so forth. This was a small move that was actually quite radical since in most conventional social science models people are assumed to be more or less the same: multiple copies of a single representative person.

Following these experiments, contemporary researchers are creating cybermodels of the ancient Native Americans who occupied Colorado's Mesa Verde and computational reconstructions of the Anasazi people in Long House Valley in Arizona; virtual Polynesian societies and digital Mesolithic foragers. They are growing crime waves and racial segregation in

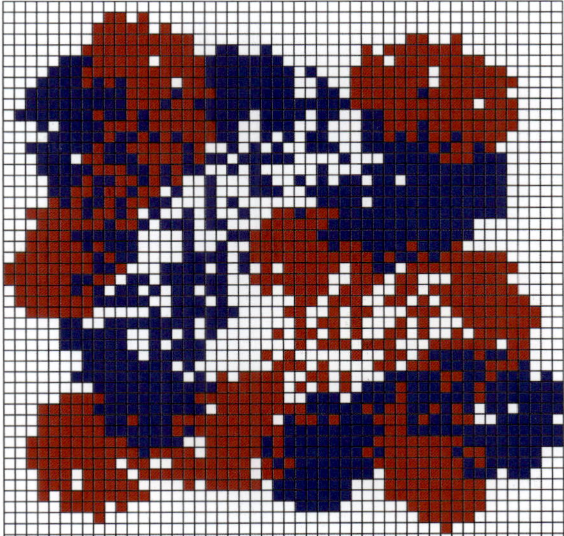

artificial neighborhoods, epidemics caused by bioterrorism and artificial genocides. Growing long-vanished civilizations and modern-day genocides on computers will probably never enable us to foresee the future in detail—but we might learn to look for small interventions that can have large, discontinuous consequences. The desire to use computers as civic thermostats to program societies, as was already imagined by Marshall McLuhan, is partially realized nowadays through "reality mining" and feeding data to statistical modeling programs, the terrifying consequence of which is the increasing surveillance of our lives.

One of the most recent applications of emergence has been the research of complexity scientists into the resolution of intractable conflicts. Conflicts become intractable because of collective trauma, or social identity, or a history of humiliation. By definition, these are the conflicts that are resistant to all the mainstream techniques of dispute resolution. Typically they are plagued by a history of "fixes that fail," peace agreements that collapse within days or weeks because they don't necessarily get at the underlying dynamics fuelling conflict. Conflict researchers have therefore been pushing for a fresh approach—one that views intractable conflicts as dynamic, complex systems similar to cells, ant colonies, or cities, and analyzes them with the mathematical and computational tools developed over the past thirty years.

Psychologists Robin Vallacher and Andrzej Nowak, both at Florida Atlantic University, have studied how the human sense of self emerges, and how feelings about others can switch from positive to negative. Using a mathematical tool known as dynamical systems theory to analyze their results, they created "agent-based" simulations that contain thousands of digital robots, each of which embodies some of the simple behaviors that social psychologists believe have a role in conflict. One such model features agents that vary in how competitive or cooperative they are and adjust those proclivities according to how much

Above: In 1971, the American economist Thomas Schelling created an agent-based model to explore the dynamics of segregation. Placing individuals (or "agents") of two different colors on a checkerboard, Schelling provided them with different parameters regarding their preference for living near agents of the other color. The simulations started with random distribution of blue and red agents, all of which were given migration options that they could use to leave their neighborhood if it did not have the required minimum frequency of agents of their own color. Schelling showed that relatively small changes in preference parameters could produce dramatic changes in levels of segregation. The image at left shows the relatively heterogeneous distribution produced when the agents are assigned a preference for a neighborhood in which at least 20 percent of the population is the same color. What is surprising is that increasing the preference criterion to only 30 percent, as shown in the image at right, creates a disproportionate level of segregation. Schelling thus showed that rules applied on a micro level produce macro effects wholly unintended from the agent's point of view.

hostility or aggression they experience from the other agents. In this simulation, small conflagrations flare up and die down much as they do in real communities. Occasionally, however, the conflicts expand until they lock the whole virtual community into a cycle of recrimination—the classic sign of intractability. Simulations suggest that seemingly intractable conflicts can be transformed or reduced by disruption of local constraints (e.g., movement through free travel). Working with Dean Pruitt of the School for Conflict Analysis and Resolution at George Mason University in Arlington, Virginia, Nowak has also developed models showing how what mathematicians call "attractors" can explain how conflicts can escalate and tip over into an intractable state. Now he and his colleagues are working on the next step: comparing the evolution of communities in these simple models with data from real-world conflicts such as the Israeli–Palestinian standoff.

The observation of certain phenomena appearing in nature and culture allows us to imagine a creative AI emerging from a collective intelligence of humans. Artificial intelligence researchers often ask if artistic creativity is computable and whether AI can produce artworks. Scientists have in fact made certain gains in computational or algorithmic creativity over the past two decades. One of the more interesting examples is the work of David Cope, professor at the University of California, Santa Cruz, who used AI to generate classical compositions by modeling the styles of great composers such as Bach and Mozart. His algorithms, which have produced music ranging from single-instrument arrangements to full symphonies, have at times fooled people into believing that the works were composed by humans. Another example is AARON, a computer program created by Harold Cohen in the 1970s. Written in LISP programming language, AARON produces large, colorful paintings that embody a highly conventional, corporate idea of art. None of these advances, however, have produced genuinely creative results.

Meanwhile, the observable erosion of singular authorship and its replacement by complex collective forms makes it increasingly apparent that the concept of "the author" is, to a large extent, a construct created by cultural industries and the art market in order to appropriate the labor of the multitude of the dispersed and networked creative process. Digital culture has accelerated the production of memes, which are examples of works without authors. They resemble the monuments of human creativity, such as the Bible and various cultural mythologies, that were created collectively and anonymously. Memes, especially Internet memes, behave like living organisms or viruses; they circulate and mutate within culture at a historically unprecedented rate and scale. Contemporary production, based on crowd creativity, is bound up with

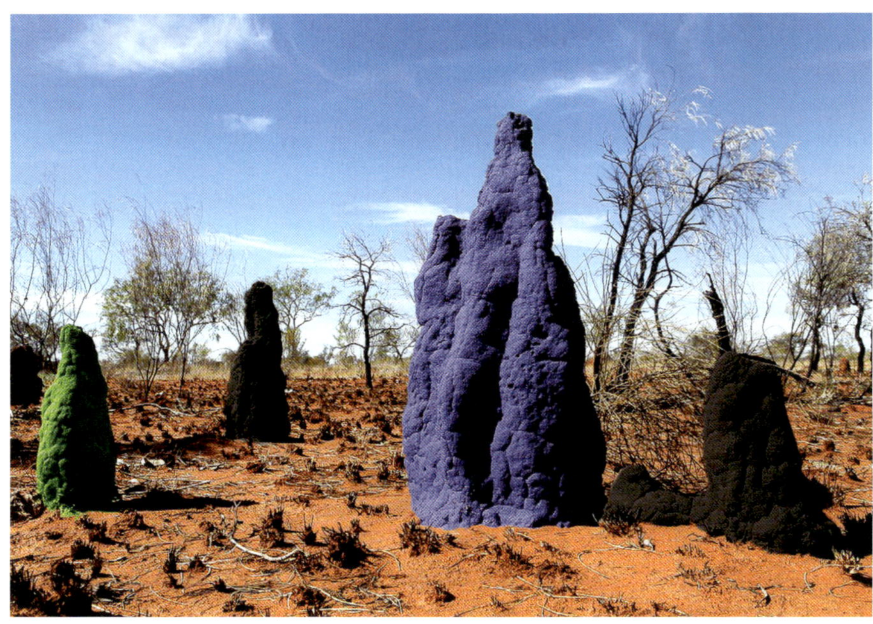

Agnieszka Kurant, *A.A.I.*, 2014. A work whose title references the concept of "artificial artificial intelligence," *A.A.I.* was created through outsourcing the artistic labor to another species: "Working with entomologists at the University of Florida, I employed an entirely unaware population of millions of termites—one of the few species other than humans that has evolved to form complex worker societies—to create their mounds using alternative building materials such as vividly colored sands, gold, and broken crystals." Courtesy Tanya Bonakdar Gallery.

circulation and acceleration. In a world in which information is nearly free, social capital is going to play a far more significant role than financial capital. Today, we no longer know when our labor or social capital is being stealthily harvested. This concealed exploitation of the energies of the social collective intelligence materializes in the phenomenon of "playbor," where value is harvested unbeknownst to the worker through labor masked as play. What was once viewed as natural social behavior, as pleasure seeking, has now been turned into labor. Consumption of digital media by audiences produces content in the form of behavioral data, social network data, and personal data that is commodified and sold to advertising clients. For example, an average Facebook user in the US and Canada brings the corporation around $36 a year through the sale of his or her personal data to advertising firms. At the time of its sale to Facebook for around a billion dollars, Instagram had exactly thirteen employees, since much of its value came from the millions of users who were contributing to the network.

In the same way that the co-creation of certain products' value is outsourced to customers, the co-creation of the value of artworks is outsourced to art audiences. Duchamp's idea of the viewer completing the work of art should now be updated to reflect the fact that the viewer now completes *the value* of the artwork. Visitors contribute to the increase in the value of artworks exhibited at various institutions by circulating images of them on social media. Viewership has become a form of invisible labor.

Meanwhile, a new working class is being born. Platforms such as Amazon's Mechanical Turk or Taskrabbit are outsourcing various microjobs to hundreds of thousands of people working online all over the world. These digital workers receive micropayments for simple tasks. Very often these are tasks that computers cannot do, which is why this process was named "artificial artificial intelligence" by Amazon's founder Jeff Bezos. This notion refers to simulating artificial intelligence through distributed human computation for those tasks that so far cannot be carried out by computers. The structure of these kinds of outsourcing platforms based on collective intelligence could potentially be harnessed in the future to solve problems to the benefit of the public good, much like Wikipedia does today. For the moment, however, with the exception of a number of social experiments,

the tasks posted on Amazon's platform are mostly corporate and often exploitative. The so-called Turkers, earning on average less than one dollar an hour, become a new working class with no protections, and no means of unionizing. The system has found a perfect worker.

Perhaps the artificial intelligence artist should be imagined as an emergent complex system of "artificial artificial intelligence," since using the collective intelligence of crowdsourcing to simulate the non-linear complex system of billions of neurons in a human brain is the closest we can get at this point to simulate the emergence of a single thought or of consciousness in general. Artworks, much like memes, often behave like living organisms, with their own agency and agenda, and my recent experiments show that the phenomenon of emergence can be applied to art production. *Production Line*, realized in collaboration with the artist and computer programmer John Menick, explores the crossover between collective intelligence and artificial intelligence. It draws on the political economy of social creativity often based on invisible and harmless exploitations. The piece applies human collective intelligence to produce artworks, the proceeds from the sale of which will be distributed using a profit-sharing model. A series of drawings was outsourced to thousands of online workers of the Amazon Mechanical Turk platform. The Turkers were asked to each contribute a single line drawn with a computer mouse. No Turker could see other Turkers' contributions or know that he or she was participating in the production of an artwork. After a predefined number of lines was completed, a simple algorithm assembled the hundreds of individual lines into one composite drawing. The result was then outputted to an ink pen plotter. If the drawing is sold on the art market, the Turkers will also share in the profits via a bonus system. By crowdsourcing art production, *Production Line* attempts to divert the flow of surplus capital from the art market to online workers. Because each Turker works in isolation, the final drawing's inchoate composition is emergent and unplanned, questioning whether online labor can cohere into a collectivity.

———————

Opposite: Agnieszka Kurant, *Production Line (Serial 1)* and *Production Line (Serial 2)*, in collaboration with John Menick, 2016. Courtesy Tanya Bonakdar Gallery.

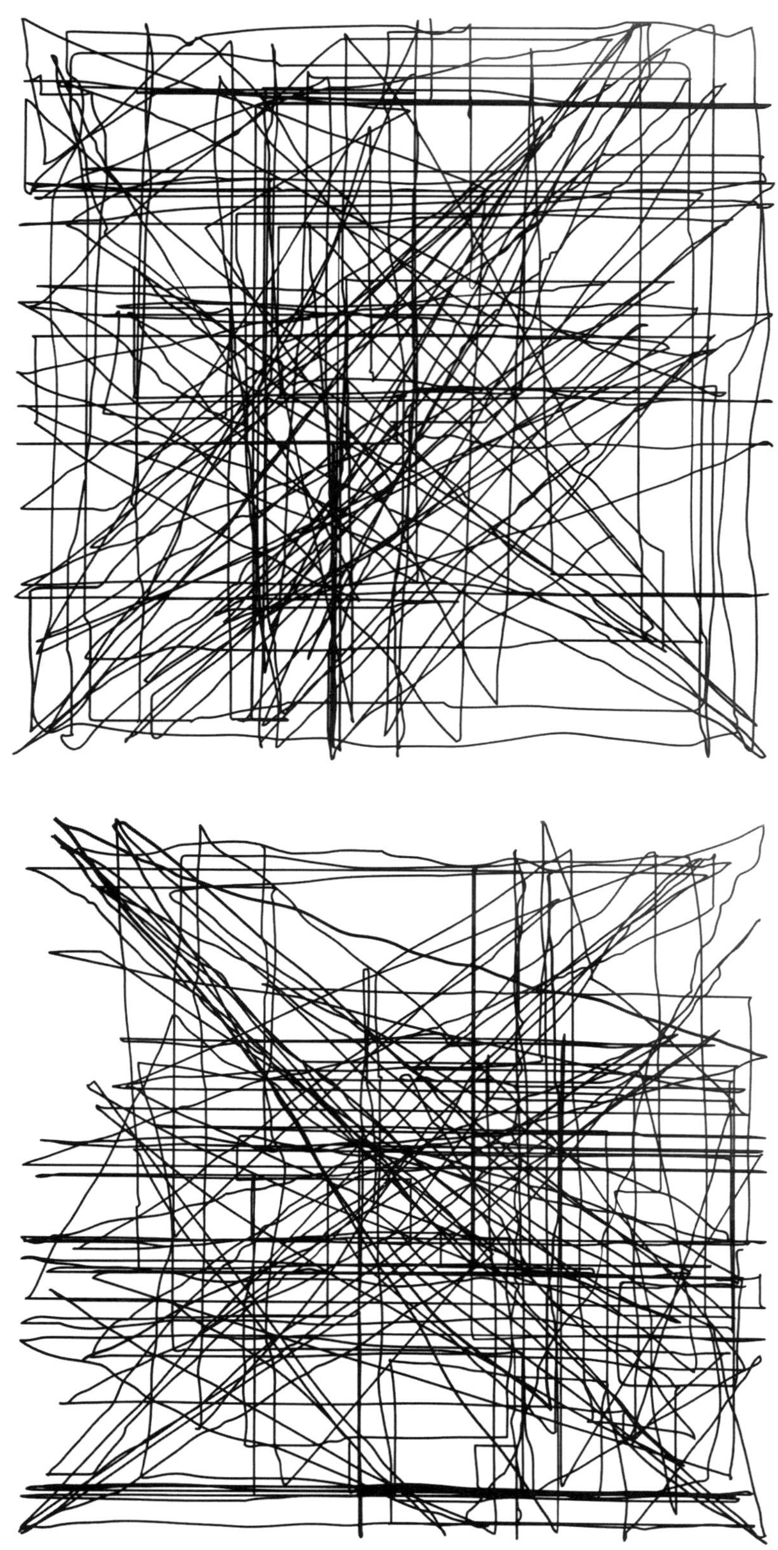

PACKING MY LIBRARY, OR, THE MELANCHOLY OF DEPARTURE
Allen S. Weiss

Years have passed since the wild dogwoods bloomed on Dogwood Ridge. The property, my own, thus no longer merits its name, as only oaks and some stray evergreens remain. For various reasons of little literary interest, I have decided, after four decades, to move. Many things now take on a crystalline presence, knowing that they will never be seen again. Yet other than the surrounding landscape and certain moons, a particular quality of silence, and three or four splendid trees plus a lavender azalea that should be a national treasure, I shall only miss the proximity of owls.

I have long feigned nomadism, claiming to live in four or five different places (Dogwood Ridge, Paris, Nice, Kyoto, and a remote farm in the Aubrac region of France), but in fact I am serially sedentary. With a library of ten thousand volumes, it would be difficult to exist otherwise, and one's psyche adapts accordingly. Furthermore, since I prefer to define myself by my writing, rather than by race, nationality, gender, sexuality, or any other form of self-identification, it is obvious that my library is the matrix of my identity, expressing the lineaments of my soul. Wherever I am, I settle in to write, with whatever handful of volumes accompanies me, and an entire phantom library in mind. Might I go so far as to say that bibliography is destiny?

The two spaces I have always cherished above all others are the library and the museum, which I have recreated in a hybrid form, *my* library-museum, where the archaeology of acquisition, the scenography of display, and the progression of discourse not only offer clues to my systems of belief and knowledge (the complexities and contradictions of which, of course, I myself can never hope to fathom), but also afford serendipitous juxtapositions of objects that sometimes shine forth like a surreal collage, sometimes clash to the point of fracturing preconceived ideas, but always break down the distinctions that I am accustomed to make between art, craft, artifact, and symptom. This space may well be termed a "study," in the varied senses of a room reserved for reading and writing, a preparatory stage of a finished work, and a particular genre, as when artists speak of "a study in ...."

Because of the impending move, this space is slowly being dismantled: the bonds that keep the books together are loosened, which etymologically means that they are *analyzed*. The initial calculation is mathematical, a simple division: I will need approximately 250 wine boxes to transport my library. (It's amazing how migratory libraries can become, given their bulk and heft.) I should mention, so that this essay not be misleading, that work on my library is being interspersed with numerous other activities relating to the move, which I find to be mostly distractions, but necessary ones. Packing also means unpacking. Just the other day I was sorting out the contents of a drawer that had probably not been opened once during the forty years I have lived here, and to my great surprise, well protected in its shroud, I found my first, and most beloved, teddy bear. Teddy! I thought him somewhat disheveled, but what can one expect after a hibernation of forty years! A Rip van Winkle of the Ursidae family! It was a heartwarming reunion.

I love making lists, and the analysis of my library inspired several sorts: favorites rediscovered, and immediately reread; outcast books, not cast out, but rather retained on a special shelf as a reminder of my bibliophilic blunders (out of courtesy to these authors, I won't reveal these titles); rarities, books that took on value with age, but as I am not a bibliophile proper, nor particularly avaricious, these offer no special pleasure; and a list of the essential hundred books of my life—the result of a long epistolary exchange with my dear friend and former editor PF, concerning one's sense of one's library, and of one's self—a small selection harbored against fear of loss, something that has haunted me since I first read Elias Canetti's only novel, *Auto-da-Fé*, which culminates in the conflagration of a great private library. By the time of that reading I already knew of the famed historic precedents, such as the burning of the great library of Alexandria—erased not only from the earth but also nearly completely from memory—so well described by Luciano Canfora in *The Vanished Library*; and of course, still in living memory, the terrible holocaust (literally: *burnt whole*) of twenty thousand books destroyed by the Nazis in a single night, 10 May 1933, on the Bebelplatz in Berlin. Among

the authors so honored by this bonfire was Walter Benjamin. Heinrich Heine's terribly prescient claim continues to resonate: *Dort wo man Bücher verbrennt, verbrennt man auch am Ende Menschen* ("Where they have burned books, they will end up burning human beings"), and I can't reread Benjamin's "Unpacking My Library" without thinking of what role the loss of his beloved library played in his suicide. (Or rather, as was the case of Vincent van Gogh and Antonin Artaud, one should more properly say that he was "suicided by society.") Holocaust, burnt whole: one only thinks of the totality of a library when it is depicted, catalogued, moved, sold ... or burned. This totality has no immediate use value to reader or writer, and generally remains an indifferent abstraction. Being a child of survivors as well as a book lover, I am deeply moved by the memorial to that horrid night, *Bibliotek,* created in 1995 beneath the Bebelplatz by Micha Ullman—a subterranean library consisting of enough empty shelves to hold those twenty thousand vanished volumes—which I visit without fail each time I travel to Berlin, alone and at night, led from afar by the dim shaft of light arising from the empty vault.

Teddy emerged with an assurance that surprised me, seeing daylight again after forty years of darkness. His suppleness, swiftness, and determination belied his physical condition which was, to be honest, piteous. (The serious damage to his left eye was uncanny, as I had just suffered an operation for a detached retina.) He immediately created for himself a throne composed of a ski bonnet filled with intricately woven galloons, which he ominously set under a restrike of one of Goya's last engravings, *The Little Prisoner,* an enchained man dehumanized to a blotch of ink. I soon realized that Teddy's gesture was mocking, sardonic, vengeful, certainly an expression of his deep resentfulness and furor at his incarceration.

I find it difficult, as do many authors, to differentiate between reading and writing. I read with pencil in hand, and write with book in hand. I totally empathize with Walter Benjamin's claim, in "Unpacking My Library," that certain authors fundamentally write because they are dissatisfied with all the books they have read, which suggests that one more list must be added to those above, to enumerate the contents of the shelves that contain my own publications. Of the citations, footnotes, and allusions found therein, 99 percent of the sources can be found within my library,

thus my own works are a sort of distillation or sublimation of their surroundings: books, art, ceramics, and memories combined.

One morning I awoke to find that Teddy had found a companion (or was it a familiar, or a servant, or a slave?): a most bizarre, somewhat disquieting pincushion doll that was obviously hidden in another drawer, a sort of miniature Pulcinella from what performance of the *commedia dell'arte* I cannot say. Teddy-Punch. Their relationship seemed rather sinister, and it evoked bad memories. When I was four, I suffered what must have been the first trauma of my life: upon returning home one night, asleep in my mother's arms, I awoke to find that Teddy had disappeared. Frantically, my parents enlisted a group of friends to search for him, as I wept, inconsolable. About an hour later, he was found sitting on the curb in front of our apartment, an odd grin on his face. Only now do I realize the profound cruelty of his disappearing act.

The wonders of juxtaposition are manifest in libraries. So are the vagaries of categories. Books can be arranged by author, title, subject, language, publisher, date of publication, even the color of the binding (the latter far more common, for decorative reasons, than one may think). Each possibility follows a certain logic, and each one has interesting consequences. I wonder whether my current system of classification will survive the voyage, however brief. I wonder about the effects of unpacking my library.

The next day I discovered Teddy surrounded by a *sloth* of plush bears. (I can't help laughing at this collective noun, sloth, given Teddy's decades-long inertia, but I am beginning to feel that he is not to be laughed at.) I hadn't imagined that there were so many, and I suspected him of bringing in outsiders to make a point. They soon disappeared, but events took a more distressing turn, as I realized that he was assembling and organizing all the inanimate creatures in sight: a roly-poly Daruma doll, who seems to be his confidant; a pile of trilobite fossils and assorted anthropod exoskeletons; numerous porcelain beans representing the infant Jesus, left over from Twelfth Night cakes (did Teddy know that I have done an object theater performance, *My Dolls,* using the very same beans that he has now appropriated?); a miniature porcelain figurine of Frozen Charlotte (inspired by the nineteenth-century poem of decidedly necrophiliac connotations, "A

Corpse Going to a Ball") somehow reminiscent of the
young women in Yasunari Kawabata's *House of the
Sleeping Beauties*, evincing a strange eroticism, a veri-
tably bearish bestiality.

Bruno Bettelheim, in *The Uses of Enchantment*,
argued that one should never read fairy tales to children from illustrated books, so as to leave every child
the free rein of their imagination to flesh out the characters and form their own fantasies in relation to the
tale. I would say the same thing in regard to private
libraries, since every one is by definition idiosyncratic,
if not eccentric. This is why, in a text all about books, I
have referred to so few titles. These few will soon join
all the others in the obscurity of their boxes, for exactly
how long I do not know.

I awoke just before dawn to find Teddy at the
window, speaking in a lugubrious and incomprehen-
sible language to the owls.

Opposite: Teddy and friend keep the author company as he
packs up his library. Photo Allen S. Weiss.

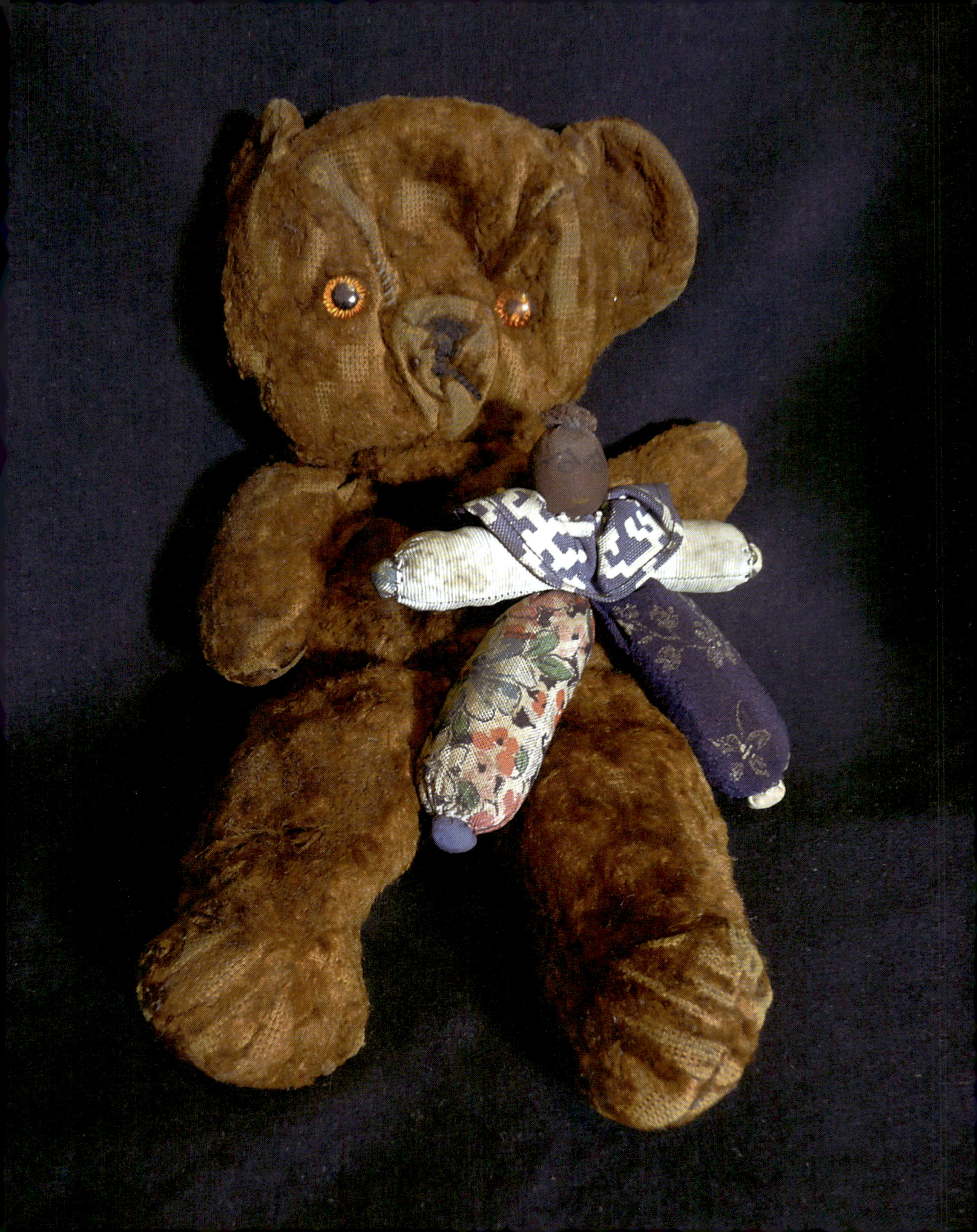

CALENDARS

CALENDARS

LABOR DAYS
Tony Wood

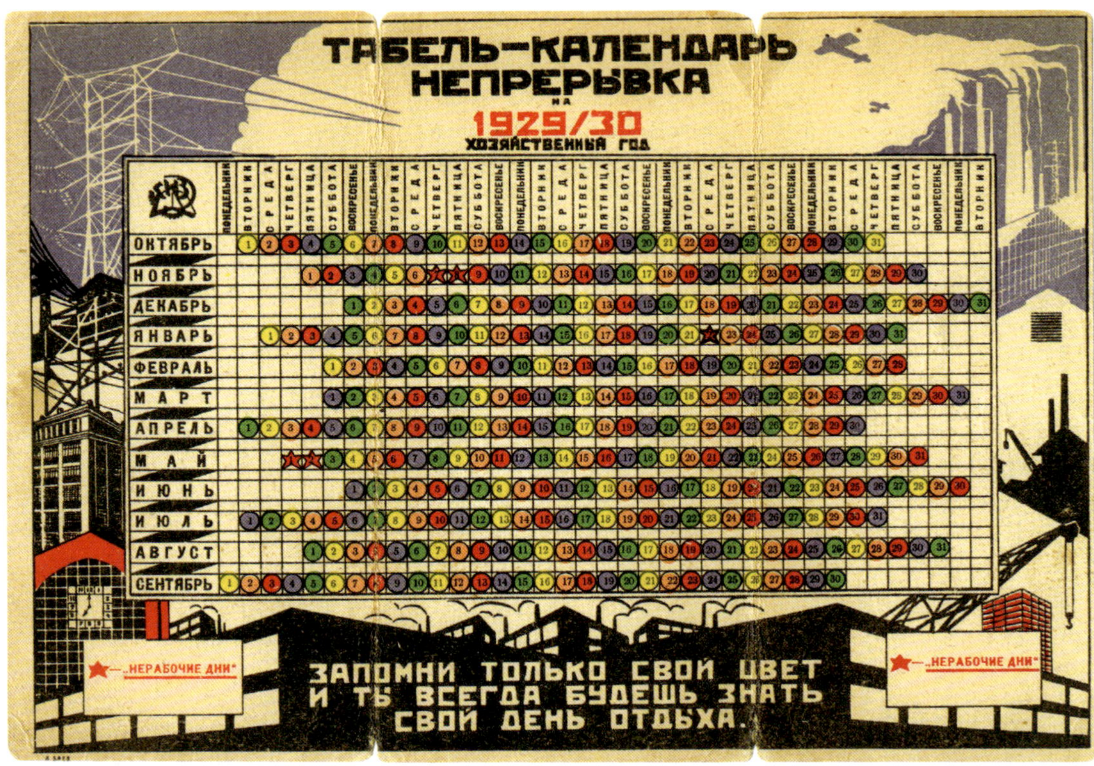

Among the many things to disappear during the world-shaking turmoil of the Russian Revolution—along with czarism, the aristocracy, private banks, landownership—were the first thirteen days of February. On 24 January 1918, Lenin signed a decree ordering the country to switch from the Julian calendar, used by the Orthodox Church, to the Gregorian, bringing revolutionary Russia into line with the rest of Europe. The two systems had been drifting more and more out of alignment since the sixteenth century, so much so that by 1918, making the change meant skipping directly from 31 January to 14 February. From then on, anyone referring to events that took place before this interregnum had to be clear whether the date they were using was Old Style or New Style. The shift also explains why the anniversary of the Great October Revolution was always celebrated in November, which often puzzled visitors to the USSR.

The 1918 calendar reform was an abrupt, one-off change, designed to signal the irreversibility of the leap from the *ancien régime* to the new. Undoing the revolution would now mean literally turning back time—which is what some upper-crust characters attempt to do in Sigizmund Krzhizhanovsky's 1929 novella *Memories of the Future* when they ask the inventor of a time machine to take them back to the days of serfdom. Pushing the calendar forward was only one part, however, of a much broader campaign to sweep away backwardness and superstition and, in particular, to loosen the grip of religion on everyday life. Early on, the Soviets invented a series of ceremonies designed to replace Orthodox rituals: in addition to secular weddings and funerals, the government

---

Above: Calendar for 1929–1930 showing rest days for each of the five worker groups, designated here by different colors. In this version of *nepreryvka*, the continuous workweek, workers had every fifth day off. The text at bottom reads: "Just remember your color and you'll always know your rest day." The five days with red stars indicate official holidays on which no one worked. Courtesy Erast Butakov.

introduced "Octobering," a Leninist alternative to baptism. There was also a weekly paper called *Bezbozhnik*—"Atheist," "Godless One"—and, from 1925, a League of the Militant Godless. Yet, as the Bolsheviks found over the course of the next decade, much of the country was still deeply attached to religion, and still attuned to rhythms set by Church feasts, saints' days, and the like. Even the names for the days of the week harbored a stubborn godliness: the Russian for Saturday is *Subbota*, from "Sabbath," while the word for Sunday is simply "Resurrection," *Voskresen'e*.

In August 1929, the Soviet government decreed a second calendar reform, which ostensibly had aims different from those of the 1918 switch. By the end of the 1920s, the country was in the midst of a frantic push to industrialize, spurred by the adoption of the first Five-Year Plan in 1928. A fever of construction seized hold of the nation, as bridges, factories, and even entire cities began to sprout across the landscape. The plan set a welter of ambitious targets that nations with more solid industrial bases would have struggled to meet; Soviet newspapers, posters, and films exhorted workers to ever-greater feats of industrial prowess by printing reams of statistics and glowing reports of "socialist competition" between factories seeking to outdo each other in "over-fulfilling" the plan. Valentin Kataev's 1932 novel *Time, Forward!* describes one such struggle, focusing on a single day in which a factory tries to break the record for poured concrete. Surprisingly, the story manages to create quite a bit of suspense, its sentences racing forward in line with the quickening tempo of society as a whole. (The book even begins by getting out ahead of itself, opening with the words: "The first chapter is omitted for the time being.")

This was the context in which Yuri Larin, a Bolshevik economist, began agitating for a plan that would allow factories to operate every day of the year. At the Fifth Congress of Soviets in May 1929, he advocated for what became known as the *nepreryvka*, the "continuous working week."[1] This entailed dividing the workforce into groups and allocating each different rest days. In effect, the plan proposed to transfer the concept of a shift system to the days of the week. At first, Larin's colleagues were unenthusiastic—especially the Commissariat of Labor, which was dubious about the logistics of running so many factories continuously. (It was hard enough getting supplies and workers for them to run at all: bottlenecks

were a constant curse of the Soviet economy, and rates of absenteeism were especially high in the early stages of the industrialization drive.)[2] But Larin apparently managed to get Stalin's ear, and by June, a proposal that weeks before had barely been discussed was being hailed in the press as "the great socialist idea."

Larin's plan involved more than a shift to a continuous workweek, however; it also meant switching the workforce from a seven-day to a five-day pattern. Until 1929, Soviet citizens worked for six days and rested on Sundays; from now on everyone would work for four days with one day off. Everyone would be getting more time off, but Larin clearly convinced the planners that the gains made from running factories continuously would more than compensate for the lost working hours. The workforce would be divided into five groups, each with a different rest day. The five shifts were often numbered. In many cases, they were color coded—red for 1, green for 2, and so on—and sometimes even symbols, such as hammer, sickle, red flag, airplane, and party membership card, were used to represent the different groups. The particular color scheme or symbols used varied from one workplace to another. Though the Soviet economy was centrally planned, many of the details of day-to-day life in the USSR depended on the individual enterprise where one worked; the same was true of the *nepreryvka* calendars, which could look quite dissimilar even for people employed in the same sector. Although the underlying principle was the same, the profusion of schedules must have been pretty disorienting. The benefits for industry of Larin's new arrangement were obvious enough, but the workers themselves were less enthused. Even though it actually meant that everyone's day off came around more quickly, family members and friends could not be guaranteed to have the same rest days, and as early as October 1929, *Pravda* was publishing letters of complaint from disgruntled (or bored?) workers:

What is there for us to do at home if our wives are in the factory, our children at school, and nobody can visit us, so that there is nothing left but to go to a State tearoom? What sort of a life is it if we are to rest in shifts and not together as a whole proletariat? It is no holiday if you have to have it alone.[3]

Larin's scheme did allow for some days when the entire workforce could take a break—five, to be precise

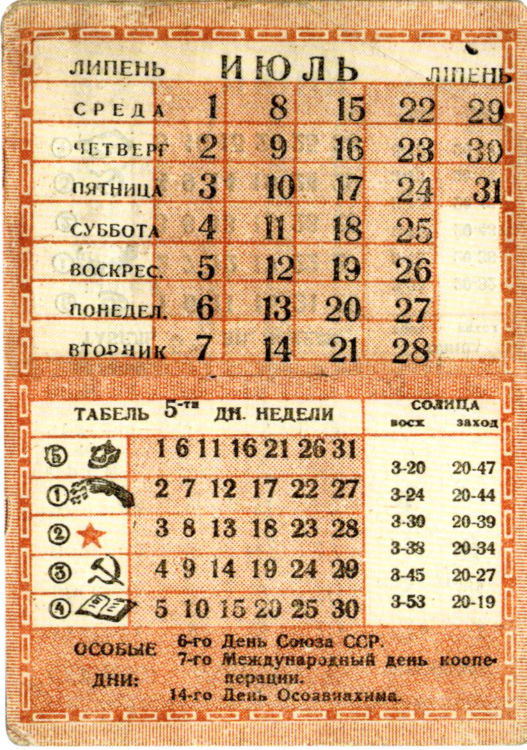

(which is why one of the pamphlets he published to explain how the *nepreryvka* would expand the number of workdays was titled *360 instead of 300*). The new holidays everyone would share were 22 January, commemorating both Lenin's death and the anniversary of Bloody Sunday, when czarist troops gunned down participants in a peaceful workers' march in 1905; 1 and 2 May, to mark International Workers' Day; and 7 and 8 November, to celebrate the October Revolution. But these aside, there was to be little opportunity for collective rest—the new Soviet calendar was decidedly short on mass festivities, with nothing like the stream of civic ceremonies the French Revolutionary calendar had envisaged.

The continuous five-day week wasn't just designed to reorganize industrial labor patterns and squeeze more hours out of the workforce. For most of the population, perhaps more significant was the *nepreryvka*'s implied assault not just on rest days per se, but on weekends specifically. The 1929 reform hadn't totally done away with the seven days of the week: calendars laying out the five-day schema continued to refer to individual days by their traditional names, but now the workweek would begin on different days depending on one's number or color. What had happened, then, was that the population's working rhythm had been uncoupled from the standard seven-day cycle. Where the French revolutionaries had done away with the old days and months altogether, instituting an entirely new calendar instead, the Soviet *nepreryvka* was not so much a calendar reform as an *attempt* to subtract meaning from the existing calendar by overwriting it with another one. Since a worker's rest day would keep falling on different days, surely no day could hold more significance than any other. Of course, there

---

Left: The months of April (top) and July from a 1931 worker's pocket calendar. Here, the five different work groups are represented by five symbols—a sheaf of wheat, a red star, the hammer and sickle, a book, and a *budenovka*, or wool military cap. Courtesy Erast Butakov.

Page 68: Soviet poster linking church holidays with drunkenness, 1920s. Courtesy Hoover Institution, Stanford University.

Page 69: Out with the old. Poster from 1930 advocating for *nepreryvka*, which is pictured as a hammer expelling the influence of religion from the calendar. The text at the bottom is a satirical poem by Dem'ian Bednyi. Courtesy Hoover Institution, Stanford University.

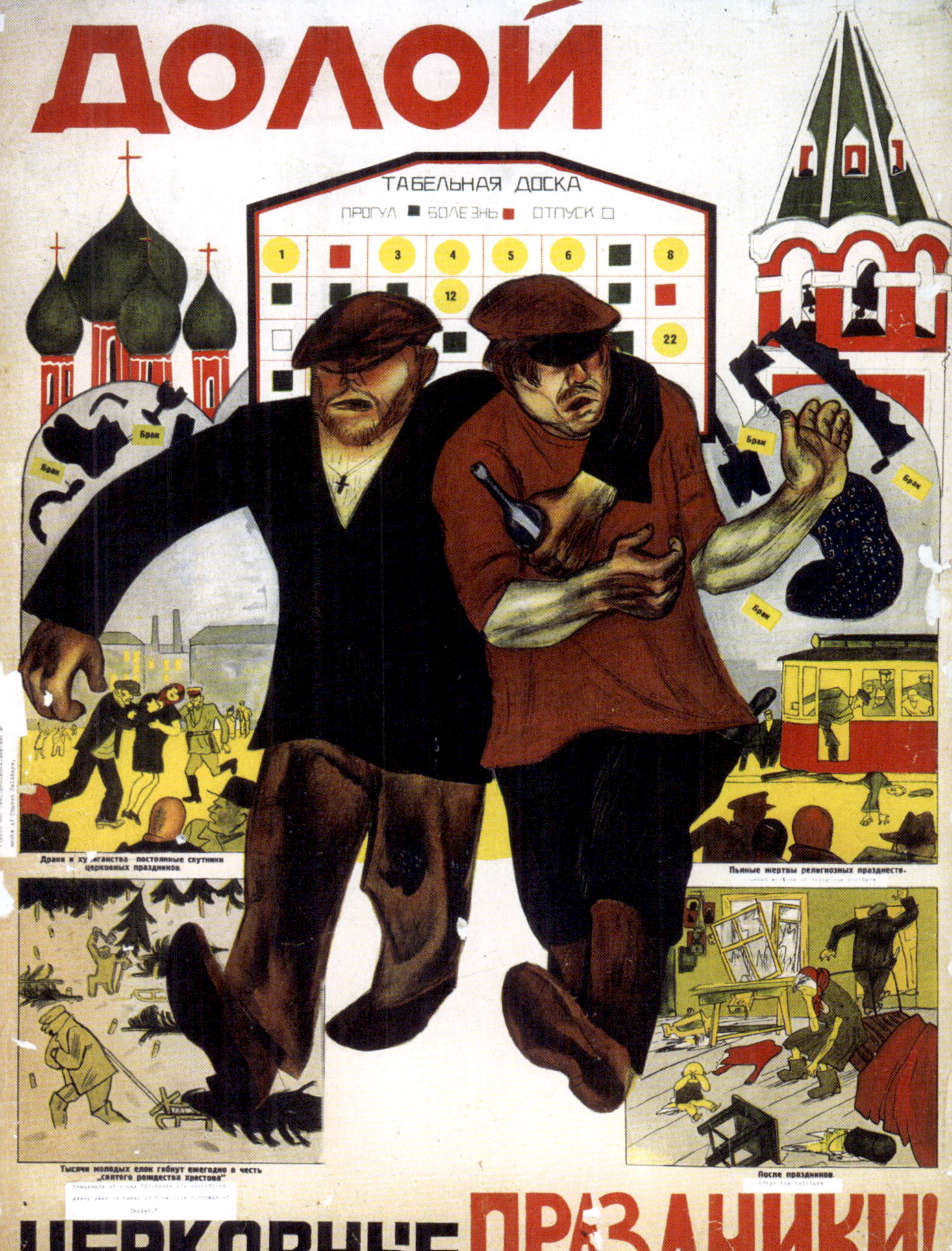
ДОЛОЙ
ТАБЕЛЬНАЯ ДОСКА
ПРОГУЛ БОЛЕЗНЬ ОТПУСК
1 3 4 5 6 8
12
22
Брак
Драка и хулиганства — постоянные спутники
церковных праздников
Пьяные жертвы религиозных празднеств
Тысячи молодых елок гибнут ежегодно в честь
"святого рождества христова"
После праздников
ЦЕРКОВНЬЕ ПРАЗДНИКИ!

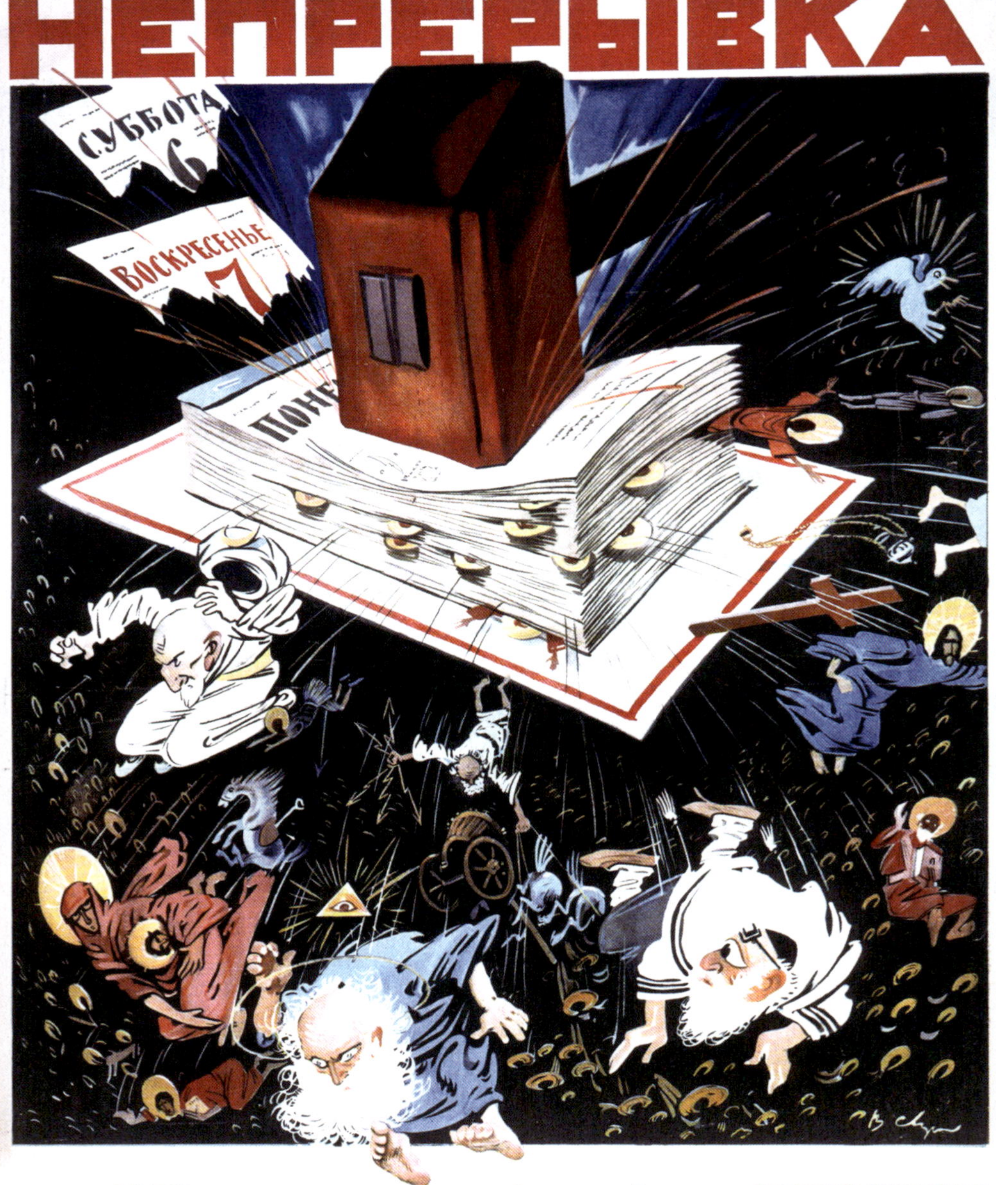

НЕПРЕРЫВКА

„БУДЯ"

Календарь есть штука не вечная,
Морока с ним бесконечная.
Смешно читать календарную историю:
Кто считал по Юлию, кто по Григорию.
В Расее до Питера, до царя,
Новогодничали с сентября,
При царе Петре
Стали год начинать в январе.
Против такого начала
Старина, как всегда, ворчала.
Наш год православный ехал, одначе,
На старенькой кляче.
Европа вперед рвалася
А Расея за нею плелася
В календаре ковыляла за ней
С опозданием в несколько дней.
После октябрьского переворота
Мы добились с Европою равного счета.
Нынче настал наш черед
Рвануться вперед,
Составить календарь поумнее,
Умнее? дельнее:
Исключить воскресение—
Рюмкоподнесение,
Уйти от субботы
С перерывом работы,
Убрать из календаря
Устаревшую выдумку, бога-царя,
Святых разгильдяев-Митяев,
Преподобных Лентяев
Не святцы нужны нам, нам встарь,
А трудовой календарь.
Мы тысячу лет по святцам молились
Да чуть и провал не провалились.
Мы не любим за делом гоняться:
Мастера мы большие безделья
                 слоняться,
Бросив дело, часами калякать,
Хлестануть без толку, без толку
                 поплакать,
А по части упорного,
Плодотворного,
Целевого труда:
Не годимся мы никуда:
Рванем во всю мочь, надорвем себе жилы
И кряхтим до могилы.
От старого порядка не было добра.
Переходить к новому пора.
Браться по-новому за работу,
По новому календарному счету:
Четыре дня — трудовые дни.
В пятый день — разумно отдохни
Не с колокольным звоном,
Не с самогоном.
Тот враг своей жизни и последний неряха,
У кого все уповы — церковь да кабак.
Жили мы гнусно, только землю паскудя.
Помолимся! Попили! Будя!

ДЕМЬЯН БЕДНЫЙ

was one particular day this would affect more than others: in theory, the reform made it impossible for the population to properly observe religious holidays or to regularly attend church.

Eviatar Zerubavel, in his book on the history of the week, sees the *nepreryvka*'s anti-religious element as a key part of its appeal to the Soviet leadership, and its introduction as a continuation of the government's earlier atheistic offensive: weekend rest days, "these two weekly bastions of Judeo-Christian religious sentiments, were clearly the main targets."[4] It's true that early on, the state propaganda announcing the benefits of the five-day week stressed its importance in combating piety; religious festivals also tended to encourage heavy drinking among workers. A propaganda poster from 1930 proudly announces, in rather clunky rhyming verse, that: "In the name of economic efficiency / Sundays have been burned off like rotten stumps: / There is no all-round festive idleness anymore! Everyone has his own days off!" The poster depicts a worker calculating how many days off he gets per year (the answer is seventy-two); perhaps it was this nationwide arithmetic test that entitled the poster to claim that the *nepreryvka* "raises the cultural level of the worker."

Although it was meant to be confined to industry and implemented gradually, the new five-day, continuous workweek spread rapidly. Within a year, the overwhelming majority of industrial enterprises reported that they had shifted to the new regimen, and large numbers of workplaces in other sectors had joined them, including many government offices, shops, cinemas, and restaurants.[5] The *nepreryvka* had brought a profound alteration to the rhythms of everyday life and leisure for the entire workforce. In that sense, Zerubavel's argument that it was principally an anti-religious reform might be exaggerating its godless credentials: if anything, the five-day *nepreryvka* was not

---

Below: Poster contrasting frivolous celebrations of Easter in the past with the commitment of the new Communist worker, 1920s. Courtesy Duke University Libraries.

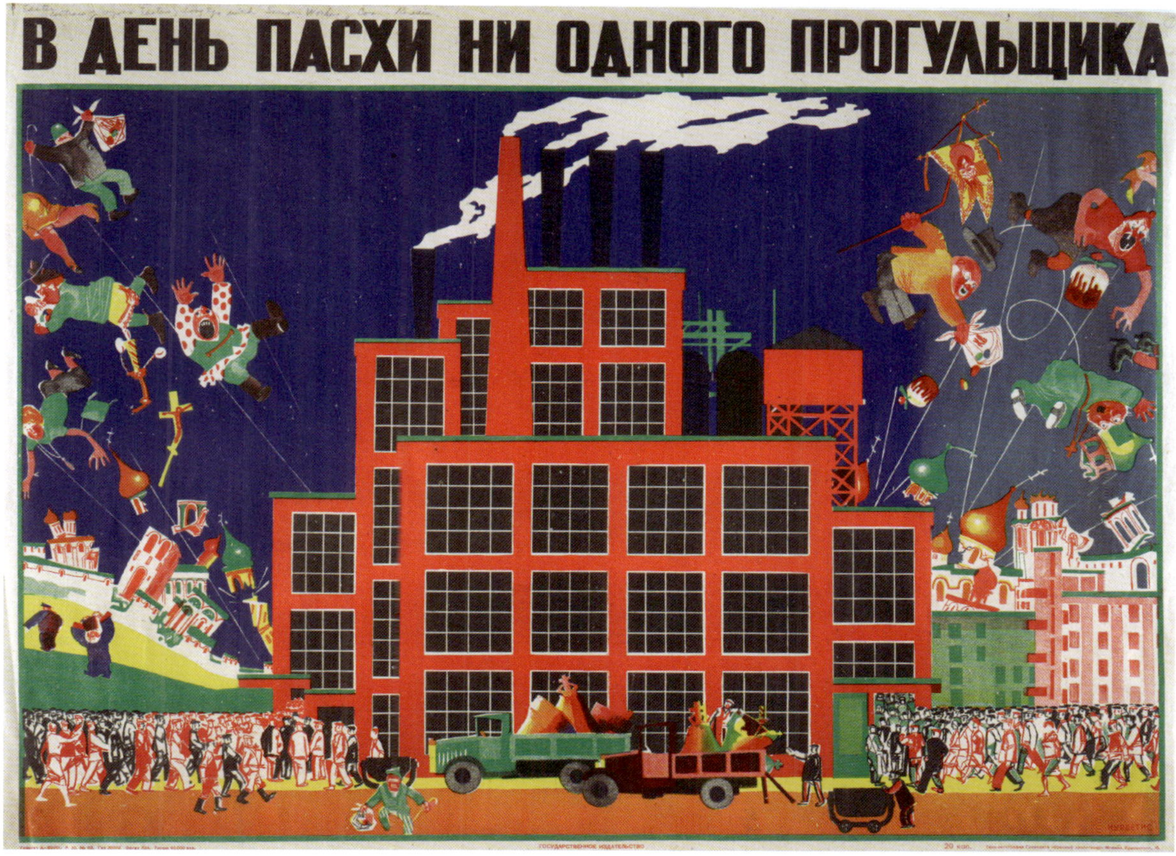

so much a destructive anti-Orthodox move as a gesture of secular faith in industrialization, an attempt to bring daily life in line with the demands of the machine age.

It wasn't long, though, before the continuous five-day week ran into fairly predictable problems: breakdown of machinery through overuse, malcoordination of shifts, more frequent supply bottlenecks, grumbling from employees who never saw their families. In June 1931, Stalin made a speech in which he complained that "some of our comrades were a little hasty in introducing the uninterrupted working-week, and in their hurry distorted it and transformed it into a system of lack of personal responsibility."[6] The system was then substantially changed by switching to a six-day pattern—five days on, one day off—and, crucially, giving everyone the same sixth day off. Rest days were now fixed on the sixth, twelfth, eighteenth, twenty-fourth, and thirtieth days of each month; Sundays were shorn of their regular place as the week's endpoint. Indeed, the six-day week, or *shestidnevka*, was, like its five-day predecessor, designed to inhabit and gradually displace the seven-day week, like a cuckoo's egg laid in another bird's nest. Calendars from the late 1930s show months divided into six-day cycles, with the traditional names of the weekdays now replaced by ordinal numbers: first, second, third, etc. Months consisted of five six-day weeks, plus, in some cases, a thirty-first day that stood alone, and which was generally a "bonus" workday.

This revised version of the reform proved much more durable, lasting until 26 June 1940. Zerubavel argues that, over the course of the 1930s, the calendar reform in effect split the Soviet population into "two distinct societies," an urban industrial segment operating on a six-day, secularized cycle and the residents of the rural hinterlands, who completely disregarded the new calendars devised in Moscow and continued to follow the seven-day "beat"—carrying on with their peasant markets and going to church on Sundays.[7] In this respect, the abolition of the *shestidnevka* could be seen as a victory for the old seven-day cycle and for the deep, rural past, which eventually reasserted itself despite the secularizing ambitions of the Soviet state.

But this view may rest on too stark an opposition between the industrial, urban realm and a foot-dragging agrarian world. What took place during the 1930s was often a paradoxical fusion of the two. In that decade, the USSR experienced one of the most rapid and extensive processes of urbanization the world had ever seen; at the same time, the human flood from the countryside was so enormous that it ended up "ruralizing" the cities—hence the oxymoronic title of David Hoffmann's portrait of Moscow in the 1930s, *Peasant Metropolis*.[8] Factory work, too, was partly ruralized. Soviet sources are rife with complaints about the failure of newly arrived migrants to shed their old work habits, in particular the tendency to slack for long periods of time only to compensate in a frantic rush as deadlines neared—a pattern of "storming" that remained a feature of the Soviet economy till the end. The whole character of the Soviet system, in other words, was shaped by the collision and conflation of rural and urban rhythms. Rather than seeing one as having ultimately defeated the other, you could call it a draw: while much of the population did continue to observe religious traditions on the sly, the country that returned to the seven-day pattern in 1940 had been transformed into an industrial superpower. When it was put to the test in World War II, the USSR ultimately outmatched the German industrial machine—and there the outcome was definitely not a draw. The most important public holiday in Russia is still Victory Day, commemorating the final German surrender of 1945. Here again, though, Russian and Western calendars differ: the other World War II Allies mark the occasion on 8 May, when the act of surrender was drawn up; the Russians, following the Soviets, choose instead to remember 9 May, when the documents were actually signed, in the small hours of a Wednesday morning in Berlin.

1 For an early account of the origins and implementation of the *nepreryvka*, see [n.a.], "The Continuous Working Week in Soviet Russia," *International Labour Review*, vol. 23, no. 2, February 1931; see also Eviatar Zerubavel, *The Seven Day Circle: The History and Meaning of the Week* (New York: The Free Press, 1985), pp. 35–43.

2 R. W. Davies, *The Industrialisation of Soviet Russia*, vol. 3, *The Soviet Economy in Turmoil, 1929–1930* (London: Macmillan, 1989), p. 85.

3 Quoted in [n.a.], "The Continuous Working Week in Soviet Russia," p. 176.

4 Eviatar Zerubavel, *The Seven Day Circle*, p. 36.

5 See [n.a.], "The Continuous Working Week in Soviet Russia," pp. 164–166.

6 Joseph Stalin, "New Conditions—New Tasks in Economic Construction," speech delivered on 23 June 1931. Published in Joseph Stalin, *Works*, vol. 13 (Moscow: Foreign Languages Publishing House, 1954). Available at <marxists.org/reference/archive/stalin/works/1931/06/23.htm>.

7 Eviatar Zerubavel, *The Seven Day Circle*, p. 42.

8 David L. Hoffmann, *Peasant Metropolis: Social Identities in Moscow, 1929–1941* (Ithaca, NY: Cornell University Press, 1994).

ANARCHIST CALENDRICS
Byron Ellsworth Hamann

What calendar system should date the masthead of an anarchist newspaper? In late nineteenth-century Kansas, editor Moses Harman experimented with several possibilities.

Harman was born in West Virginia on 12 October 1830. Over the next few years, his parents slowly moved the family west, finally settling in Crawford County, Missouri, in 1838. Harman would stay in this part of the country (the tristate area of Missouri, Illinois, and Kansas) for the next seven decades, until a winter spent in Los Angeles convinced him to move to southern California. He spent the last two years of his life there, and died in 1910.

After graduating from high school in 1851, Harman tried a number of professions: farmer, teacher, circuit-riding preacher, and, during the Civil War, hospital nurse. (Problems with one of his legs prevented him from enlisting for the Union.) Married in 1866, and widowed in 1877, Harman left Missouri for Kansas in 1879. There, in the riverside town of Valley Falls, he embarked on a new career as radical journalist and chronological agitator.[1]

Three years earlier, in 1876, the National Liberal League was founded in Philadelphia. A coalition of various organizations across the United States, its initial aim was the total separation of state from church, including a repeal of Sunday laws and an end to religious instruction in public schools. Soon after moving to Valley Falls, Harman became involved in the local League chapter. In 1880, he was elected coeditor of the chapter's new monthly periodical, the *Valley Falls Liberal*. The paper's goals were outlined in a front-page prospectus: "To support the cause of LIBER-ALISM in its effort to break the chains which have been riveted upon the minds and souls of men and women by that religion of Fear and Hate, misnamed Christianity..."

Inspired by this manifesto, Harman quickly moved to replace the paper's *Anno Domini* dating with a new chronology, apparently of his own design. Starting in November 1880, the masthead of the *Valley Falls Liberal* carried the American Nation (A.N.) count, its Year 1 corresponding to 1776. As Harman explained in the January, A.N. 105 issue:

1881.

The year 1880 since the Christian Era, came, and is now just gone to keep company with the "years beyond the Flood." But when that Flood was, and when that Era commenced, authentic history does not inform us. Christian scholars are very much divided on these questions. It is pretty generally admitted, however, that the Chronology with regard to the latter is wrong—some placing the error at four, and some at eight or nine years. Thus we ought to call the year now commencing 1885 or 1889 instead of 1881. Then again, it is conceded generally that Jesus of Nazareth was not born in winter but in spring; and hence the year should commence, not in January but in April or May. In view of these difficulties and for other reasons that will readily present themselves, we prefer to reckon time from a date concerning which there is no dispute: and, as Americans, we choose to date our little paper from our National Birthday.

Readers of the January issue might have been surprised that its A.N. date was still 105, as it had been in December—but this was because the new year in Harman's system did not begin until July. And so when midsummer arrived, the masthead (finally) read: "Valley Falls, Kansas, July, A.N. 106."

Two months later, in September—having just celebrated the paper's one-year anniversary—Harman changed its name from the (local-sounding) *Valley Falls Liberal* to the (statewide) *Kansas Liberal*. He also updated the masthead mission statement: "Total Separation of the State from Supernatural Theology. Perfect Equality before the Law for all Men and Women. No privileged classes or orders—No Monopolies." The renamed paper continued to be dated with the A.N. system for the next seven months. But in April 1882, at the same time the *Kansas Liberal*'s headquarters were temporarily moved to Lawrence, Harman reverted to mainstream chronology: April 13, 1882. The paper was back in Valley Falls by October, and early in 1883 chronological experimentation also returned. The 12 January issue was dated E.M. 283: in the Era of Man.

This system had been promulgated the previous fall at the sixth annual National Liberal League convention. Held in St. Louis from 29 September to 1 October 1882, the convention turned to the topic of calendar

reform on its third and final day. A detailed article on the proceedings appeared in the 25 October 1882 issue of the *Boston Investigator*:

After this business was concluded, Mr. George Chainey, of Boston, arose and said that several resolutions and suggestions relative to a new secular calendar had been referred to the Committee on Resolutions, and that they desired him to report the following, which he read: —

THE MODERN ERA.

Whereas, The uncertain and mythical origin of the Christian calendar now in general use commits those who use it, to some extent, at least, to the Christian theology; and,

Whereas, It would be relief to many and a great convenience to have a more certain, modern, and purely secular date for recording time,

Resolved, That we earnestly recommend all those who do not wish so [to] express their adherence to the Christian theology to unite in all parts of the world upon a common, secular, universal date as the year *one* of a modern era; and,

Whereas, Three great events common to the whole human race, and which gave mankind a new heaven and new earth, point to the year known as "A.D. 1600," making our present year 282, as the proper beginning of the modern era, we call special attention to those facts, viz.:—

1. The general publication and acceptance of the new or Copernican system of astronomy.
2. The discovery of the unity of the human race (i.e., humanity in its solidarity and continuity) by the extension of commerce and European civilization to Asia, Africa, and Australia, and the recognition of progress in the success of the ages and generations of the human race.
3. The foundations of International Law by Hugo Grotius (begun in 1600 and published in 1625); and,

Whereas, These events, which changed the face of the world, are fitly consecrated by the martyrdom of the great Liberal of his age, Giordano Bruno, who was burned to death by the Christian Church at Rome, on the 16th day of February, 1600, for proclaiming the new astronomy, the true solar system, the infinity of the heavens and of worlds; and,

Whereas, This modern date may be most conveniently used to succeed the old era, having its last two figures the same, and being capable of a familiar contraction to '82 for 282, just as the old date, 1882, is contracted to '82; therefore,

Resolved, That the National Liberal League adopt this date, and earnestly recommend its general use.

The resolution was adopted unanimously and with applause.

Then followed a discussion of what to name the new chronology. The system's creator, George N. Hill (secretary of the Investigator Hall Society in Boston), pushed for *Anno Scientia*—the Era of Science, or E.S. Another proposal was for "Age of Reason." But in the end, "Era of Man" (E.M.) won out, "passed by so large a majority that it was almost a general consent."

Back in Kansas, in late August 1883 (E.M. 283)—eight months after introducing Era of Man dating—Moses Harman rebooted the *Kansas Liberal*. He changed its name to *Lucifer the Light-Bearer* ("the name applied by the ancients to the morning star, the Herald of Dawn") and expanded its content. An ad for *Lucifer* printed in the 11 June 1884 issue of *Liberty* (a radical paper from Boston) announced a wide range of controversial topics—and Harman's interest in anarchism, which he had already voiced in the *Kansas Liberal*, was asserted at the start:

A fortnightly free thought, anarchistic journal, devoted to the fearless discussion of all questions of human interest, including the land question, the money question, the question of the relations of the State to the Individual, the question of prohibition vs. temperance, the marriage question, heredity, etc., etc. LUCIFER discusses all these and other subjects from the standpoint of Individualism, holding that no true Socialism is possible where the rights of the individual man and woman are not regarded as the only rights there are, and respected accordingly.

LUCIFER repudiates the imposed authority alike of gods and states, and holds in infinite scorn the prurient meddlesomeness of society.

LUCIFER carries with it the sparkling light and invigorating breezes of the wide-sweeping prairies of the West. It preaches the gospel of reciprocal Rights and Duties, and sounds a trumpet-call to ACTION.

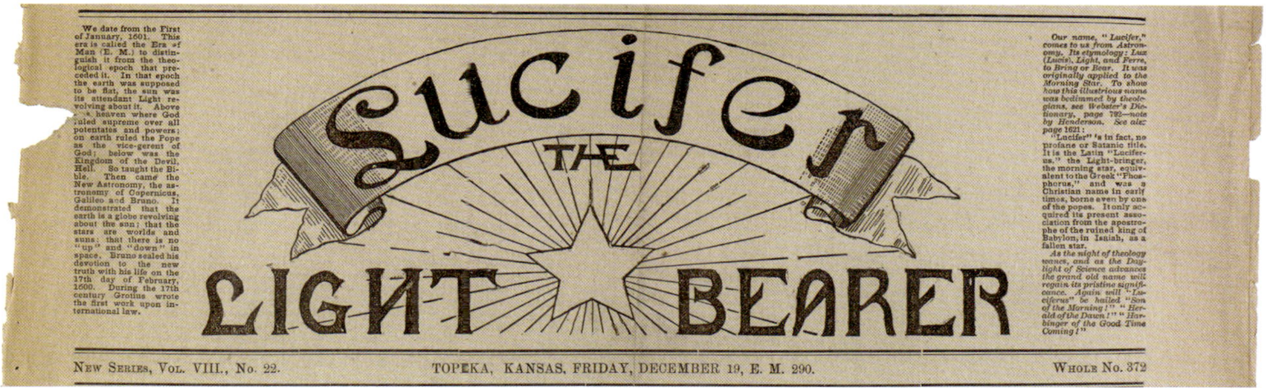

NEW SERIES, VOL. VIII., No. 22.　　　　TOPEKA, KANSAS, FRIDAY, DECEMBER 19, E. M. 290.　　　　WHOLE No. 372.

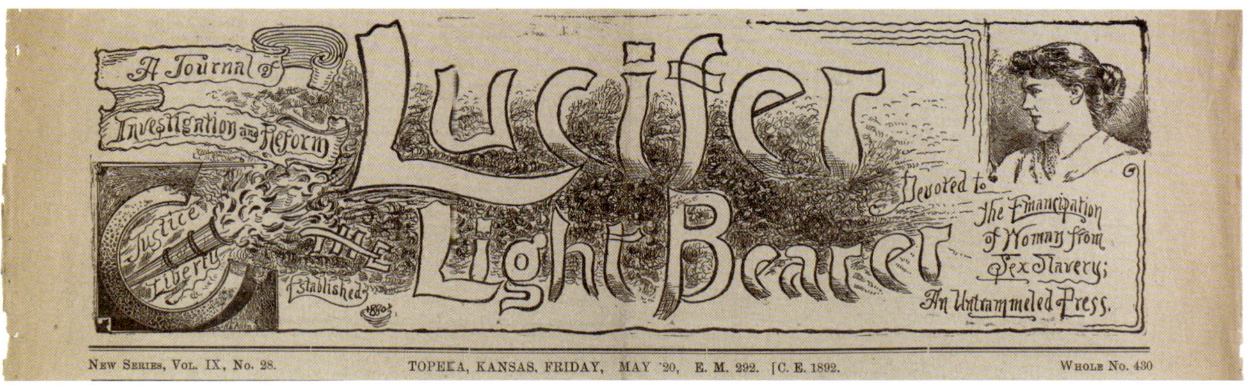

NEW SERIES, VOL. IX, No. 28.　　　　TOPEKA, KANSAS, FRIDAY, MAY '20, E. M. 292. [C. E. 1892.　　　　WHOLE No. 430.

Two mastheads from Moses Harman's newspaper *Lucifer the Light Bearer*—one giving the year as E.M. 290 (top) and the other noting both the E.M. year, 292, and the C.E. year of 1892.

Throughout these changes of title and themes—and across various updates in design—the E.M. system stayed in the masthead. Not all of Harman's readers understood what the abbreviation meant, and so from time to time he offered them an explanation. The 8 January E.M. 286 issue included this extended commentary:

OUR CALENDAR

A St. Louis correspondent (whose name we have mislaid) asks:

"What do you mean by 'E.M. 285' at the head of your title page?"

To save trouble and time in answering this frequently recurring question, we will here give a brief résumé of what we have frequently before stated in these columns, in regard to the matter.

The abbreviations "E.M." mean Era of Man, and are used instead of, or in contradistinction from "A.D."—Anno Domini, or Era of Christianity; and for these among other reasons:

1st. We object to the popular or Christian Chronology because of its lack of historical foundation, or starting point. In other words, we object to it because it bears upon its face an acknowledged falsehood. No scholar, be he Christian or non-Christian, will dare to maintain that Jesus of Nazareth was born on the 25th of Dec., eighteen hundred and eighty-five years ago. Every historian of any note agrees that the true date of the Nazarene's birth, both as to day and year, is shrouded in the obscurity of tradition; and, if candid, he will also agree that the very existence of the man Jesus, as an historical personage, cannot now be established.

2d. As Rationalists we object to the use of A.D. (year of our Lord) because we acknowledge allegiance to no lord or master, whether temporal or spiritual. The so-called Christian Era began during what may be aptly be termed the theologic era, or Era of gods and superstitions. It was the age of belief in the supernatural—of belief in the subordination of man to the arbitrary will of a deity or of many deities. Man, as such, had no rights that the gods were bound to respect. Rights belonged to the gods and to their representatives, the kings, princes and priests.

3d. The revolt against the rule of the gods as represented by priests and kings is of comparatively recent date. Not until about three hundred years ago—not until the circumnavigation of the globe had determined the true shape of the earth—not until modern science,

telescope in hand, turned her gaze upon the dome of heaven and showed to mortals that there is no dome there! no thrones there! no gods there!—Not till the new cosmology of Copernicus and Galileo began to take the place of the mythological cosmogony, did the true Era of Man begin.

4th. The immediate and necessary result of this destruction of the old cosmogony—the cosmogony which made the earth the center and chief fact of the universe—was a radical reconstruction of the methods of thought and investigation. Instead of referring to Authority for the truth of any theory—in morals, in government, in religion—all theories were subjected to the remorseless crucible of scientific investigation, which takes nothing for granted. The result of this investigation, thus far, is that there is nothing outside of or beyond Nature, and that chief fact or product of nature is MAN. *And though kings and priests, in the name of their gods, still hold sway over the greater part of humankind, they no longer refer to their deities alone as the source of their power. They are now willing to admit that the people have rights that must be respected, even by the viceregents of the gods themselves.*

The number 286 that we place on our title page to represent the year now just begun, refers to the death of Giordano Bruno, a distinguished martyr to science, which event took place in Rome, Feb. 1601; of the Christian chronology.[2] We use this number,

(a) Because it records a well-known fact in modern history, and for this reason there is not likely to be any dispute in regard to the initial point of the new calendar.

(b) The martyrdom of Bruno was a most memorable event in the history of the struggle between Science and Theology—between Reason and Superstition—between the Rights of Man and the assumed rights of gods, kings, and priests.

(c) The centuries reckoned from the death of Bruno correspond with the centuries of Christian chronology. Hence the two calendars are easily referable to each other.

For these reasons, besides others that might be named, we place E.M. at 286 at the mast-head of LUCIFER *to designate the current year.*

Overleaf: The so-called Biccherna 72, 1582–1583. The image, one of a series created to decorate the registers of the treasury (the *biccherna*) of the Republic of Siena, depicts Pope Gregory XIII presiding over the council considering the reforms that would result in the institution of his eponymous calendar in the autumn of 1582.

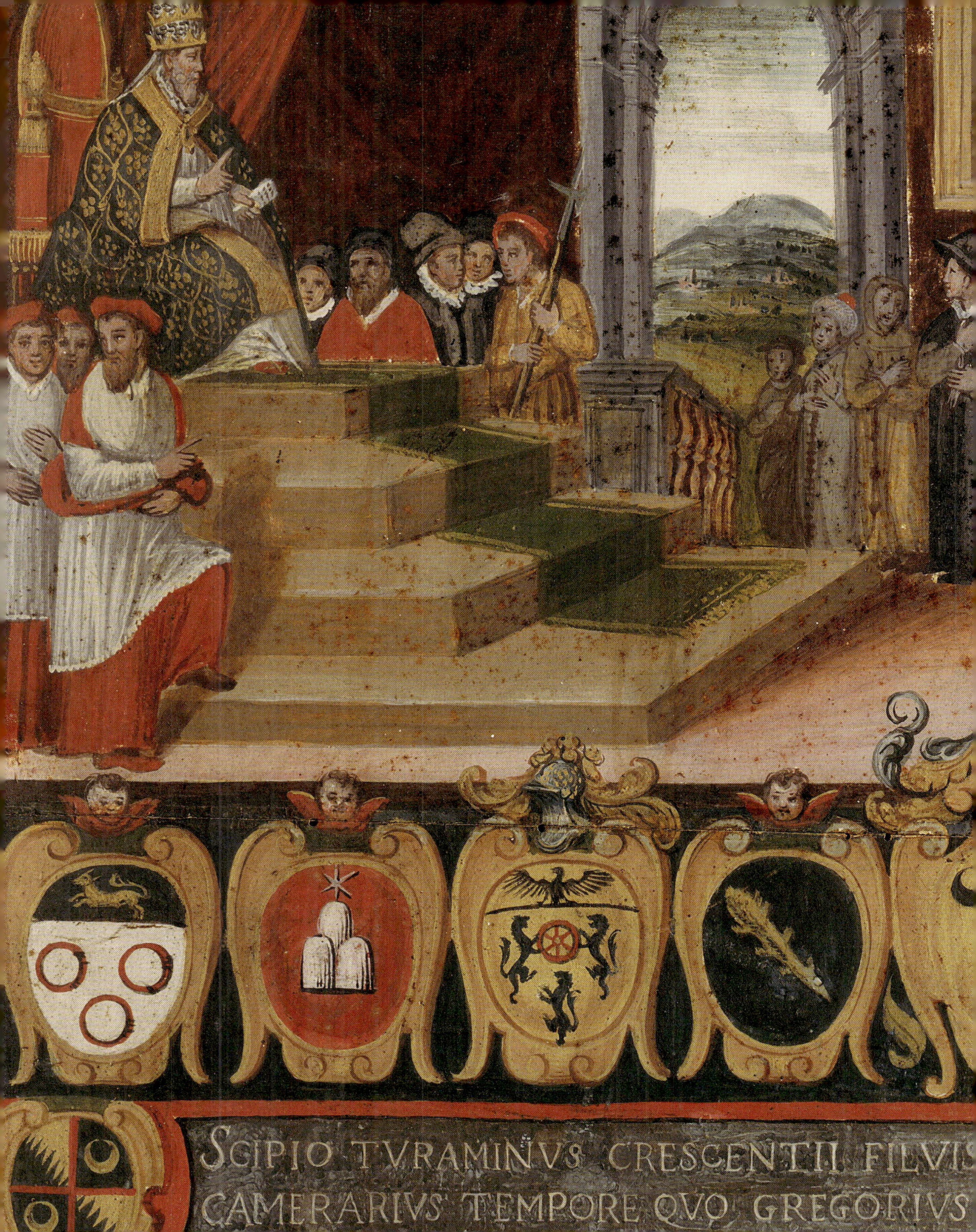

SCIPIO TVRAMINVS CRESCENTII FILVS
CAMERARIVS TEMPORE QVO GREGORIVS

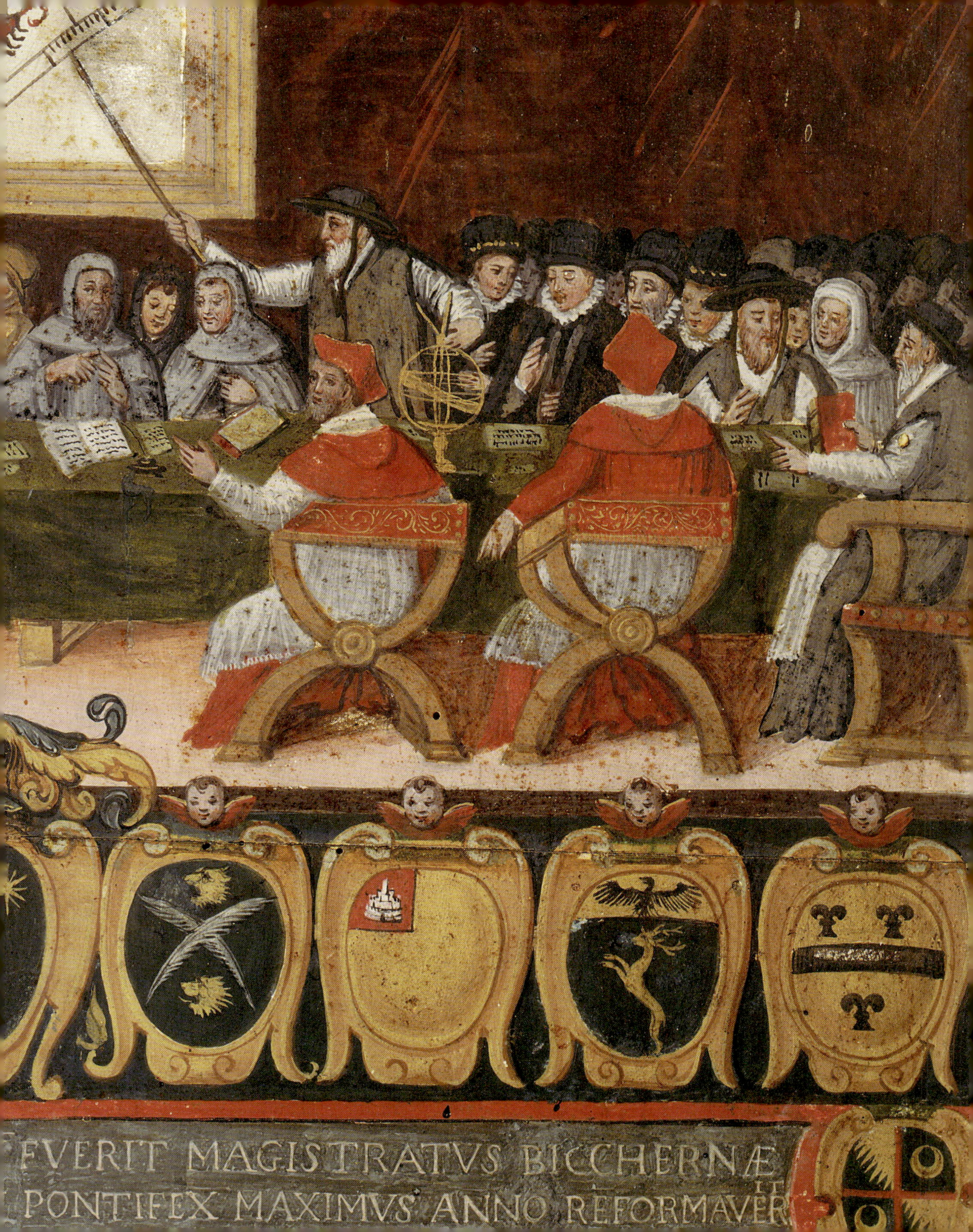
FVERIT MAGISTRATVS BICCHERNAE
PONTIFEX MAXIMVS ANNO REFORMAVER

Harman's last foray into chronological experimentation took place at the start of 1892, when he adopted a dual-dating system for *Lucifer*'s masthead. The day of the week, month, and day were still followed immediately by the E.M. year. But that number was now followed by a bracketed C.E. date. The inaugural example read: "Friday, January 1, E.M. 292 [C.E. 1892]."

We might be tempted—following twenty-first century conventions—to interpret this abbreviation as an early appearance of the "Common Era" or "Current Era" phrasing that exploded into popularity circa 1989. Ironically, however, this is not what C.E. meant for Moses Harman. Instead, C.E. meant "Christian Era."[3]

It is certainly true (as Early English Books Online reveals) that the phrases "common Aera" and even "before the common Aera" had been around since the 1600s. But they were often qualified by an appended "of Jesus" or "of Christ." And they do not seem to have been linked to any abbreviations: the use of a phrase is one thing; the baptism of a chronological system quite another. The chronological markers C.E. and B.C.E. emerged in the middle of the nineteenth century—and when they did, their *C* stood for "Christian." Moses Harman's apparently perverse insistence on stressing the Christian origins of the C.E. was not idiosyncratic: it was a common interpretation of a new abbreviation.

Perhaps the earliest and highest-profile use of these twin abbreviations was in the title of Morris J. Raphall's *Post-Biblical History of the Jews; From the Close of the Old Testament, about the Year 420 B.C.E. Till the Destruction of the Second Temple, in the Year 70 C.E.* This two-volume work was a bestseller. First published in Philadelphia in 1855, it was reprinted the next year in both New York and London, followed a decade later by another New York printing in 1866. Vexingly, Raphall never provides a "Note to the Reader" explaining how to interpret his titular B.C.E. / C.E. abbreviations. But a look at his prose is revealing. Across nine hundred pages, Raphall never uses the phrases "Common Era" or "Current Era." Instead, like Harman, he refers to the *Christian era*: "It must be borne in mind that, from Josephus, who wrote in the first century of the Christian era"; "others assume the third century of the Christian era as the probable date..."[4] Raphall was a rabbi at New York's Greene Street Synagogue in Greenwich Village, and so was well aware that the *Anno Domini* system was provincially Christian: neither common, nor necessarily current.

All of which raises rather devastating problems for current uses of B.C.E. / C.E. dating. As abbreviations, their full-length referents are open to interpretation. Attempts to use these abbreviations as secularized alternatives to B.C. and A.D. propose that their strings of letters be read as "[before the] Current Era" or "[before the] Common Era." But those same B.C.E. / C.E. strings of letters had been around for over a century before they became fashionable in the late 1980s, and in that earlier history, the *C* was neither "Common" nor "Current," but "Christian." Tragically, recent attempts at historical secularization were doomed from the start by their own historical naiveté.

This naiveté extends to the very rereadings of *C* as "Common" or "Current." Asserting the renamed *Anno Domini* system as "Common" throughout the world ignores the violent history by which this system became global: the conquests and missionizations that, over the past five centuries, imposed the Christian-Julian and (after 1582) Catholic-Gregorian calendar on people throughout the world—often demanding that their own calendars be forgotten. At the same time, it is important to remember that the Catholic-Gregorian calendar never became truly Common to all people everywhere, something quickly revealed by newspaper mastheads in many parts of today's world, from Tehran to Pyongyang to Taiwan to, say, Chicago, where the Chinese-language *World Journal* is dated with multiple non-Gregorian calendar systems.[5] A few months ago, Bolivian president Evo Morales even called for a national revival of pre-Hispanic Andean calendars. Are people who do not use the C.E. calendar trapped in the past—excluded from the "Current Era" like the living fossils of nineteenth-century evolutionism?

Early in this millennium, anthropologist Michel-Rolph Trouillot diagnosed something he called North Atlantic universals: "Words that project North Atlantic experience on a universal scale that they themselves have helped to create. ... North Atlantic universals are always prescriptive inasmuch as they always suggest a correct state of affairs—what is good, what is just, what is sublime or desirable. That prescription is inherent in the very projection of a historically limited experience on the world stage. North Atlantic universals are always seductive, at times even irresistible, precisely because they manage to hide their specific—localized, and thus parochial—historical location."[6] Moses Harman's attempts at calendrical reform were, of

course, just as political as more recent attempts to assert a Current or Common Era. Yet despite living in late nineteenth-century Kansas, Harman's chronological radicalism was not provincial. The American Nation system was explicit about its limited, nationalist framework for time. The Era of Man was grounded in an early modern horizon of European expansion well aware of religious conflicts within Europe itself. And Harman's last experiment for *Lucifer*—the use of multiple calendars, one of them explicitly Christian— was far more sophisticated than simply renaming the Christian Era as Common or Current, and then proclaiming it a secular and (North Atlantic) universal standard for world history.

· · ·

The last issue of *Lucifer the Light-Bearer* was published on 6 June E.M. 307 [C.E. 1907]. A month later, it was redesigned and launched as the *American Journal of Eugenics,* a word defined on the front cover as "the doctrine of progress or evolution, especially in the human race, through improved conditions in the relations of the sexes." Moses Harman was still editor, and the new journal continued to explore themes that had been central to *Lucifer.* Articles in the premiere issue included "Opposition to Freedom of the Press," "Marriage as a Business Proposition," and "Medical Interest in Sexual Problems." But chronological radicalism had been abandoned. The new masthead featured a disappointingly singular, unmarked date: July 1907.

1 On Moses Harman, see William Lemor West, "The Moses Harman Story," *Kansas Historical Quarterly*, vol. 37, no. 1 (Spring 1971). Available at <kshs.org/p/the-moses-harman-story/13209>. Also see Philip Ray Michael, "Moses Harman, *Lucifer, the Light Bearer,* and the Trials of Kansas Free Thought at the End of the Nineteenth Century" (master's thesis, Emporia State University, 2009). For publication details on Harman's newspapers, and their relation to other radical newspapers in the United States, see Ernesto

A. Longa, *Anarchist Periodicals in English Published in the United States (1833–1955): An Annotated Guide* (London: The Scarecrow Press, 2010).

2 Harman here revises the Liberal League's starting date of 1600 (the actual year of Bruno's death) to 1601. Technically, if 1600 were counted as Year 1 of the E.M. system, the E.M. system would always be one year "off" from the *Anno Domini* system: 1600 would be E.M. Year 1, 1601 would be E.M. Year 2, and so on.

3 Harman's dual-dating system was explained for readers on

page two of every issue starting (at least) from 15 February 1895: "OUR DATE: A correspondent asks, 'What do you mean by E.M. 294, and C.E. 1894?' Ans. The first means Era of Man, and dates from the Burning of Bruno in 1601. 'C.E.' means Christian Era."

4 Morris J. Raphall, *Post-Biblical History of the Jews; From the Close of the Old Testament, about the Year 420 B.C.E. Till the Destruction of the Second Temple, in the Year 70 C.E.* (Philadelphia: Moss and Brother, 1855). The quotations are on page 14 of volume one and page

75 of volume two, respectively.

5 For details, see my "How to Chronologize with a Hammer, Or, The Myth of Homogeneous, Empty Time," *HAU: Journal of Ethnographic Theory*, vol. 6, no. 1 (Summer 2016).

6 Michel-Rolph Trouillot, "North Atlantic Universals: Analytical Fictions, 1492–1945," *South Atlantic Quarterly*, vol. 101, no. 4 (Fall 2002), pp. 847–848.

SHUFFLING THROUGH THE YEAR
Adam Jasper

What is a deck of cards? The standard "French deck" has fifty-two cards—divided into four suits of thirteen cards each—plus two jokers. The suits are hearts, spades, clubs, and diamonds. Each suit has an ace, nine number cards (from two to ten) and three face cards: a jack, a queen, and a king. On one side, cards are designed to be recognized as quickly as possible, and on the other, to be indistinguishable from all the other members of the deck. It is universally acknowledged that cards are for playing.

The familiar competitive games, such as poker, depend on a tension between meaningful patterns—arrangements of cards such as a flush, a straight, or a full house—and the actual distribution of cards in the deck. It is widely repeated in scholarship that the earliest games were likely to be trump-based and involved trick taking, like the medieval game *karnöffel*, whose rules were so convoluted that they required writing down, and so have survived. It's also well documented that cards were used for gambling very early on. Card playing appears in paintings as a pastime of soldiers, and as an un- or even pre-Christian activity, as in the game that is interrupted by the risen Christ in Jerg Ratgeb's Herrenberg Altarpiece (1519). The first public record we have of the existence of cards consists of attempts by various city authorities to have them banned (starting with Bern in 1367). Taken all in all, it makes sense to assume that cards were always a profane activity, a trivial pastime that perfectly complements getting drunk and losing money.

Look again. There are fifty-two cards in four suits. Not unlike the year, with its fifty-two weeks and four seasons. Can playing cards be read as a kind of calendar? In total, there are twelve face cards, which correspond to the number of months in a year. And the lunar months? Well, there are thirteen of them, and there are thirteen cards in a suit. Weeks, months, lunar months. It's a striking correspondence, but proves nothing on its own. The way to test the depth of this relationship is to see if any of these seemingly arbitrary features of the deck can be explained by reference to the annual calendar. And this turns out, in the most surprising ways, to be the case.

Adding up the total value of all the cards in a suit, from one to thirteen, yields 91. The total value of all

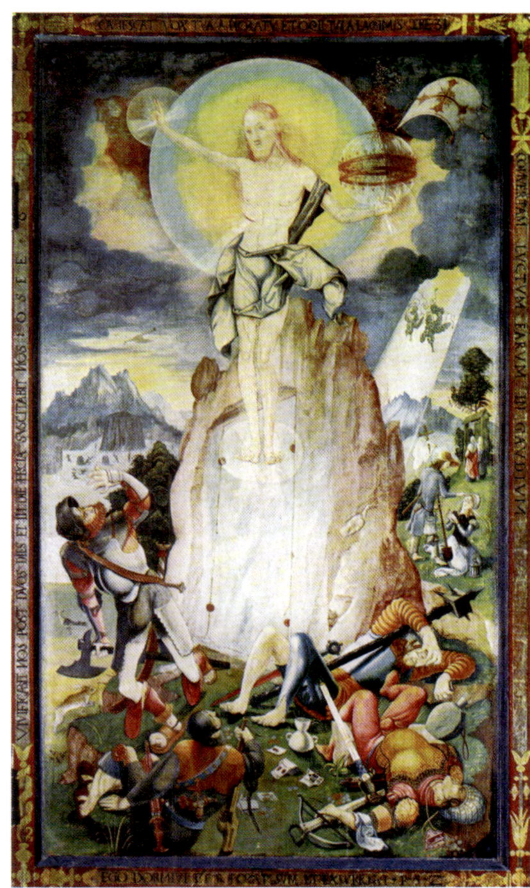

One of the panels of Jerg Ratgeb's Herrenberg Altarpiece (1519) depicting a card game interrupted by the resurrected Christ. By examining the cards and noting the fact that the soldier at lower right seems to be suffering from an inguinal hernia, at least one scholar has suggested that the game being played is *karnöffel*.

the number cards in a deck is 364. The length of a year, minus one day. But then, what else is the joker for? The joker, in cards as in myth, represents the element of disorder that stops the world from lining up, from running smoothly. (The word *karnöffel* itself means inguinal hernia, or, in the poetic logic of the Middle Ages, an extra testicle, an unwelcome guest.) And every year requires at least one day that defies the cosmic order, whether it be the climax of the Saturnalia, carnival, or the winter solstice disguised as Christmas. The joker can play the role of that residual day. So, 365. And there is a second joker for the leap year. An obvious objection: the joker first becomes a standard inclusion in every deck in the nineteenth century through the popular game of euchre. But the concept of the fool card is older. The fool in the tarot deck, which dates back to the fifteenth century, has no fixed position within the arcana, and it is usually marked with the Arabic numeral 0—the placeholder that alone means nothing, but means magnitudes in context.

Compared to the tarot, the standard deck is ancient. Although there have always been variants, the basic set of fifty-two cards divided into four suits, with three court cards, is a constant. The famous defense of cards written in 1377 by Johannes of Rheinfelden (ten years after they were banned in Bern) describes a fifty-two-card deck. It could be argued that the division has other meanings, such as the four quarters of the world, or various social classes. The symbolism of French suits—hearts, clubs, diamonds, spades—can, for example, be mapped onto social strata: the nobility, the clergy, the bourgeoisie, and the peasant. However, the German deck, which has suits of hearts, acorns, hawk-bells, and leaves, seems more clearly seasonal. Acorns appear in autumn, and hawking—hunting for rodents with birds—is traditionally practiced in winter.

But can a deck of cards easily *function* as a calendar, regardless of whether or not there are enough coincidences to suggest that it might have been modeled on one? Take a deck. Take all the cards of one suit out of it—say, hearts. That's thirteen cards. Then take all the number cards belonging to the other suits (the cards from 2 to 10), that's twenty-seven more cards. If you count out all the possible combinations of hearts, either on their own, or combined with a number card from one of the other three suits, the total is 364 (13 + 13 × 27). So the first day of the year could be represented by the king of hearts, the second day by the queen of

hearts and the two of clubs, the third day by the jack of hearts and the three of clubs, and so on, until every possible combination of hearts and number cards from the other three suits is exhausted, all 364 of them. If you repeat the process with the other three suits taking turns in the role we've assigned to hearts, you can unambiguously represent every day in a period of four years with one or two cards, with every card in the deck used at least once.

This permutational approach to representing time has precedents. In *The Anthropology of Time*, Alfred Gell describes a cyclical Balinese calendar that relies on what mathematicians call modular arithmetic.[1] In Bali, which lies close to the equator, where the twilight is always brief and the sun varies its path much less noticeably, a solar calendar makes less sense. Days are, rather, identified through the interaction of independent five-, six-, and seven-day weeks. Like our own days and months, their calendar is cyclical, but it consists of much shorter interlocking cycles, rather like the changes of bell ringing. So the day that comes after 5/1/7 is 1/2/1, the one after it is 2/3/2, and so on. The entire pattern takes 210 days to repeat. Such a calendar is not designed to allow for the easy measurement of duration, but rather for distributing rituals and communal activities. Quoting Clifford Geertz, Gell argues that the purpose of such a calendar is not to tell you what day it is, but rather, "what *kind* of day" it is.[2]

Our calendar is also algorithmic, and has been since Julius Caesar made the length of a month a standard number of days, rather than based on a priest's observation of a new moon. (This not only deprived some Roman priestly offices of carefully cherished political powers, but also immediately caused the dates of the full moon to drift from their traditional position. The soothsayer's warning "Beware the Ides of March" can therefore be understood as a multilayered threat, a reference not only to Caesar's personal peril but also to one of the reasons for it, namely that his dictatorial rule had put the political and celestial orders out of alignment). However, the Balinese calendar is overflowing with patterns. To delve deeper into Geertz: "The outcome of all this wheels-within-wheels computation is a view of time as consisting of ordered sets of thirty, thirty-five, forty-two, or two hundred and ten quantum units ('days'), each of which units has a particular qualitative significance of some sort indexed by its trinomial or binomial name: rather like our notion of

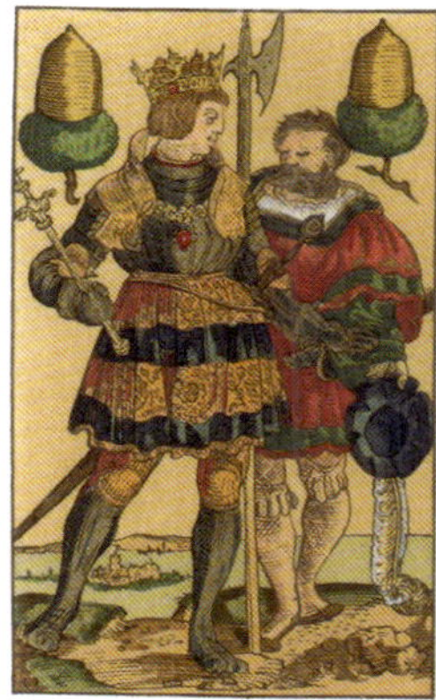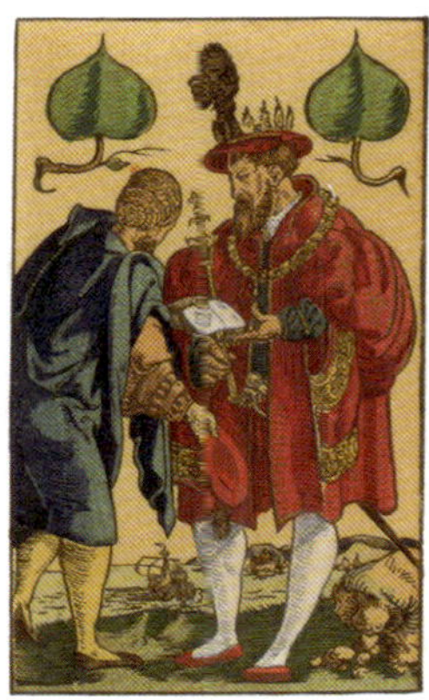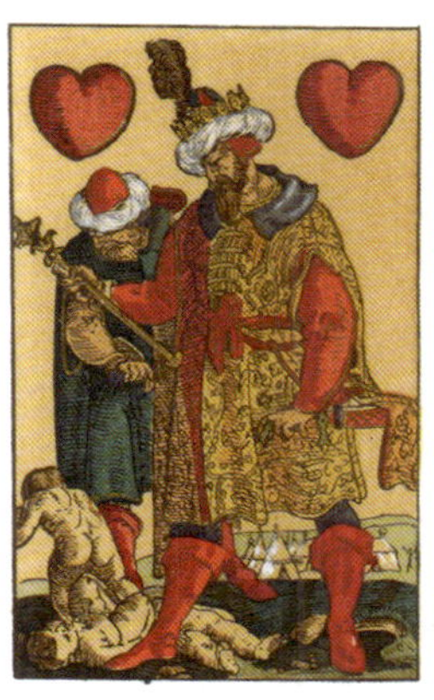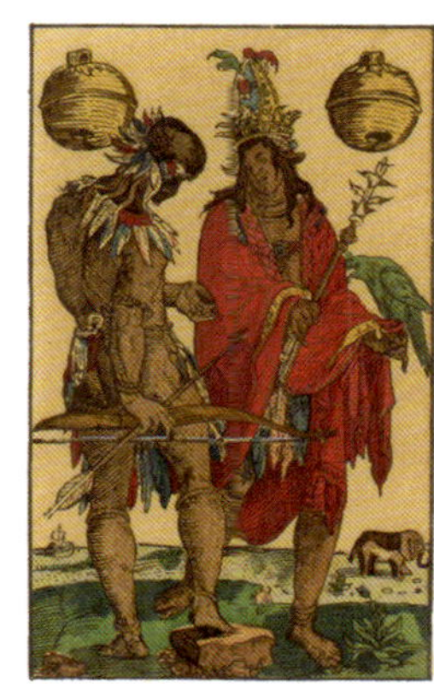

All the two-spots from a sixteenth-century German satirical deck.

the unluckiness of Friday-the-Thirteenth. … To identify a day in the thirty-five-day set, one needs its place and name in the five-name cycle (for example, *Klion*) and in the seven-: for example, *Boda-Klion*—this is *rainan*, the day on which one must set out small offerings at various points to 'feed' the gods."[3] One cycle might determine an appropriate day to begin an activity; another, whether the activity should be undertaken in the village or the fields, and so on—the entire society is thus synchronized. As Geertz writes, "There are good and bad days on which to build a house, launch a business enterprise, change residence, go on a trip, harvest crops, sharpen cock spurs, hold a puppet show, or (in the old days) start a war, or conclude a peace."[4] The coincidence of certain cycles determines festivals, work, and religious observances with the same syncopated perfection as a gamelan orchestra. Furthermore, the Balinese calendar, thanks to its complexity, is an excellent system for meddling with the distribution of chance. Even the position of birds in cockfights is

determined: "You fight a small, headstrong, speckled brown-on-white cock with flat-lying feathers and thin legs from the east side of the ring on a certain day of the complex Balinese calendar, and a large, cautious, all-black cock with tufted feathers and stubby legs from the north side on another day, and so on."[5] This makes intuitive sense: once you have a calendar, it immediately makes itself indispensable when it comes to envisioning the future, and predicting events—some days are auspicious for certain activities, others are not. Insofar as some events (such as the eternal return of Mondays) are socially synchronized, the future is under collective (but sadly, not individual) human control. It is understandable that this social control very quickly reifies into a cosmic order. If the calendar is a grid that can foretell the future, why shouldn't it be a model in games that negotiate the relationship between subjective and objective chance?

Which brings us to Gell's ingenious explanation for why seven-day weeks are so common, even outside of cultures emanating from the Middle East. Gell notes that the Umeda people of lowland Papua New Guinea make use of seven days articulated around the word for "today," "i.e., the day before the day before yesterday/the day before yesterday/yesterday/today/tomorrow/the day after tomorrow/the day after the day after tomorrow."[6] That's the length of time that is communicable without any mensuration needed. Talking about longer spans of time, especially in the case of reported speech, requires a system of measurement that synchronizes speakers with reference to an external framework, but until a calendar provides that framework, seven days is an intuitive scope for temporal reckoning—time cut to the scale of individual experience. That is why if you want to know what day it is, the answer is simple: today is always Thursday.

Is our theory true? Almost everything that is believed about the earliest history of playing cards is conjecture. Take, for instance, a pair of charming theories from the nineteenth century: H. Wilkinson's belief

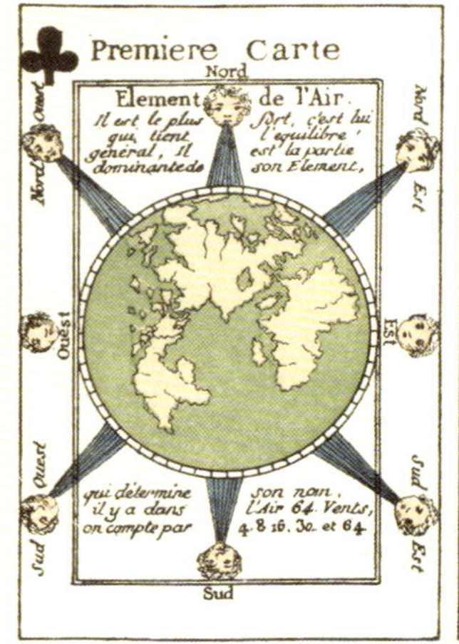

Première Carte
Nord
Ouest
Est
Sud
Nord Ouest
Nord Est
Sud Ouest
Sud Est
Element de l'Air.
Il est le plus   fort, c'est lui
qui tient   l'équilibre,
général, Il   est la partie
dominante de   son Element,
qui détermine   son nom,
il y a dans   l'Air 64. Vents,
on compte par   4. 8. 16. 30. et 64.

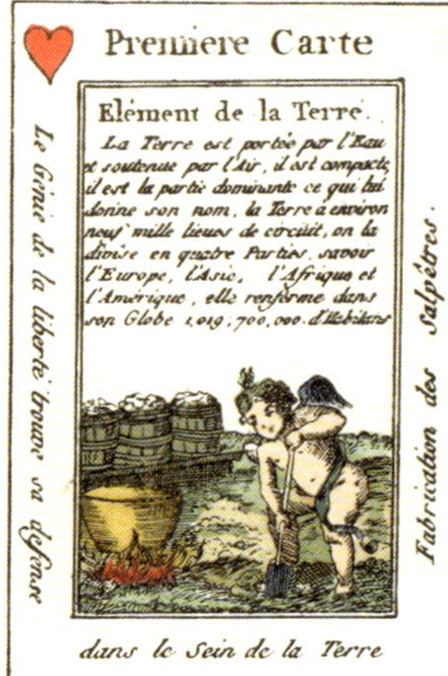

Première Carte
Le Génie de la liberté trouve sa défense
Fabrication des Salpêtres.
Element de la Terre.
La Terre est portée par l'Eau
et soutenue par l'Air, il est compacte,
il est la partie dominante ce qui lui
donne son nom, la Terre à environ
neuf mille lieues de circuit, on la
divise en quatre Parties, savoir
l'Europe, l'Asie, l'Afrique et
l'Amérique, elle renferme dans
son Globe 1.019.700.000. d'Habitans
dans le Sein de la Terre

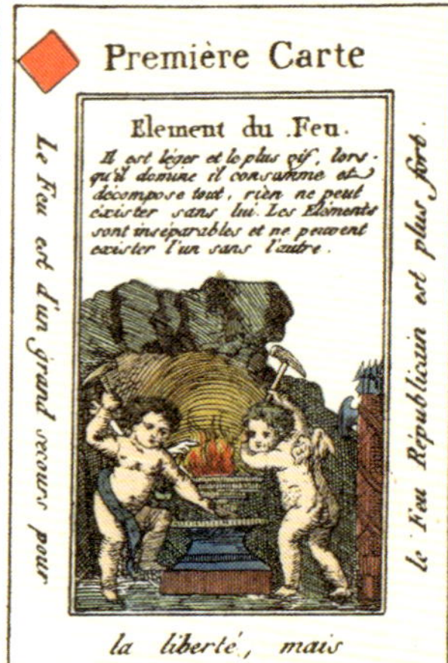

Première Carte
Element du Feu.
Il est léger et le plus vif, lors
qu'il domine il consume et
décompose tout, rien ne peut
exister sans lui. Les Elémens
sont inséparables et ne peuvent
exister l'un sans l'autre
le Feu Républicain est plus fort
la liberté, mais

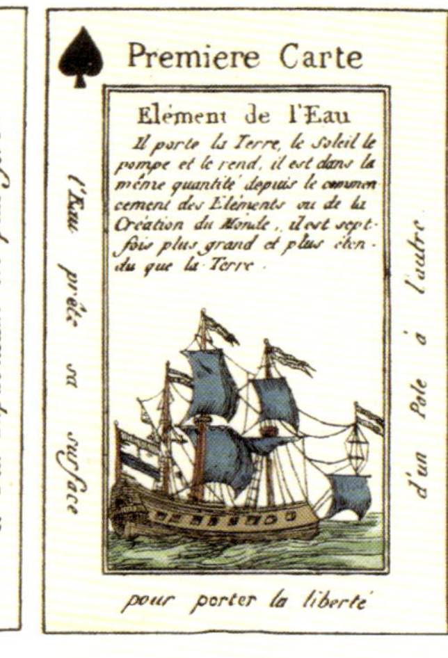

Première Carte
Element de l'Eau.
Il porte la Terre, le soleil le
pompe et le rend, il est dans la
même quantité depuis le commen-
cement des Elémens ou de la
Création du Monde, il est sept
fois plus grand et plus éten-
du que la Terre
l'Eau près ou sa surface
d'un Pole à l'autre
pour porter la liberté

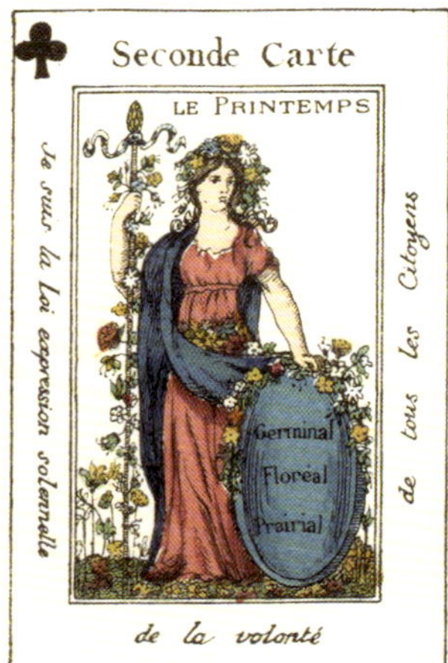

Seconde Carte
LE PRINTEMPS
Je suis la Loi expression solennelle
de tous les Citoyens
Germinal
Floréal
Prairial
de la volonté

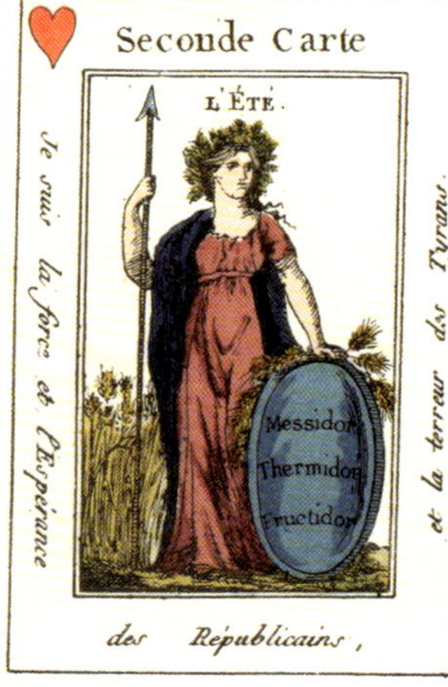

Seconde Carte
L'ÉTÉ.
Je suis la force et l'Espérance
et la terreur des Tyrans.
Messidor
Thermidor
Fructidor
des Républicains,

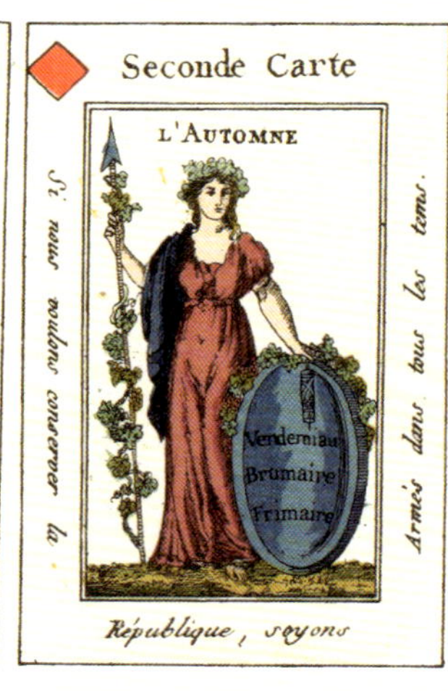

Seconde Carte
L'AUTOMNE
Si nous voulons conserver la
Armés dans tous les tems.
Vendémiaire
Brumaire
Frimaire
République, soyons

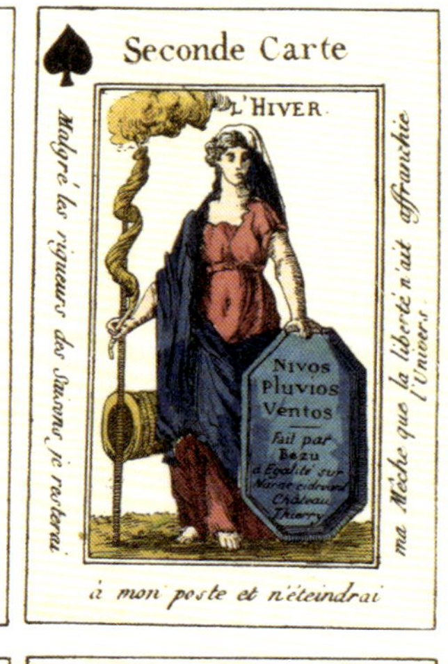

Seconde Carte
L'HIVER
Malgré les rigueurs des Saisons, je resterai
ma Mèche que la liberté n'ait affranchie l'Univers.
NIVOS
PLUVIOS
VENTOS
Fait par
Bezu
à Egalité sur
Marne cidevant
Château
Thierry
à mon poste et n'éteindrai

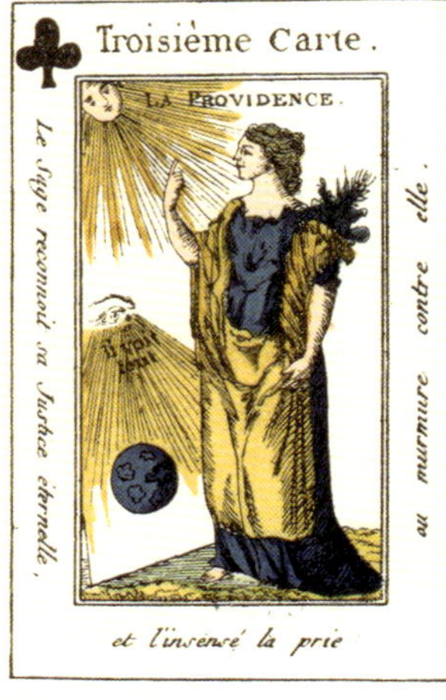

Troisième Carte.
LA PROVIDENCE.
Le Sage reconnoit sa Justice éternelle,
ou murmure contre elle.
Il voit tout
et l'insensé la prie

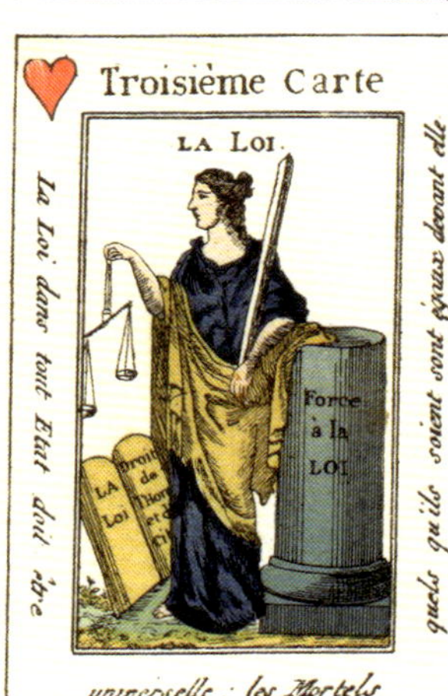

Troisième Carte
LA LOI.
La Loi dans tout État doit être
quels qu'ils soient sont égaux devant elle
Droit
de
l'Hom
et
LA
Loi
Force
a la
LOI
universelle; les Mortels

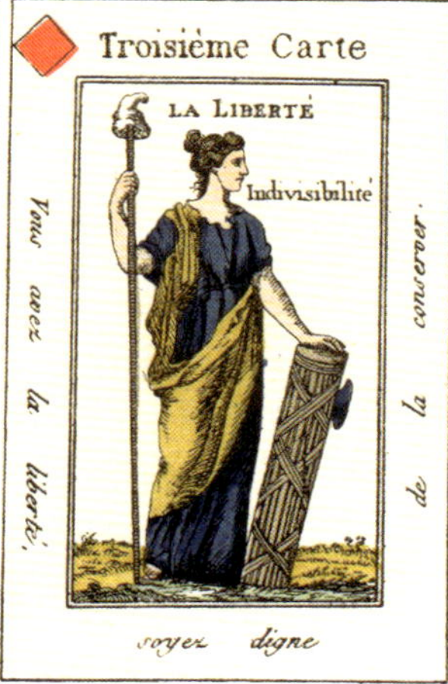

Troisième Carte
LA LIBERTÉ
Indivisibilité
Vous avez la liberté,
de la conserver.
soyez digne

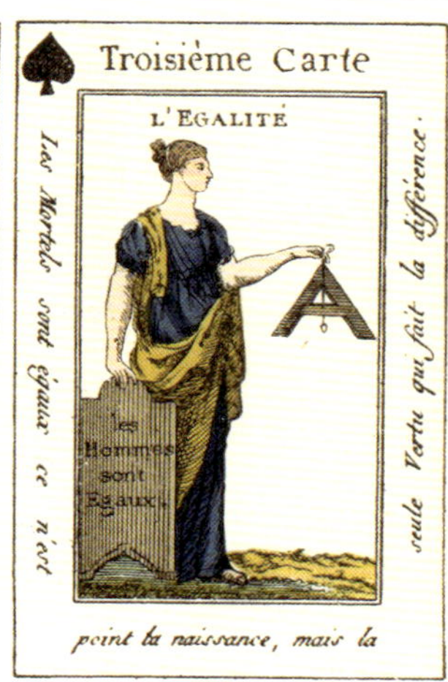

Troisième Carte
L'EGALITÉ
Les Mortels sont égaux ce n'est
seule Vertu qui fait la différence.
A
les
Hommes
sont
Egaux.
point la naissance, mais la

that the Italian suit known as "cups" comes from a Chinese character being read upside down, or Stewart Culin's proposal, reported in the *Journal of American Folklore* in 1895, that cards had descended from decorated arrow shafts, which had at one time been used in games of chance. We do know that the deck is an extremely socially conservative artifact. Once established, motifs—which determine, for example, the appearance of the king of hearts—remain almost unchanged for centuries. This preservation of motifs might have something to do with familiarity and ease of recognition, but it also reinforces the way in which we experience the cards' ornamentation as integral to their function: the sense that a player has that the cards have a legitimacy much like currency, or even that the way they fall expresses an agency beyond mere chance. (This is not insignificant when the time comes to pay up for a lost bet). Much of the scholarship on playing cards that is still cited dates to the nineteenth century, and has hardly been updated since. This is not least because new finds in the field are so scanty. Because creased or dirty cards cannot be used in gambling, and are usually thrown out when worn, old playing cards are incredibly rare, even in proportion to other mass-produced woodcuts. Those that have been preserved were usually saved unintentionally—by being used as scrap paper in the binding of books.

The conservative nature of card design means that when innovations appear, they are usually introduced under the pretext of a return to a more ancient tradition. But the latent calendrical qualities of decks can become visible when traditional forms are blocked or rejected. The best example of this can be seen in decks produced during the French Revolution. Needless to say, monarchs were not welcome in France during this period, and so decks were issued in which the kings were replaced with the four elements: air, earth, fire, and water. Jacks, in turn, were displaced by revolutionary virtues: providence, the law, liberty, and equality. And the unloved queens? They became the seasons—spring, summer, autumn, and winter—and the twelve new republican months were listed on their shields: the spring months of Germinal, Floréal, and Prairial on one, summer's Messidor, Thermidor, and Fructidor on another, and so on. In a striking moment of convergent evolution, the revolutionary government tried to simplify and harmonize the months to thirty days each—to make them, so to speak, as regular as a deck of cards.

So what is the oldest game? *Karnöffel* might be the oldest game for which we have written rules, but the very fact that the rules were sufficiently complex that they needed to be recorded suggests that it is not the first. Consider that the biggest difference between a deck of cards and a calendar is that the deck of cards can be shuffled, whereas the relationships between days on a calendar are in a fixed order. There is a game that is based, almost entirely, on moving from one condition to the other, that involves sifting through a randomly shuffled deck and restoring the lost order of the whole. This game plays a much deeper, and more reassuring, role than the nerve-racking competition of poker. It is, rather, a game that beguiles time and seemingly reverses its chaotic effects, a kind of time machine. Solitaire, also called patience, strips away all the extrinsic factors (money, other people, etc.) and leaves the core bare for us to see. The goal of the game is to reverse the entropy of the shuffle, expressing the tension between random event and sought-for symmetry that characterizes the human experience of time—and we spend billions of hours a year playing it.[7] As Johan Huizinga wrote in *Homo Ludens* (1938), playing games "creates order, *is* order." The deepest secrets of the world come very lightly disguised. We may not know what the oldest card game is, but it seems only fair that the most fundamental of all card games should be one in which cards in a random sequence are demonstrated, piece by piece, to belong to a cosmic order.

1 Alfred Gell, *The Anthropology of Time* (Oxford: Berg, 1992), p. 72.

2 Clifford Geertz, "Person, Time, and Conduct in Bali" in Clifford Geertz, *The Interpretation of Cultures: Selected Essays* (New York: Basic Books, 1973), p. 397. My italics.

3 Ibid., p. 393.

4 Ibid., p. 396.

5 Clifford Geertz, "Notes on the Balinese Cockfight," in Clifford Geertz, *The Interpretation of Cultures*, p. 427, footnote 13.

6 Alfred Gell, *The Anthropology of Time*, p. 88.

7 Computer scientist Luis von Ahn has estimated that in 2003 some nine billion hours were spent playing the game on Microsoft Windows alone. See Jim Rossignol, *This Gaming Life: Travels in Three Cities* (Ann Arbor: The University of Michigan Press, 2008), p. 103.

THE LENS OF TIME
Adam Herring

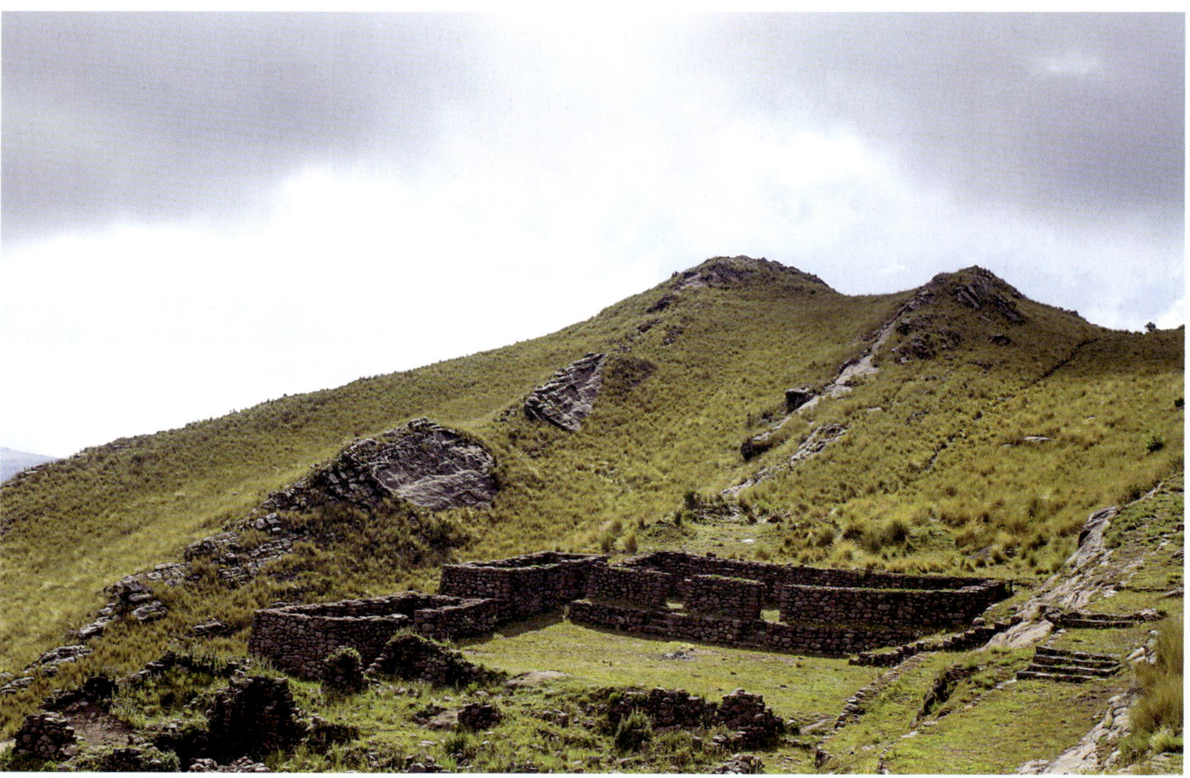

The founders of the Inca dynasty, so their descendants recalled, were birthed from a cave in the high Andes. They were a group of eight siblings—four male-female couples. Emerging into daylight, the founders wandered Peru's southern highlands. In time and after many episodes of conflict, the siblings came to stand on a tall mountain along the southern rim of the Cuzco basin—Mount Huanacauri. It was here that the first Inca were given to behold a series of divine apparitions, not least the wide valley-prospect itself, framed beneath a rainbow across the sky. This narrative of coming-into-vision—from the darkness of the cave to the rainbow's colors—traced the Inca founders' rise to power. They moved into the valley, and there they set to the principal duties of Inca lordship: a domestic life of social obligation and maize cultivation.

In later centuries, the Inca leadership did not recall the year of their dynasty's foundation, nor how long the first siblings had wandered the highlands before they settled in Cuzco. Nor to our knowledge did the mature Inca state mark the date of its foundation on an annual calendar. In Mexico, the Aztec of Tenochtitlan marked the events of their dynastic history with great temporal exactitude; they recalled that a world-creation before their own came to an end on a specific day with a catastrophic flood, and the day that a world-creation before that was extinguished with a rain of fire. They commemorated the dates of two even earlier apocalypses (of hurricane winds and ravenous jaguars, respectively). And they prophesied the date of their own world's destruction, by earthquake. Among the Maya dynasties of southern Mesoamerica's lowlands, the present era was understood to come to full completion on the day-count of 13.0.0.0.0—21 December 2012 in the Gregorian calendar. Scholars today do not know what event was prophesied for that completion date; a seventh-century AD hieroglyphic inscription recovered from Mexico's Tabasco State records that a supernatural entity named B'olon Yookte', "9-Root,"

Above: Mount Huanacauri, along the southern rim of Cuzco basin. Photo Adam Herring.

would "descend" (*yeem-*) on that day—though the text is fragmentary and poorly understood. The Maya lords of Calakmul's Snake Dynasty employed an eccentric, nonstandard calendrical system to record the reigns of their most ancient kings. Across Mexico's highlands and the Isthmus of Tehuantepec, nobles of many ethnicities took their birthdate as their proper name: that day-position in the Mesoamerican 260-day divinatory calendar foretold the story of their lives. The same divinatory calendar remains in use among Maya healers in highland Guatemala today. The very word Maya likely derives from a Yukatek Mayan expression that can be translated as "keepers of calendric prophecy" or "those bound by time's fate." By contrast, South America's Inca, the rulers of the largest empire in the pre-contact Americas, kept no count of days to reckon their history, nor did they parse each year into strictly observed calendrical cycles.

All that said, the Inca did carefully observe the passage of time. They recognized the monthly cycles of the moon, and the repetition of lunar cycles over and across the solar year. The calendar of lunar months (*quilla*) seems to have provided the basis for the Inca state's annual ceremonial. The Inca leadership marked each month with a particular ceremonial: Camay in January, a period of fasting during the onset of the highland rainy season; Chacra Ayaqui in the dry month of August when maize was sown. They observed important movements in the sky that took place over these months: the rise of the Milky Way in the night sky in the month they knew as Uma Raymi (October), and the progressive change of a dark formation within it, the Black Llama (Yacana). Solar phenomena marked the most significant passages of the year: the ceremonies of the Inca state were keyed to the sun's movement and position in the sky. The planting season was commenced when the sun moved past upright gnomons placed along the skyline of the Cuzco basin. The solstices (*raymi*), the days marked by the longest and shortest periods of solar energy, were the highpoints of the ceremonial calendar: June solstice (Inti Raymi), when the austral sun was most weak and short-lived, and December solstice (Capac Raymi), when the sun was hottest and longest in the sky.

Capac Raymi was the Inca state's ritual high season, a month-long cycle of ceremonial actions. The month's activities reached their climax at the day of solstice, when the sun was understood to be "seated" directly

over Cuzco. On that day, thousands of Inca gathered in Cuzco's main space of public ceremony. The rite began early, with drumming and singing commencing in the dawn hours. The intensity of song and noise increased as the sun rose into the sky. At midday, the assembled Inca were loudest and most active. The crowd's activity peaked as the sun passed directly overhead. The Andean nobleman Felipe Guaman Poma de Ayala illustrated the ritual in his manuscript of 1615. His face turned to the sun, the Inca emperor leads the ceremony.

The Inca chose, however, not to record much else. They do not appear to have kept any elaborate almanacs of temporal periods or astronomical movements, nor counts of days or months that could amount to historical annals. It is an irony that Western specialists are keen to redress: The lost Inca systems of calendrical and historical reckoning are the holy grail of Inca Studies. No lost Inca calendars or dynastic annals have been recovered so far. Even so, there is abundant evidence that the Inca devised masterful schemes of systematized knowledge. The life of the Inca capital was nothing if not regulated: social identity and organization, water rights, and sacred landscapes were all comprehended within elaborate systems of hierarchy and relation. Meanwhile, Inca administrators stood over the empire's subject peoples, counting the goods and labor those provincials gave up in tribute. Those managers committed this actuarial data to memory, keeping their knowledge fresh and accurate by means of knotted-string documents, *quipu*; "cord-keepers" (*quipucamayocuna*) those functionaries were called. Such annual tribute-cycles were a form of calendar—an ordered reckoning of time's durations and cycles—which is to say that the Inca state imposed a calendar on hundreds, even thousands of subaltern communities across the Andes. The Inca were hated for it, or so indicates the rapid defection of so many of the Incas' subjects to Spanish authority after 1532.

Inca governance did not want for intellectual acumen or systematic thought, but Inca reckoning of historical time and the annual cycle was remarkably vague by European standards. In the early 1570s, Spanish viceroy Francisco de Toledo sought to impose some kind of recognizable chronology on the Inca dynastic past. He commissioned many histories from longtime Spanish settlers and churchmen in Peru. Interviews of aged Inca nobles were conducted. The settlers and clerics sounded off, as did the Inca elders

and their *quipu*-bearing servants. Quills scratched paper, depositions were recorded and archived. Competing accounts were suppressed. The result was a fiction, a king list with its own trumped-up timeline. It was a useful contrivance nonetheless; it met the exigencies of crown administrators and jurists insofar as it served as the colonial power's official history of its Inca subjects. An imperial chronotype was imposed on the descendants of the Inca: the mythic structure of European temporality displaced the Andean cosmology of time that had been there before. The king list and timeline imposed by Spanish viceregal decree remains in use among many academic specialists: it humanizes the Inca, endowing that distant, foreign society with a sense of historical depth and temporal relation.

If the Inca leadership did not keep close account of historical time nor closely regulate the yearly cycle, they were acutely time-conscious. The Inca state did not regiment and report time so much as manipulate it as a medium of human experience. Time's linear sequence was revised, for instance, so as to produce a new and more logical past. As new kings came to power, new eras were inaugurated. Previous history was redacted. Old modes of being were revised, historical inheritance was shifted, new identities and social roles were vested with ancient pedigree. Pachakuti Inka, "Lord Cataclysm," was the Inca dynasty's model king: dynastic usurper, aggressive conqueror, purger of the Inca nobility, master builder, administrator of change. There is no evidence of that dynast's actual, factual existence. Whatever transpired during the time of his supposed reign—a period of decades in the mid-fifteenth century, or so Viceroy Toledo decreed—Pachakuti Inka came to be an idea, a memory that served his descendants as a principle of Inca governance. He embodied a tenet of Inca kingship, the ruler's prerogative to change what was and had been.

Inca leaders understood that there was little use in marking time too closely, for its intervals could be compressed or dilated, or else revised and restaged. Time took place in absolute measure, certainly, though it was also a felt happening: spans of time constituted states of being, modes of consciousness. The forward flow of time was a fact, but so was the plasticity of its instants and the complexity of its sequential patterns. As but one aspect of human experience, time could be governed by other logics of consciousness. Time always transpired in particular physical places, for instance, and so those physical places possessed their own time. Time was an experiential phenomenon, a social event, a set of cosmological relations. To narrow time's identity to counts or cycles of days was to fail to comprehend time's cosmological, social, and experiential intricacies.

Calendars could serve the Inca state, and so the Inca state observed time's patterns. This said, the state had other, more effective servants. The Inca dynasty did not keep almanacs that might have helped predict eclipses of the sun and moon, for instance. There was no need, as the Inca state could cope with those emergencies as they arose. Mass action was enough: the populace was assembled, the ritual protocols were observed. The darkened celestial beings (sun or moon) were strengthened. The clamor of public ritual (optical, sonic, kinetic) generated restorative cosmological energy: bright colors of costume, the sound of voices and drums, dance and procession. Dogs were whipped—their high-pitched whine produced needed vitality as well. Eclipses are unusual though not extraordinary events. Their effects were reversed over and again. Eclipses happened, like bad weather, the uprising of subject peoples, or the loss of animal stock in the high grasslands. All were unforeseen emergencies, and all were the occasion for effective social action coordinated by the Inca leadership.

Other events repeated themselves, and could be theatricalized on a regular timetable. As December solstice approached, noble Inca boys were readied for their induction to adulthood. They endured a cycle of ritual cleansing, hazing, feasting, and harangue. They retraced their dynastic ancestors' climb to the peak of Mount Huanacauri. At the peak, they were subject to more teaching: from their position overlooking the Inca dynastic center, the boys were told to recall the omens first witnessed by the Inca dynasty's founding siblings. They were asked to recall the primordial sibling who turned to stone on the mountain and so transformed the alien landform into kinsman and brother. The peak on which they stood was their living brother as well. They were given to remember the golden lance that the siblings cast into the valley, and how the glinting projectile buried itself in the thick loam of the valley bottom. That spear was a sunbeam, its arcing flight an act of conquest, its essence the male principle. The view from the peak made these facts plain to their eyes. (Noble girls were with the boys on the mountain

as well, though set off at a distance, busied with the symbolic duties of sisters and wives.)

The noble Inca boys were to witness all this, and also to recall the rainbow, the omen that marked the founder-siblings' ancestral coming-into-vision. Rainbows unfurl in a sweeping, ordered luminosity— suffused in sunlight and deeply unnatural in the purity and strength of their colors. They assumed quite specific meanings in the Andean tradition. Rainbows signaled the advent of new cosmic and social order, a "turning-about" both calamitous and transformative. (The rainbow was the chosen sign of the ruler Pachakuti Inka, the Inca dynasty's paradigmatic disruptor.) They were also the signs of dynastic and sacral translation, their traverse across the sky understood as a transferal of sacred energies from one watery locale to another.

Western science reminds us of two important facts. First, rainbows are an effect of sunlight. They always appear at the anti-solar point in the sky, for they are reflections of the sun's rays. Second, rainbows exist only in the individual beholder's consciousness. They are an optical trick occasioned by sunlight's refraction through the lens-like surfaces of airborne water droplets. Rainbows thus claim no objective presence in nature in and of themselves, other than as a set of preconditions for a certain perceptual process. Rainbows thus manifest the twofold reality of human existence. They are at once solar—the manifestation of the most powerful physical entity encountered in human experience—and egocentric, an experience of individual human psychology. Rainbows underscore the cosmological axiom of life on earth: they are the objective fact of the sun. They also reveal the perceptual basis of all human experience: they are the truth of subjective experience.

At the nexus of these two truths lies a third verity: the truth of social experience. Vision, like all sensory perception, hardly atomizes the individual psyche, for it is a principal means of subjective connection to the world of shared experience. It is the basis for the social commonality of *intersubjectivity*. As human perception is embodied and performed, so too is it tied to interpersonal contexts, instants, situations. It is a complexly externalized, inherently social form of human psychology. Sensory perception is founded in social life: and so perception is the basis of society's foundation. The rainbow above Cuzco marked the

foundation of the Inca dynasty. In mythological terms, its witnessing effected the institution of human (Inca) society all told.

There was no rainbow before the boys' eyes, of course. Rainbows cannot be summoned up, even by the Inca state. Though the idea was enough. After all, there was the mature dynastic center of Cuzco underneath where the rainbow would have been. The rainbow was not there but the urban center it portended was. When was a rainbow ever present, given its strangeness as a natural phenomenon? The rainbow's absence was just one more perceptual anomaly attendant upon its invisible presence. For the boys at the top of the mountain, time folded back on itself, time stood still, and time never was.

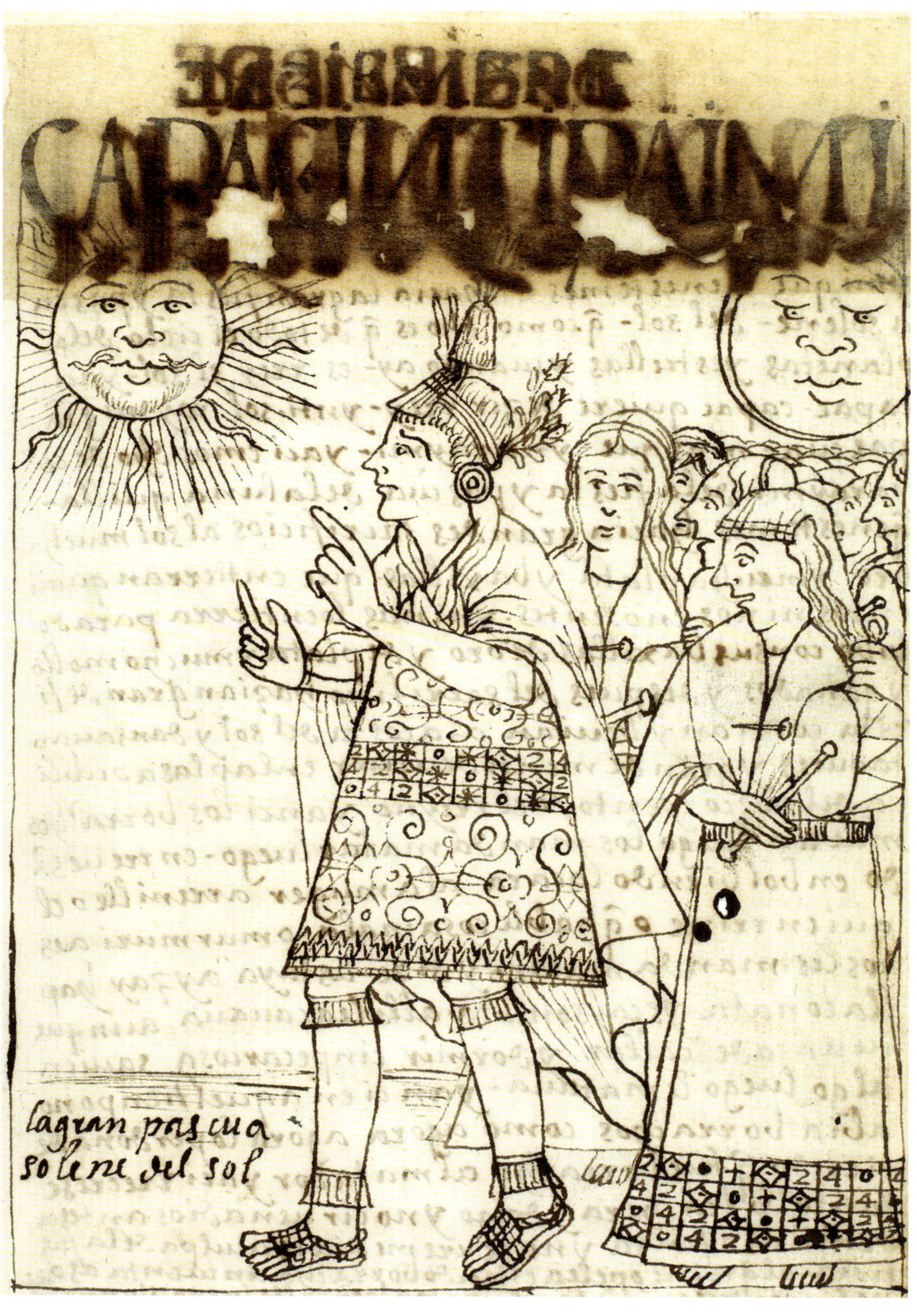

lagran pascua
solene del sol

Some time ago, *Cabinet* made the institutional decision to systematize the way the magazine denoted years. Up until then, we had for the most part used BC and AD ("before Christ" and "Anno Domini"), when necessary, to designate dates. We imagined—like many others—that adopting BCE and CE instead (which we understood to mean "Before the Common Era" and "Common Era") signaled a politically enlightened shift away from an explicitly Christian chronological terminology to one that was more neutral. Lo and behold, while researching the thematic of this current issue, we bumped into Byron Ellsworth Hamann's excellent essay "How to Chronologize with a Hammer, or, The Myth of Homogeneous, Empty Time," which sets out a persuasive argument that the BCE/CE system, though perhaps well intentioned, is in fact even worse than what it replaced. For him, "the fatal flaw of attempts to rebaptize the BC/AD dating system with BCE and CE," is that it "tries to secularize and naturalize a framework that is profoundly religious and artificial." Even worse, "if BCE and CE are used as abbreviations for 'Before Common Era' and 'Common Era,' they are also condemned to complicity with a (superficial and unconvincing) denial of European conquest and colonization—which was the process by which a very provincial, originally Catholic model of timekeeping was enforced as a 'common' standard throughout the world. Alternatively, if the abbreviations are understood as referring to a 'Current Era,' this relegates other calendrical systems (such as the Hijri) to an outdated past (a far too common rhetorical move where Islam is concerned)." Hamann's contribution to this issue, which looks at how nineteenth-century American anarchists addressed these problems, chastened us still further. Following this political enlightenment, we have in fact changed our style sheet back to what it used to be! So we can now say that we are writing this in 2016 AD, according to the Catholic calendrical system—now commonly known as the Gregorian calendar—mandated by the Council of Trent in 1563. We are also writing it in 1438, according to the Islamic calendar; in 4714, according to the Chinese calendar; in 1394, according to the Indian Civil calendar, and so on.

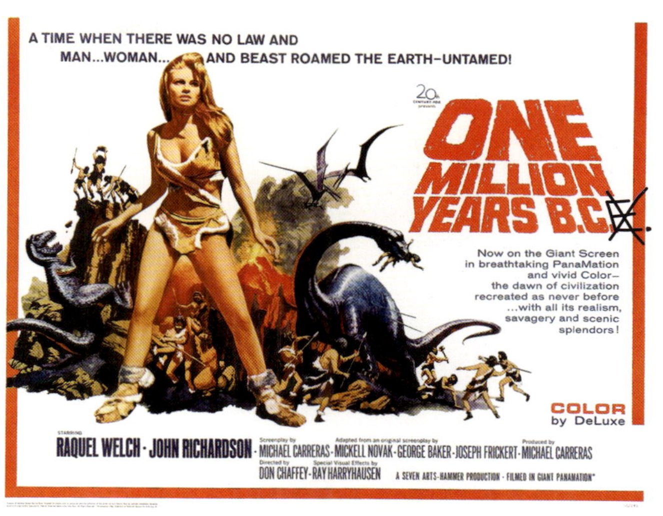

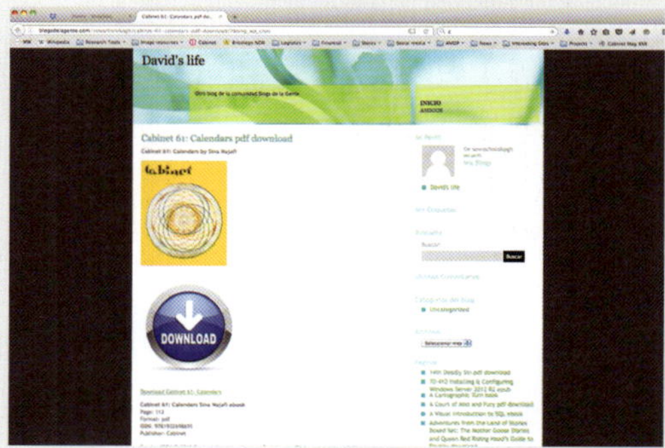

And so it came to pass that in the Year of Our Lord 2016, the stable chronology promised by our (and any) calendar was once again brought to its knees by the spatiotemporal hallucination that is the Internet. As faithful readers will remember, a website was offering our last issue for download long before we had even begun to edit it. So it seemed only fitting that this, our "Calendars" issue, would suffer the same fate. As we were informed by a Google Alert on 15 August, a site called "David's Life" had this very issue on offer for download. And for free! David seemed like a pleasant enough fellow, and so in an effort to expedite the production process and get you your issue earlier, we went ahead and downloaded it. It was good—at times, even great—certainly good enough for us to pass off as our own work. The only hitch was that it was only 96 pages, rather than the 112 pages that we typically produce. Since we've made catching up on our production schedule a priority, we poked around further and discovered that issue 62 was also available for download, and seemed to have been edited in a similarly passable fashion. It is coming your way soon and it too will be slimmer than the typical issue.

Such a nice number, 96. So superior to ungainly old 112. It can be easily rotated into 66, 69, and even 99! There's more. According to Neil Sloane's *On-Line Encyclopedia of Integer Sequences* (see Margaret Wertheim's interview with Sloane in issue 57), it is also an octagonal number (hooray!), a refactorable number (yay!), an untouchable number (whoa!), and a semiperfect number. This last quality is especially appealing to us, since semiperfection is precisely what we aim for with each and every issue.

Numbers are important. Say you want to paint your apartment. You're a Jeffersonian and you enjoy a touch of presidential nostalgia, so you go to the hardware store and you decide on a paint color from Benjamin Moore's so-called Classics line: 018, aka Monticello Peach. But when the clerk writes down the number, he writes 180 by mistake. Now, that number designates a paint color called Beverly Hills, which, not surprisingly, is the color of gold. You come home and instead of finding shelter in Jeffersonian restraint, you end up in an apartment showcasing Trumpian excess. Some version of this mishap occurred during the production of our last issue, where a simple transposition of numbers by our printers resulted in the subdued, matte varnish we normally use on our cover being replaced by a very flashy, high-gloss finish. It is so damn shiny. The printers offered to remove every cover by hand and redo them, but the delay would have added an extra season to the issue (see previous page). Only European newsstand copies were finally redone. Readers: do not imagine that this cover was a prescient nod in the direction of the world we are slouching toward as of 9 November 2016 AD (Anno Domini), or, perhaps what will come to be known as 9 November 1 AD (Anno Donaldi).

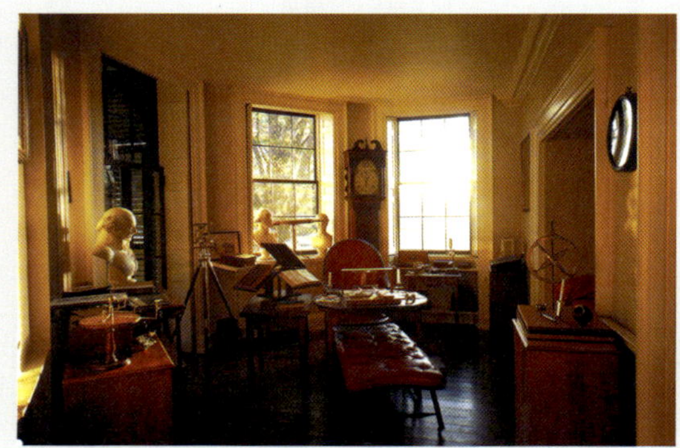

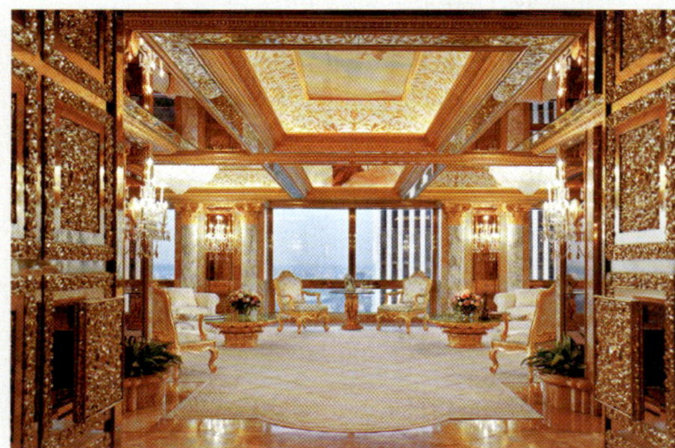

Our only hope is that our next president finds the charms of fishing sooner rather than later. No need to wait for retirement, like Herbert Hoover and others! (See Justin E. H. Smith's essay in this issue.) The charms of the stream await; the trout are eager to be caught and eaten by a powerful man. We have ordered a copy of Hoover's *Fishing for Fun, and To Wash Your Soul* to be delivered to 1600 Pennsylvania Avenue, Washington, DC, on Friday, 20 January 2 AD.

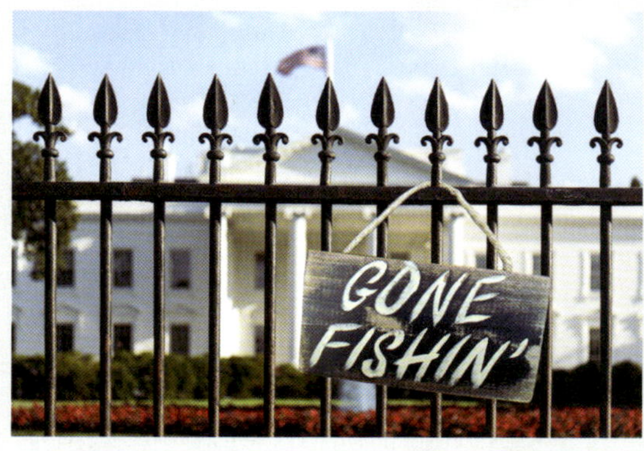

The MIT Press

Fantasies of the Library

edited by Anna-Sophie Springer and Etienne Turpin

"When we think of the library we often focus on its systems of order—the even-spaced rows of shelves, the discrete call numbers on the spines of books. But *Fantasies of the Library* reveals that our experience of the library is instead one of chaotic discovery and unexpected interconnections, a true reflection of the often nonlinear and dreamlike state of our own minds."

—**Dan Cohen**, Executive Director, Digital Public Library of America

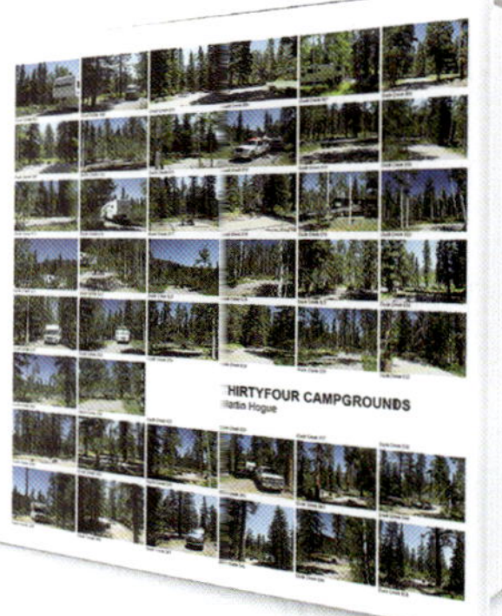

Thirtyfour Campgrounds

Martin Hogue

". . . an engaging and provocative commentary on leisure as many people know it today."

—**Richard Longstreth**, George Washington University

". . . a work of landscape photography and land art, uncannily integrating site, nonsite, website, and campsite."

—**Matthew Coolidge**, Director, Center for Land Use Interpretation

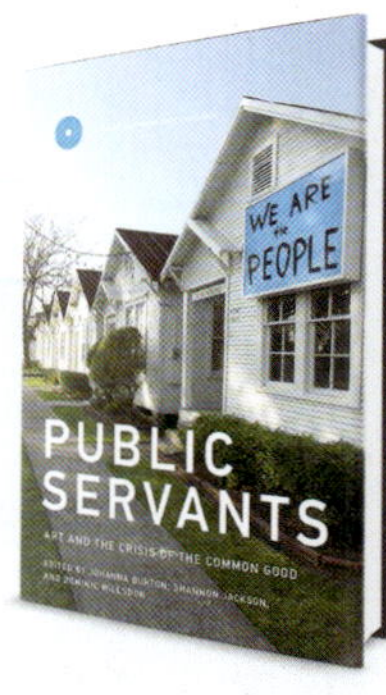

Public Servants

Art and the Crisis of the Common Good

edited by Johanna Burton, Shannon Jackson, and Dominic Willsdon

Essays, dialogues, and art projects that illuminate the changing role of art as it responds to radical economic, political, and global shifts.

Critical Anthologies in Art and Culture
Copublished with the New Museum, New York

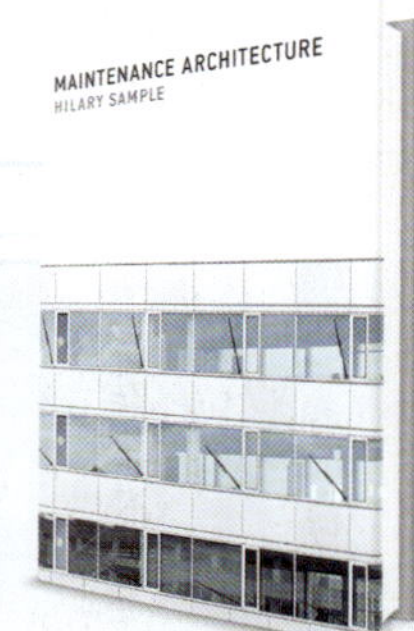

Maintenance Architecture

Hilary Sample

"The timing of this marvelous book couldn't be better. . . . Insofar as maintenance is a public concern—ranging from social justice to visible beauty—street cleaners and squeegees get their due, also works of art, and the topics that underpin current discussions of experimentation, performance, and sustainability."

—**David Leatherbarrow**, Professor of Architecture, University of Pennsylvania

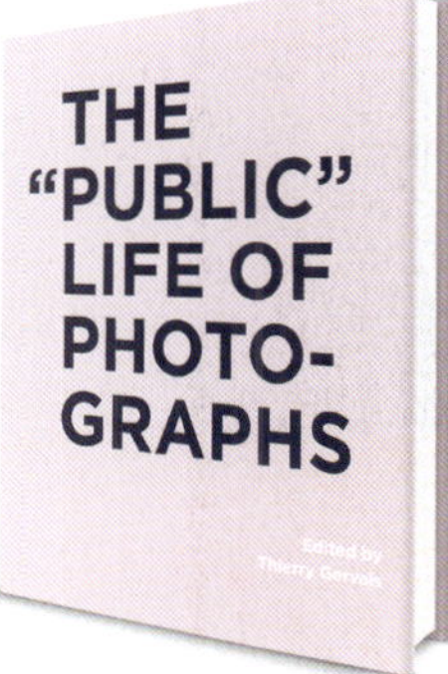

The "Public" Life of Photographs

edited by Thierry Gervais
foreword by Paul Roth

An exploration of the relationship between how photographs are made available to the public and how they are received and understood.

RIC Books | Copublished with Ryerson Image Centre, Ryerson University, Toronto

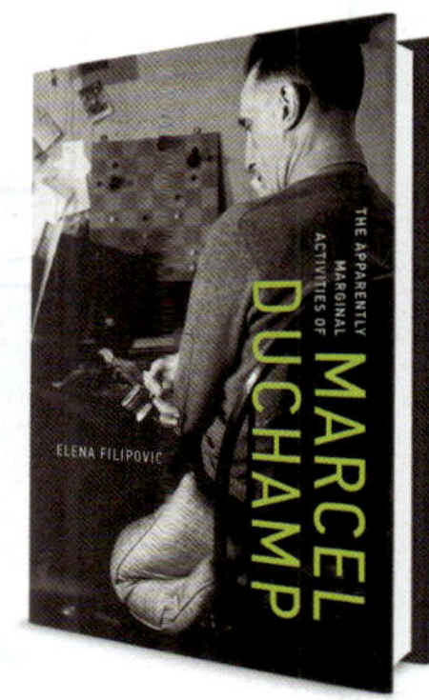

The Apparently Marginal Activities of Marcel Duchamp

Elena Filipovic

"Rather than see [Duchamp's] activities as ancillary to his life as an artist, Filipovic locates them, brilliantly, at its center; they are indeed only 'apparently marginal.' This is just the book to reanimate discourse around Duchamp."

—**Hal Foster**, Princeton University, author of *Compulsive Beauty* and *Prosthetic Gods*

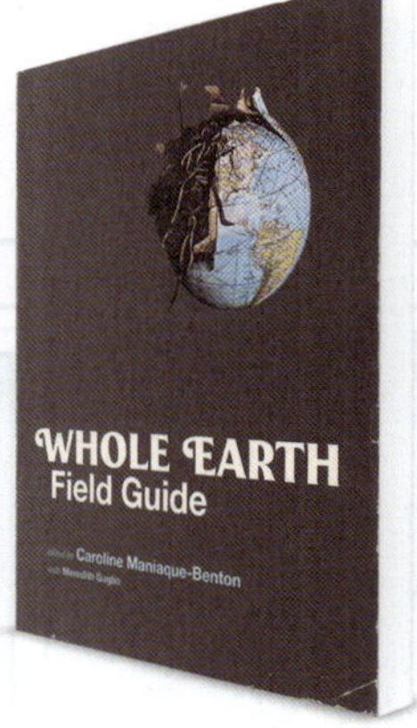

Whole Earth Field Guide

edited by Caroline Maniaque-Benton with Meredith Gaglio

". . . Caroline Maniaque-Benton brilliantly unveils the universe the *Whole Earth Catalogue* opened for the eyes of its readers around 1970. Spanning the extended field of knowledge in which today's digital practices have found their roots, her anthology provides an indispensable documentation for the contemporary reader."

—**Jean-Louis Cohen**, Institute of Fine Arts, New York University

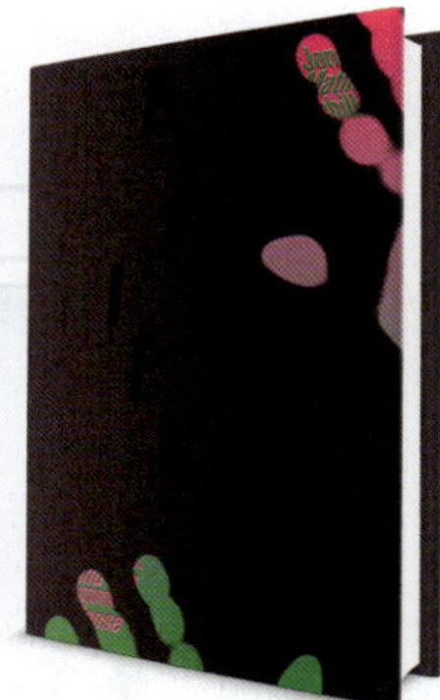

Experience

Culture, Cognition, and the Common Sense

edited by Caroline A. Jones, David Mather, and Rebecca Uchill

A book that produces sensory experiences while bringing the concept of experience itself into relief as a subject of criticism and an object of contemplation.

Copublished with the Center for Art, Science & Technology (CAST), MIT

mitpress.mit.edu

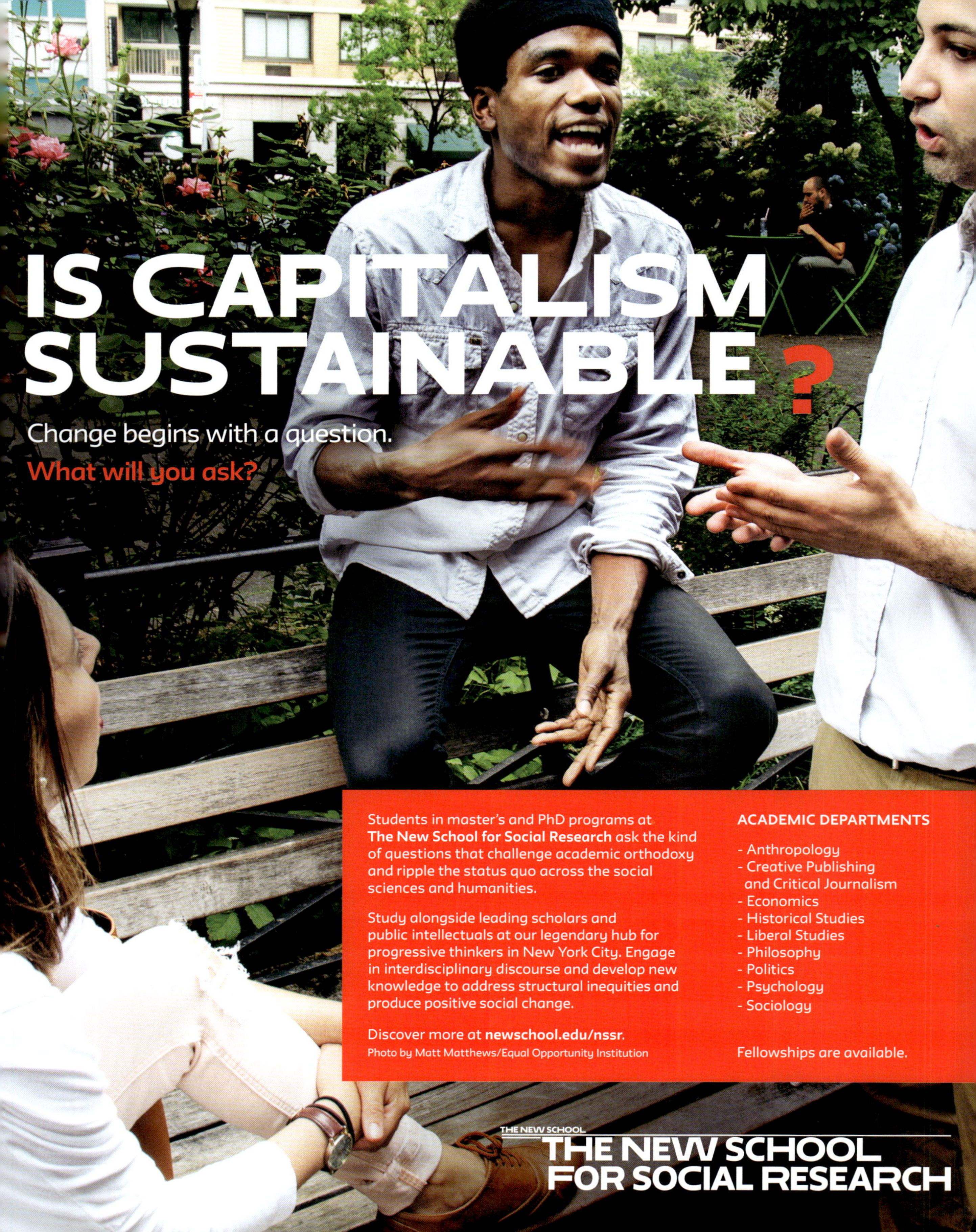
IS CAPITALISM SUSTAINABLE?
Change begins with a question.
What will you ask?

Students in master's and PhD programs at The New School for Social Research ask the kind of questions that challenge academic orthodoxy and ripple the status quo across the social sciences and humanities.

Study alongside leading scholars and public intellectuals at our legendary hub for progressive thinkers in New York City. Engage in interdisciplinary discourse and develop new knowledge to address structural inequities and produce positive social change.

Discover more at newschool.edu/nssr.
Photo by Matt Matthews/Equal Opportunity Institution

ACADEMIC DEPARTMENTS

- Anthropology
- Creative Publishing
  and Critical Journalism
- Economics
- Historical Studies
- Liberal Studies
- Philosophy
- Politics
- Psychology
- Sociology

Fellowships are available.

THE NEW SCHOOL
THE NEW SCHOOL
FOR SOCIAL RESEARCH

e-flux

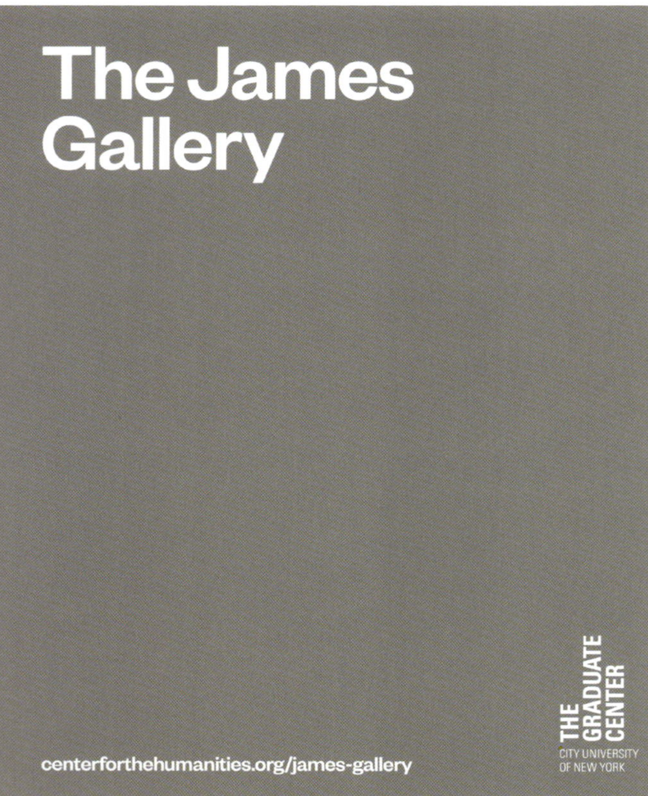

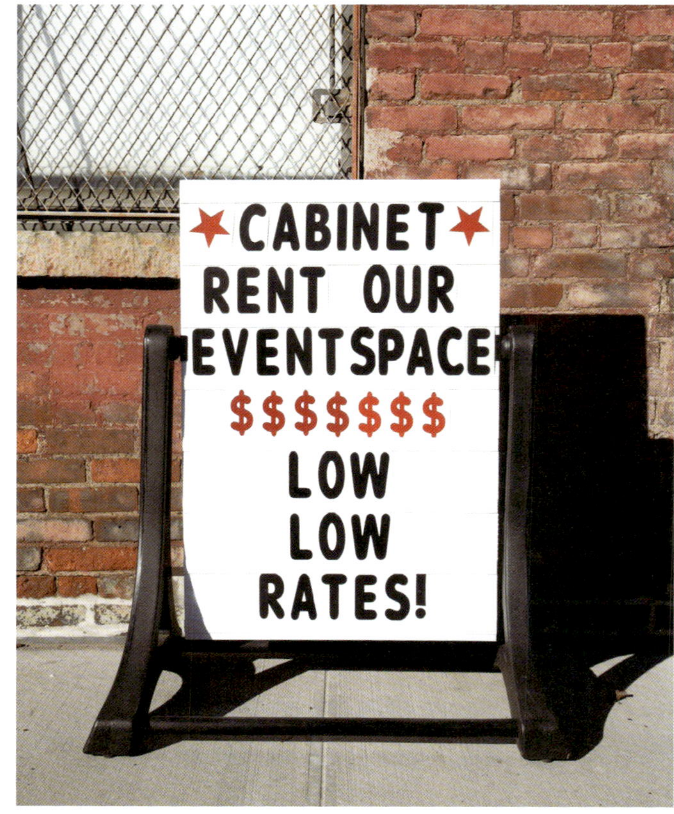

UNITED STATES POSTAL SERVICE ®

Statement of Ownership, Management, and Circulation
(All Periodicals Publications Except Requester Publications)

1. Publication Title Cabinet	2. Publication Number 0 2 0 – 3 4 8	3. Filing Date 10/5/2016
4. Issue Frequency quarterly	5. Number of Issues Published Annually 4	6. Annual Subscription Price $32

7. Complete Mailing Address of Known Office of Publication *(Not printer) (Street, city, county, state, and ZIP+4®)*

181 Wyckoff Street, Brooklyn NY 11217

Contact Person
Sina Najafi
Telephone *(Include area code)*
718 2228434

8. Complete Mailing Address of Headquarters or General Business Office of Publisher *(Not printer)*

181 Wyckoff Street, Brooklyn NY 11217

9. Full Names and Complete Mailing Addresses of Publisher, Editor, and Managing Editor *(Do not leave blank)*

Publisher *(Name and complete mailing address)*

Immaterial Incorporated, 181 Wyckoff Street, Brooklyn NY 11217

Editor *(Name and complete mailing address)*

Sina Najafi, 181 Wyckoff Street, Brooklyn NY 11217

Managing Editor *(Name and complete mailing address)*

none

10. Owner *(Do not leave blank. If the publication is owned by a corporation, give the name and address of the corporation immediately followed by the names and addresses of all stockholders owning or holding 1 percent or more of the total amount of stock. If not owned by a corporation, give the names and addresses of the individual owners. If owned by a partnership or other unincorporated firm, give its name and address as well as those of each individual owner. If the publication is published by a nonprofit organization, give its name and address.)*

Full Name	Complete Mailing Address
Immaterial Incorporated	181 Wyckoff Street Brooklyn NY 11217

11. Known Bondholders, Mortgagees, and Other Security Holders Owning or Holding 1 Percent or More of Total Amount of Bonds, Mortgages, or Other Securities. If none, check box ▶ ☒ None

Full Name	Complete Mailing Address

12. Tax Status *(For completion by nonprofit organizations authorized to mail at nonprofit rates) (Check one)*
The purpose, function, and nonprofit status of this organization and the exempt status for federal income tax purposes:
☒ Has Not Changed During Preceding 12 Months
☐ Has Changed During Preceding 12 Months *(Publisher must submit explanation of change with this statement)*

PS Form **3526**, July 2014 *[Page 1 of 4 (see instructions page 4)]*   PSN 7530-01-000-9931   **PRIVACY NOTICE:** See our privacy policy on www.usps.com

13. Publication Title	14. Issue Date for Circulation Data Below
Cabinet	2/15/2016

15. Extent and Nature of Circulation			Average No. Copies Each Issue During Preceding 12 Months	No. Copies of Single Issue Published Nearest to Filing Date
a. Total Number of Copies *(Net press run)*			8594	7995
b. Paid Circulation (By Mail and Outside the Mail)	(1)	Mailed Outside-County Paid Subscriptions Stated on PS Form 3541 (Include paid distribution above nominal rate, advertiser's proof copies, and exchange copies)	2446	2309
	(2)	Mailed In-County Paid Subscriptions Stated on PS Form 3541 (Include paid distribution above nominal rate, advertiser's proof copies, and exchange copies)	0	0
	(3)	Paid Distribution Outside the Mails Including Sales Through Dealers and Carriers, Street Vendors, Counter Sales, and Other Paid Distribution Outside USPS®	4325	3966
	(4)	Paid Distribution by Other Classes of Mail Through the USPS (e.g., First-Class Mail®)	292	62
c. Total Paid Distribution *[Sum of 15b (1), (2), (3), and (4)]* ▶			7063	6337
d. Free or Nominal Rate Distribution (By Mail and Outside the Mail)	(1)	Free or Nominal Rate Outside-County Copies included on PS Form 3541	0	0
	(2)	Free or Nominal Rate In-County Copies Included on PS Form 3541	0	0
	(3)	Free or Nominal Rate Copies Mailed at Other Classes Through the USPS (e.g., First-Class Mail)	13	15
	(4)	Free or Nominal Rate Distribution Outside the Mail (Carriers or other means)	175	94
e. Total Free or Nominal Rate Distribution *(Sum of 15d (1), (2), (3) and (4))*			188	109
f. Total Distribution *(Sum of 15c and 15e)* ▶			7521	6446
g. Copies not Distributed *(See Instructions to Publishers #4 (page #3))* ▶			1343	1549
h. Total *(Sum of 15f and g)*			8594	7995
i. Percent Paid *(15c divided by 15f times 100)* ▶			97.41	98.31

17. Publication of Statement of Ownership

☒ If the publication is a general publication, publication of this statement is required. Will be printed in the January 2017 issue of this publication.   ☐ Publication not required.

18. Signature and Title of Editor, Publisher, Business Manager, or Owner	Date
Sina Najafi (signature) Sina Najafi, Editor-in-chief	10/5/2016

I certify that all information furnished on this form is true and complete. I understand that anyone who furnishes false or misleading information on this form or who omits material or information requested on the form may be subject to criminal sanctions (including fines and imprisonment) and/or civil sanctions (including civil penalties).

PS Form **3526**, July 2014 *(Page 2 of 4)*

HOW TO ORDER

1. Mail a check to Cabinet, 181 Wyckoff Street, Brooklyn, NY 11217, USA.
2. Shop online at <cabinetmagazine.org/shop>.
3. Call +1 718 222 8434.
4. Fax +1 718 222 3700.

Checks, made out to "Cabinet," must be in USD and drawn on a US bank. We also accept Visa, MC, AmEx, Discover, and Paypal (paypal@cabinetmagazine.org). Prices valid till 1 May 2017. Visit <cabinetmagazine.org> to view our limited and unlimited editions, posters, and other tchotchkes.

A SELECTION OF OUR BOOKS.
VISIT OUR ONLINE SHOP FOR MORE.
Prices include postage.

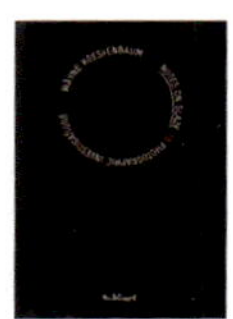

Notes on Glaze
A collection featuring all 18 of Wayne Koestenbaum's "Legend" columns, as well as an introduction by the author.

US $25
Elsewhere $28
(Subscriber discount: -$7)

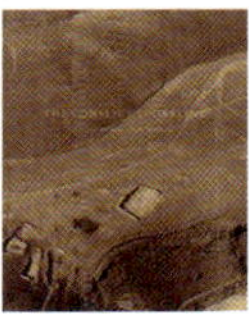

The Conflict Shoreline:
Colonialism as Climate Change
Eyal Weizman's analysis of climate change as a political tool used to displace the Bedouins in the Negev Desert.

US $33
Elsewhere $40
(Subscriber discount: -$7)

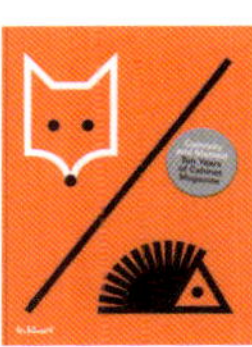

Curiosity and Method:
Ten Years of Cabinet Magazine
An encyclopedia with entries culled from the first 10 years of *Cabinet*.

US $41
Canada & Europe $57
Elsewhere $63
(Subscriber discount: -$5)

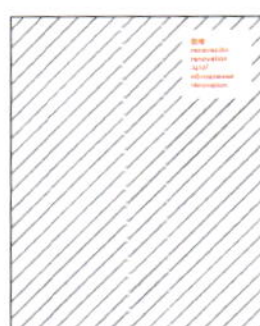

Renovation
Photographer Nancy Daver port's visual meditation on the recent overhaul of the United Nations' headquarters.

US $32
Elsewhere $48
(Subscriber discount: -$7)

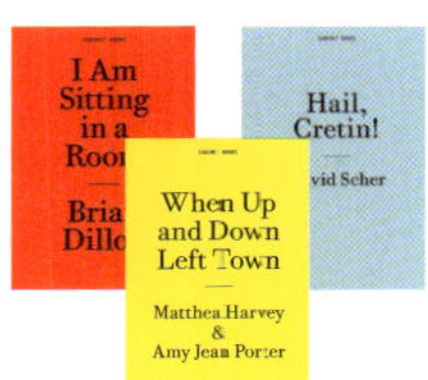

The first 3 volumes in our "24-Hour Book" series: *I Am Sitting in a Room* by Brian Dillon; *Hail, Cretin!* by David Scher; and *When Up and Down Left Town* by Matthea Harvey & Amy Jean Porter.

US $15 (Harvey & Porter: $12)
Canada $16 (Harvey & Porter: $14)
Elsewhere $20 (Harvey & Porter: $17)
(Subscriber discount: -$2)

A SELECTION OF OUR BACK ISSUES.
VISIT OUR ONLINE SHOP FOR MORE.
Available back issues are $10 each plus postage. Postage rates: US $2 per issue; Elsewhere $7 per issue, $17 for 3 issues.

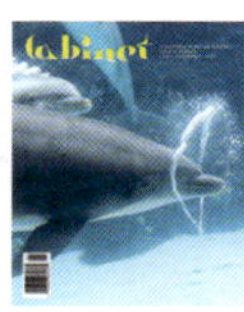 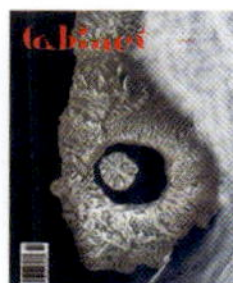 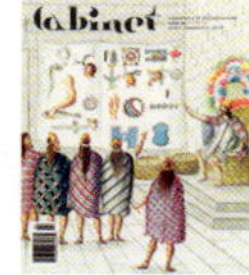 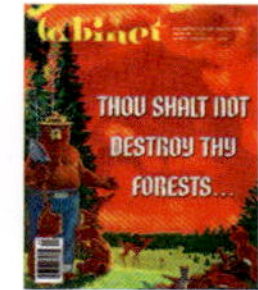

Issue 37
Bubbles

Issue 38
Islands

Issue 39
Learning

Issue 40
Trees

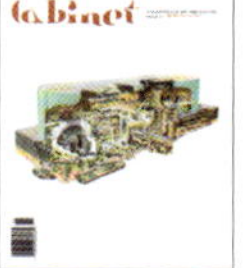 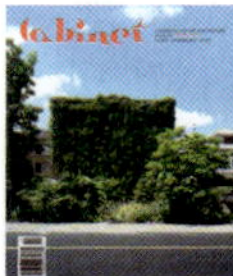 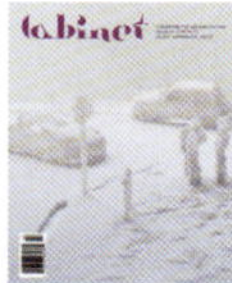 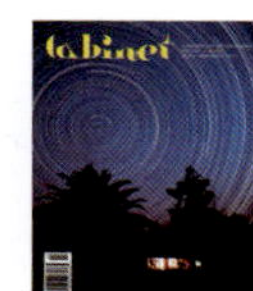

Issue 41
Infrastructure

Issue 42
Forgetting

Issue 43
Forensics

Issue 44
24 Hours

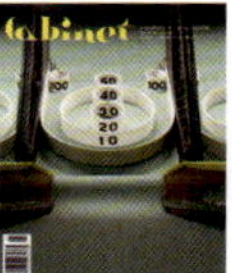 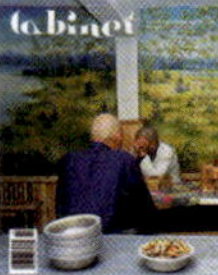 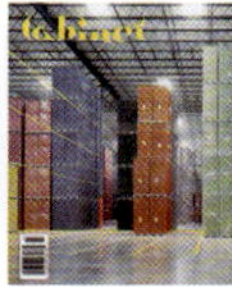 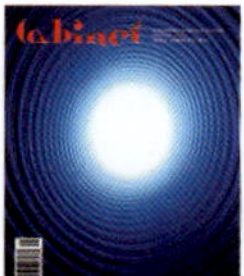

Issue 45
Games

Issue 46
Punishment

Issue 47
Logistics

Issue 49
Death

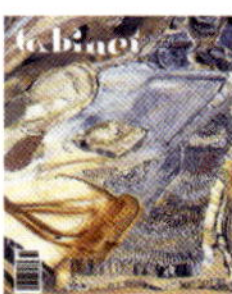 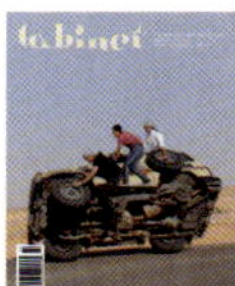 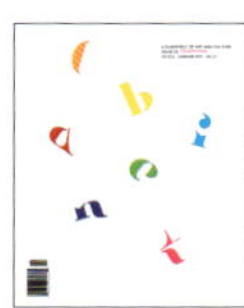 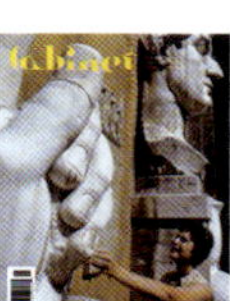

Issue 50
Money

Issue 51
Wheels

Issue 52
Celebration

Issue 53
Stones

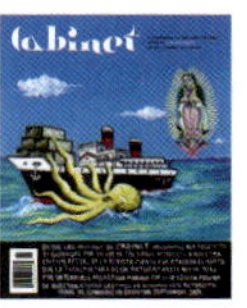 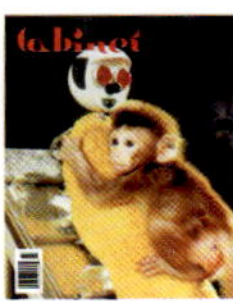 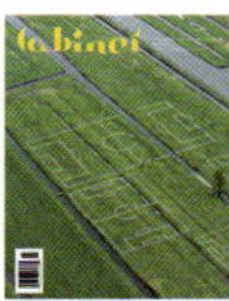 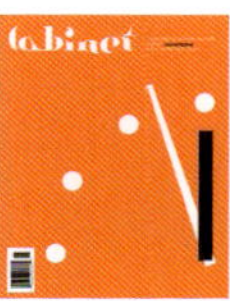

Issue 54
The Accident

Issue 55
Love

Issue 56
Sports

Issue 57
Catastrophe

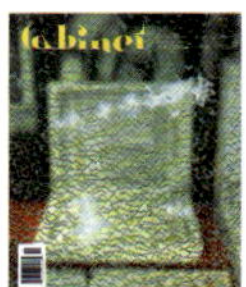 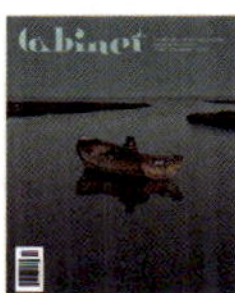 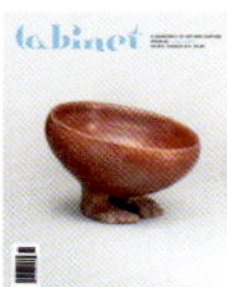 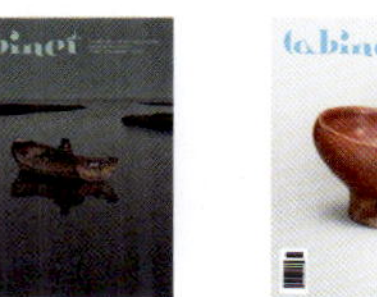

Issue 58
Theft

Issue 59
The North

Issue 60
Containers

CABINET
181 Wyckoff Street
Brooklyn, NY 11217 USA
phone + 1 718 222-8434
fax + 1 718 222-3700
info@cabinetmagazine.org
www.cabinetmagazine.org

Issue 57, Spring 2015

Cover: Founded in 1945 by University of Chicago scientists who had helped develop the first atomic weapons, the *Bulletin of the Atomic Scientists* created the Doomsday Clock two years later to convey the urgency of threats to humanity and the planet. The decision to move (or to leave in place) the minute hand of the clock is made every year by the *Bulletin*'s Science and Security Board in consultation with its Board of Sponsors, which includes seventeen Nobel laureates. When the clock debuted in 1947, it was set at seven minutes to midnight. In 1953, when the US and the Soviet Union began testing hydrogen bombs, it was moved to its most extreme position to date—two minutes to midnight. In 1991, after the two countries signed the Strategic Arms Reduction Treaty, the clock was set to seventeen minutes to midnight. In 2015, after three years of remaining at five minutes before midnight, the clock was moved ahead two minutes as a result of "unchecked climate change, global nuclear weapons modernizations, and outsized nuclear weapons arsenals."

POSTMASTER
Please send address changes to Cabinet, 181 Wyckoff Street, Brooklyn, NY 11217.

Cabinet (USPS # 020-348, ISSN 1531-1430) is a quarterly magazine published by Immaterial Incorporated, 181 Wyckoff Street, Brooklyn, NY 11217. Periodicals Postage paid at Brooklyn, NY, and additional mailing offices.

Printed in Belgium by Die Keure, our final defense against catastrophe.

ADVERTISING
phone + 1 718 222-8434
advertising@cabinetmagazine.org

DISTRIBUTION
Cabinet is available in the US and Canada through Disticor, which distributes both using its own network and through Ingram, Ubiquity, Hudson News, Media Marketing Research, Small Changes, Cowley Distribution, Kent News, MSolutions, the News Group, Chris Stadler, and Don Olson Distribution.

To carry Cabinet through one of these distributors, contact Melanie Raucci at Disticor: phone + 1 631 587-1160, mraucci@disticor.com

Cabinet is available in Europe and elsewhere through Central Books, London: orders@centralbooks.com

Cabinet is available worldwide as a book, with an ISBN, through DAP: phone + 1 212 627-1999, dap@dapinc.com

For further information, contact: circulation@cabinetmagazine.org

INDIVIDUAL SUBSCRIPTIONS

1 year (4 issues):	2 years (8 issues):
US $32	US $60
Canada $38	Canada $72
Western Europe $40	Western Europe $76
Elsewhere $50	Elsewhere $96

Please send a check in US dollars made out to "Cabinet," or mail, fax, or email us your Visa/MC/AmEx/Discover info to:

181 Wyckoff Street
Brooklyn, NY 11217 USA
phone + 1 718 222-8434
fax + 1 718 222-3700
subscriptions@cabinetmagazine.org
www.cabinetmagazine.org/subscribe

INSTITUTIONAL SUBSCRIPTIONS
Institutional subscriptions are available through library agencies such as EBSCO, or directly from Cabinet:
www.cabinetmagazine.org/subscribe

SUBMISSIONS
We only accept submissions via email. Guidelines available at:
www.cabinetmagazine.org/information/submissions.php

Editor-in-chief
Sina Najafi

Senior editor
Jeffrey Kastner

Editors
D. Graham Burnett, Christopher Turner

UK editor
Brian Dillon

Art director
Everything Studio

Operations manager
Nora Rodriguez

Editorial assistants
Juli Brandano, Margherita Peliti

Website directors
Ryan O'Toole, Luke Murphy

Editors-at-large
Saul Anton, Sasha Archibald, Mats Bigert, Brian Conley, Christoph
Cox, Jeff Dolven, Leland de la Durantaye, Jesse Lerner, Jennifer Liese,
Ryo Manabe, Alexander Nagel, George Prochnik, Frances Richard,
Daniel Rosenberg, Aaron Schuster, David Serlin, Debra Singer,
Justin E. H. Smith, Margaret Sundell, Allen S. Weiss, Eyal Weizman,
Margaret Wertheim, Gregory Williams, Jay Worthington, Tirdad
Zolghadr

Contributing editors
Molly Blieden, Eric Bunge, Pip Day, Charles Green, Adam Jasper,
Srdjan Jovanovic Weiss, Lytle Shaw, Cecilia Sjöholm, Carl Michael
von Hausswolff, Sven-Olov Wallenstein

Events
Bryony Quinn (London)

Cabinet national librarian
Matthew Passmore

Cabinet is a non-profit 501(c)(3) magazine published by Immaterial
Incorporated. Our survival depends on support from generous
foundations and individuals. Please consider supporting us at whatever
level you can. Donations are tax-deductible for those who deal with
Uncle Sam. All gifts are acknowledged online. Contributions of $25 or
more will be acknowledged in the next possible issue; those above $100
will be noted in four issues. Checks to "Cabinet" can be sent to our
office; please write "To delay the inevitable!" on the envelope.

Cabinet wishes to thank the following visionary foundations and
individuals for their support of our activities during 2015. Additionally,
we will forever be indebted to the extraordinary contribution of the
Flora Family Foundation from 1999 to 2004; without their support,
this publication would not exist. We would also like to extend
our enormous gratitude to the Orphiflamme Foundation and the
Opaline Fund for their generous support.

$100,000
The Lambent Foundation

$50,000
The Warhol Foundation for Visual Arts

$15,000
The New York City Department of Cultural Affairs

$10,000
The National Endowment for the Arts

$8,000
The New York State Council on the Arts

$3,000
The Danielson Foundation

$1,500–$2,500
Stina & Herant Katchadourian, Steven Rand and Nancy Wender,
Terry Winters

$501–$1,000
Anonymous, Martha & Thomas G. Armstrong, Sara Clugage, Spencer
Finch, Alexander Nagel, Sandy Tait & Hal Foster, The Edward C.
Wilson and Hsu Coue Wilson Family Fund

$500 or under
Pamela Cederquist, Steven Igou, Deborah Lovely, Case Randall,
Maisie Martin Siegel, Meredith Martin & Joshua Siegel, Lenore &
Richard Niles, Sal Randolph, Margaret Sundell and Reinaldo Laddaga

$250 or under
Cameron Allan, Defne Ayas, Tauba Auerbach, Jeff Beall, Freya Cooper
Kiddie, Mia Enell & Nicholas Fries, George Ganat, Jair Gonzalez, Alex
Goodfriend, Cynthia Hansen, Peter Jaszi, Craig Kalpakjian, James
Katzenberger, Scott LeBouef, Paul McConnell, Elizabeth Merena,
Helen Mirra, Andrew Pederson, Paul Ramirez Jonas, Eric Schmid,
Pooja Shah & Rebecca Ward, John Sherburne, James Siena, Debra
Singer & Jay Worthington, Jude Tallichet & Matt Freedman

$100 or under
Simon Albrecht, David Altman, James Baker, Temple Burling, Crystal
Carter, Brian Cohen, Claire Connelly, Ed DeCarbo, Cooper Downs,
Alan Dudley, Elizabeth Finch, Heather Galbraith, Susan Harris, Lucy
Hogg and Blake Gopnik, Annene Kaye-Berry, Esben Krohn, Carin
Kuoni & John Oakes, Jim Martin, Julia Meltzer, Tommy Moorman,
Marguerite Perret, Roman Podkolzine, Privat Club, Kathleen Rooney,
John Sargent, David Serlin & Brian Selznick, Andrea Simitch, Rick
Skibinski, Benjamin Terrell, Pamela Tibbetts, Margery Thomas-Mueller,
Owen Walton, Marina Warner

CONTRIBUTORS

Sasha Archibald is an editor-at-large of *Cabinet*, and Curator of Special Projects at Clockshop in Los Angeles.

Walter Benjamin (1892–1940) was a German theorist and writer. His radio broadcasts were recently collected in *Radio Benjamin* (Verso Books, 2014).

D. Graham Burnett is an editor of *Cabinet* and teaches at Princeton University. He, Jeff Dolven, and Asad Raza are organizing the Tivoli Park Workshop at this year's Ljubljana Biennial.

Stassa Edwards is a Miami-based writer. She is a contributor at the website Jezebel and has written for *Lapham's Quarterly*, *Aeon*, and the *Public Domain Review*. She is currently writing a book about the history of hysteria.

William Firebrace is a London-based writer and teacher. He is the author of *Things Worth Seeing* (Black Dog Publishing, 2000), *Marseille Mix* (Architectural Association, 2010), and *Memo for Nemo* (Architectural Association, 2015).

Maria Golia, a long-time resident of Egypt, is the author of *Cairo, City of Sand* (Reaktion Books, 2004) and *Photography and Egypt* (Reaktion Books, 2010). *Meteorite*, a cultural history, will be published by Reaktion Books in autumn 2015.

Patrick Lyons is a PhD candidate in the French Department at University of California, Berkeley, currently working on projects on literary friendship and on the phenomenology of annotation. He has written reviews for *Critical Theory*, among other publications.

Adam Morris is a writer and translator in San Francisco. His translations from the Portuguese include Hilda Hilst's novel *With My Dog-Eyes* (Melville House, 2014), and João Gilberto Noll's *Quiet Creature on the Corner* and *Atlantic Hotel* (Two Lines Press, forthcoming in 2016 and 2017, respectively). He is writing a book on American messianic movements (Liveright, forthcoming).

George Pendle is a writer based in Washington, DC, who contributes to the *Financial Times*, the *Economist*, *frieze*, and *Atlas Obscura*. His books include *Strange Angel: The Otherworldly Life of Rocket Scientist John Whiteside Parsons* (Harcourt, 2005), *The Remarkable Millard Fillmore* (Crown, 2007), and *Happy Failure* (Karma, 2014). He is the founder of <carpetsforairports.com>.

George Prochnik has written for the *New York Times*, the *New Yorker*, *Bookforum*, and the *Los Angeles Review of Books*, among other publications. His most recent book *The Impossible Exile: Stefan Zweig at the End of the World* (Other Press, 2013) received the National Jewish Book Award for Biography/Memoir in 2014. He is also the author of *In Pursuit of Silence: Listening for Meaning in a World of Noise* (Doubleday, 2010) and *Putnam Camp: Sigmund Freud, James Jackson Putnam, and the Purpose of American Psychology* (Other Press, 2006).

Anson Rabinbach is a professor of history at Princeton University and co-founder of *New German Critique*, which he continues to co-edit. He recently co-edited, with Sander L. Gilman, *The Third Reich Sourcebook* (University of California Press, 2013).

George Scheer is the cofounder and executive director of Elsewhere, a living museum and residency set in a former thrift store. He is also project director of South Elm Projects, a series of site-specific art commissions in Greensboro, North Carolina, produced with support of ArtPlace America. In 2012, he co-curated Kulturpark, a six-week research residency and public art production in Spreepark, an abandoned amusement park in East Berlin.

Stephanie Sherman is an art director, curator, and writer currently working between San Diego and London. She is the cofounder of Elsewhere, a living museum and residency set in a former thrift store, and codirector of Common Field, a new visual arts organizing network. Her most recent book, *A Manual for Urban Projection*, coauthored with Ali Momeni, will be available in fall 2015. See <stephaniesherman.net> for more information.

Neil Sloane is a mathematician who worked for over forty years at AT&T. In 1964, he founded the Encyclopedia of Integer Sequences, which is now online and contains more than 260,000 sequences. He lives in New Jersey.

Matthew Spellberg is a graduate student in comparative literature at Princeton University. His work has appeared in the *Yale Review*, the *Southwest Review*, the *Los Angeles Review of Books*, *Guernica*, and other journals and magazines. He is completing a study of the sculptor William Kent and a book about dreaming.

Margaret Wertheim is the director of the Institute For Figuring, a Los Angeles nonprofit dedicated to the poetic and aesthetic dimensions of science and mathematics. Her latest book, co-authored with Christine Wertheim, is *Crochet Coral Reef* (Institute For Figuring, 2015); it documents the institute's project in which thousands of women worldwide have joined in making a woolly archipelago of handicraft reefs as a collective artistic response to global warming.

Hayden Williams is a New York–based writer originally from Glasgow. He is finishing a novel about a picklemaker from Idaho who comes to Brooklyn and becomes an artisanal legend.

Carmen Winant is an artist and writer. Currently a professor of visual theory and feminist art history at Columbus College of Art and Design, she is at work on an experimental book about the nature of practice.

AF328630

COLUMNS

INVENTORY /
GOOD BOY
George Pendle

*"Inventory" examines or presents a
list, catalogue, or register.*

———

It was not the first time N.U.R.P.38.
EGU.242 had parachuted into
German-occupied France. He hadn't
minded the nighttime plummet, the
cold air slapping at his face. It was
getting back that worried him. Look
what had happened to Mary the last
time; half her body had been ripped
apart by shrapnel, probably from their
own side's bloody bombs. When was
that? Yesterday? Two weeks ago? He
couldn't remember. He never could.
He shivered inside his down coat.
How he longed to get home, back
to Sussex and Sid. Ah, Sid. No one
better. Sid always looked after him,
kept him watered and fed, cooed
sweet nothings into his ear each
morning. But Sussex was a long way
away. N.U.R.P.38.EGU.242 knew the
numbers: fewer than one in eight of
his kind ever returned. There were
marksmen waiting all along the coast
for him. Falcons too. He flinched as
the cold metal canister was strapped
to his leg. Suddenly the sock was
whisked off his head and the fingers
holding him loosened. With one snap
of his wings, he was away, up and up,
rising through the night air. He took
one large circle over the men below,
felt the tug of the earth's magnetic
field on his beak, and headed for
home.

    During World War II, N.U.R.P.38.
EGU.242, a red checker pigeon
better known as Commando, was
airdropped into occupied France
over ninety times. Carried into the
war zone by British secret agents, or
parachuted in by himself in a special
container to be retrieved by members
of the Resistance, Commando trans-
ported crucial messages—concerning

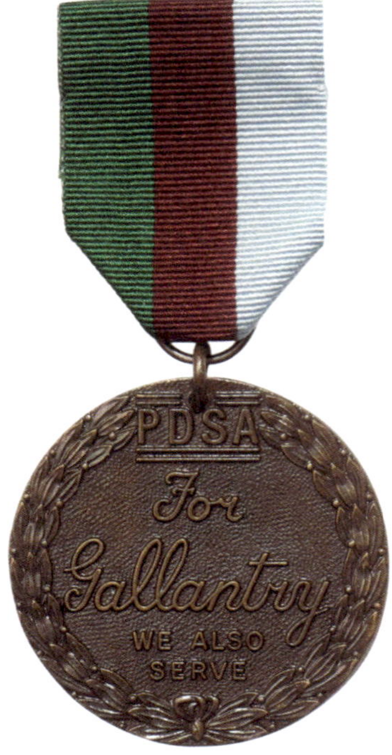

The PDSA Dickin Medal.

enemy troop movements or potential
bombing targets—back to England
in a tiny cylinder strapped to his
leg. Since being caught in possession of a radio could get you
tortured and executed by German
troops, pigeons like Commando
provided a far safer means of covert
communication. Donated to Great
Britain's National Pigeon Service by
prominent pigeon fancier Sid Moon,
Commando survived bombs, bad
weather, sharpshooters, and Nazi
falconers in pursuance of his mission.
For his courage under "exceptionally
adverse conditions," he was awarded
the highest honor that a non-human
combatant can receive—the Dickin
Medal.

    First instituted in 1943 by the
British animal welfare pioneer Maria
Dickin, the Dickin Medal—awarded
by the People's Dispensary for
Sick Animals—is a bronze medal-
lion inscribed with the words "For
Gallantry" and, in smaller letters, "We
Also Serve." Intended to honor the
work of animals in wartime, the medal

was awarded to Commando and
thirty-one other pigeons—the species
with the most recipients. (Mary of
Exeter, a pigeon who survived severe
shrapnel wounds, falcon eviscera-
tion, and having part of her wing shot
off, was another.) Dogs have been
awarded the medal twenty-nine times,
horses three times, and, surprisingly,
considering its supercilious nature, a
cat once. Selection criteria are strict
and require eyewitness reports and
the recommendation of a commanding officer, but once these have been
satisfied, an animal can seek to enter
the pantheon of such heroic fauna
as Rifleman Khan, the Alsatian dog
who saved a soldier from drowning while under heavy enemy fire, or
Upstart, a police horse who remained
unperturbed while directing traffic as
flying bombs exploded around him,
or Simon, the feline outlier who was a
ship's cat aboard the HMS *Amethyst*
and received his medal for raising
morale and killing off a rat infestation
during the infamous Yangtze incident
of 1949.

    It has long been taken for granted
that animals are brave. In Plato's
Laches, Socrates states without
hesitation that the lion, the leopard,
and the boar all display an innate
courage. Charles Darwin too thought
animal bravery was self-evident, writing in *The Descent of Man* (1871)
that a simple observation of his own
dogs—Bran, Dash, Nina, Pincher,
Pointer, Polly, Sheilah, Snow, Spark,
and Sappho—showed that animals
not only displayed courage but also
enacted a whole range of human
emotions. "The fact that the lower
animals are excited by the same
emotions as ourselves is so well
established," he wrote, "that it will
not be necessary to weary the reader
by many details." Yet against this
unquestioning belief in feral fortitude
runs a less cuddly strand of thinking that states that animals are not
being brave at all. René Descartes,
in *Passions of the Soul* (1649),
held that animals were non-sentient

"natural automata," lacking language and self-consciousness, and thus capable of only an unthinking fearlessness rather than true bravery. When the Soviet army trained suicide dogs to carry explosives underneath enemy tanks, were they creating plucky heroes of the Motherland or drooling four-legged drones? Was Commando the pigeon a real war hero, or was he a Pavlovian Candidate?

Of course, Descartes was writing before the discovery that many animals share the same brain structures as humans and appear to undergo many of the same chemical changes during emotional states. But even if animals could be categorically proven to display an emotional equivalent to human courage, this does not necessarily explain our willingness to bestow medals upon them. Honors are traditionally intended to ennoble the recipient, and while biological innovations may make it easier to ascribe courage to an animal, it seems willfully anthropomorphic to assign the emotion of pride to an animal with no conception of time or sense of self.

In *Some Thoughts Concerning Education* (1693), John Locke lamented the cruelty of children to animals, "for the custom of tormenting and killing of beasts will by degrees harden their minds even towards men, and they who accustom themselves to delight in the suffering and destruction of inferior creatures, will not be apt to be very compassionate or benign to those of their own kind." While Locke did not weigh in on whether animals displayed human emotions, he did suggest that they are intrinsically bound to human sentiments—if we are cruel to animals, we will be cruel to others; if we are good to animals, we will be good to others.

This bond has allowed animals to carry with them a particularly pliable symbolic power, especially in the case of dogs. As the most widespread household pet, dogs hold within them connotations of domesticity and family. Thus, when a dog is awarded a medal for wartime courage—and increasingly they are the favored recipients of the Dickin Medal—it also spreads a favorable light of kindness and loyalty on the personnel with whom the dog has been working. The Dickin Medal, then, acts as a strange form of moral propaganda in which the animal is being used to humanize the soldier. That is not all, for as well as helping the British Armed Forces pilfer an animal's symbolic value, the Dickin Medal also seems to be acting as a form of atonement. In the past century, nearly the entire animal kingdom has been co-opted into humanity's conflicts. Eight million horses died in World War I, approximately the same number as the combined casualties of all human armies. Since then, pigs have been trained to find mines, bats have been airdropped from planes with incendiary devices stitched to their bellies, and, more recently, donkeys have been used as (presumably) unsuspecting suicide bombers in both Iraq and Afghanistan. No corner of the animal kingdom has evaded the draft. To date no insect has won the Dickin Medal, but in the 1960s the US Army did try to use lice, ticks, and fleas to detect ambushes by recording the increasingly frenzied sounds these creatures make when they sense humans nearby. Lice, it turned out, were the best at sensing nearby humans, but moved so quietly that their agitation was not loud enough to hear. Subsequent attempts to fit them with shoes, the better to hear their footsteps, ended in failure.

But are awards such as the Dickin Medal really just devices for abetting and expiating the bad behavior of humans, or can we really learn something about animals by ascribing human emotions to them? For many years, the field of ethology—the study of animal behavior—railed against anthropomorphism and rejected Darwin's free attribution of emotions to animals. In the 1940s, a fierce spat broke out among entomologists after one researcher claimed to have discovered that mosquitoes emitted "distress calls." The use of the word "distress," with its implicit suggestion of a complex range of emotions, caused controversy to rage until the phrase was changed to the less leading "warning call." However, in the past quarter century, anthropomorphism has increasingly being seen not only as a benefit but an inevitability. "[Anthropomorphism] has presumably also been 'pre-programmed' into our hereditary make-up by natural selection," writes the animal behaviorist John S. Kennedy in *The New Anthropomorphism* (1992), "perhaps because it proved to be useful for predicting and controlling the behavior of animals." Awarding medals to animals is thus a way of shoring up our implicit anthropomorphic beliefs and of asserting our interspecific links. Anthropomorphism is good for us because it is good for our relations with them.

Perhaps too there is something else, something that transcends both the presenter of the medal and its recipient. For there, floating free in furry, feathered, or fetlocked form, is the sight of a human ideal uncorrupted by human baseness, pinned as if under glass, forever showing us the right way to behave.

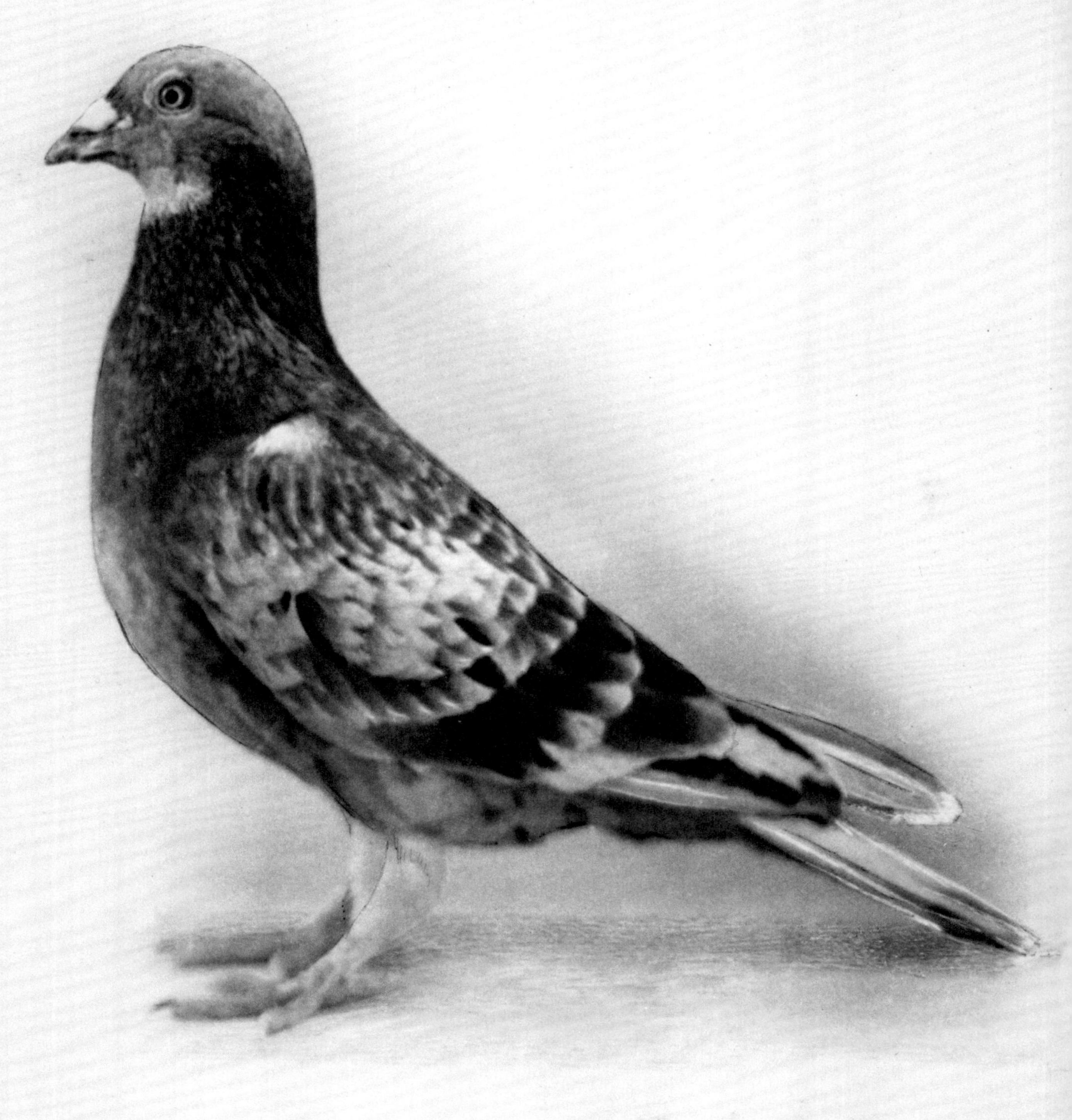

Recipients of the PDSA Dickin Medal

Dogs

Bob (mongrel)
6th Battalion, Royal West Kent Regiment
Date of award: 24 March 1944
"For constant devotion to duty with special mention of patrol work at Green Hill, North Africa, while serving with the 6th Battalion of the Queen's Own Royal West Kent Regiment."

Jet (German shepherd)
Ministry of Aircraft Production serving with Civil Defence Services
Date of award: 12 January 1945
"For being responsible for the rescue of persons trapped under blitzed buildings, while serving with the Civil Defence Services of London."

Irma (German shepherd)
Ministry of Aircraft Production serving with Civil Defence Services
Date of award: 12 January 1945
"For being responsible for the rescue of persons trapped under blitzed buildings, while serving with the Civil Defence Services of London."

Beauty (terrier)
PDSA rescue squad
Date of award: 12 January 1945
"For being the pioneer dog in locating buried air-raid victims, while serving with a PDSA rescue squad."

Rob (collie)
Special Air Service
Date of award: 22 January 1945
"Took part in landings during North African campaign with an infantry unit and later served with a special air unit in Italy as patrol and guard with small detachments in enemy territory. His presence with these parties saved many of them from discovery and subsequent capture or destruction. Rob made over twenty parachute descents."

Thorn (German shepherd)
Ministry of Aircraft Production serving with Civil Defence Services
Date of award: 2 March 1945
"For locating air-raid casualties in spite of thick smoke in a burning building."

Rifleman Khan (German shepherd)
6th Battalion, Cameronians (Scottish Rifles)
Date of award: 27 March 1945
"For rescuing Lieutenant Corporal Muldoon from drowning under heavy shell fire at the assault of Walcheren, November 1944, while serving with the 6th Cameronians (SR)."

Rex (German shepherd)
Ministry of Aircraft Production serving with Civil Defence Services
Date of award: April 1945
"For outstanding good work in the location of casualties in burning buildings. Undaunted by smouldering debris, thick smoke, intense heat, and jets of water from fire hoses, this dog displayed uncanny intelligence and outstanding determination in his efforts to follow up any scent that might lead him to a trapped casualty."

Rip (mongrel)
Stray picked up by Civil Defence squad at Poplar, London E14
Date of award: July 1945
"For locating many air-raid victims during the blitz of 1940."

Sheila (collie)
Date of award: 2 July 1945
"For assisting in the rescue of four American airmen lost in the Cheviot Hills in a blizzard after an air crash in December 1944."

Peter (collie)
Ministry of Aircraft Production serving with Civil Defence Services
Date of award: November 1945
"For locating victims trapped under blitzed buildings."

Judy (pointer)
Date of award: May 1946
"For magnificent courage and endurance in Japanese prison camps, which helped to maintain morale among her fellow prisoners and also for saving many lives through her intelligence and watchfulness."

Punch and Judy (boxers)
Date of awards: December 1946
"These dogs saved the lives of two British officers in Palestine by attacking an armed terrorist who was stealing upon them unawares and thus warning them of their danger. Punch sustained four bullet wounds and Judy a long graze down her back."

Ricky (collie)
Date of award: 29 March 1947
"This dog was engaged in cleaning the verges of the canal bank at Nederweert, Holland. He found all the mines, but during the operation one of them exploded. Ricky was wounded in the head but remained calm and kept at work. Had he become excited, he would have been a danger to the rest of the section working nearby."

Brian (German shepherd)
13th Battalion, Airborne Division
Date of award: 29 March 1947
"This patrol dog landed with his battalion in Normandy in June 1944 and having done the requisite number of jumps by war's end, became a fully qualified 'paratrooper.'"

Antis (German shepherd)
Date of award: 28 January 1949
"Owned by a Czech airman, this dog served with him in the French Air Force and Royal Air Force from 1940 to 1945 both in North Africa and England. Returning to Czechoslovakia after the war, he substantially helped his master's escape across the frontier when, after the death of Jan Masaryk, he had to flee from the communists."

Tich (mongrel)
1st Battalion, King's Royal Rifle Corps
Date of award: 1 July 1949
"For loyalty, courage, and devotion to duty under hazardous conditions of war, 1941 to 1945, while serving with the 1st King's Rifle Corps in North Africa and Italy."

Gander (Newfoundland)
Royal Rifles of Canada
Date of award: Awarded posthumously on 27 October 2000
"For saving the lives of Canadian infantrymen during the Battle of Lye Mun on Hong Kong Island in December 1941. On three documented occasions, Gander, the Newfoundland mascot of the Royal Rifles of Canada, engaged the enemy as his regiment joined the Winnipeg Grenadiers, members of Battalion Headquarters 'C' Force, and other Commonwealth troops in their courageous defence of the island. Twice Gander's attacks halted the enemy's advance and protected groups of wounded soldiers. In a final act of bravery, the war dog was killed in action gathering a grenade. Without Gander's intervention, many more lives would have been lost in the assault."

Apollo (German shepherd)
New York Police Department
Date of award: 5 March 2002, on behalf of all the search and rescue dogs that worked in the aftermath of 11 September 2001
"For tireless courage and unstinting devotion to duty during the search and rescue operations at Ground Zero and the Pentagon. Faithful to words of command and undaunted by the task, the dogs' work and unstinting devotion to duty stand as a testament to those lost or injured."

Salty and Roselle (Labrador retrievers)
Date of awards: 5 March 2002
"For remaining loyally at the side of their blind owners and courageously leading them down more than seventy floors of the World Trade Center to a place of safety following the terrorist attack on New York on 11 September 2001."

Sam (German shepherd)
Royal Army Veterinary Corps
Date of award: 14 January 2003
"For outstanding gallantry in April 1998 while assigned to the Royal Canadian Regiment in Drvar during the conflict in Bosnia-Herzegovina. On two documented occasions, Sam displayed great courage and devotion to duty. On 18 April, Sam successfully brought down an armed man threatening the lives of civilians and service personnel. On 24 April, while guarding a compound

harbouring Serbian refugees, Sam's determined approach held off rioters until reinforcements arrived. This dog's true valour saved the lives of many servicemen and civilians during this time of human conflict."

Buster (spaniel)
Royal Army Veterinary Corps
Date of award: 9 December 2003
"For outstanding gallantry in March 2003 while assigned to the Duke of Wellington's Regiment in Safwan, southern Iraq. Buster, an arms and explosives search dog, located an arsenal of weapons and explosives hidden behind a false wall in a property linked with an extremist group. Buster is considered responsible for saving the lives of service personnel and civilians. Shortly after the find, all attacks ceased and troops replaced their steel helmets with berets."

Lucky (German shepherd)
Royal Air Force Police
Date of award: Awarded posthumously on 6 February 2007
"For the outstanding gallantry and devotion to duty of the RAF Police anti-terrorist tracker dog team, comprising Bobbie, Jasper, Lassie, and Lucky, while attached to the Civil Police and several British Army regiments, including the Coldstream Guards, 2nd Battalion Royal Scots Guards, and the Gurkhas during the Malayan Emergency. Bobbie, Jasper, Lassie, and Lucky displayed exceptional determination and life-saving skills; the dogs and their handlers were an exceptional team, capable of tracking and locating the enemy by scent despite unrelenting heat and an almost impregnable jungle. Sadly, three of the dogs lost their lives in the line of duty; only Lucky, who served from 1949 to 1952, survived to the end of the conflict."

Sadie (Labrador)
Royal Army Veterinary Corps
Date of award: 6 February 2007
"For outstanding gallantry and devotion to duty while assigned to the Royal Gloucestershire, Berkshire, and Wiltshire Light Infantry during conflict in Afghanistan in 2005. On 14 November 2005, military personnel serving with NATO's International Security Assistance Force in Kabul were involved in two separate attacks. Sadie and Lance Corporal Yardley were deployed to search for secondary explosive devices. Sadie gave a positive indication near a concrete blast wall and multinational personnel were moved to a safe distance. Despite the obvious danger, Sadie and Lance Corporal Yardley completed their search. At the site indicated by Sadie, bomb disposal operators later made safe an explosive device. Sadie's actions undoubtedly saved the lives of many civilians and soldiers."

Treo (labrador)
Royal Army Veterinary Corps
Date of award: 24 February 2010
"On 15 August 2008, while acting as forward protection for 8 Platoon, the Royal Irish Regiment, Treo located a 'daisy chain' IED—an improvised explosive device designed to trigger a series of bombs—on a roadside where soldiers were about to pass. It was subsequently confirmed that the device uncovered was new to the area and would have inflicted significant casualties. On 3 and 4 September 2008, Treo's actions were reported as saving 7 Platoon from guaranteed casualties, again as the result of an IED. Without doubt, Treo's actions and devotion to his duties, while in the throes of conflict, saved many lives."

Theo (spaniel)
Royal Army Veterinary Corps
Date of award: Awarded posthumously on 25 October 2012
"For outstanding gallantry and devotion to duty while deployed from September 2010 to March 2011 with 104 Military Working Dog Squadron during the conflict in Afghanistan."

Sasha (Labrador)
Royal Army Veterinary Corps
Date of award: Awarded posthumously on 21 May 2014
"For outstanding gallantry and devotion to duty while assigned to 2nd Battalion, The Parachute Regiment, in Afghanistan 2008."

Pigeons

SURP.41.L.3089, a.k.a. White Vision
Date of award: 2 December 1943
"For delivering a message under exceptionally difficult conditions and so contributing to the rescue of an air crew, while serving with the Royal Air Force in October 1943."

NEHU.40.NS.1, a.k.a. Winkie
Date of award: 2 December 1943
"For delivering a message under exceptionally difficult conditions and so contributing to the rescue of an air crew, while serving with the Royal Air Force in February 1942."

1263 MEPS 43, a.k.a. Tyke or George
Date of award: 2 December 1943
"For delivering a message under exceptionally difficult conditions and so contributing to the rescue of an air crew, while serving with the Royal Air Force in the Mediterranean in June 1943."

NPS.41.NS.4230, a.k.a. Beach Comber
Date of award: 6 March 1944
"For bringing the first news to this country of the landing at Dieppe under hazardous conditions in September 1942, while serving with the Canadian Army."

NPS.42.31066, a.k.a. Gustav
Date of award: 1 September 1944
"For delivering the first message from the Normandy beaches from a ship off the beachhead, while serving with the Royal Air Force on 6 June 1944."

NPS.43.9451, a.k.a. Paddy
Date of award: 1 September 1944
"For the best recorded time with a message from the Normandy operations, while serving with the Royal Air Force in June 1944."

NURP.36.JH.190, a.k.a. Kenley Lass
Date of award: March 1945
"For being the first pigeon to be used with success for secret communications from an agent in enemy-occupied France, while serving with the National Pigeon Service in October 1940."

NPS.41.NS.2862, a.k.a. Navy Blue
Date of award: March 1945
"For delivering an important message from a raiding party on the west coast of France, although injured, while serving with the Royal Air Force in June 1944."

NPS.42.NS.44802, a.k.a. Flying Dutchman
Date of award: March 1945
"For successfully delivering messages from agents in Holland on three occasions. Went missing on fourth mission, while serving with the Royal Air Force in 1944."

NURP.41.A.2164, a.k.a. Dutch Coast
Date of award: March 1945
"For delivering an SOS, from a ditched air crew close to the enemy coast, over a distance of 288 miles in 7½ hours under unfavourable conditions, while serving with the Royal Air Force in April 1942."

NURP.38.EGU.24, a.k.a. Commando
Date of award: March 1945
"For successfully delivering messages from agents in occupied France on three occasions—twice under exceptionally adverse conditions—while serving with the National Pigeon Service in 1942."

NURP.40.GVIS.453, a.k.a. Royal Blue
Date of award: March 1945
"For being the first pigeon in this war to deliver a message from a force-landed aircraft on the Continent, while serving with the Royal Air Force in October 1940."

NPS.43.29018, a.k.a. Ruhr Express
Date of award: May 1945
"For carrying an important message from the Ruhr Pocket in excellent time, while serving with the Royal Air Force in April 1945."

NPS.42.NS.15125, a.k.a. William of Orange
Date of award: May 1945
"For delivering a message from the Arnhem Airborne Operation in record time for any single pigeon, while serving with the Army Pigeon Service in September 1944."

**NPS.42.21610,
a.k.a. Scotch Lass**
Date of award: June 1945
"For bringing thirty-eight
microphotographs across the
North Sea in good time, although
injured, while serving with the
Royal Air Force in Holland in
September 1944."

NU.41.HQ.4373, a.k.a. Billy
Date of award: August 1945
"For delivering a message from
a force-landed bomber, while in
a state of complete collapse and
under exceptionally bad weather
conditions, while serving with
the RAF in 1942."

**41.BA.2793,
a.k.a. Broad Arrow**
Date of award: October 1945
"For bringing important
messages three times from
enemy-occupied country,
viz. May 1943, June 1943, and
August 1943, while serving
with the Special Service on the
Continent."

NPS.42.NS.2780, unnamed
Date of award: October 1945
"For bringing important
messages three times from
enemy-occupied country,
viz. July 1942, August 1942,
and April 1943, while serving
with the Special Service on
the Continent."

NPS.42.NS.7524, unnamed
Date of award: October 1945
"For bringing important
messages three times from
enemy-occupied country,
viz. July 1942, May 1943, and
July 1943, while serving with
the Special Service on the
Continent."

NPSNS.42.36392, a.k.a. Maquis
Date of award: October 1945
"For bringing important
messages three times from
enemy-occupied country,
viz. May 1943 (Amiens), February
1944 (Combined Operations),
and June 1944 (French Maquis),
while serving with the Special
Service on the Continent."

NURP.40.WCE.249, a.k.a. Mary
Date of award: November 1945
"For outstanding endurance
during war service in spite of
wounds."

**NURP.41.DHZ56,
a.k.a. Tommy**
Date of award: February 1946
"For delivering a valuable
message from Holland to
Lancashire under difficult
conditions, while serving with
the National Pigeon Service in
July 1942."

**NURP.39.SDS.39,
a.k.a. All Alone**
Date of award: February 1946
"For delivering an important
message in one day over a
distance of four hundred
miles, while serving with the
National Pigeon Service in
August 1943."

42WD593, a.k.a. Princess
Date of award: May 1946
"Sent on a special mission to
Crete, this pigeon returned to
her loft (Royal Air Force,
Alexandria) having travelled
about five hundred miles,
mostly over sea, with highly
valuable information. One of
the finest performances in
the war record of the Pigeon
Service."

**NURP.37.CEN.335,
a.k.a. Mercury**
Date of award: August 1946
"For carrying out a special task
involving a flight of 480 miles
from northern Denmark in July
1942, while serving with the
Special Section, Army Pigeon
Service."

NURP.38.BPC.6, unnamed
Date of award: August 1946
"For three outstanding
flights from France while
serving with the Special Section,
Army Pigeon Service, 11 July
1941, 9 September 1941, and 29
November 1941."

USA43SC6390, a.k.a. GI Joe
Date of award: August 1946
"This bird is credited with
making the most outstanding
flight by a US Army pigeon
in World War II. Making the
twenty-mile flight from
British 10th Army HQ in the
same number of minutes, it
brought a message that arrived
just in time to save at least a
hundred Allied soldiers from
being bombed by their own
planes."

**NURP.41.SBC.219,
a.k.a. Duke of Normandy**
Date of award: 8 January 1947
"For being the first bird to arrive
with a message from 21st Army
Group behind enemy lines on
D-Day, 6 June 1944, while serv-
ing with Army Pigeon Service."

NURP.43.CC.1418, unnamed
Date of award: 8 January 1947
"For the fastest flight with mes-
sage from 6th Airborne Division,
Normandy, 7 June 1944, while
serving with Army Pigeon
Service."

DD.43.T.139, unnamed
Date of award: February 1947
"During a heavy tropical storm,
this bird, in the service of the
Australian Army Signal Corps,
was released from Army Boat
1402 which had foundered on
Wadou Beach in the Huon Gulf.
Homing forty miles to Madang,
it brought a message which
enabled a rescue ship to be sent
in time to salvage the craft and
its valuable cargo of stores and
ammunition."

DD.43.Q.879, unnamed
Date of award: February 1947
"During an attack by the
Japanese on a US Marine
Corps patrol on Manus Island,
pigeons in the service of the
Australian Army Signal Corps
were released to warn headquarters of an impending enemy
counterattack. Two were shot
down but DD.43.Q.879 reached
HQ despite heavy fire directed
at it, with the result that enemy
concentrations were bombed
and the patrol extricated."

**NURP39.NPS.144,
a.k.a. Cologne**
Date of award: unknown
"For homing from an aircraft
that disappeared over Cologne,
although seriously wounded,
while serving with the RAF in
1943."

Horses

Olga
Date of award: 11 April 1947
"On duty when a flying bomb
demolished four houses in
Tooting and a plate-glass
window crashed immediately in
front of her. Olga, after bolting

for a hundred yards, returned
to the scene of the incident and
remained on duty with her rider,
controlling traffic and assisting
rescue organisations."

Upstart
Date of award: 11 April 1947
"While on patrol duty in Bethnal
Green, a flying bomb exploded
within seventy-five yards, show-
ering both horse and rider with
broken glass and debris. Upstart
was completely unperturbed and
remained quietly on duty with
his rider, controlling traffic, etc.,
until the incident had been dealt
with."

Regal
Date of award: 11 April 1947
"Was twice in burning stables
caused by explosive incendiar-
ies at Muswell Hill. Although
receiving minor injuries, being
covered by debris, and close to
the flames, this horse showed no
signs of panic."

Cats

Simon
Date of award: August 1949
"Served on HMS *Amethyst*
during the Yangtze Incident,
disposing of many rats though
wounded by shell blast.
Throughout the incident, his
behaviour was of the highest
order."

*The data above has been supplied by
the PDSA. We have in some cases
amended the information for consistency and clarity. It has, however,
not always been possible to confirm
certain specifics, including the exact
dates of some of the awards.*

LEFTOVERS / SURPLUS MEANING
George Scheer & Stephanie Sherman

"Leftovers" investigates the cultural significance of detritus.

———

By 2003, downtown Greensboro, North Carolina, was so sleepy that on Sundays you could play tennis in the middle of the street. The turn-of-the-century buildings—three stories high in short blocks along Elm Street, the main drag—were mostly vacant. During the weekdays, however, there was still some activity. Mr. Kindley took orders from his desk at his office furniture showroom. Bill at Coe's Grocery and Seed sold tomato plants, Cheerwine soda, 40s, and cigarettes for under three dollars. Every morning at 6:30 on the dot, Jack Wagner picked up a copy of the *News and Record* from the box on the corner. Around 10:30, Ralph and his son Mike dragged their used appliances onto the street corner. Blumenthal's neon signs still advertised an old deal: a chance to win a free pack of cigarettes with the purchase of work wear. Occasionally around noon, a truck pulled up to deliver a piano to John Foy's shop for repair. By 5:30, the owners of the antique stores and picture galleries were on their way home, and Juanita at Deal Printing was closing up her offices. People shuttling to and from the nearby Urban Ministries shelter in the late evening kept an eye on the otherwise empty streets.

It wasn't always this way. In 1939—the year that a tornado touched down on the 600 block—Sylvia and Joe Gray bought a three-story building at 606 South Elm Street in the heart of a bustling downtown. Joe was a playful New Yorker who took up the family business, driving his father on sales

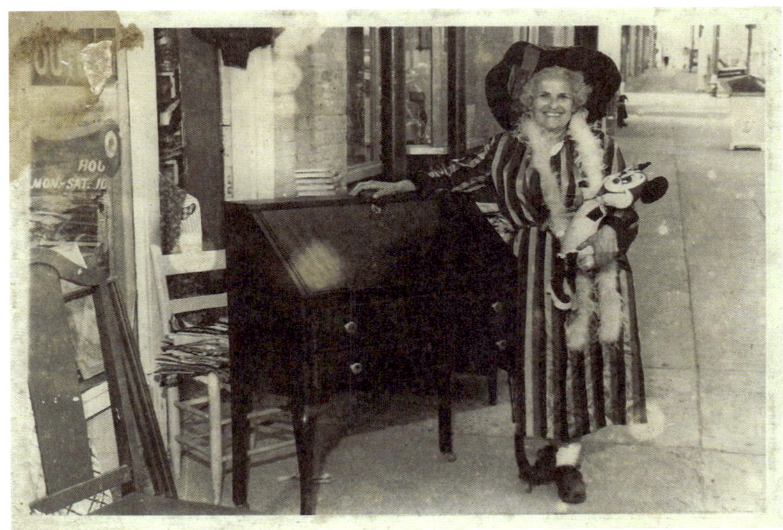

Sylvia Gray in front of her surplus store, ca. 1978. All images courtesy George Scheer.

excursions between New York and Raleigh. Realizing delivery trucks full of new North Carolina furniture were returning from New York empty, Joe began buying up repossessed furniture and shipping it to North Carolina for repair and resale. That's how Joe had ended up resettling his father, mother, and brother Mel in the South, where he met Sylvia, a Southern Jewish beauty from Mt. Airy, North Carolina. The two courted, married, and their love took shape through their surplus store, the Carolina Sales Company. At first, they sold furniture, and later work wear and Army-Navy surplus, on the first floor; they kept a boarding house on the second, and, for a short time, lived on the third beside the business office and repair shop. They worked as a team. He played the front man, corresponding with customers, merchants, wholesalers, and dealers. She kept to the margins—managing the books, inventories, and accounts of shipping costs, CODs, lot payments, and sales contracts. His name was signed to every invoice; her chicken scratch covered the surface of every receipt.

The young couple had their first child, a daughter, as World War II reached its height. Their second, a son, arrived just as the war was coming to a close. At this time, manufacturing industries across the country began transitioning from war production to domestic markets. Sylvia and Joe's business shifted to accommodate the vast quantity of surplus flowing freely as postwar salvage from the War Department. Leftover gear from training depots at military bases in Pennsylvania, Georgia, and North Carolina was sold in wholesale lots by bid. War suppliers, such as the Georgia Shoe Manufacturing Company in Flowery Branch, Georgia, converted to national retail, selling paratrooper boots under the name "Pair-A-Trooper" for the consumer market. The surplus store served as a storefront and storehouse for pup tents, outfits, mess kits, canteens, wool mummy sleeping bags with poplin covers, jungle hammocks, rucksacks with metal frames, entrenching shovels, boots, pistol belts, and musette bags. On the third floor of 606 South Elm Street, Joe and Sylvia cut and pasted product illustrations to make catalogues for distribution to scoutmasters, hospitals, and hotels throughout the nation.

The surplus store developed in a period of economic transition from

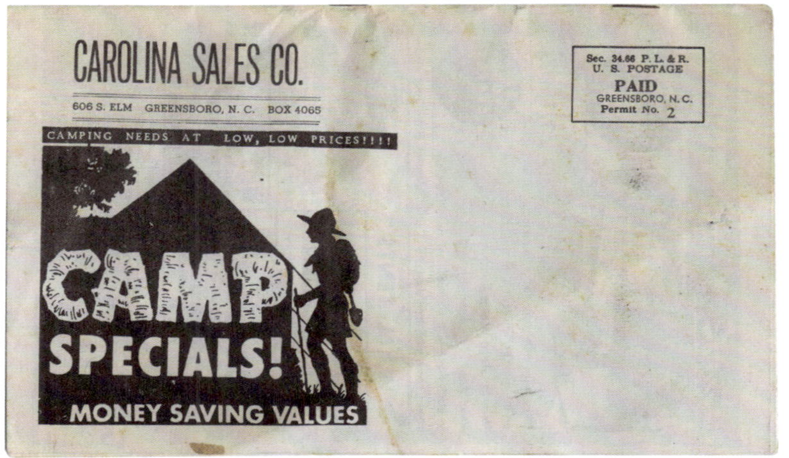

From war materiel to camping gear. Undated sales catalogue from the Carolina Sales Co.

the leftovers of post-Depression war production to the 1950s boom of newness and domestic convenience. From 1945 to 1955, the American economy avoided post-war woes by spilling its war excess into the domestic market. Joe and Sylvia joined a predominantly Jewish network of national and international suppliers, manufacturers, and wholesalers participating in the Army-Navy surplus trade. They purchased blind lots and seconds—defective or imperfect merchandise—as well as wholesale goods and novelties for resale to Boy Scout troops around the country. A litany of competing catalogues, trade magazines, and advertisements attested to the growth of a leisure market based on naturalist adventures.

Joe's unexpected heart attack in 1955 left Sylvia with three children. His death marks a rupture in the surplus store's business archive. Invoices give way to condolence cards, the flurry of correspondence and sales of military inventories slows. In 1959, she's still purchasing window card advertisements for the surplus store from Deal Printing a few doors down. The tradition of buying surplus inventories would be continued under her watch, albeit in a multitude of forms. The war surplus shifted to textiles, thousands of bolts of fabric and upholstery, notions, buttons, ribbon cuttings, and threads, all bought from factory floors. Then women's wear, including Sunday hats, gloves, dresses, blouses, blazers, shoes, costume jewelry, suits, and ties. Some appliances, some kitchenware, some housewares. And then dolls, toys, books, and games. She brought in knickknacks and curios, everything really, one of everything, sometimes two or three, all somewhere between thrift and antique. When she died in 1997, her mountains of things filled the three-story building, leaving only a small footpath. The downtown store was locked up in the mostly abandoned city center. There, the flotsam and jetsam of economic overproduction and industrial excess—its materials, fantasies, and fictions—remained.

. . .

Greensboro sits in the Piedmont Triad, a regional flatland containing a cluster of cities three hours' drive from both the mountains and the coast. The city was founded as the county seat in 1808 on a swampy plot of land poorly chosen for its exact geographical centrality within both Guilford county and North Carolina. Settled by Quakers, Presbyterians, and eventually Jews, the city celebrated progressive growth through new educational institutions, most no more than a mile from the downtown city center. Guilford College was founded by the Quakers in the 1830s, followed by Bennett College, an African American women's college founded in 1873; the Agricultural and Mechanical College for the Colored Race (today known as North Carolina A&T), a land-grant institution, opened in 1891; and 1892 saw the establishment of another women's college, the University of North Carolina at Greensboro. Though it had no river or other distinguishable natural features promoting trade and exchange, the creation of an east–west rail line in 1865 across the state facilitated Greensboro's push to become a hub of commerce and industry.

Though textiles, cotton, and tobacco had long been staples in the region, it was Moses and Caesar Cone, Jewish brothers from Baltimore, who established Cone Denim at Proximity Mills in 1895 and quickly made Greensboro the world leader in denim production. It wasn't just manufacturing that made Greensboro a production and distribution hub. Between 1943 and 1946, over three hundred thousand soldiers received basic training at the Overseas Replacement Depot (ORD) before being shipped to the European and Asian theaters. For a brief three years, Greensboro became a global stopover for departures and, less frequently, returns. Shortly after the war, those same warehouse facilities and bases, located on a train spur off East Market Street, were purchased by Lorillard Tobacco, which grew into a national brand by packaging and selling the local crop.

On the south side of Greensboro, Joe and Sylvia's surplus store was part of a growing sector of jobbing houses (a manufacturers' distributor) with new national and international reach. Joe bought wholesale from a diverse set of suppliers, accessing

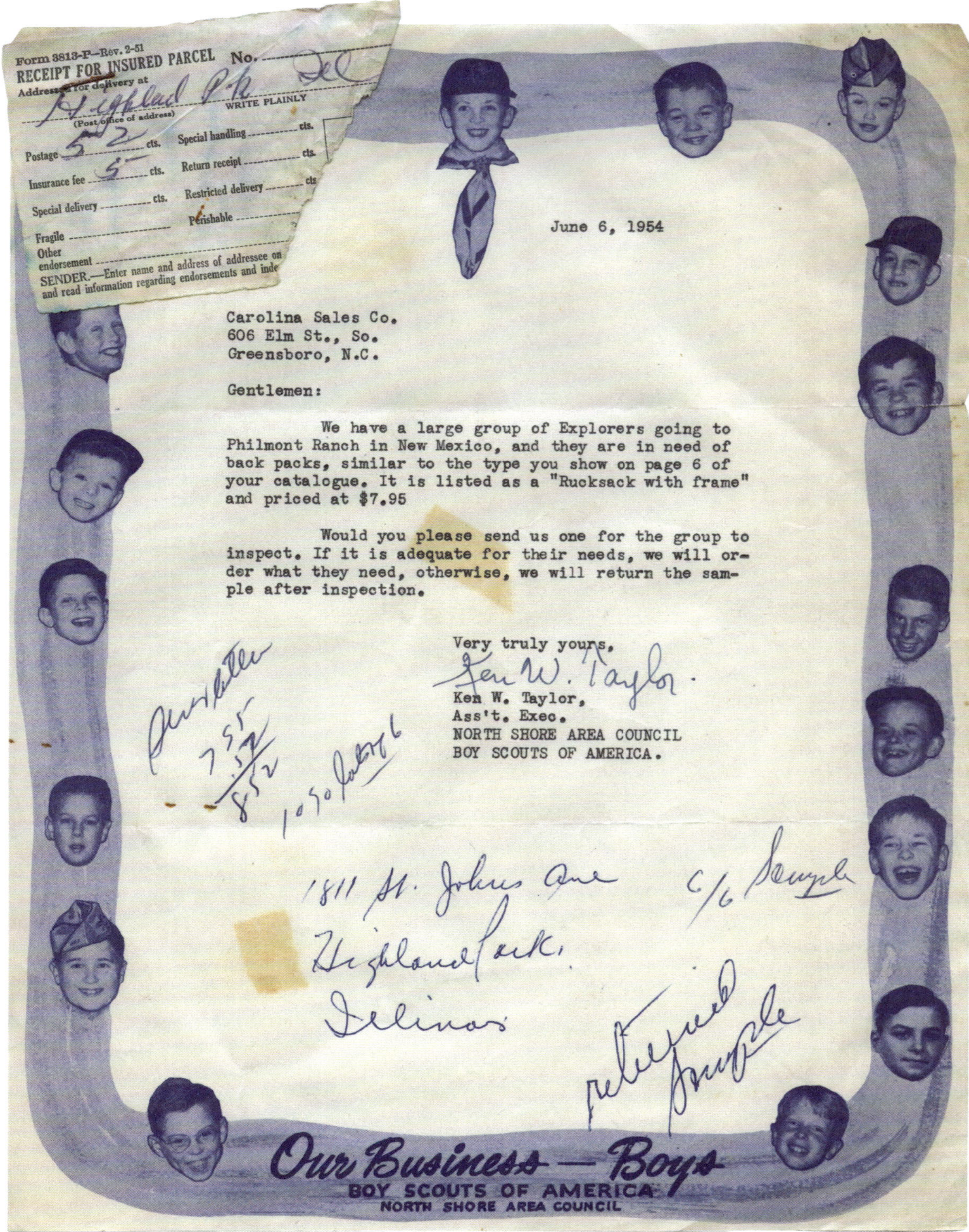

1954 letter from an Illinois council of the Boy Scouts of America asking for a sample rucksack.

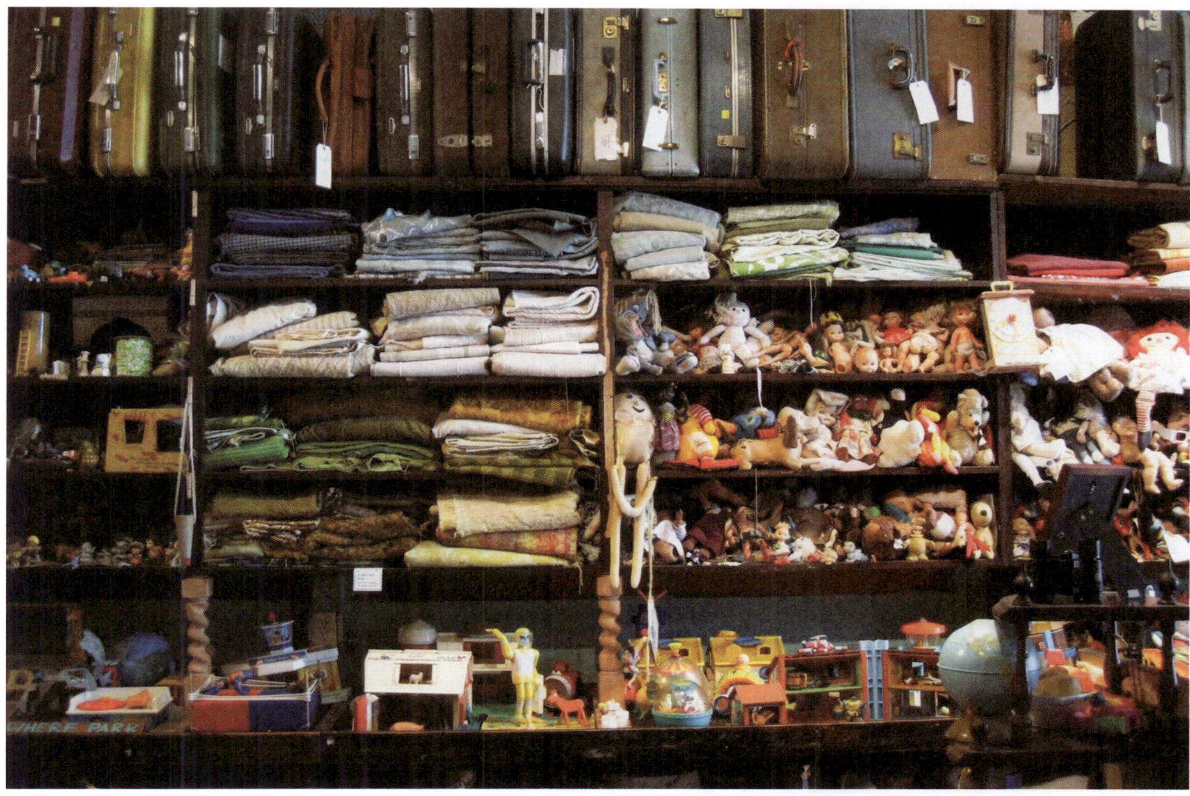

Nothing for sale. The store's inventory, rearranged after Sylvia Gray's death to become the material basis for Elsewhere.

global goods for a new generation of rugged adventurers pursuing nature with the spoils that the war industry had left behind. He monitored listings of government sales, public auctions, and surplus bids, and kept the addresses of disposal and salvage officers at naval bases in Quonset, Rhode Island; Charleston, South Carolina; Norfolk, Virginia; Memphis, Tennessee; and Parris Island, South Carolina. On 3 March 1949, for example, the quartermaster at Fort Bragg, North Carolina, issued him an invitation to bid on the "sale of property and waste material." In June of that year, Joe purchased a "lot of watches, clocks, and miscellaneous" from the salvage officer at Fort Belvoir, Virginia. Joe also bought goods directly from manufacturers: thirteen pairs of Pair-A-Trooper boots for $78 from Georgia Shoe Manufacturing Company, and $22.50 for six dozen sateen cargo pocket

fatigue trousers from Brooks-Miller in Chicago. Colonial Knife Company in Providence invoices him for several dozen pocket knives. Meanwhile, he is also collecting the catalogues, advertisements, and illustrations of dozens of competing surplus businesses: H. Rosenberg at the Broadway Mercantile Co. at 647 Broadway "near Bleecker Street" buys and sells army surplus, work clothes, and camping equipment, while Robert Goldberg at Hoosier Tarpaulin & Canvas Goods in Indianapolis lists over thirty sizes of "DeLux Tarpaulins." A repair-and-resell spirit championed the durability of American-made originals and promised any small town businessperson a voice in the market. The Grays' surplus store took up this commercial call in its motto: "Pay Less for More."

Joe fielded hundreds of letters from scoutmasters requesting orders and merchandise samples.

Ken Taylor, assistant executive of the North Shore Area Council of the Boy Scouts of America, writes, "We have a large group of Explorers going to Philmont Ranch in New Mexico, and they are in need of back packs." He wants to order one Brooks-Miller Co. "rucksack with frame" for the troop to inspect. Hundreds of similar requests pour in from small towns throughout the country. Scoutmaster Floyd Young of Troop 98 in Mendon, Ohio, scrawls an order for outfits, tents, mess kits, canteens, and sleeping bags, including tax to total $30.35. "Well pleased with the goods," Young makes an additional request less than a month later. Reports of sales of the "Scout Knife," "Scout Knapsack," and "Scout Ax" reach the desk of Arthur McKinney, assistant to the Chief Scout Executive, at 2 Park Avenue in New York City, who demands Joe and Sylvia cease using the term. In his letter, he reminds

them that "when the Congress of the United States incorporated the Boy Scouts of America, it gave to us the sole right to the use of such terms as Scout, Scouter…"

Sylvia continued to run her downtown store after Joe's passing. Over the next twenty years, the city would undergo tremendous disinvestment through white flight and suburbanization. Cone had begun selling off the mill villages as early as the 1940s. The third generation of mill children, who grew up in the villages and walked downtown for treats and entertainment, watched as their houses were sold and carried away by trucks. Warnersville, a historically black neighborhood built by ex-slaves in 1867 on land sold to them by a Quaker, gave way to housing projects for the low-income elderly, set along an overbuilt highway designed to become a gateway into the city center. In 1970, Murrow Boulevard, another five-lane, underutilized, inner highway—named for the esteemed newsman Edward R. Murrow, who was born in Greensboro—effectively divided East Greensboro, a predominantly African American neighborhood, from the downtown core. The roadway cut through and segregated the once-dense urban landscape that the A&T Four walked through toward their famous Woolworth's lunch counter sit-in. Everywhere, shopping centers with inflated roadways built to accommodate suburban mobility progressively recentered business activity in an ever-widening radius outside of downtown. As each shopping center was anchored by a supermarket, the downtown core became a food desert. Despite this catastrophic decline, a few businesses managed to maintain life downtown, but most of the dedicated corner shopkeepers, small business owners, food vendors, antique dealers, and resident and neighborhood associations folded during this period. Aside from Blumenthal's,

Deal Printing, and Schiffman's Jewelry, no other business spanned the decades from war to millennium.

By the 1980s, the store—known by her grandchildren as "GG's store"—was a little-regarded and intermittently patronized mountain of surplus within the "Old Greensborough" arts and antique district. Sylvia was a child of the Depression, so everything had use, reuse, or resale value. She shopped every day at the Salvation Army and Goodwill down the street, and collected leftovers from the local Jewish community and estate sale remains. Perhaps she shopped to remember what she had, or to fulfill some quest. Inside the store, inventories were everywhere. Things were stacked and piled, or preserved inside plastic bags tied with ribbon and strung one to the next. She would cut buttons off clothes and string them together and put them in jars because they were worth more that way. Everywhere, hangers were hung with three or more items, every shelf was heaped with things, as far up as she could reach. She preferred you didn't browse. Instead, she asked what you wanted and would scurry off to find it. If Sylvia liked you, it would be cheap. If she didn't, she wouldn't sell. If you tried to haggle, she would refuse. She knew where everything was. When the fire marshal planned to conduct his annual visit, he would call ahead, and Mrs. Gray's sons would come over to clear a three-foot aisle. She sat by the front, reading, sitting, talking on the phone, keeping the books. Sylvia went to work until the day before she died, three days after her eightieth birthday, on 23 April 1997.

For six years, the store sat. Every Thanksgiving, the family came together and visited it. Every now and then, someone who had come to retrieve a piece of furniture or gather what they needed for a Halloween costume would wander through the musty labyrinth of recollections, but

it remained a time capsule. Sylvia's children didn't know what to do with it. The overwhelming amount of materials, the memory of their mother, and limited demand for downtown real estate prevented them from taking action. And of course it was possible that amid the seeming junk lay exceptional antiques and vintage artifacts. On closer inspection, this turned out not to be the case. Instead, the store contained a multitude of misprints, kitsch relics, and reproductions, each item a particular oddity and a special case. The store was in fact a cultural treasure, an imperfect archive of everyday materials from across the decades.

In 2003, Sylvia's grandson George and his friend Stephanie, writers of collaborative fictions and co-authors of this text, resettled the old store with a group of artists and musicians. We began with a simple declaration, "nothing for sale," and set out to explore different orders of value through the endless arrangement of Sylvia's puzzle. In the old store, we camped, cooked, played, thought, sorted, moved things around. We untangled decades of cultural detritus, discovering the myriad characters, stories, and histories hidden in the collection. This world beyond words delivered an unfolding storybook written with objects. More and more people—artists, shoppers, neighbors, and visitors—passed by and through. As Greensboro began to benefit from the national urban turn and from a developing cultural economy in its downtown, the old store took on new meaning as project space, anchor, and destination. The place, which we named Elsewhere, is a living museum, endlessly reinvesting its surplus in new ideas and formations built from the same old things.

INGESTION / FISHING FOR VITAMIN A
Sasha Archibald

"Ingestion" is a column that explores its topic within a framework informed by history, aesthetics, and philosophy.

———

The currency of the Cook Islands depicts the goddess Ina, who, during a long journey on the back of a shark, suffered a lapse of manners and relieved herself without dismounting. Ina's urine, the myth explains, is the cause of the pungent odor and foul taste of shark flesh. Indeed, a California shark fisherman remembers that whenever his boat arrived in the harbor, "people would fall down," so nauseating was the smell.[1] No wonder that aside from the Asian delicacy of shark's fin soup (which is said not to taste of shark at all), sharks are rarely eaten: monsters and trophies *par excellence*, but rarely offered as dinner plate fare.

Yet, for a brief period in the 1940s, sharks became a prized catch, their innards destined for human consumption. Independent fishermen dropped tuna, salmon, and cod and took up "sharking," while existing fisheries adapted their assembly lines and new ones sprang up, hastily built on spindly wooden piers. Sharks rarely venture as far north as Alaska, but in all other major fishing towns of the American Pacific coast—San Pedro, Santa Barbara, Tomales Bay, San Francisco, Astoria, and Seattle—as well as in the Scottish New Hebrides, shark hauls between 1943 and 1949 fetched legendary prices.

The princely profits came not from fillets or fins, but from oil extracted from the shark's liver, an expansive hunk of viscera rich in vitamin A. Comprising up to a quarter of a shark's weight and 90% of its body

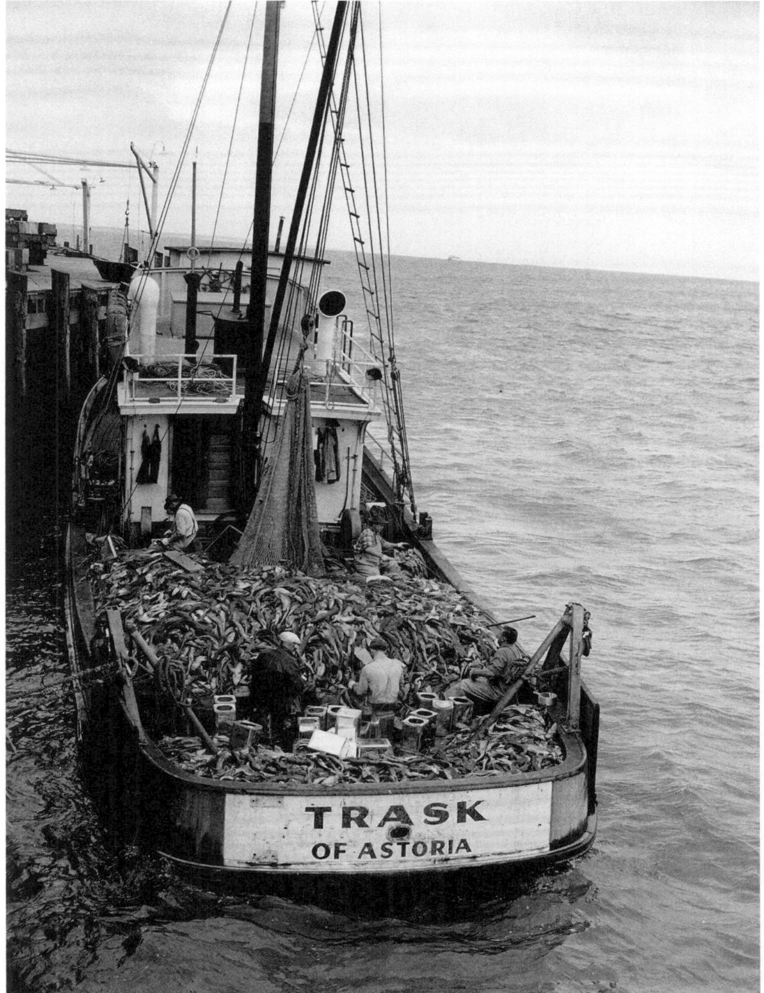

George Moskovita and his crew with a haul of soupfin sharks aboard the *Trask of Astoria*, Astoria, Oregon, 1948. Courtesy Columbia River Maritime Museum.

cavity, a shark's liver is proportionally the largest in the world, gorged with lipids that keep the animal buoyant and supply it with energy during migratory journeys. It is because of its extraordinary liver that the giant basking shark is able to glide along the ocean surface, mouth agape, for miles at a stretch—a prehistoric sea monster skimming plankton with a maw as tall as a child.

The self-published memoir of George Moskovita, a lifelong fisherman born in the San Juan Islands to an Irish mother and a Yugoslav father, describes his 1940s shark liver business.[2] Moskovita operated

out of Astoria, a fishing town at the northwestern tip of Oregon. Situated directly on the mouth of the Columbia River, Astoria was at the time teeming with industrious fishermen and Chinese- and Scandinavian-born fish packers. Moskovita began his career catching soupfin shark, sometimes called dogfish, by laying out cotton netting, about a mile's worth, and suspending the vertical nets roughly fifty feet below the water surface using a combination of weights and submerged aluminum or glass floats.[3] (Fishermen in this era contended with few restrictions except the territorial ire of other fishermen; Moksovita's

underwater floats allowed boats to pass overhead, unencumbered by his equipment.) The nets were pulled up after a storm—pods of soupfin cover more territory during foul weather—and otherwise once a week. On a bad day, the catch was small, or eels had found it first. Consuming only the livers, eels could quickly worm their way through a bulging net. A hundred sharks, Moskovita remembers, was a decent haul. When the catch was large, the fishermen worked through the night, winching the nets by hand to heave their fortune on board.

A second memoir about 1940s shark fishing, Gavin Maxwell's *Harpoon Venture*, details a very different process. The setting is the Scottish New Hebrides, where the industry was confined to the Herculean efforts of Maxwell himself. Whereas Moskovita was a pragmatic fisherman, Maxwell was a hunter casting about for a capitalist venture that might justify his appetite for killing large sharks. His obsession was seeded by a momentous encounter with a basking shark in 1944: after a brief moment of awe, Maxwell opened fire with a Breda light machine gun, discharging three hundred rounds "straight into the huge expanse of the flank," while his helmsman gouged the shark's fin for good measure.[4] Nonetheless, the shark managed to swim away, seemingly impervious to an automatic weapon. The animal that foils the hunter is often the same on which the hunter fixates, and Maxwell, true to rule, spontaneously sank his substantial inheritance into opening a shark fishery. Lured by an oil buyer who promised £50 for a ton of shark oil—a price that would more than double in the following two years—Maxwell purchased the entire island of Soay, and proceeded to outfit a fleet, construct a factory, design equipment, and enlist the (dubious) local workforce.[5] Killing the sharks was no easy matter but transporting the carcasses from sea to factory proved equally formidable; an early

attempt to lift a seven-ton shark by crane seemed to work until the animal abruptly tore in two, its back half dangling in the air as its front crashed down in a shower of entrails. (Maxwell described the sound as that of a rotten stick snapping in half, except much louder.) Eventually, Maxwell developed a system for laying out rows of dead sharks along the tide line until the harbor's concrete pilings were "swimming in oil and blood and littered with gigantic piles of offal."[6] He never, however, managed to make his processing plant profitable; *Harpoon Venture* reads as a case study of industrial failure.

Moskovita, on the other hand, made a decent living. A soupfin liver weighs about five pounds, and the price per pound leaped from twenty cents in 1937 to eighteen dollars in 1949.[7] At peak market value, the liver of a single shark would be worth nearly one thousand dollars today. The livers were packed into five-gallon cans, which were tested for potency in a process called "stovepiping." Drilling down the center of the can, stovepipers sent a sample

of the contents off for analysis. The darker the livers, the more valuable the can; light-colored livers were often discarded for fear they would degrade the price of the entire lot. Based on the lab results, the price was fixed and the livers sold. The cans were frozen and shipped to various processing plants where the raw livers were centrifuged to yield squalene, the technical term for shark liver oil.

It is tricky to put a definitive dollar value on the shark liver industry, given that market prices were volatile and catches unrecorded. An exhibit at the Columbia River Maritime Museum, however, suggests that in 1943 in the state of Oregon alone, some 270,000 pounds of shark liver, or about 65,000 sharks, were taken, representing a value of 5 million dollars, or in today's currency, something like 68 million dollars.[8] The sum is difficult to square with today's Astoria: a faded town, desolate in the winter rain, the relics of its waterfront industry corroded by salty winds or dissipated in spectacular fires. Only oblique hints remain of Astoria's one-time splendor,

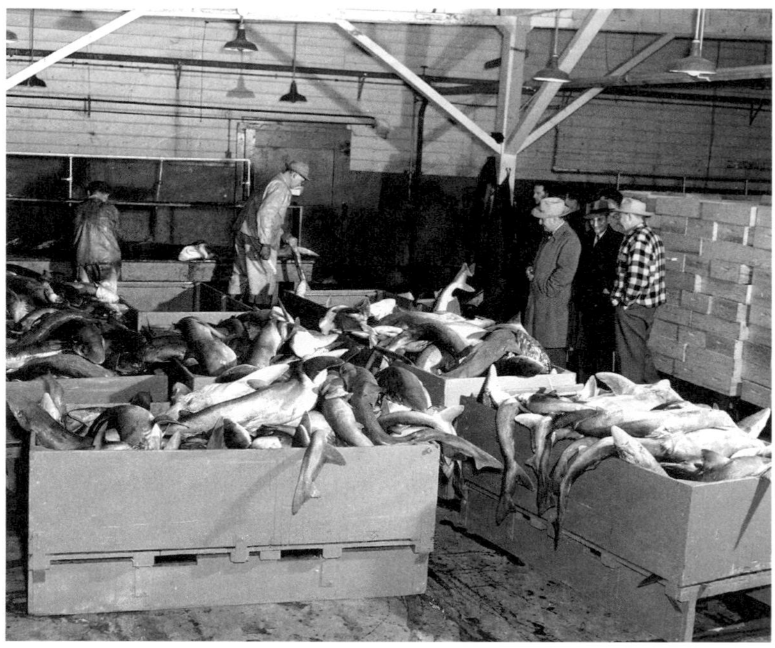

Soupfin sharks being processed in Astoria, Oregon. Courtesy Columbia River Maritime Museum.

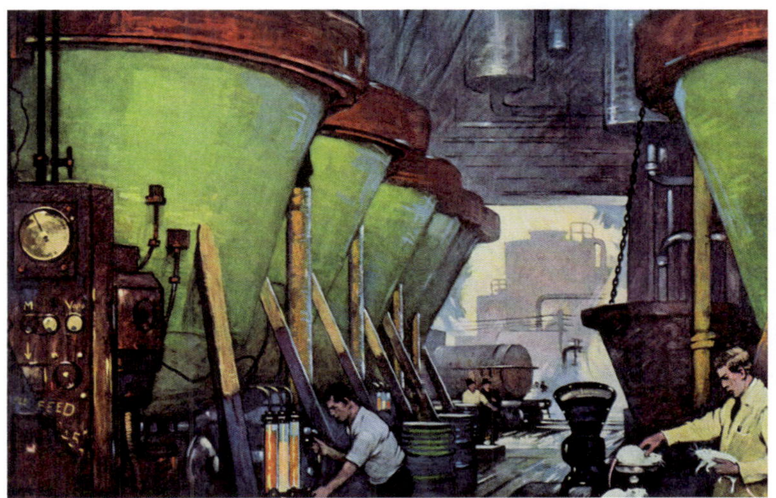

National Geographic depiction of a factory separating vitamin A from shark liver oil, 1945. Note the rats on which the vitamin A is tested. Illustration by Thornton Oakley.

a near-mythical era of prosperity paid for by old-growth timber and loads of fish so heavy fishermen had to be wary of sinking their own boats. The explorers Lewis and Clark, however, wouldn't have been surprised. Astoria was the final endpoint of their westward journey and their makeshift home for several months. They described the area with wonder as a place where the inhabitants subsisted on fish, but never actually went fishing, so amply could they be fed by the sturgeon, whale, and salmon that serendipitously washed up on shore.[9]

Moskovita and Maxwell agreed that the profit to be made from a shark was all in the liver —"The shark's liver is the elephant's ivory," wrote Maxwell.[10] Shark industry enthusiasts suggested markets for the residuals—the skin could be made into shoes; the backbones into walking sticks; the eyes, varnished and lacquered, into trinkets; the flesh into dog food—but the demand for livers was at such a pitch that there was little incentive to use the whole animal.[11] Astoria fishermen managed to sell some shark to local Oregon mink farms—minks happily eat shark entrails—but generally the liver-stripped carcass was returned to the water. In the usual routine, fishermen

ended their workday sitting on overturned buckets amid mounds of putrid flesh, knife in hand for the "livering." Each shark was handled one by one: white belly slit, liver removed, carcass tossed overboard. A photo shows Moskovita—his nickname was "Musky"—standing amid piles of shark, their livers ghoulishly draped over his open palms.

The surge in shark prices was an effect of World War II. A dose of Norwegian cod liver oil was a US household routine in the 1930s and 1940s and war interrupted America's imports. (Britain responded to the crisis by diluting their existing stock with whale oil.[12)] Wartime rhetoric and a credulous zeal for vitamins turned the shortage into a crisis. Scientists had begun to discover vitamins in the first decades of the century, and it didn't take long for American "vitamania" to take hold. Mothers supplied their children with supplements, the government supplied its military, and employers supplied their workers. Articles in the popular press claimed that vitamin A was particularly crucial for pilots, who needed superior vision to execute nighttime bombing missions. The novelty of vitamins combined with American war jingoism to create the impression that

shark-derived vitamin A worked like a magic tonic. It seemed plausible to readers of *National Geographic* and *Popular Mechanics* that a vitamin pill could turn a sluggish worker into a gleaming robot and an ordinary pilot into a bionic-vision superhero.

Such hyperbole contained a grain of fact. It had been known for centuries that liver oil could instantly cure night blindness. A mid-nineteenth-century medical text describes nyctalopia, which disproportionately afflicted soldiers, sailors, and prisoners, as one in which the patient "is unable to discriminate the largest objects after sunset or by moonlight; he gropes his way like a blind man, stumbles against any person or thing placed in his footsteps."[13] Traditional remedies included administering liver oil directly to the eye—in Chinese medicine the raw liver was squeezed to yield medicinal eye drops—or preparing a liver feast, or a combination of both: Ancient Egyptians ate liver, but also prescribed pressing roasted ox liver to the eye. Inhabitants of Newfoundland were instructed to lean over the frying pan as their liver dinner sizzled.[14] Cod liver oil worked equally well; long before vitamin A was isolated in 1920, studies that tracked the incidence of night blindness (and the associated corneal lesions, diarrhea, and leathery skin) among impoverished children in Russia, Japan, Denmark, and various countries in Africa suggested that the affliction could be miraculously healed, sometimes in a few hours, by a single dose of foul-smelling oil.

Perhaps World War II pilots were truly at risk of suffering from vitamin A deficiency, or perhaps the American public was duped into believing that the gains of vitamin A were commensurate with the dosage—an enduring quackery that has sold many vitamins. Vitamin A has a wondrous effect in cases of nutritional deficiency, but in most instances it has none at all, the placebo effect notwithstanding. There is even the danger of adverse

results. All except the most exorbitant doses of water-soluble vitamins—vitamin C and the multiple forms of vitamin B—can be eliminated through urine and perspiration, whereas excess amounts of vitamin A are simply banked in the liver. The liver has a limited capacity, however, such that it is possible to become ill or even die from liver cirrhosis induced by vitamin A poisoning. Eskimos knew to avoid the liver of a bear or arctic fox—a dose of vitamin A so potent it could be fatal—but such wisdom was lost amid twentieth-century vitamania. In 1974, a London health fanatic, Basil Brown, died of what the coroner described as "carrot juice addiction."[15]

The shark liver oil boom was also a consequence of chemical companies—prototypes of today's pharmaceutical firms—who were aggressively forging relationships with food manufacturers via the "discovery" of vitamins. "Vitamin research," writes historian Kendra Smith-Howard, "transformed the way in which Americans evaluated foods' health value."[16] Food companies jumped to use vitamin science to promote their products, an understandable hook that quickly veered into more questionable territory. Declaring the vitamin content of a food segued into tampering with the food product itself—using additives to enhance the vitamin load—until, eventually, even concocted foodstuffs could acquire the sheen of vitamin-rich wholesomeness. Margarine was a case in point. In the early decades of the twentieth century, margarine was considered a poor man's substitute for butter, less tasty and less healthful than the real thing. No one who could afford butter ate margarine, and several states even required that margarine be dyed pink so as to prevent accidental consumption of the counterfeit. Margarine fortified with vitamin A, however, proved a horse of a different color. Entering the market in 1938 and widely endorsed by nutritionists, the same hydrogenated lard now radiated health. Real butter, especially that made from cows fed alfalfa, is also resplendent in vitamin A, and yet the perceived value of the additive trumped the product that needed no additive, and margarine sales soared.

Ventures in vitamin marketing were immeasurably helped by the development in 1947 of synthetic vitamin A. The invention may have been compelled by the food industry—no one could find a way to rid shark oil of its stink—or perhaps it was a quick response to a dwindling supply of sharks. Indeed, anecdotal reports suggest that the Pacific coast soupfin had been nearly fished to

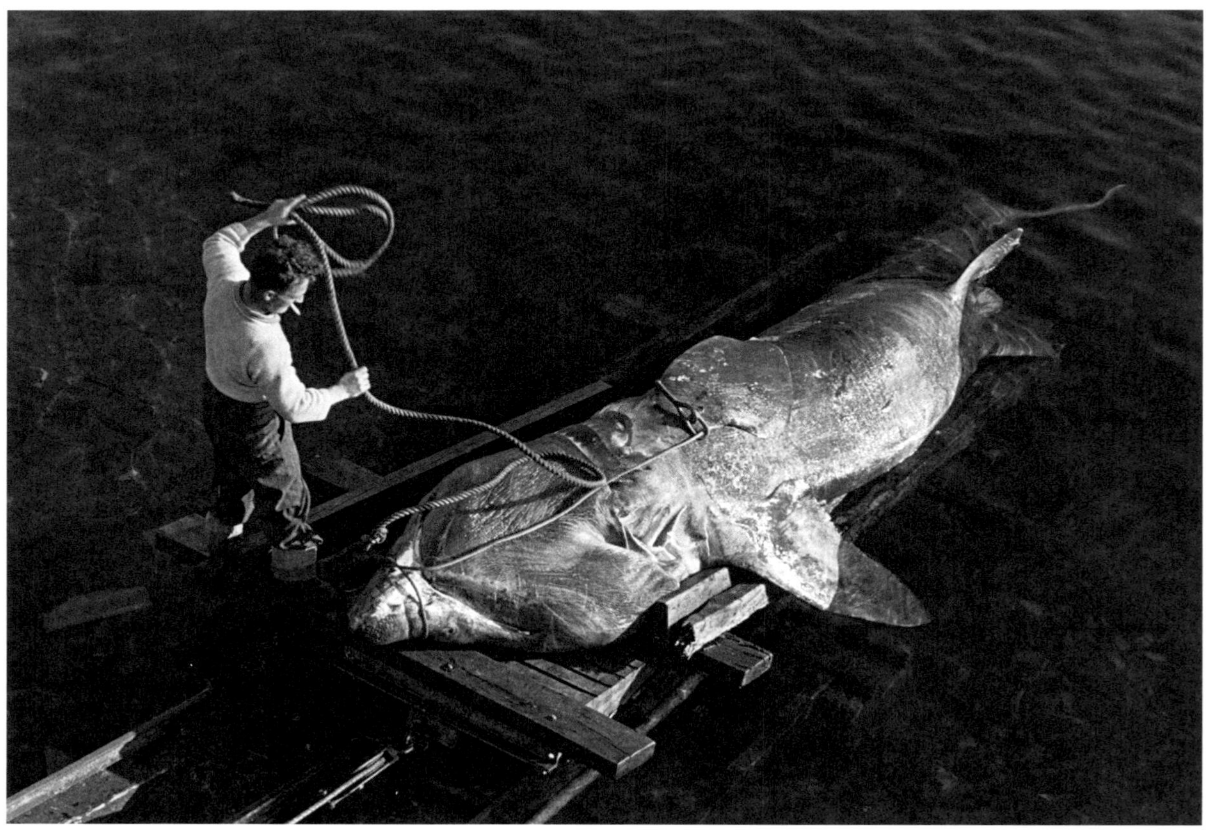

Gavin Maxwell basking in the glory of a shark kill, 1946. Photo Raymond Kleboe.

exhaustion in less than a decade. In any case, synthetic vitamin A flooded the market, cod liver oil was back on American grocery store shelves, and sharking became a thing of the past.[17] The price of shark liver plummeted: $18 a pound in 1949 to $1.80 a pound a year later. A report in June 1950 by the Oregon Fish and Wildlife Commission found not a single fisherman pursuing shark.

Maxwell abandoned his Soay basking shark operation the same year Oregon fishermen turned to other prey. His book about the venture became a bestseller, and launched Maxwell's career as a writer of natural history. Of what he tenderly called "my pathetic ruined little factory," Maxwell wrote: "I remember it with nostalgia for something beautiful and lost, the Island Valley of Avalon to which there can be no true return, no second spring."[18] Indeed, Maxwell's shark fishery, like Astoria's "movie-star incomes," proved to be an evanescent flicker.[19] "We were wrecked on the sheltering rock of our own harbor," lamented Maxwell, but his wistfulness earns no sympathy.[20] Only a fool mistakes a slaughtered animal for a sheltering rock.

1 Ethan Steward and Nick Welsh, "World War II, Santa Barbara's Waterfront, and 2,000 Shark Livers a Day," *The Santa Barbara Independent*, 14 August 2008.

2 George Moskovita, *Living Off the Pacific Ocean Floor* (Astoria, Oregon: self-published, 2000). The book, which is out of print, has just been reissued by Oregon State University Press.

3 Moskovita purchased discarded nets on the cheap from Astoria's salmon packers; an average-sized salmon could slip through gaps that would ensnare a soupfin. Such driftnets were subsequently nicknamed "the curtain of death." Moskovita writes that it was a nuisance when the nets pulled up anything besides soupfin, including other shark species. The catch was only as good as what could be sold on the dock, and everything else was discarded.

4 Gavin Maxwell, *Harpoon Venture* (New York: Lyons & Burford, 1996), pp. 14–15. See also Robert Macfarlane, "Shark Attack: Gavin Maxwell's Harpoon at a Venture," *The Guardian*, 19 July 2014.

5 Gavin Maxwell, *Harpoon Venture*, p. 27. The price may seem low, but two of Maxwell's large basking sharks would yield close to a ton of oil.

6 Gavin Maxwell, *Harpoon Venture*, p. 155.

7 Sigurd J. Westrheim, "The 1949 Soupfin Shark Fishery of Oregon," *Fish Commission Research Briefs*, vol. 3, no. 1 (September 1950), p. 40. Special thanks to Carmel Finley for sharing her research.

8 Figures from Columbia River Maritime Museum exhibition text. The museum has based this calculation on a price of $18.50 per pound of oil. It is unclear why they have done so as Sigurd Westrheim's official report for the Fish Commission of Oregon asserts that prices peaked at $18 per pound in 1949. The statistics on pounds of liver caught in 1943 does comport with the Fish Commission report, however; see Sigurd J. Westrheim, "The 1949 Soupfin Shark Fishery of Oregon," p. 39. Currency translation calculated by the author at <www.measuringworth.com>.

9 "Their food is principally fish that is thrown on the Shores by the Seas & left by the tide." William Clark, journal entry of 8 January 1806, in *The Journals of the Lewis and Clark Expedition*, University of Nebraska Press / University of Nebraska-Lincoln Libraries-Electronic Text Center. Available at <lewisandclarkjournals.unl.edu>. The tribes built boats, but used them only to bury their dead at sea.

10 Gavin Maxwell, *Harpoon Venture*, p. 85.

11 "Boom in Shark Fishing: Source of Vitamins," *The Science News-Letter*, vol. 42, no. 9 (29 August 1942), pp. 131–132. Special thanks to Juli Brandano for directing my attention to this article.

12 H. C. H. Graves, "Price of Cod-Liver Oil," *The Lancet*, vol. 235, no. 6072 (13 January 1940), pp. 97–98. Graves was presumably referring to whale oil made from blubber as opposed to whale liver oil, but this could not be verified.

13 Jean-Baptise Fonssagrives, cited in Richard D. Semba, *The Vitamin A Story: Lifting the Shadow of Death* (Basel: Karger Medical and Scientific Publishers, 2012), p. 3.

14 The Orthodox Russian Church made liver an exception to the Lenten ban on animal products, perhaps because without it, observers would otherwise feel the effects of vitamin A deficiency.

15 True, Brown drank a gallon of fresh carrot juice a day, but he was more likely killed by the concentrated synthetic vitamin A tablets he munched as a snack. "Can Carrot Juice Kill?," *New Scientist*, 21 February 1974, p. 452.

16 Kendra Howard-Smith, *Pure and Modern Milk: An Environmental History Since 1900* (New York: Oxford University Press, 2014), p. 58.

17 In an odd coincidence, vitamin A's longstanding link to vision was echoed in its manufacturing history; the first company in the US to market a synthetic version was Distillation Product Industries, a division of Eastman Kodak.

18 Gavin Maxwell, *Harpoon Venture*, p. 252.

19 "Fishing for Vitamins," *Popular Mechanics*, vol. 77, no. 6 (June 1942), p. 2.

20 Gavin Maxwell, *Harpoon Venture*, p. 251.

COLORS / BLACK
Hayden Williams

"Colors" is a column in which a writer responds to a specific color assigned by the editors of Cabinet.

———

Hello, *Cabinet* editors! I've never met you, all the back and forth for this column having been conducted by email, but I wish I could see your faces as you read this for the first time. I guess I should say how pleased I was at first to be asked to contribute to your magazine, which I've read, from time to time, over the past few years. And I've seen some of the previous Colors columns. In fact, I have in my hand issue 36, from Winter 2009. Do you remember that issue? It's got some excellent things in it. I especially enjoyed the Georg Simmel essay on Grülp, a non-existent color. Simmel being Simmel, he manages to pull it off with bravura.

Also lurking in that issue, close to the front of the magazine, is Paul La Farge's Colors column, which I equally admired. In fact, I found it extremely memorable, though you apparently did not. You told me that every writer gets their own color, but La Farge has already written about black, for Chrissake! Of course, we've all read Kierkegaard on repetition, but that's not what's going on here. None of this was intentional on your part. The relevant essay here is Freud on repetition compulsion. I suggest you read it, lying down, on a comfortable couch, preferably with an expensive analyst nearby. It'll open up many avenues of your mind for you to explore. And they won't be beautiful Parisian avenues, with nice trees in the middle. They will be more like Avenue C in the late '70s. Do you remember *that*?

But enough about you. Let's talk about me. What did you see in me that made you assign, or try to assign, the color black to me? In your first email you wrote: "The color we will assign you will sit productively to the side of your writerly sensibility." What the fuck does that mean? Do sensibilities have sides? And how can anything sit productively? I don't know about you, but the only time I sit productively is on the loo. So,

I ask again: why black? Did you detect a wee darkness in me that you felt the assignment would, as you might say, elicit and amplify? I bet you felt very satisfied when you sent me the email telling me "my" color. And to go back to Freud: in all these years, have you ever had one moment when you thought, "Maybe all these color assignments are not about our writers but about ourselves." Here's an exercise for you to do in your spare time. Take all the colors you've ever assigned and put them in a long line. Then take out your diaries and see if the color you assigned at any one time can be "productively" matched to what was going on in your lives. It'd be good to have that analyst nearby.

So here is your Colors column. You can publish it, or not. I, meanwhile, will start working on an essay for you that I actually would like to write, one I don't believe you've published before. I'm going to contact all your Colors writers of the past fifteen years and ask them to tell me what color *you* should be assigned. I suggest you read that Freud before I send you their responses.

WATER FOUL
Stassa Edwards

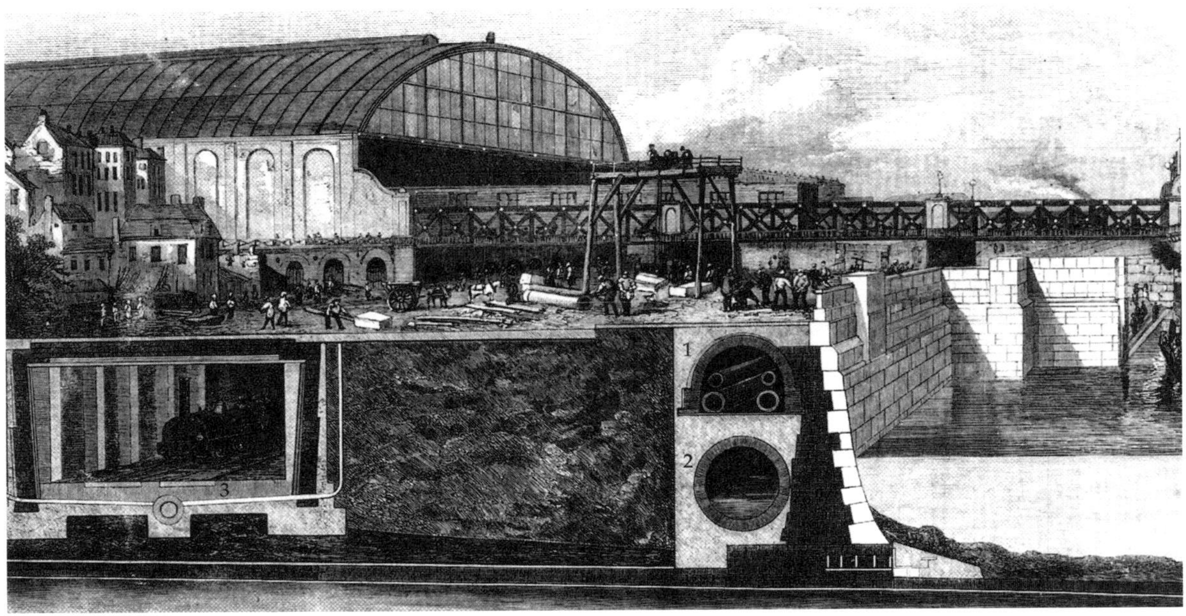

By the summer of 1858, the stench in London was unbearable. The River Thames, long the dumping ground of human, animal, and industrial waste, could no longer bear the refuse of London's nearly two million residents. The river had always been dirty—even today its stale smell is synonymous with London. Its meandering form must have made it seem like the perfect dump site and, from the time of the Roman founding of the city some eighteen hundred years prior, Londoners had thought little of tossing their rubbish in the river. Perhaps they thought no one would notice, or that the waste would be pulled to sea; perhaps they didn't think. But in the summer of 1858, the Thames itself finally noticed. That summer was unusually hot—some estimate the hottest on record—and the layers of shit stewed in the sun. In protest, the river overflowed and released an odor so unbearably fetid that Londoners dry-heaved and vomited in the streets: that summer was dubbed "The Great Stink."

The Great Stink drove the business of England to a malodorous halt. Newspapers described "men struck down with the stench, and all kinds of fatal diseases, up-springing on the river's banks" and Parliament, sitting in its posh new building on the Thames, turned entirely to solving the smell. The

Great Stink was a potent reminder of the frailty of Britain's power—London was Europe's largest metropolis and the edges of Britain's empire were ever expanding, and yet the business of empire could be interrupted by a downright primitive system of waste removal.

But the Great Stink also spoke to the very limits of urban modernity. Only seven years prior, in 1851, England had held the Great Exhibition where it showcased its expansive power and knowledge. Visitors to the exhibition were reassured that Victorian England alone held the monopoly on the greatest advances in science and medicine. Now, as Charles Darwin was frantically working on *The Origin of Species*, racing against competitors to get the book to press, and Henry Gray was publishing his compendious anatomy book, Londoners were gagging at the smell of their own refuse. The Great Stink was, perhaps, an unwelcome metaphor for

Above: Section view of the Thames Embankment depicting London's underground infrastructure. The tunnel for the Metropolitan District Railway is at left (3); Joseph Bazalgette's sewer system (2) runs beneath the "subway," a horizontal shaftway built to house gas and water pipes (1). From the *Illustrated London News*, 22 June 1867.

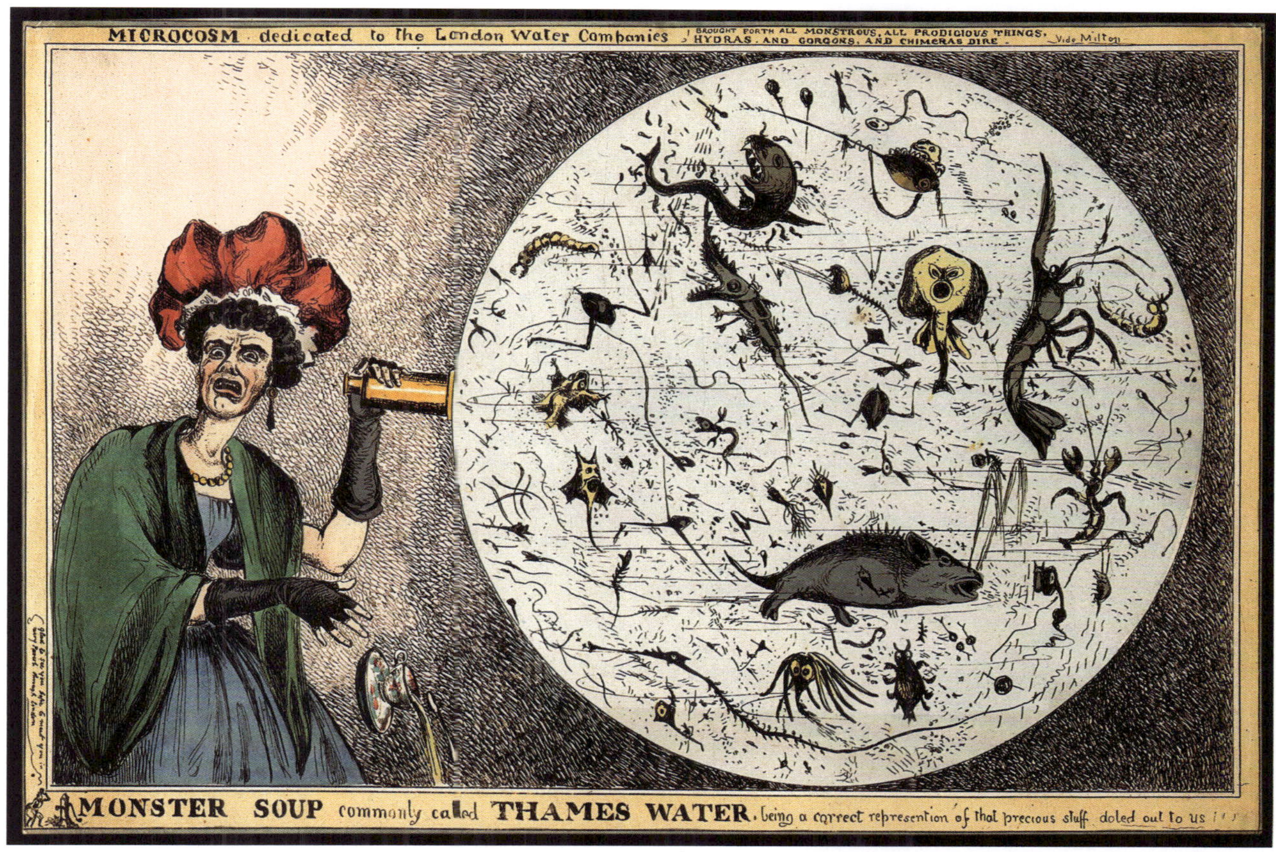

1828 etching by William Heath depicting a woman
dropping her teacup in horror on discovering the
monstrous contents of a magnified drop of water from
the Thames. Courtesy Wellcome Images.

London's paradoxical modernity: it was the epicenter of a world power, its citizens could fundamentally change human knowledge, but all of this could be ended by a plumbing problem. And that is exactly what the Great Stink was: an epic plumbing catastrophe nearly two thousand years in the making.

. . .

Ever since the city was a tiny Roman outpost, garbage was laid to rest in its river. But the population of Londinium was small; the empire's citizens never quite took to the harsh weather or the unwelcoming population. And the Romans knew better than to live too close to the water. As London grew, it expanded beyond the boundaries of the Roman settlement and towards commerce on the Thames. Fish traps and millers' weirs were built on the river, forever altering its geography and tidal flow. Commerce had such a profound effect that it turned parts of the Thames into a stagnant pool, quite literally stemming the river's tide. The Magna Carta outlawed the weirs and traps—but the document, though powerful enough to rein in the king, was ignored by London's merchants and proved ineffective in restoring the river's flow. Commerce reigned over the river, not the king.

Around the 1500s, there was a general sense that the Thames was too dirty and that something should be done, but who should do it was a question that remained unanswered. Henry VIII was too busy beheading wives, his daughters too busy executing heretics. Besides, the murkiness of the Thames must have seemed like a spectacular backdrop for the condemned as they were paraded down the waterway toward the executioner's axe. In good British fashion, it was decided that the problem should be bequeathed to future generations. Over the following centuries, there were some haphazard attempts to fix the Thames; some tinkering here and there. Among the ousting of kings and Protestant rebellions, private companies played with the river, adding an occasional waterwheel or drainage grate. But as the population of London surged, the Thames alone bore the weight of unplanned expansion.

Every decade or so, a monarch or politician would mutter something about the dirtiness of the river and suggest that someone should really do something. Heads would nod in agreement, but no one, of course, ever did anything. The health of the Thames had little effect on the city's wealthy. Besides, much of their waste didn't even make it to the river; private hauling companies came late at night, spiriting away the contents of some of the thousands of open cesspools to the countryside, where they were used to fertilize the nation's crops. The many who couldn't afford the spare shilling to have their cesspools emptied waited for heavy rains, which cleaned them out by flooding what they held into open drains designed to carry the rainwater to the river. It was in that same current that Londoners washed their clothes and from which they drew their household water.

. . .

By 1815, there were more than two hundred thousand cesspools throughout the city. Full of livestock, covered with horse manure, overcrowded, and with open cesspools on every street, London must have reeked with the toxic smell of shit. That year, Parliament outlawed cesspools, but they also repealed the laws that prevented direct dumping into the Thames. *Everyone* began pouring their waste into the public drains.

It's impossible to say why the smell of cesspools began to bother wealthy Londoners more in the nineteenth century than any time prior. Perhaps it was the shift toward privatization in this period—the emergence of family and familial intimacy—that demanded the domestication of waste. Or it might have been that the migration into cities produced the desire to find beauty in those spaces and differentiate them from the familiar farm smell of the countryside. "Smell," Dominique Laporte wrote in his genealogical meditation *History of Shit*, "the antinomy of order and hygiene, is equally incompatible with beauty." Or, perhaps, it was simply the sense that urban spaces are more pleasing, or are at least more bearable, if they are not littered with shit. Whatever it was, nineteenth-century Londoners demanded a safe distance from bodily discharge and its odors.

If the bourgeois sought refuge from the offending smell of human waste, they also wanted to banish those whose livelihood depended on that very waste. As Londoners began discarding their privy's contents into the river, an entire subculture

dedicated itself to digging through shit to find treasure. The poorest of the city's poor scavenged the
waste, sifting out food, change, and "pure" dog shit
to be sold to leather cleaners. Social observer Henry
Mayhew sketched the taxonomy of the lowly laborers in his serialized 1840s classic of muckraking,
London Labour and the London Poor. Describing the
"subterranean city of sewerage," Mayhew identified
the "toshers" who rummaged in the sewers for precious objects that might have slipped through the
drains. And there were also "mudlarkers," usually
boys, who picked through the mudflats and drainage entrances of the Thames at low tide. Those who
relied on the Thames for their daily bread were
the least skilled of England's unskilled labor, men
unable or unwilling to work factory jobs and abandoned boys too artless for Fagin's gang.

Though disdained and discarded by London's
middle classes, the subterranean dwellers were vital
figures in the city's waste management—their unofficial labor kept the drains flowing and freed proper
Victorian families from the offensive odors of their
own bodies. The Thames scavengers were a strange
metaphor for the river: fetid animals who crouched
in dung, morally toxic yet bounteously providing. It
was a paradox that seemed to be the material reality
of modernity itself.

Like their metaphorical counterpart, toshers and
mudlarkers were overburdened by the weight of
urban refuse. It's estimated that by 1857, some 250
tons of human, animal, and industrial waste entered
the Thames daily. By then, the waste had killed
what little life the Thames still supported—the river
salmon that Londoners had once feasted upon were
all gone. It was in that same year that the flush toilet
was invented, and Victorians rushed to have them
installed in their homes—after all, to no longer
have to touch one's own shit was the ultimate status
symbol of modernity. But coupled with London's
swelling population, the flush toilet—like all technological advances—proved perilous. The device
and the plumbing that came with it hooked directly
to the subterranean cesspits buried throughout the
city. But the cesspits were already unable to contain
the swelling population's waste, and the added
water overburdened the outdated system, forcing
their content onto the streets and into its open drainage. The toilet, however miraculous, displaced the

problem to the middle of the Thames. The city's
refuse was too dense for the river to carry to the
ocean, and there it sat.

The celebrated scientist Michael Faraday published a call to arms of sorts in 1853, writing in the
Builder that "the flood is now on, below London
Bridge, bad as poetical descriptions of the Stygian
Lake, while the London Dock is black as Acheron
… where are ye, ye civil engineers? Ye can remove
mountains … and fill rivers … can ye not purify the
Thames, and so render your own city habitable?"
That a river in Hades could be conjured up when
describing the Thames speaks to the murky death
trap into which the life-giving river had morphed.
But few listened to Faraday; maybe no one could
imagine London without the soot that covered its
monuments or the shit that filled its river. What
would a scientist know about commerce?

In that summer of 1858, however, an oppressive
heat wave rolled in, and modernity's waste fer-
mented in the sun. The Thames revolted and spewed
back the hundreds of years of offerings Londoners
had given to its water. It's mercifully hard to imagine
how devastating and incapacitating the onslaught of
the stink must have been. Londoners reported vom-
iting attacks, seizures, and even deaths. Language
itself seemed to fail as the noxious smell drifted off
the Thames. "Gentility of speech," wrote the *London
City Press*, "is at an end—it stinks."

. . .

It was then that everyone decided that something
should really be done. The stink was toxic; the foul-
smelling vapors that emerged from the river were
believed to be the source of cholera. The illness, this
account went, was a rot of the body that could be
caught simply from inhaling putrid air. The disease
had swept the city some four years prior and the epidemic had left nearly ten thousand dead in its wake.
But the epidemic's victims had been largely poor,
and believed to be victims of their own fetid, dirty
lifestyle. The Great Stink was different; wealth could

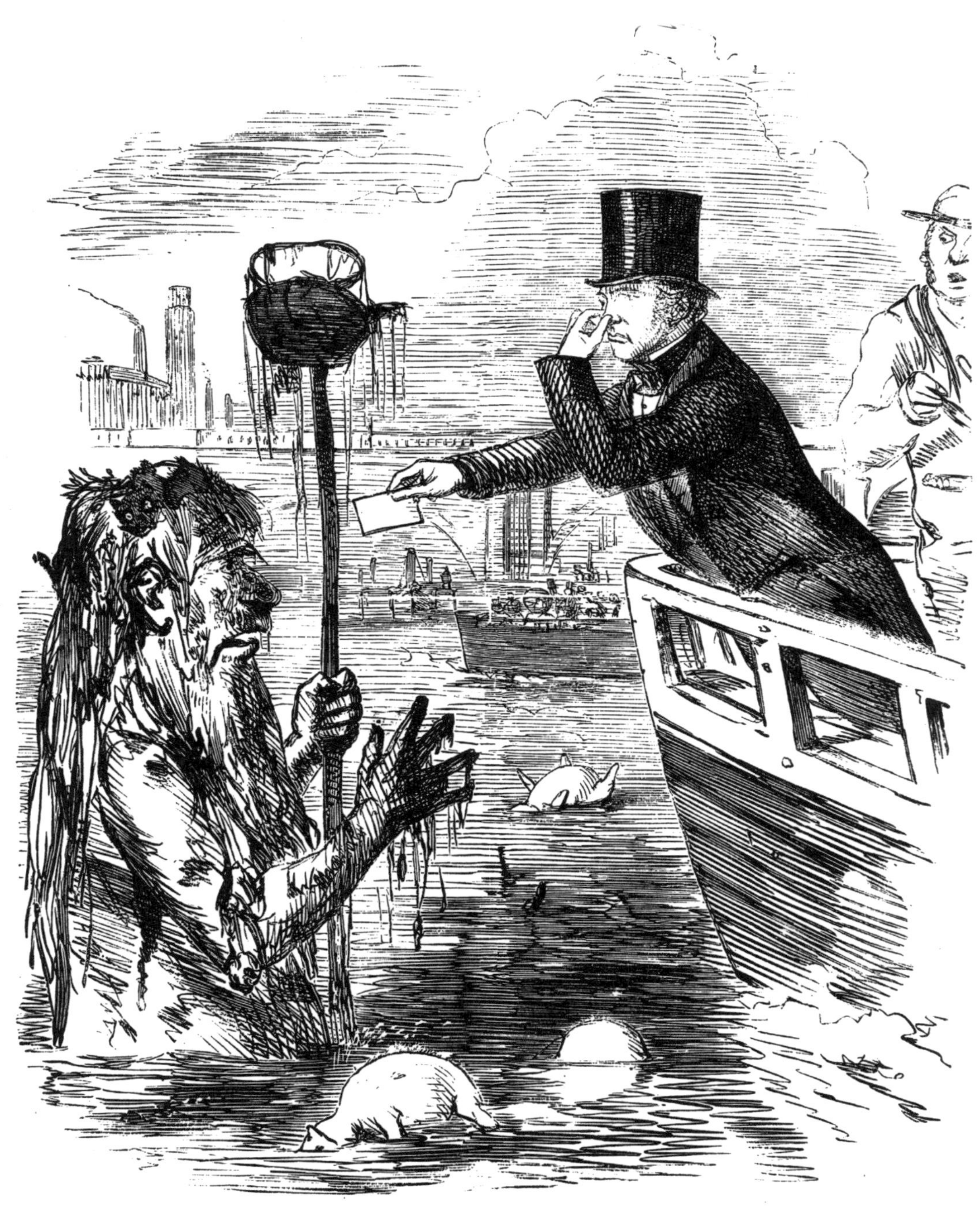

FARADAY GIVING HIS CARD TO FATHER THAMES;
And we hope the **Dirty Fellow** will consult the learned Professor.

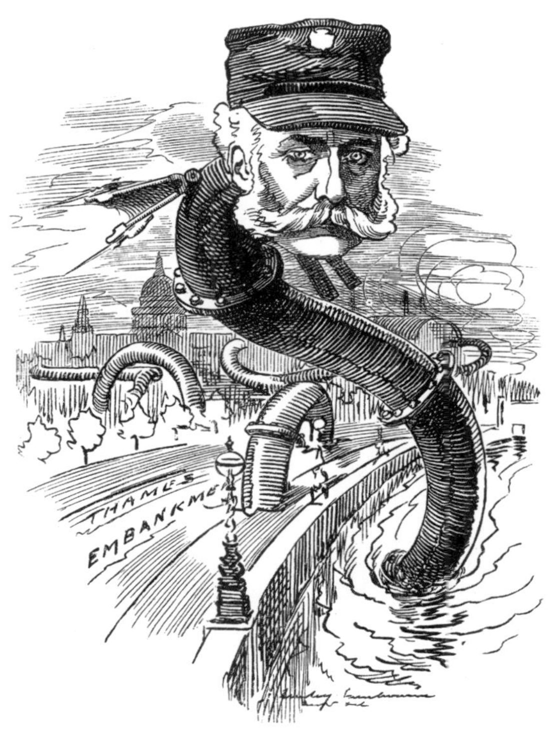

Bazalgette, master of drainage. Cartoon from *Punch, or the London Charivari*, 1 December 1883.

not protect from putrid, deadly stench. As cholera lurked, the reassuring stability of the hygienic and fragrant threatened to crumble.

Hundreds of years of arguing hadn't answered the question of just who should fix the problem. Parliament insisted it was the city of London's responsibility; the city of London claimed it was broke. The Thames was everyone's problem, and no one's responsibility.

Members of Parliament took to the chamber floor to do what they had been sent to do—give speeches. But as the *Globe* laconically recounted, "Disgust, alarm, and reasonable precautions induced members to stop away." The stink was so overpowering it muted usually long-winded orators. Parliament tried again and ordered that the windows be covered with sheets soaked in lime chloride. But the attempts to block the noxious air wafting into Parliament were futile—the ordinary work of government came to a grinding halt.

Londoners complained to newspapers; a reader of the *Morning News* described the "abominable, loathsome, and fever-breeding smells perpetually

emitted from that river which was formerly the boast of every Englishman." In return, the paper's editors demanded answers from their government, asking, "Is this atrocious state of a semi-barbarous age to continue?" The public agreed that the stink, odious and noxious, tainted the nation's image as an unsoiled beacon of modern progress.

Parliament still hemmed and hawed. They ordered sanitary crews to dump tons of lime into the river. When that didn't work, members suggested that the chamber be permanently moved. But no, they finally agreed, that would not do: their posh neo-Gothic monolith had just been completed at the cost of a few million pounds. If they abandoned their fashionable new building, then voters might raise an eyebrow come election time.

Benjamin Disraeli—then the House of Commons' minority leader—took to the floor and offered a speech that resembled the second-rate novels he had written before setting his eyes on politics. "This Stygian Pool reeking with effable and intolerable horrors," Disraeli called the Thames, warning all of a "pervading apprehension of pestilence in this great city!" The comparison to the rivers of Hades endured. Now was the time to banish the watery road to death.

Disraeli's speech came with a solution: he introduced a Metropolis Management Amendment Act that created the Metropolitan Board of Works (MBW) and gave the board unfettered authority to undertake a vast overhaul of the city's sewers. The bill was enacted into law with near-lighting speed—it took only eighteen days—and Parliament gave the board 6.5 million pounds for the undertaking. Out of shit, treasure arose: recognition that public works and infrastructure were necessary to sustain modern urban life. Almost immediately after Disraeli's bill passed, London was saved from the Great Stink in the most British way imaginable—the sun gave way to overcast weather, and it rained for days.

• • •

The MBW appointed Joseph Bazalgette as chief engineer of the overhaul. Bazalgette designed a series of large, intercepting combined sewers—their width accounted for the swelling population, and then some. Bazalgette broke ground a few days after the plan was approved. The bending shape of the

Thames presented a bit of a problem for the engineer; in order for his plan to work, the river would need to be narrowed and large pumps would have to be built throughout the city. He built the Victoria, Albert, and Chelsea embankments in a period of six years, reclaiming 3.5 miles of land from the river. The Embankment served to narrow the river, to make her tide run smoother and faster, and to keep the sewage from pooling and standing in the middle of the city. The embankments also invited Londoners to stroll along them—to walk, as it were, on the river, engaging in a conquerors' dance over filth and disease.

Bazalgette also built a series a pump houses that did the work gravity would not, forcing the waste to navigate the uneven terrain of the city. Pumping stations were erected at Abbey Mills and Crossness and, unlike the nondescript pumping stations that litter most urban landscapes, Bazalgette's were elaborately designed with intricate, organically shaped iron work. Crossness's Moorish-inspired ironwork slyly winked at the pilgrims who flocked to behold modernity's Mecca.

Bazalgette's project took nearly twenty years to complete. Cholera was to break out in the city once more, but afterward was nearly banished. His system wasn't perfect, of course; it didn't separate the sewage or recapture the river's water—it only pushed the shit out to the ocean and hoped for the best. In later years, engineers would jokingly call a quick fix a "Bazalgettianism," but for those who endured the summer of the Great Stink, he would remain a hero: a man who, according to the *Builder*, was the "deadliest foe" of "the malignant spirits whom we moderns called cholera, typhus, and smallpox." For his effort, Bazalgette would be knighted by Queen Victoria—one of many women widowed by Britain's disease-ridden water.

.   .   .

Perhaps the history of modernity can be written as our triumph over our own bodies—or at least our bodies' refuse. We have distanced ourselves from our waste as it rushes invisibly beneath our cities, and so have come to imagine that our not seeing or smelling actual waste means that it does not exist. We stroll on embankments along the Thames or the Seine, or watch our children play in parks along

the East River, and think these waterways beautiful despite their polluted realities. That is the paradox of the urban dweller's modernity, a form of denial that depends on a particular perception of the clean and hygienic, and demands a kind of sensory amnesia.

That our urban pastoral can be interrupted by unwanted odor or the bodily secretions of others speaks to modernity's otherwise safe distance from shit. We banish it at every chance, flush it underground, invoke it as insult, and police its presence in polite conversation. Its smell is terrifying because it reminds us how tenuous urban triumph is. Perhaps the Great Stink is an urban madeleine of sorts—not the sweet-smelling spongy cake that Proust envisioned, but a foul-smelling, deformed inversion of it. It invades the senses, creating memories of sensory revulsion. It reminds us of how quickly our smart city existences can devolve into primitive conditions.

Maybe it's this sensory fear that has led Londoners to begin fixing Bazalgette's fatigued sewer system before the Thames mutinies yet again. Bazalgette's system was designed to serve only four million; today the population of London numbers eight million. He designed his system to protect the comfortable corners of Victorian homes, to keep them dry and guard them from their own waste. To do so, he ensured that any overflow from the sewers would go directly to the Thames; there are nearly fifty raw sewage floods into the river each year. That the Thames—or any river—should have to bear the weight of modernity, of commerce and urban expansion, is a compromise that we're willing to bear. We only ask that it do so submissively.

Bibliography

William Cohen and Ryan Johnson, eds., *Filth: Dirt, Disgust, and Modern Life* (Minneapolis: University of Minnesota Press, 2004).

Alain Corbin, *The Foul and the Fragrant: Odor and the French Social Imagination*, trans. Miriam L. Kochan, Roy Porter, and Christopher Prendergast (Cambridge, MA: Harvard University Press, 1986).

Stephen Halliday, *Sir Joseph Bazalgette and the Main Drainage of London* (London: London Guildhall University, 1997).

Dominique Laporte, *History of Shit*, trans. Nadia Benabid and Rodolphe el-Khoury (Cambridge, MA: The MIT Press, 2002).

Henry Mayhew, *London Labour and the London Poor* (London: Penguin Classics, 1986).

THE MEANINGFUL DISAPPEARANCE
OF GERMAINE GREER
Carmen Winant

One great thing about the feminist revolution of the 1960s and 1970s was its ability to make a scene. Take the unforgettable "Dialogue on Women's Liberation," a panel that took place in New York City in 1971 in which four female delegates were tapped to speak in a discussion moderated by Norman Mailer, who had just published the decidedly un-feminist *The Prisoner of Sex*. Billed as a dialogue, the result—documented in filmmaker D. A. Pennebaker's *Town Bloody Hall*—more closely resembled a riot. The teeming crowd became unruly even before the event had started, with one heckler yelling out above the din, "Women's lib betrays the poor! Norman Mailer betrays the poor!" The audience, which included Betty Friedan and a soft-spoken Susan Sontag, came to hear about the burgeoning revolution. They came to see Mailer publicly attack, and be attacked by, the women's libbers about the politics of sex. But most of all, they came to see Germaine Greer.

She was something to be seen: clad in a black fur jacket and a glamorous floor-length sleeveless dress, the thirty-two-year-old Greer was six feet tall, angular verging on bony, and in possession of a thick crown of frizzed-out black hair. Her style on stage was less performance than poised seduction. Despite her languid manner, which noticeably awed the other panelists, Greer's responses to both Mailer and the audience were so razor sharp it's hard to believe they were delivered extempore. At one point, Greer chastens a man who inquires what he might expect of sex in the feminist age, what women are "asking for," by responding without hesitation (and more than a little unkindly), "You might as well relax. Whatever it is they're asking for, honey, it's not for you." Unabashed and wildly charismatic, Greer was the most important feminist in the world. Today, few remember her name.

Greer was born in January 1939 in Melbourne, during a record heat wave (it averaged 110 degrees Fahrenheit the week she was delivered) and in the wake of the Black Friday Fires, which burned nearly five million acres of Australian bush. She grew up in the suburbs, went to private Roman Catholic schools, and, by all accounts, was exceptionally smart. According to her rambling but occasionally moving 1990 book *Daddy, We Hardly Knew You*, Greer's World War II veteran father was an anxiety-riddled wreck who was abusive toward her mother and distant around his children. The book also alludes to abuse suffered at the hands of her mother, later described as a "terrorizing force" by Greer biographer Christine Wallace. By 1954, Greer was sixteen, five feet eleven, and having a love affair with a female classmate. By age seventeen, she was enrolled in the University of Melbourne, possessing—again, according to Wallace—an "intellectual arrogance" and a tendency to be bullying in arguments. She starting wearing long gowns, took up acting, dated a philosophy professor whom she would later describe as her most important romantic partner, and studied Lord Byron. By age twenty, she was a self-made, self-described anarchist communist.

It wasn't until moving to Cambridge, England, in 1964 to pursue her PhD in Elizabethan drama that Greer uncovered her real revolutionary ambitions and began to court public notice. Greer's various pursuits included acting on stage, where she went by the name Rose Blight; cohosting, along with the DJ Kenny Everett, the comedy television series *Nice Time*; penning satirical garden columns under the pseudonym Dr. G.; playing the sex-kittenish lead in a short film called *Darling, Do You Love Me?*, and cofounding the radical pro-pornography magazine *Suck*. (Greer herself appeared nude in its pages, as well as in *Oz*, another underground periodical based in London; a few photos, more slapstick than smutty, still live on online.) She married a construction worker and divorced three weeks later. Presumably influenced by the New York Radical Women's protest at the Miss America Pageant around the same time, she called bras "a ludicrous invention" and spoke openly against monogamy; to the then thirty-year-old Greer, both were conditions of a deeply socialized patriarchy that desperately

---

Opposite and pages 36–37: The multifaceted Germaine Greer. Studio collages by Carmen Winant, 2015.

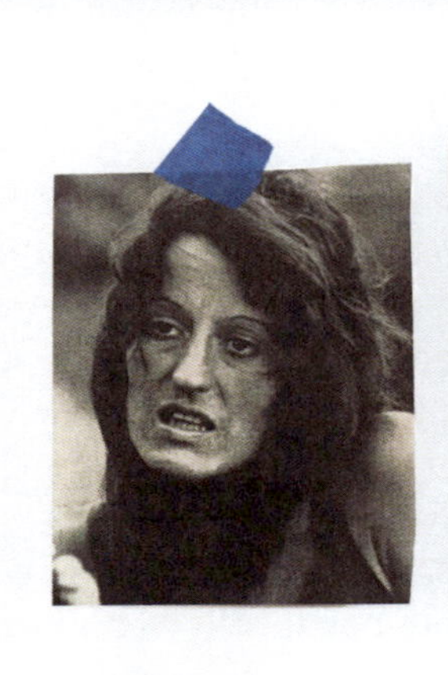
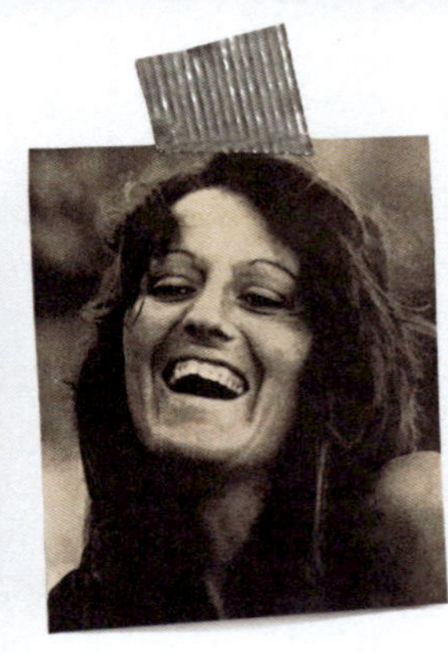
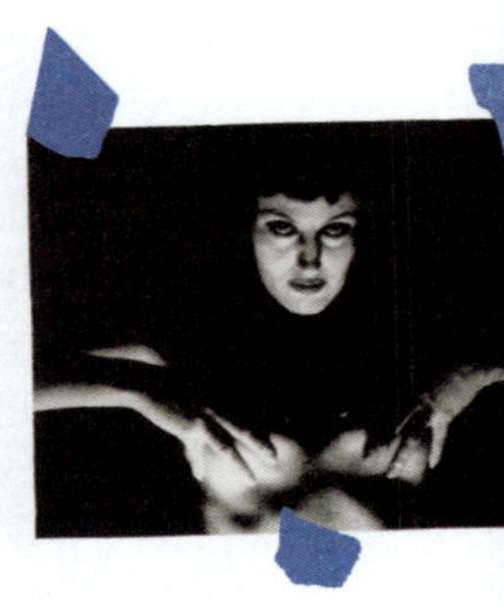
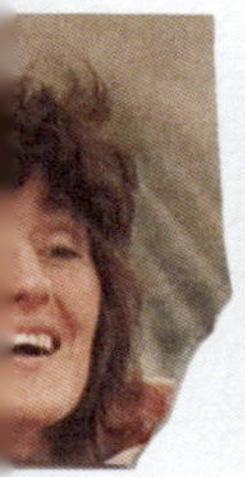
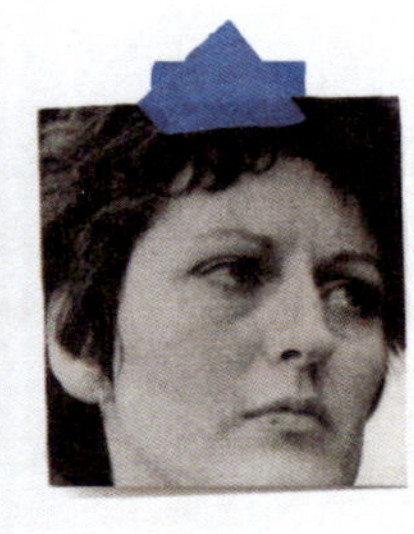
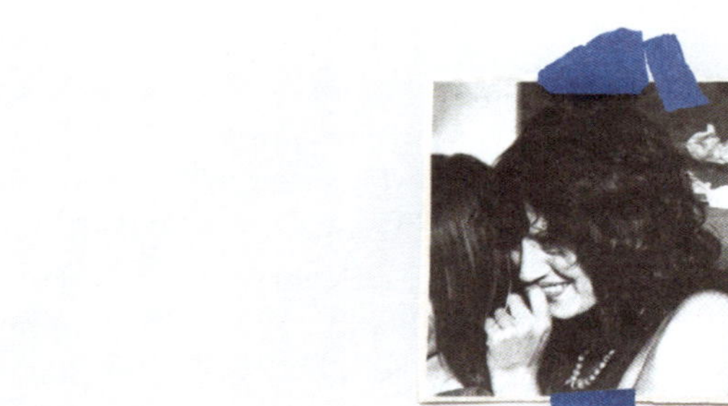
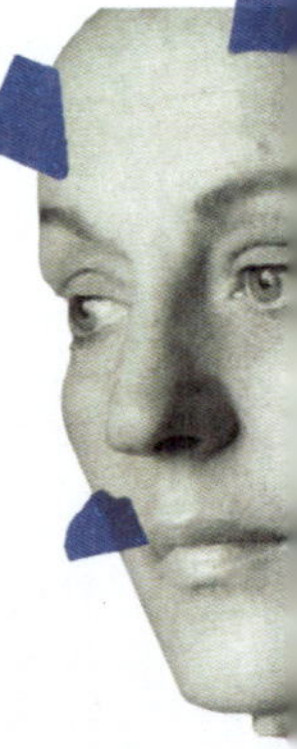
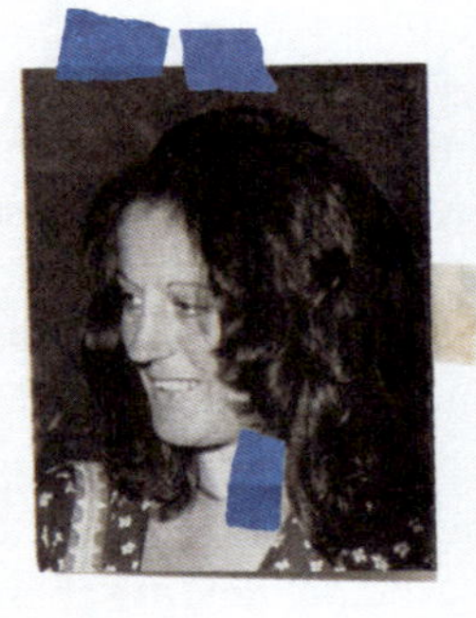
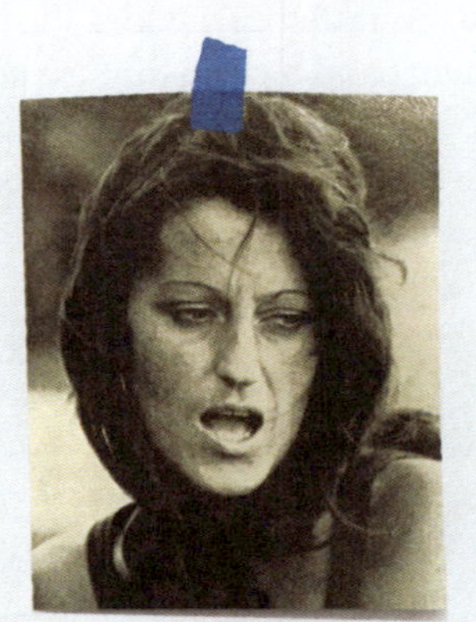
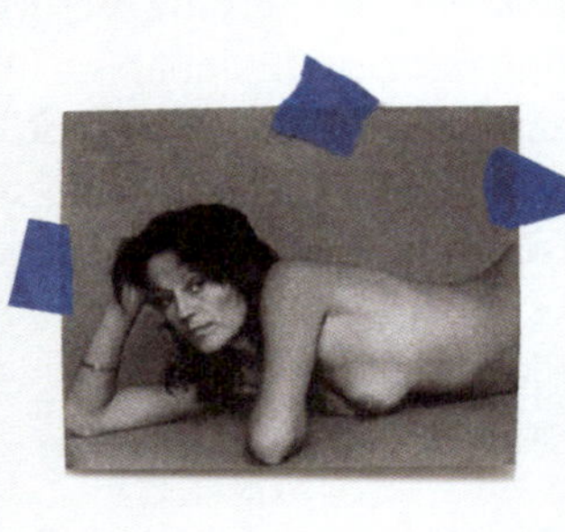

needed upending. Everyone who knew her reported that she was funny, exceedingly quick, and vulgar, using phrases like "cunt-lapping," "motherfucking," and "cocksucking" while making discursive arguments about sexual power. (She would be arrested in 1972 for using similar language during a talk in New Zealand.) Greer was wildly unapologetic about her opinions, her manner of speaking, and her commanding body. She had, to paraphrase Mailer, the gift of impossible presence.

The Female Eunuch, Greer's first book and the central node of her career, came out in 1970. It was a sensation, selling out its print run in a matter of months and establishing Greer as a leading mind in women's liberation and an international intellectual celebrity. More than other books that came out around its time, including Kate Millet's 1969 text *Sexual Politics* and Shulamith Firestone's *The Dialectic of Sex*, also published in 1970, *Eunuch* was written to be read by women who were not intellectuals, and existed outside of the movement. According to Greer, feminism was, and had to be, for everyone. This was a book written *to* women and not just *for* women. Divided into cogent sections called "Gender," "Curves," "Hair," "Sex," and "The Wicked Womb," it described the ways in which sexism was institutionalized in every woman's life, from hair products to housewifery. Even when Greer's ideas themselves were risky or rarefied, her colloquial, often-vulgar style of writing helped her to connect with common women. The book's most often quoted line gives a good sense: "If you think you are emancipated, you might consider the idea of tasting your own menstrual blood—if it makes you sick, you've got a long way to go."

The strategy worked. *Eunuch* had tremendous reach, selling out its first two runs and eventually being translated into eleven languages. The book was discussed on late-night talk shows and in middle-class living rooms. It has never gone out of print. Gloria Steinem and Letty Pogrebin founded *Ms.* magazine the year after its release; following Greer's lead, feminist activists were finding a way to popularize and disseminate their message into the mainstream.

While it touched on issues from consumerism to menstruation, *Eunuch* had a single argument at its core: gendered oppression is all-pervasive.

It argued that women were systematically subjugated to the power and will of men and too fearful, polite, or unaware to retaliate and claim authority over their own lives. "What many women mistake for happiness is in fact resignation," Greer told an Australian reporter the year *Eunuch* was published. More importantly, she made the case that this deeply inculcated sexism was the product not of fear but hostility. It was a loaded idea that would inform feminist, and eventually queer, theoretical discourse to come. In a now famous, blunt line from the book, she wrote, "Women have very little idea of how much men hate them." This societal structure, according to Greer's text, repressed women sexually and severed them from their libidos—hence the title of the book, a premise initially derived from a chapter of Black Panther Eldridge Cleaver's *Soul on Ice* entitled "Allegory of the Black Eunuch." Divorced from their sexuality, women were not self-empowered, but rather submissive, demeaned, and, in some cases, enslaved. Lacking agency of their own, they had come not only to be hated by men but by themselves. "Out of her own and her man's imagination," Greer wrote, "she will continue to apologize and disguise her … crippled and fearful self." This idea, that power was tethered not only to making money and asserting physical dominance but ownership over one's sexual desires, was novel. Just seven years prior in her book *The Feminine Mystique*, Betty Friedan had written of the malaise of the American housewife as "the problem that has no name." *The Female Eunuch*, as a title and an idea, claimed just the opposite. Greer's words cut like a precise blade; reading them one recalls just why the sexual revolution was called a war.

It was a daring thesis for a daring time, and Greer met praise and backlash in equal measure. Both responses prompted her to become the public face of women's liberation, a position she took on with gusto. Greer travelled around the world being photographed, giving lectures, granting interviews, and engaging in debates. Unlike other feminist radicals such as Andrea Dworkin, Robin Morgan, Susan Brownmiller, Sheila Jeffreys, or Mary Daly, she was fast becoming a household name, intent on delivering her message through literary and pop channels alike. Greer's contemporary Gloria Steinem was perhaps the only other figure in the movement to

become a public personality, appearing on the covers of *Newsweek* in 1971, *McCall's* in 1972, and *People* in 1974. Greer undoubtedly courted media attention; to what extent she did so because she felt it necessary to act as the ambassador of her cause, as opposed to simply desiring personal fame in its own right, remains unclear.

Several months after her book was published, the Australian Broadcasting Corporation created a short documentary about Greer on her return trip to Melbourne, which was nationally televised. In a particularly powerful scene, a group of local teenage schoolgirls describe how the book helped refashion their sense of self-worth. One pig-tailed girl states, "They are conditioning us to take the place of an average housewife." It is Greer's text, she reports, that has opened her eyes to society's attempts to "brainwash" her into submission. Greer herself is interviewed for the film while leaning against a brick wall and smoking a cigarette. Coolly self-assured, she appears custom-built to lead a modern women's revolution.

The following year, in 1971, Greer was featured on the cover of *Life* magazine reclining on a park bench under the imprudent title, "Saucy Feminist That Even Men Like." (One reader smartly wrote in to the editor, "Now that you are taking oppressed people so seriously, I am looking forward to the companion article: 'Saucy Black Militants That Even Whites Like.'") The magazine—which pictured Greer yelling at a protest; laughing at a party as she sits on the floor with a long-haired young man, their limbs entwined; carrying a bundle of branches in the countryside—attempted to create a holistic, if whitewashed, portrait of the young, pioneering feminist. With the exception of Greer's statement that "women should never marry," the article was tame; consider by comparison the titles of her pieces "I Am a Whore" and "Welcome to the Shit-Storm," contributed to *Suck* and *Oz* magazines, respectively, the same year. Within a few months' time, Greer was interviewed by *Playboy* and wrote a story for *Harper's* about George McGovern, the Democratic presidential nominee. Her name appeared much larger than her subject's on the cover.

In a 1973 debate on the resolution "This House supports the Women's Liberation Movement" at her alma mater, Cambridge University, Greer took on the American conservative William F. Buckley. In contrast to the language in her book, the debate was highly intellectual in tone—"I am not talking to this audience as I would talk to those of my sisters who are working in factories," Greer acknowledged—reminding her contemporaries that she was not just a radical, but a radical with a PhD. She triumphed so decisively that Buckley wrote in his 1989 memoir *Firing Line*: "[Greer] trounced [me]. ... Nothing I said, and memory reproaches me for having performed miserably, made any impression or any dent in the argument. She carried the house overwhelmingly." From a man who made a career of debating, facing off against public intellectuals with progressive values such as Gore Vidal, Noam Chomsky, and James Baldwin at the same Cambridge dais, among others, the defeat is telling.

During this time, Greer is said to have had trysts with Warren Beatty, Federico Fellini, Martin Amis, and, of all people, her regular sparring partner Norman Mailer. She was popular in every sense of the word. Described by her biographer as having "the youth, the charisma, the chutzpah and the media savvy" to lead the movement, Greer had managed to both radicalize and glamorize women's liberation. In her wake, more and more women were self-identifying as feminists and organizing consciousness-raising groups within their local communities. The revolution was finally being substantiated through the kind of collective ownership she had so vehemently fought for. And then, just as suddenly, Greer wasn't relevant.

Some probably saw it coming. For one thing, *Eunuch* had its problems. It did not propose concrete solutions to the questions it raised, prompting frustration within the ranks. Greer never mentioned abortion or reproductive rights in the text, failing to anticipate what many would claim as the critical feminist issue of the next four decades: *Roe v. Wade* would be written into law just four years after *Eunuch* was published. As with most second-wave leaders, Greer spoke to gender alone as a source of oppression for women, failing to acknowledge how poor or non-white women might be oppressed by other forms of socialized patriarchy. And, despite her early and progressive views on gay rights, Greer was, and continues to be, largely transphobic. In *Eunuch*, for instance, she alludes to the story of a

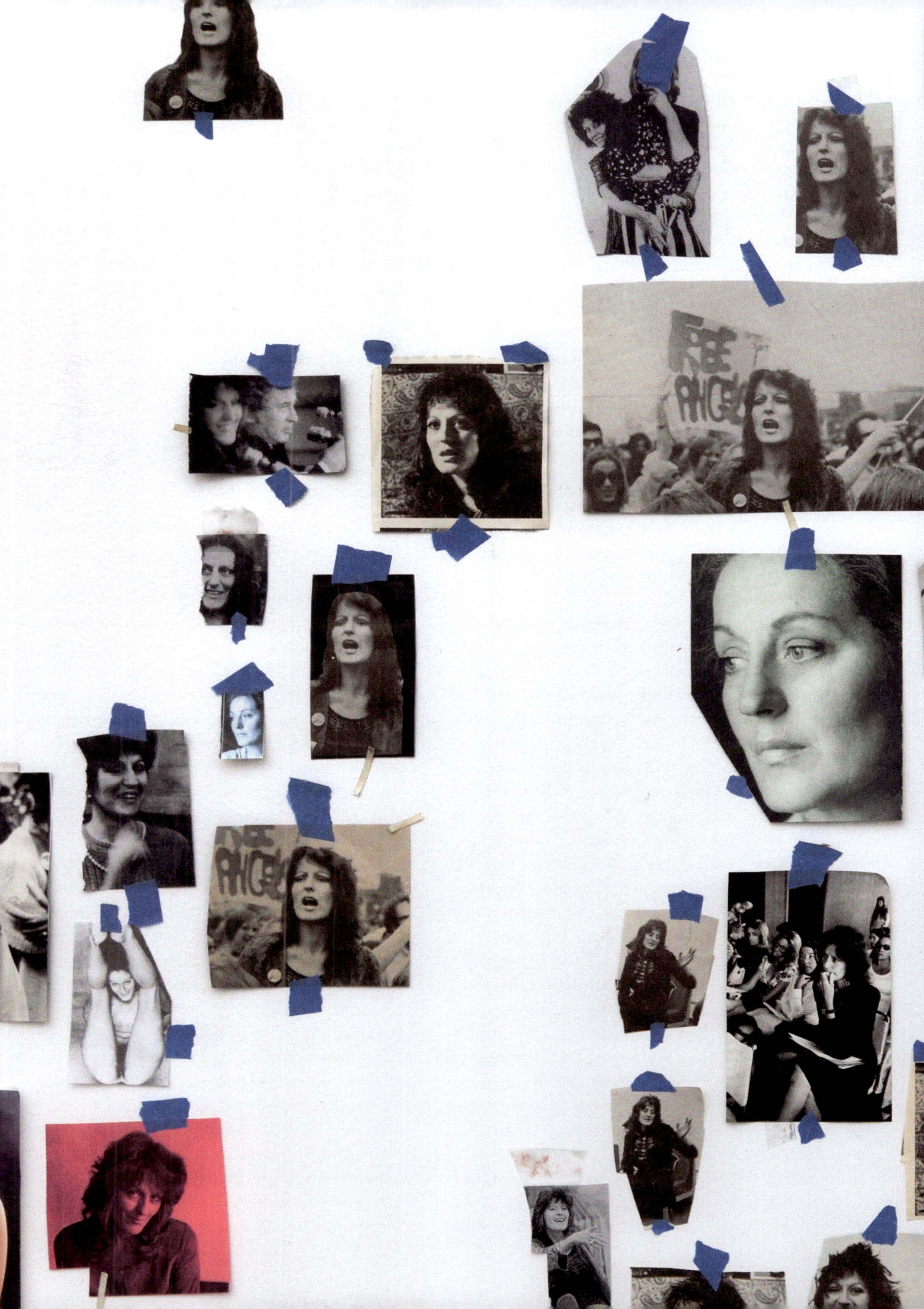

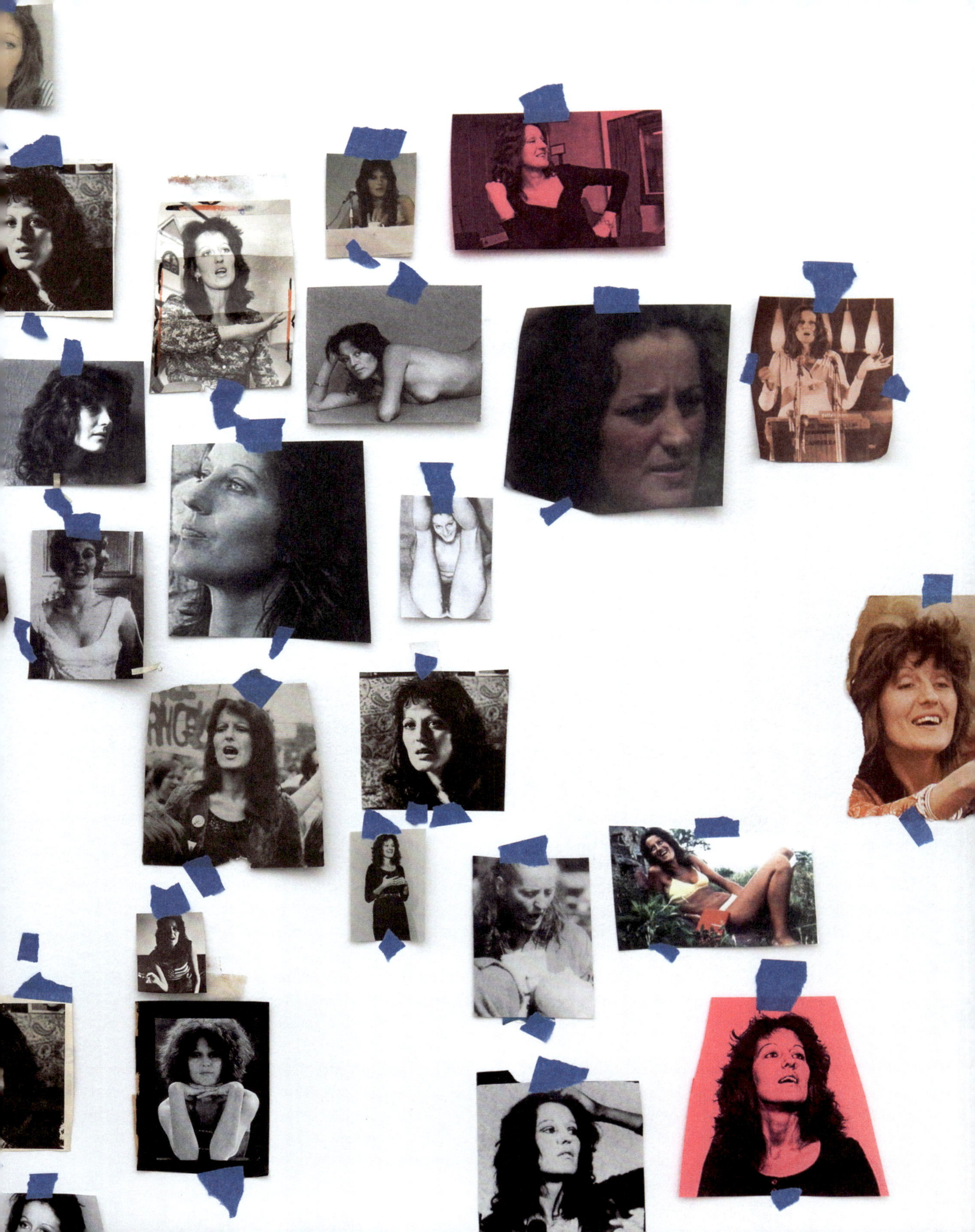

man who wants to become a woman, understanding the impulse as identification with, and craving for, feminine subjugation. This attitude persisted most notably in Greer's 1999 book *The Whole Woman*, in which, in a chapter entitled "Pantomime Dames," she chastised society's acceptance of male-to-female transsexuals, writing, "The insistence that man-made women be accepted as women is the institutional expression of the mistaken conviction that women are defective males."

Other controversial views in *Eunuch* included Greer's propositions that families raise their children communally, that testosterone "is a rare poison," and that even "the most basic assumptions about feminine normality" should be banished. It is likely that Greer was being deliberately inflammatory; the movement needed impropriety and even fury. But these provocations, no matter how strategic, don't always sit well. Phrases such as "female faggots" and "professional nigger," which make their way into the text at various points, feel misguided and derogatory. Ultimately, this kind of prodding radicalism, which had initially propelled Greer into the limelight, was her popular undoing. By the early 1980s, *Eunuch* came to be viewed as largely hyperbolic and out of date.

Greer was, in some important ways, always out of step with herself and her party. She chastised women who allowed men to define their image, but posed nude herself in the pages of sex-positive magazines. She plucked her eyebrows to oblivion despite calling upon women not to spend worthwhile energy "keeping themselves pretty [as it] reflects a dissatisfaction with the body as it is," and generally self-presented as a sex icon. (Her sexiness was, undoubtedly, part of her charismatic appeal.) Greer supposedly had an affair with Norman Mailer, who was notoriously anti-contraception, anti-abortion, homophobic, and, according to many, anti-feminist; nicknamed "a male chauvinist pig" by the writer Kate Millett, was he not in some sense the very man that Greer was talking about when she wrote that "men hate women"? And, despite her loathing of publicity outside of her control—Greer does not grant interviews under any circumstances and described her unauthorized biographer as "flesh eating bacteria" (what she would think of this piece I can only imagine)—in 2005, after having published

twelve other books and taught in various universities, Greer appeared as a cast member on Australia's edition of *Big Brother*, a lowbrow reality television show that constrains contestants to a house and films round the clock. If the personal is indeed political, as the second-wave feminists of her era championed, it's hard to reconcile Greer's decisions with her credo.

Most importantly, there are real philosophical contradictions within Greer's own inveterate dogma. In her 1984 book *Sex and Destiny*, Greer—a woman who made the persuasive case that women had been alienated from their potential sexuality as a source of independence—suggested chastity as a desirable method of prevented unwanted births and "conserving energy." In *The Whole Woman*, which even many of her devoted followers felt went too far, Greer critiqued, among other things, contraception ("Male interference with conception and birth"), medical screenings for cervical and breast cancer ("Many times more likely to destroy a woman's peace of mind than it is to save her life"), abortion ("The masculine medical establishment and the masculine judiciary"), and Western efforts to counter female genital mutilation in Africa ("An attack on cultural identity"). For someone who indirectly helped pave the way for these advances in women's heath—reproductive, sexual, and otherwise—it's a series of confounding postures that ultimately prompt one to wonder if Greer has always been more interested in provocation than solidarity.

More than anyone else in the feminist leadership, Greer was, and is, rife with contradictions. Unlike her peer Gloria Steinem—a figure that, like any good politician, was rarely inconsistent in her actions or rhetoric, and far outlasted her for this reason—Greer was highly unpredictable, behaving like a feminist who, as she herself put it, did "not represent any organization." While Steinem founded the Ms. Foundation for Women, the Feminist Majority Foundation, National Women's Political Caucus, Women's Action Alliance, Choice USA, and the Coalition of Labor Union Women, Greer was a lone wolf. (She was a regular contributor to *Oz* and *Suck*, and would go on to found *Tulsa Studies in Women's Literature*, but was never part of particularly influential or inclusive collectives.) It's a position that allowed Greer to speak for herself but ultimately left

her vulnerable to attack. Years later, this behavior would prompt Helen Lewis, the deputy editor at *The New Statesman*, to describe Greer as the movement's "arsonist." In other words, women's liberation had needed the incendiary rhetoric of someone willing to burn things down—including, quite possibly, herself.

Though her fame began to seriously wane in the late 1970s, Greer has not entirely dropped out of sight—she remains a vaguely public intellectual. Greer has taught at various institutions, including the University of Tulsa in Oklahoma, Newnham College, Cambridge, and Warwick University. She continues to write books that range in topic from menopause to aboriginal disenfranchisement to Shakespeare's wife, Anne Hathaway. Her latest, *White Beach*, about rainforest reclamation, was published in 2014. Greer consistently pens articles for UK-based magazines and periodicals like the *Guardian* and the *Sunday Times*. "On Rage," from 2008, was turned into a short book. She has written collections of poems and branched into art criticism. As a quasi-celebrity, Greer has appeared on numerous TV shows in addition to *Big Brother*, such as *Extras* (2006) and *The Female of The Species* (2006), decisions that recall the on-screen, performative pursuits that predated her writing.

No text or cultural shape-shift by Greer has come close to matching the influence and persuasion of *Eunuch*. That is a tall order; with the exception of the encyclopedic, collectively written *Our Bodies, Ourselves*, published in 1971, no other book of that decade took such an accurate reading of the cultural temperature. It's not an extended slump; Greer's scholarship and popular journalistic and critical pursuits have veered miles away from the contemporary zeitgeist that she once so perceptively had helped to form. "The Greer I was reading was so different from the one I remembered and liked," wrote Margaret Talbot of *The Whole Woman* in a 2014 essay for *The New Yorker*. It's a sentiment echoed by nearly every feminist of that generation.

The possibility of rehabilitating Greer's public image is not, at this point, interesting or even viable. What remains compelling about Greer is the question of what her irrelevancy reveals about the state of contemporary gender politics, or feminism as we know it. As with any party, who is pushed out

the door is just as telling as who's allowed in. If we understand Greer to be in the way, what exactly do we consider her to be in the way of?

It's a difficult question to approach, much less answer. As our female pop stars so readily demonstrate, contemporary feminism is a messy, complex, and often bewildering affair. Look no further than Katy Perry declaring herself not to be a feminist despite "believ[ing] in the strength of women" in a recent acceptance speech for *Billboard*'s Woman of the Year award, or Madonna notoriously electing to call herself a "humanist" instead of a feminist. Or think of Selena Gomez decrying fellow pop star Lorde for not being "very feminist" in attacking her lyrics as sexist and regressive: "That's not feminism. [Lorde is] not supporting other women." Gomez may have confused feminism for a sleepover party. In any case, it's a confusing time to be a liberated woman.

Understood as a symptomatic clue, Greer's marginal status points to some obvious features of today's popular feminism: it champions women's reproductive health as a central concern; is aligned with trans and gender self-identification rights; does not privilege sexual pleasure as much as sexual power, believing in a woman's freedom to wield her sex and sexuality as a vehicle of authority and intervention. And, a few non-obvious ones: it is reluctant to embrace plucky leadership or stake potentially divisive positions within culture (the movement ultimately objected to Greer's stances, yes, but also to her divisive radicalism itself). The closest thing to popular leadership we have at the moment might be Sheryl Sandberg, the chief operating officer of Facebook, whose ongoing campaign discourages the labeling of ambitious girls as "bossy." It's a virtuous cause, if a little safe and a lot elitist. The success of Sandberg's "lean in" strategy demonstrates, if anything, that current feminists wish to co-occupy conditions that *The Female Eunuch* posits as fundamentally irreconcilable—to be both polite and liberated, at once. Is such a thing possible? Greer would likely argue not, and it's hard to disagree.

Germaine Greer wasn't right or wrong but both, and better: she was a productively destructive force, intent on razing male dominance. She embodied the profound contradictions of her time. Unlike some more cautious, prudent, and arguably effective

second-wave feminists, she didn't have a single
cause and her actions and opinions often clashed.
It has become fashionable to discredit Greer as the
crazy aunt of women's liberation, but this is not her
due. The early 1970s needed a blunt, unapologetic
radical unafraid to jolt the movement alive. (It was a
time, let's remember, in which women could not get
a mortgage without a male cosigner.) Talbot, again
writing in *The New Yorker*, confessed to missing
"Greer's swagger." Coupled with her intelligence, it
was, perhaps, the source of her potency.

While Greer is undeniably at odds with the goals
and rhetoric of today's complex and often convoluted feminism, women's liberation as we know it
would not exist without her daring in the first place.
As Helen Lewis wrote in tribute, "a softer, sweeter,
more accommodating woman wouldn't have written *The Female Eunuch*. Today's feminists shouldn't
airbrush her legacy into something we find more
palatable—particularly when the movement still so
often demands that its pioneers also be saints." We
should resist discrediting Greer, who would have
been unsuccessful if she hadn't been defiant, flawed,
abrasive, and, to use Lewis's word, "un-sisterly."
Selena Gomez, take note. Greer was the catalyst.
Let's remember that as we rightfully tell her to get
out of the way.

TIMBER!
Adam Morris

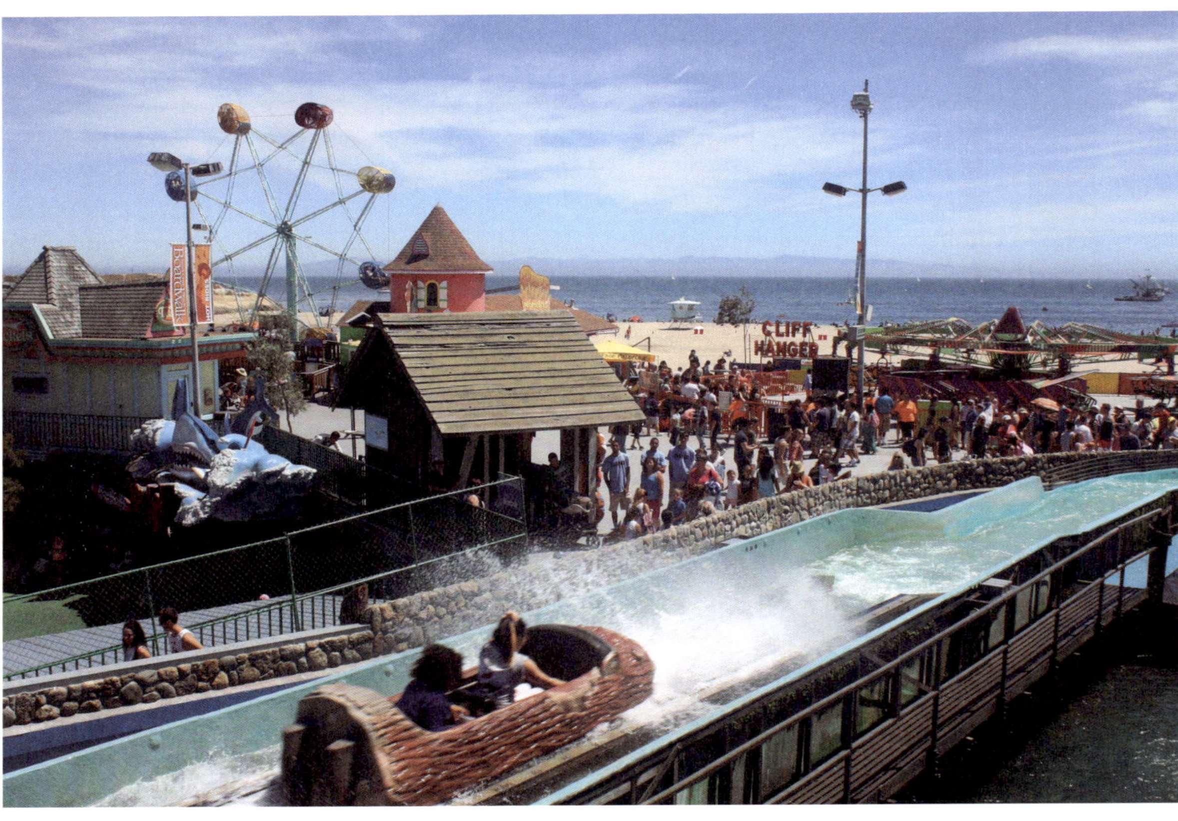

Pioneered in the 1960s, the flume, or "log ride," has spent the past fifty years conquering the world of amusements. Created to commemorate triumphalist narratives of the American West and offer a few minutes of simulated participation in rugged frontier life, rides modeled on logging flumes are found in nearly every state in the US, as well as across Europe and Asia. They typically feature a multi-person boat in the shape of a dugout canoe that is carried up an incline by conveyor belts before meandering through winding half-pipes of heavily chlorinated water. The final plunge into a log pool generates a spray for riders and bystanders, and is now usually captured on camera for the purpose of souvenir photos. Variants for children cultivate a taste for the ride from an early age.

The flume is perhaps the most iconic vestige of Arrow Development, a small design firm founded by a pair of US Navy technicians named Ed Morgan and Karl Bacon. The two principals had met as wartime engineers for Westinghouse in suburban San Jose, California, an area now part of Silicon Valley, which was (and remains) a hub for military-industrial manufacturing.

Theme parks did not yet exist when Arrow was incorporated in 1943. There were "kiddielands," carnivals, and seaside boardwalk parks. But the metals required for the modern theme park—born with the opening of Disneyland in 1955—were reserved for the war effort. The fledgling company roped in whatever contracts it could manage from nearby clients, including the Stanford Linear Accelerator, Hewlett-Packard, and a local crop duster company.

After designing a few playground apparatuses for local parks, Arrow was contracted to develop a twenty-foot merry-go-round for Alum Rock Park in San Jose. Morgan and Bacon still knew more about

Above: Logger's Revenge, Santa Cruz Beach Boardwalk Amusement Park. Photo Adam Morris.

fighter planes than carousels, but a friend in the carnival business in nearby Palo Alto let them study his
merry-go-rounds. Their innovation—a steel, rather
than wood, carousel—was the first in a series of
revolutionary Arrow inventions. The firm parlayed
its carousel success into a brand specialty, landing
a contract for a mechanized boat ride on Oakland's
Lake Merritt called Lil' Belle. Before long, they had
developed a rotating airplane ride that found buyers
at parks across the country. When they heard about
plans for Disneyland, Morgan and Bacon got permission to take Lil' Belle to Burbank for Walt Disney's
personal inspection. Disney loved the ride, and commissioned the firm to design several more for the
park, including four of the park's five opening-day
attractions. Disney would prove a scrupulous overseer, often turning up unannounced to test Arrow's
prototypes.

Collaboration between the two firms lasted into
the 1970s, and was instrumental in the creation of
the amusement park as we know it today. Morgan
and Bacon became legendary figures in the industry,
and Arrow is credited with having "transformed the
technology of amusement."[1] Small but mighty, the
firm went on to develop not only the flume ride, but
also invented the modern steel-tube roller coaster.

Walt Disney wished to maintain a degree of
control over the availability of the ride designs he
commissioned for Disneyland, and after observing
Arrow's wavering finances for several years, Disney
decided to buy a one-third stake in the company
in 1963. In particular, he acted to prevent former
Disney consultant and theme park impresario C. V.
Wood from purchasing the firm. At the time, Wood
was in the employ of Six Flags Over Texas, which
had opened in 1961. Unable to copy the popular
Disney rides outright, the flamboyant and fortuitously named Wood instead snapped up a different
Arrow design for Six Flags. The result was the first
modern flume ride, born of this flurry of innovation
and incipient competition.

Arrow had already begun prototyping the flume
in 1962; its first model opened at Six Flags Over
Texas in 1963. Disney, meanwhile, remained preoccupied with incorporating audio and animatronics
into new attractions for Disneyland. These techniques premiered in primitive form at the World's
Fair in 1964 with the launch of the It's a Small World
ride. Arrow was enlisted to help design the ride's
mechanics, which required a simple, less-thrilling
flume structure more suited to the sensory spectacle
that surrounded the riders. Sponsored by Pepsi and
dedicated to UNICEF, the ride offered passengers
a river cruise past world landmarks and singing

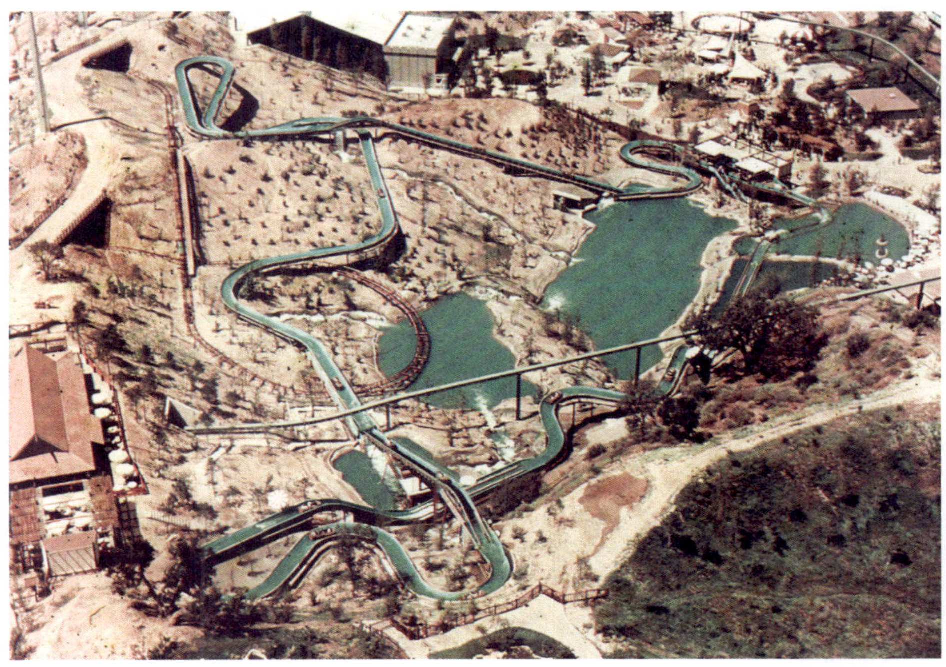

The Log Jammer flume ride at Magic Mountain in Valencia, California. This photo was taken in 1971, the year the amusement park (now known as Six Flags Magic Mountain) opened. The ride was closed in 2011.

children in regionally themed costumes. After the fair, the ride relocated to Disneyland and was later replicated for Disney World, Tokyo Disneyland, and Disneyland Paris. It also resulted in a spin-off attraction, Pirates of the Caribbean, which seized on riders' desire for a more exciting experience by incorporating flume-like dips and a final plunge.

Water rides have been a feature of amusement parks since the late nineteenth century. By 1897, New Yorkers could enjoy the Shoot-the-Chutes ride at Coney Island's Sea Lion Park. To ride the chutes, passengers climbed stairs to a loading platform for a quick descent in ten-person flat-bottomed boats. When Sea Lion Park was demolished in 1903 to make way for Luna Park (itself destroyed by fire in 1944), the old mill ride was the one attraction that was retained. Mountain Torrent followed in 1906: this improvement on the original ride was the first boat-coaster combination, which guided riders through mountain scenery before the final splashdown in an "alpine lake." Even in these early models, water rides always involved a spectatorial component: watching the terror and delight on the faces of those descending.

Arrow introduced sophisticated hydrodynamic engineering to these primitive water attractions, resulting in faster and longer rides—and a much bigger splash. The executives at Six Flags were at first dismayed that riders actually got wet descending the Texas flume, and demanded a redesign. However, they reversed course after a "dry" redesign of the boats resulted in the ride's unpopularity. Following the success of the flume at Six Flags, a second flume called Mill Race was built at Ohio's Cedar Point. A third opened at Knott's Berry Farm in 1969. Continuing with the logging thematics, Knott's called their flume the Timber Mountain Log Ride. To promote its opening, the first to plunge down Timber Mountain were Western film star John Wayne and his son Ethan.

The ride became a runaway hit for Arrow, selling wildly across the world. In a late interview, Bacon recalled selling over a hundred flume rides to parks across the US and Europe before selling the company in 1973. Early flumes were only thirty feet high, but it wasn't long before this height doubled. Arrow also designed a portable flume ride, but discontinued the model after predictable complications ensued:

hurried carnival operators were less than careful with the ride's complicated hydraulics, and slapdash assembly led to disastrous leaks.

Roller coasters are themed according to the demands of the park that commissions them, drawing on motifs as diverse as animals, pirates, and outer space. Generally, these themes are incorporated superficially, being restricted to ride names, color schemes, sound effects, and some surrounding landscape features. Similarly, boat rides might also adopt any sort of thematics. And although the flume ride can occasionally deviate from the thematics of logging—for instance, substituting battleships or rafts for ersatz hollowed logs—they tend to resist this thematic fungibility. The name of the first flume at Six Flags Over Texas, El Assadero, is in fact a misspelling of the Spanish term for "sawmill," *el aserradero*. The Timber Mountain ride at Knott's embellished El Assadero's original logging theme with a scenic lumber mill and forest populated by various stuffed animals, and redwood timbers were sent to New York for the It's A Small World ride. The most accessible flume ride from where I live in San Francisco, the Logger's Revenge at Santa Cruz Beach Boardwalk, sends its queue through a small mill, complete with a functioning (if technically inaccurate) watermill. Tellingly, the flume ride I grew up riding at Hersheypark, on the fringe of Pennsylvania coal country, adapts the ride to a more local form of resource exploitation: called the Coalcracker, this flume features boats shaped like small coal barges. But by and large, the flume is faithful to its historical roots. From the kinetically dubbed Log Jammer at Kennywood, outside of Pittsburgh, to the flatly named Flumeride of the Liseberg theme park in Gothenburg, Sweden, the timber mill is a persistent motif. This is because the concept and design of the flume derive directly from the grand logging flumes used in the Sierra Nevada and Cascade mountains of California and the Pacific Northwest.

Crude lumber flumes were used for transporting logs in the forests of Michigan as early as the mid-nineteenth century. But it wasn't until the San Francisco gold rush created a drastic shortage of lumber on the West Coast that flumes were implemented widely for mountaintop logging. Approximately 300,000 settlers and speculators arrived in California between 1850 and 1860,

making it one of the largest and fastest voluntary mass migrations in history.[2] The new towns needed lumber quickly. But due to a relative shortage of sawmills, lumber had to be imported from as far away as Norway, China, and Australia, as well as the eastern United States, making it a hugely expensive commodity. Boomtown fires compounded shortages with tragic loss: San Francisco burned, and was rebuilt, six times in eighteen months between 1849 and 1851.

Fortunately for the forests, efficient technology for mountaintop logging had not yet been invented. Loggers instead turned their attention to the coastal forests of Douglas fir (there known as Oregon pine). Writing in 1900, conservationist John Muir remarked that it had "cost less to go a thousand miles up the coast for timber, where the trees came down to the shores of navigable rivers and bays, than fifty miles up the mountains."[3] But already by the late 1850s, loggers were mowing down the coastal forests at untenable rates, and soon Civil War–era sawmills in the foothills of the Sierra Nevada mountains were also facing depleting supplies. Ancient mountaintop forests beckoned from the peaks of the Sierras. Innovation came in the form of train logging, hydraulic V-flumes, and powerful "steam donkey" engines used to winch log chains—three inventions which by the end of the century had eliminated much of the need for the slow and costly animal and human labor then required to transport huge redwood logs from mountain forests to sawmills. These technologies finally made mountaintop logging practical and profitable.

The lumber boomlet was an era unto itself. As logging historian Hank Johnston described it in his book *The Whistles Blow No More*, although flume and railroad logging on the slopes of the Sierra Nevada lasted only sixty-eight seasons, the practice "typified nearly everything that was exciting about steam logging out West."[4] Like other aspects of the frontier, imagined profits from the mountain lumber boom invited deceit and treachery. Facing shortages, lumber companies from Maine and the Great Lake states bought up land on the cheap in California. Others shrewdly paid only for "stumpage," the right to clear timber off private or government land. Crooked speculators also paid locals to file homestead or mining claims on government land, then kick back the land use to loggers. Between 1874 and 1942, nearly

five billion board feet of lumber were sent by flume and rail down the Sierras to lumber markets around the world. By Johnston's reckoning, the Sierra lumber boom generated "more than 500 miles of railroad track, 170 miles of lumber flumes, 28 locomotives, 16 sawmills," and employed "thousands of boomer lumberjacks."[5] Most of this activity took place on the strip of the Sierras between Sequoia and Yosemite National Parks.

The need for flume and rail logging was twofold. In the first place, some felled trees in the Sierra Nevada were so large that they needed to be blasted apart with dynamite or gunpowder before they could be divided and transported. In a group portrait taken of the entire population of a Sierra logging camp in 1888, all 126 inhabitants are seen standing on the stump of a single tree.[6] There was never any question of bringing the best logs down intact. Instead, mountain sawmills rough-cut the trees to be sent down the mountain. But areas with the best lumber were at high elevations, and timber would need to travel long distances and down steep grades from mountaintop sawmills to finishing mills in the company towns that sprang up in the San Joaquin Valley. Oxen wagons were costly and slow, and oxen-powered lumber chutes still functioned only with difficulties. The steam donkey engine sped things up and reduced dependence on animals and feed. Trains were effective on main routes, but also expensive to build. Fuel for mountaintop trains also needed to be sent up existing steam-powered inclines.

The most creative solution to the problem was the V-flume, which according to Johnston was "undoubtedly the most unconventional form of lumber transport ever conceived."[7] Box-shaped flumes already existed since pioneer days, but long pieces of wood would get stuck in them and wedge the flume closed. As the name indicates, V-flumes were shallow V-shaped troughs constructed from boards only 1.25 to 1.5 inches thick and 32 to 48 inches wide, placed on a continuous series of trestles that ran anywhere from ground level to spans ninety feet high over creeks and gorges.

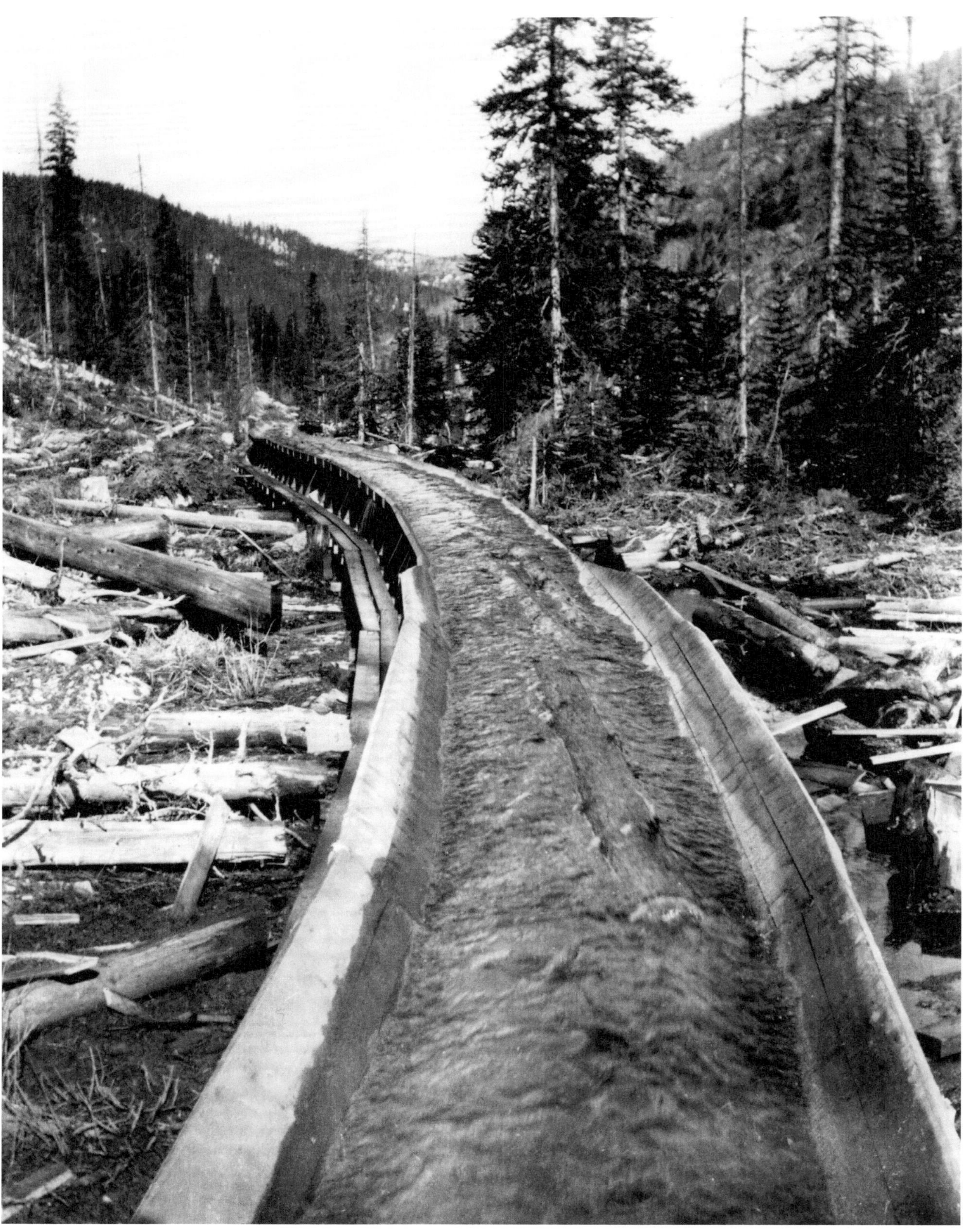

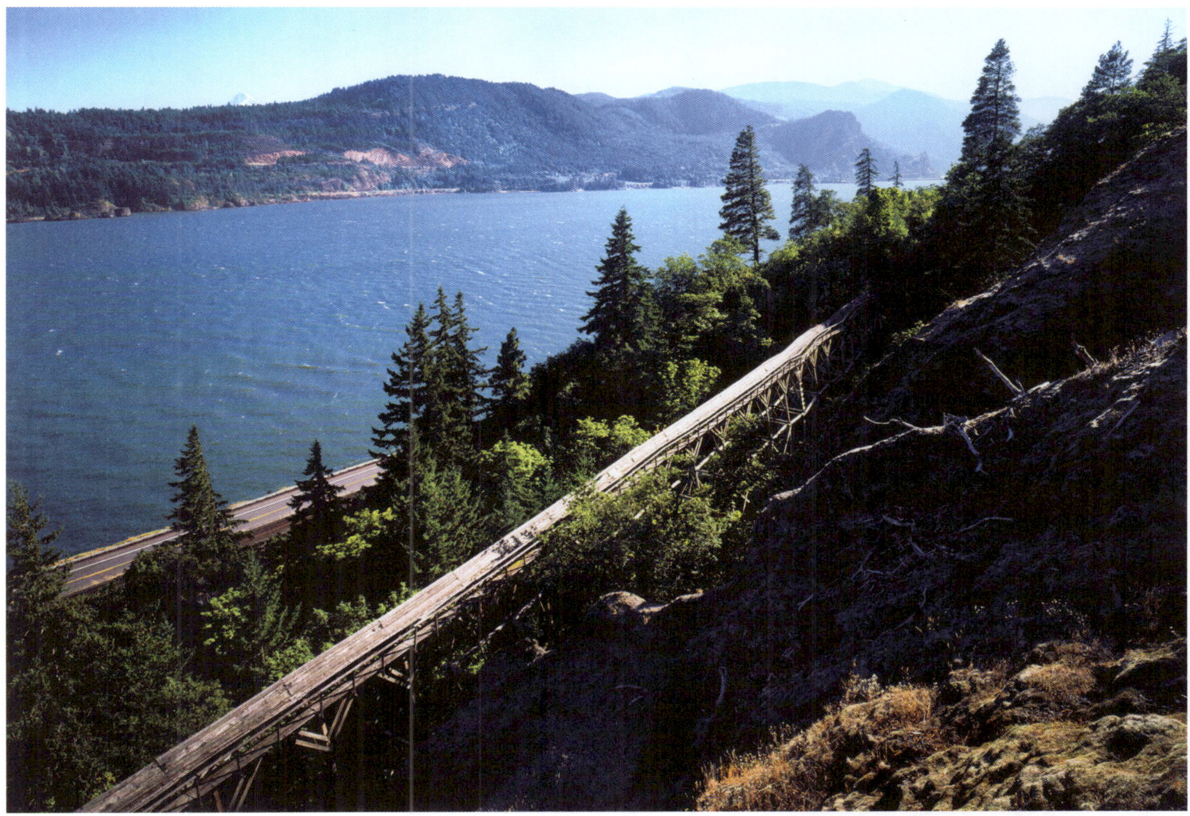

J. W. Haines is generally given credit for inventing the first successful V-flume, a twelve-mile chute from the east side of the Sierras to the Carson Valley and the Comstock Lode in Nevada in 1859. Mines like Comstock had an insatiable need for lumber, which was used to build scaffolding supports inside the tunnels. Comstock alone gobbled up so much timber—millions of board feet each year—that it was called the "tomb" of the Sierra forests.[8]

Haines's success was copied, but only imperfectly, throughout the northern Sierra in the 1870s and 1880s. In the southern Sierra, lumber companies were much more successful: flumes ranging from forty to sixty miles long meandered through forests, over trestles, along canyon walls, and down mountain slopes to the valley mills. The advantages of flumes were clear: they used no energy, required far less labor than railroads or oxen carts, and doubled as irrigation supply. Between 1874 and 1894, three of the world's longest flumes were built within a few miles of each other in the Sierras. Of the five major Sierra lumber companies, three were fluming operations: Madera Sugar Pine Lumber Company, Fresno Flume and Lumber, and Sanger Lumber each had flumes over forty miles long. Except for one year in 1912, the five major loggers were never all operational at the same time, but at least one of the great flumes was in use every season from 1876 to 1931.

Though faster and cheaper than railroads, flumes still required year-round maintenance and constant monitoring. Flume "herders" lived in company shacks stationed every few miles along the route. Herders were responsible for tying together bundles of logs, preventing jams, and spotting leaks. Even through ice and rain, herders ran along narrow catwalks to straighten jams with a tool called a picketoon, occasionally plunging to an early death.

Above: Broughton flume, Washington, 2000. Spanning nine miles between a lumber mill in Willard and a finishing mill in Hood, this flume—in use from 1923 to 1986—was one of the last to operate in the United States. Since this picture was taken, this portion of the flume has been removed. Photo Jet Lowe. Courtesy Library of Congress.

Herders and National Forest Service workers also traveled along the flumes in homemade boats. Though sometimes forbidden by the companies, lumberjacks often celebrated the end of the work-week with joyrides down the flumes to valley towns.

Company families also took guests for thrill rides on the flumes. Describing one such outing, Mrs. J. C. Forkner, daughter of one of the principals of the Fresno Flume and Irrigation Company, recalled that her father organized flume party rides for up to eight people at a time.[9] Owners of the Bonanza company flume in Nevada decided to inaugurate their "river in a box" with a celebratory ride, inviting *New York Tribune* reporter H. J. Ramsdell to accompany them down the relatively short fifteen-mile flume. The experience terrified Ramsdell, not least because the two boats carrying the five-man party collided with each other on the way down.[10] Though rides were sometimes just for kicks, flumes were also useful rapid transit in emergencies. On some occasions, the bodies of dead herders and lumberjacks were even strapped to boats and floated down to the coroner in the valley.

Amusement park flumes tend to leave out some of the more lurid, if historically accurate, details surrounding lumber flumes. Logging camps were dangerous and dirty, and entertainment for lumberjacks largely consisted of what Johnston calls the "three Bs": booze, brawling, and brothels. Though an essential component of Western boomtowns, gambling and prostitution do not feature prominently in the version of the Wild West depicted at many amusement parks. Period photographs of logging camps also reveal the utter destruction they left across the pristine Sierra Nevada—a consequence usually omitted by park landscape designers. Instead, amusement park flume rides concentrate on less unsavory aspects of the West: rugged adventure, quick riches, and natural beauty. As amusement

parks and rides grow ever more expensive, technologically integrated, and adrenaline-pumping, the flume still trundles on, despite the demands it places on park space and water supply. The flume's function at the amusement park is now one of cultivating nostalgia for different, more hopeful times.

In today's era of resource insecurity, climate change, and American imperial decline, however, this sentimental narrative is difficult to sustain. The thematics of the flume ride are tainted by awareness of the environmental atrocity it naively celebrates. Indeed, the threat of climate change had already been presaged by the naming and launch of the original Assadero flume in 1963. In a twist of historical irony, the ride's name is far closer to the term *asadero*, than it is to *aserradero*. *Asadero* is Spanish for "rotisserie," "grill," or "roaster"—a brutal accident of translation that mars the flume's whitewashed ecocidal legacy by suggesting the inevitable consequences of mass-scale lumbering. But perhaps even more damning is the way amusement seekers gleefully line up to be slotted into the hollowed boats. Packaged snugly as sausages, they assume the position of raw material awaiting processing in the vast industrial regimes of accumulation and exploitation that most credible scientists identify as the causes of global climate change.

1 Robert R. Reynolds, *Roller Coasters, Flumes, and Flying Saucers: The Story of Ed Morgan and Karl Bacon, Ride Inventors of the Modern Amusement Parks* (Jupiter, FL: Northern Lights Publishing, 1999), p. 13.
2 Hank Johnston, *The Whistles Blow No More: Railroad Logging in the Sierra Nevada* (Glendale, CA: Trans-Anglo Books, 1984), p. 9.
3 John Muir, "The Forests of the Yosemite Park," *The Atlantic*, vol. 85, no. 510 (April 1900). Available at <theatlantic.com/national/archive/2013/04/going-to-the-woods-is-going-home/275179>.
4 Hank Johnston, *The Whistles Blow No More*, p. 7.
5 Ibid.
6 The photo is reproduced in Hank Johnston, *The Whistles Blow No More*.
7 Hank Johnston, *The Whistles Blow No More*, p. 87.
8 Thomas J. Straka, "Timber for the Comstock," *Forest History Today* (Spring/Fall 2007), pp. 5–6. Available at <foresthistory.org/publications/FHT/FHTSpring-Fall2007/FHT_2007_Comstock.pdf>.
9 Hank Johnston, *The Whistles Blow No More*, p. 88.
10 The infamous ride is recounted in Thomas J. Straka, "Timber for the Comstock," pp. 9–10.

THE FAX NUMBERS OF THE BEAST, AND OTHER MATHEMATICAL SPORTS: AN INTERVIEW WITH NEIL SLOANE
Margaret Wertheim

Everyone knows a few integer sequences: the even numbers, the odd numbers, the primes. And we've all heard about the Fibonacci sequence (1, 1, 2, 3, 5, 8, 13…), where each term is computed by adding together the two previous terms. In 1964, mathematician Neil Sloane, then working on a PhD at Cornell University, began to write down interesting sequences of numbers on file cards. His research on neural networks generated quite a few; he pressed his friends for examples and consulted mathematics textbooks. As the horde of sequences grew, he transferred them to punched cards, then magnetic tape, and eventually to the web, where today, more than half a century later, his Online Encyclopedia of Integer Sequences (OEIS) has surpassed 250,000 entries. Used widely by professional mathematicians, computer theorists, and scientists, the OEIS has been called the most influential math website in the world. In addition, the database draws a huge international audience of recreational mathematicians, people who, for pleasure, surf its delights to explore the ways in which numbers can play. As a kind of numerological version of the *Oxford English Dictionary*, the OEIS is the place to go if you want to learn what any sequence of digits might mean, if it has been discovered already, or if it is entirely new. Every entry has a formal catalogue number and is complete with technical definitions, links to a vast network of citations and references, a visualization of the sequence as a graph (oftentimes revealing elegant patterns), and the option to hear it played as a piece of music. In February, Margaret Wertheim spoke by phone to Sloane, who runs the OEIS Foundation in Highland Park, New Jersey.

CABINET: What compelled you to begin the OEIS?

SLOANE: Of course, it wasn't called the OEIS in 1964. *O* stands for "online" and that didn't happen until 1996. At the beginning, I called it a Dictionary of Integer Sequences, and in 1973, I published a small handbook that had 2,373 sequences. When I got to 10,000, I decided to put it on the Internet.

Originally the idea came from work I was doing for my PhD thesis at Cornell. I was studying neural networks, which are like artificial brains with computer simulations of neurons. When these "neurons" fire, they trigger other neurons, which in turn trigger others—you have to have a certain amount of activity before a neuron gets triggered. And the question was, "If you have a network of these configured in a particular way, and you start by making one fire, will the activity continue to propagate through the network? Will it die out, or will it saturate the network?" I was looking at models of this, and I could count the number of cells firing at any given time, and I would come up with a sequence of numbers. For instance, if you start with one neuron firing, that might trigger two others that in turn trigger six, then twenty, and so on. Then after a while, the firing might die out. So using a computer, or by hand, I could calculate the beginning of a sequence, with each configuration of the network having its own specific sequence.

I knew I was going to have a lot of sequences I needed to understand. The first one I looked at, I couldn't find in any of the books. I looked in the obvious places: John Riordan's book on combinatorial analysis, Abramowitz and Stegun's *Handbook of Mathematical Functions*, and others. There were lots of sequences there, but not the one I had. So I thought it might be helpful to make a list of sequences I came across, in my own work and also in math books and journals. I started writing them on file cards and it seemed no one had done this before. So I started the collection and it began to grow.

CABINET: Do you still have the file cards?

SLOANE: Oh, no. I threw them away years ago when I transferred it all to punched cards. That was in the late 1960s, shortly after I joined Bell Labs. In the early 1970s, I transferred the collection to magnetic tape. I don't have the punched cards or tape either. It's all on the network these days, up in the cloud. I've been doing this for fifty years and as computers have progressed, every step forward has made my life easier.

CABINET: How do mathematicians benefit from this database?

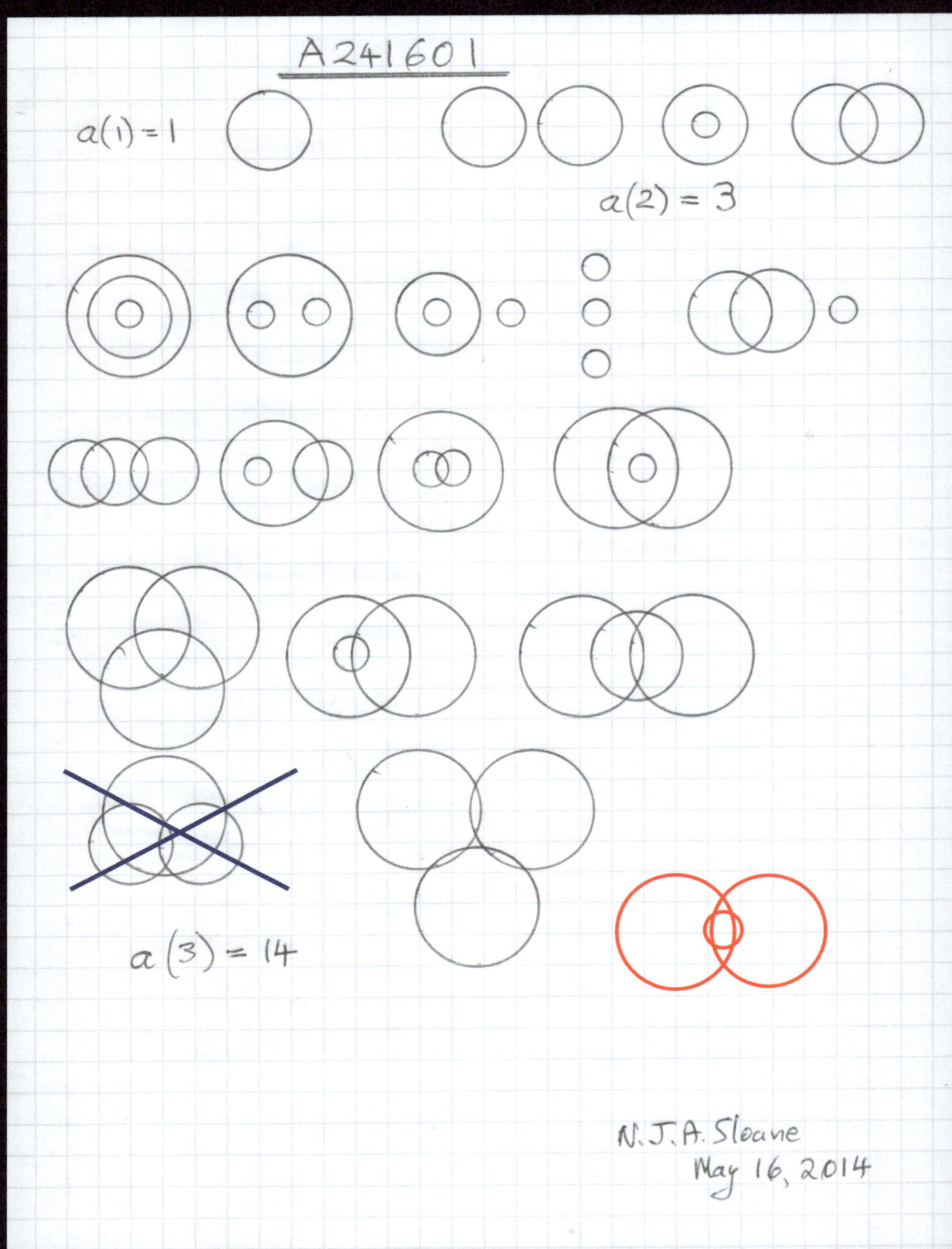

How many ways are there to draw one circle on a plane? And two, three, and so on? The circles can be any size, but aren't allowed to touch tangentially—i.e., if two circles meet, they must do so at two points, not one. For one circle, there is obviously only 1 way, but for two circles, there are 3 ways. For three circles, there are 14 ways. Neil Sloane's original drawing for this sequence had a duplicate (here crossed out) and missed one possibility (later added in red). With four circles, there are 168 unique ways to arrange them, but no one knows the answer for five circles. This sequence was initially assigned reference number A241601, but was the runner-up in the OEIS competition to see which sequence would get reference number A250000, and it is now A250001.

SLOANE: If you're a writer and you want to know how a word is used, you can look it up in the *Oxford English Dictionary* and find the record of the first person to use the word and examples of how it is used in a sentence. Well, it's the same thing with integer sequences. You come across a sequence in your work and you want to know, "Am I the first person to see this sequence, or has it been studied before?" Until my database, there was nowhere you could find that information, so it's been a great boon to mathematicians. They can look up a sequence and say, "Oh, that's something that came up in topology in the 1940s." Or, "This was a sequence that came up in chemistry in 1929." It will tell you things you didn't know about your sequence, such as, "This is also the list of the number of nodes in labeled, rooted trees." And your context might be totally different. So if my database tells you this comes up in studying the periodic table or in counting the branches in binary trees, that's very interesting to you, especially if I give you a formula or computer program so you can compute a lot more terms of your sequence.

It's also great fun. There are a huge number of recreational mathematicians—people who just love numbers—and they will browse the database looking for interesting sequences. And some will try to create new or interesting sequences themselves. So there is a lot of pleasure. It's like going to a museum or a gallery and looking at the latest artworks.

CABINET: What makes for an interesting sequence?

SLOANE: What makes for a good painting, or a good piece of music? It's the same question. The editor has to decide. I have a board of editors, a large group of people who are hard at work all the time, night and day all over the world, looking at submissions and deciding whether or not they are worth putting into the OEIS. If one of them says, "Yes, this is great," then it goes in. Or, one will say, "This is junk. This does not belong in the OEIS."

CABINET: How do you determine "junk" in this context?

SLOANE: As an example, one person tried to submit the sequence giving the number of pages in each of the seven Harry Potter books. That is not something

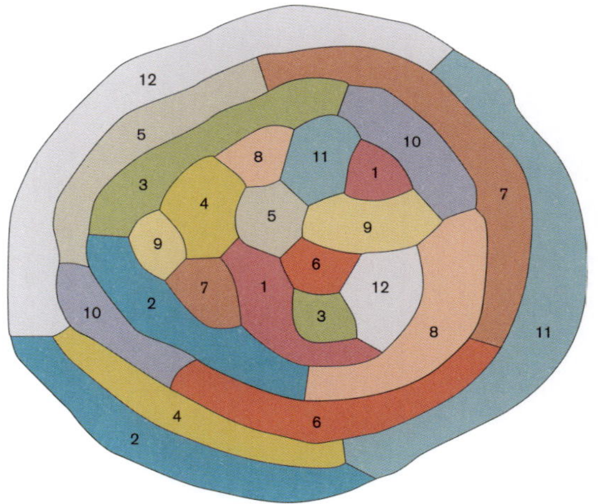

Above: A problem asks what is the maximum number of colors needed to make a planar map in which no two adjacent countries share a color. The answer turns out to be 4, no matter how many countries and what shape they are. Known as the 4-color map theorem, this is a simple case where each country consists of one contiguous territory (i.e., $n=1$). Now imagine a more complicated scenario involving imperial powers, where an "empire" is defined as consisting of two or more non-contiguous territories. For the map here (drawn by mathematician Ian Stewart) in which each empire has exactly two territories, the maximum number of colors required is 12. Mathematicians have proven that when the number of territories, n, belonging to each empire is two or greater, the maximum number of colors needed is $6n$, no matter how many empires and what shape their territories. If each empire had three territories, for example, the maximum number of colors necessary would be 18. Thus, sequence A230628 runs 4, 12, 18, 24, 30, and so on.

Opposite: Cellular automata are systems consisting of an array of squares, each of which may be either on (black) or off (white). Mathematicians model such systems on computers. For each iteration of the sequence, every square changes color according to a set of rules based on the colors of its neighboring squares. For example, a square might change from on to off if all the squares surrounding it are off. The diagrams here illustrate the first eleven steps of the so-called Fredkin replicator, a cellular automaton in which numerical patterns repeat in a mysterious way. The replicator operates according to one rule: in each new iteration, a cell will be on if, and only if, in the previous iteration an odd number of its surrounding squares were on. Thus, sequence A160239, which counts the number of on squares in each iteration of the Fredkin replicator, begins 1, 8, 8, 24, 8, 64, 24, 112, 8, 64, 64.

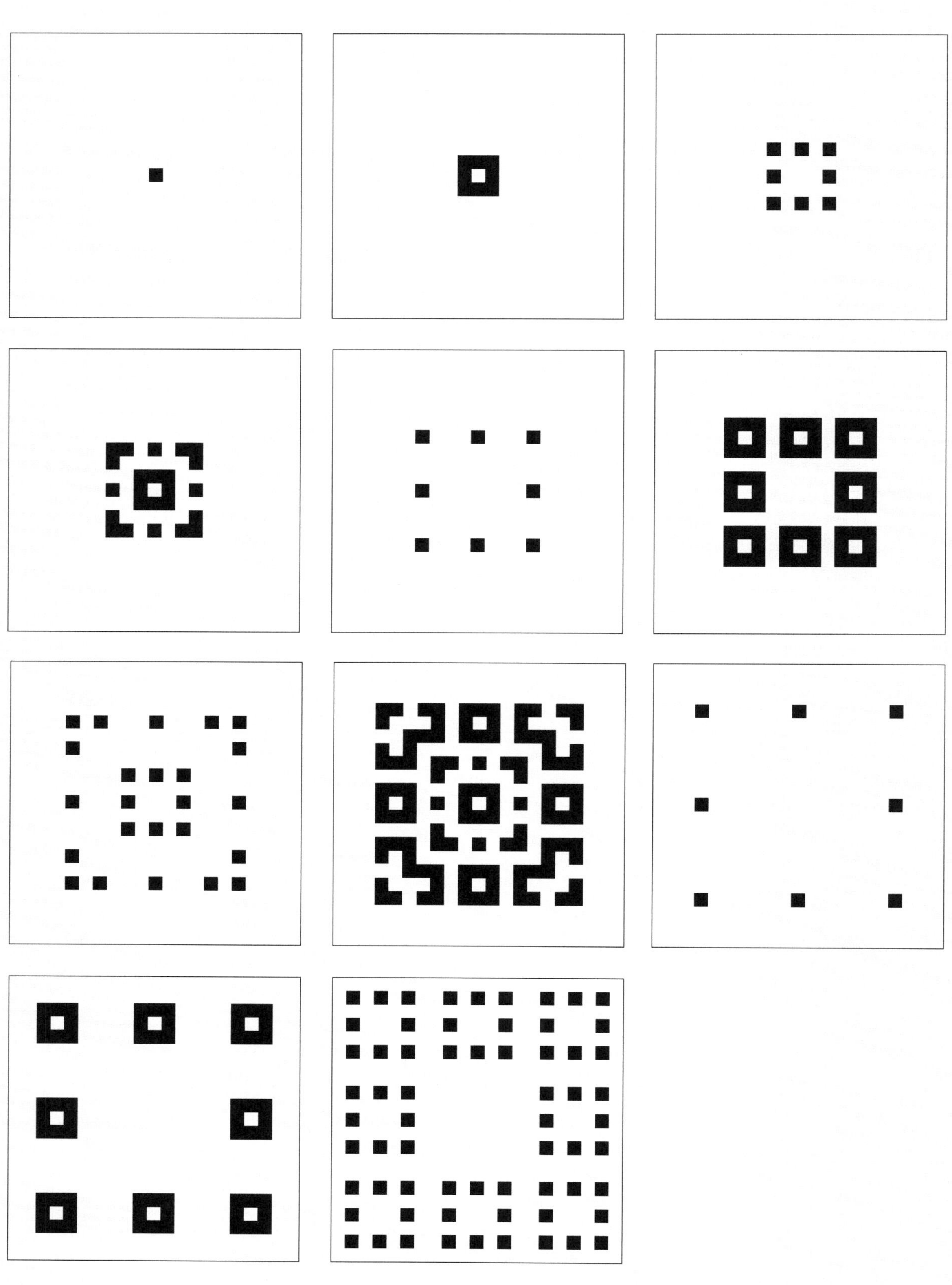

we accepted because, first of all, it depends on the edition. Are we talking about the paperback edition, the hard cover, the English edition, the American edition, the German translation? And so on. Do you include the front matter, or the stuff at the back? What do you mean by the number of pages? It's not a well-defined problem. This is a scientific database, and if I'm going to make an exception about accepting non-mathematical sequences, then it had better be something people have discussed.

For instance, subway stops in Manhattan. There are several different New York City subway lines with stops at numbered streets (12th Street, 23rd Street, 34th Street, 42nd Street, etc.), and these are famous sequences. They come up in IQ tests all the time, so they go in, no question. Or the sequence of numbers around a dartboard. There are only two or three different conventions for dartboards, so they go in; and the numbers around a roulette wheel. These are non-mathematical, but they're interesting, and in my judgment deserve to be in the OEIS.

CABINET: So it isn't just pure mathematics?

SLOANE: No. There's chemistry, physics, biology, botany, and many other things, including cultural sequences. I would regard a dartboard as a significant cultural sequence. We also include the list of years in which the eighteen King Louis of France came to the throne. Maybe this one is questionable, but I accepted it at the time. Marginal sequences having to do with dates involving, say, American politicians, those usually don't seem well defined. Things that depend on the calendar year—like the dates of Easter—some get accepted, others rejected.

CABINET: If I've got a sequence of numbers from some cultural or physical domain, can I submit it for consideration?

SLOANE: Yes. Anyone who registers and gives a real name can submit sequences. We have thousands of people submitting from all over the world.

CABINET: This parallels the making of the *Oxford English Dictionary* chronicled in Simon Winchester's book *The Professor and the Madman*, where people all over the planet contributed word entries that were vetted by professional philologists. What kinds of people submit integer sequences?

SLOANE: There's a wide spectrum: mathematicians, and also a lot of computer scientists who are typically counting the number of steps needed to carry out some sort of procedure, such as sorting a long list of words. The study of the complexity of various algorithms is a major part of computer science and these studies tend to come up with sequences of numbers. For example, if you've got a particular sorting algorithm—say you want to arrange playing cards in ascending order—what's the worst-case number of steps it would take if you have to sort five cards, six cards, seven cards, and so on. There are also people who aren't mathematicians, but maybe professionals in some other field, who send in sequences they've come across in their work. And then there are a lot of amateurs.

CABINET: Mathematics as a field encompasses a great deal of play. One thinks of Martin Gardner's wildly popular "Mathematical Games" column in *Scientific American*. I'm fascinated by the notion of amateurs sitting around dreaming up number sequences.

SLOANE: We don't want to encourage too much of that, but you know, a small amount of dreaming is fine. There are some people who try to get as many sequences as they can into the OEIS; they submit far too much stuff of marginal value. Let's take the prime numbers. You can ask: "What are all the prime numbers that begin with 7?" Okay, that's a sequence in the database. But then you could say, "What about all the prime numbers that begin with 763?" That's obviously too contrived. But if you say, "What about all the prime numbers that contain 666, the 'number of the beast'?" That's in the database; they're called "beastly primes." Then you recall how when everyone had a fax machine, the fax number was often the one following the phone number. So if my phone number was 555-4440, then my fax would be 555-4441. Well, there was a discussion about including prime numbers that contain 667, the "fax number of the beast." This is an example of going too far.

OEIS reference number A131645

6661, 16661, 26669, 46663, 56663, 66601, 66617, 66629, 66643, 66653, …

The "beastly primes"–the sequence of prime numbers that contain the substring 666, "the number of the beast."

OEIS reference number A138563

667, 1667, 2667, 3667, 4667, 5667, 6667, 6670, 6671, 6672, …

The sequence of prime numbers that contain the substring 667, "the fax number of the beast."

OEIS reference number A245045

3, 11, 17, 43, 67, 113, 131, 193, 241, 353, …

This prime sequence by Chai Wah Wu consists of prime numbers n, such that for some integer k,

$$n = \frac{(k^2 + 2)}{6}$$

Making $k=1$, 2, or 3 does *not* give a prime. But when $k=4$, $n=18/6=3$, which is a prime. Thus, 3 is the first term in the sequence. When $k=8$, $n=66/6=11$, so this is the second term, and so on.

OEIS database reference number A254337

0, 1, 8, 6, 10, 14, 12, 4, 20, 16, …

This remarkable new sequence, submitted in February 2015 by Maximilian F. Hasler–a physicist and mathematician at the Université des Antilles et de la Guyane, Martinique–is one of Sloane's all-time favorites. Here is its definition:

No term in the sequence is a prime.
No sum of 2 consecutive terms is a prime.
No sum of 3 consecutive terms is a prime.
No sum of 4 consecutive terms is a prime, and so on …
No term repeats any previous term.
For any term, always pick the next **smallest** *number that fits the above rules.*

Here is how we calculate the first few terms:

We start with 0, then 1, so the sequence begins 0, 1. The next term cannot be 2 or 3 because they are prime.
It cannot be 4 either because 1+4=5 which is prime, and so it is not 5 either.
It cannot be 6 because 1+6=7, which is prime, and so it is not 7 either.

It *can* be 8. So it *must* be 8.
Thus the first three terms are: 0, 1, 8.
What is the fourth term? Given that we always have to choose the *smallest* number possible that has *not* been used before, we see that it cannot be 2, 3, or 5 (all prime), and it cannot be 4, because 1+8+4=13 which is prime. However, it *can* be 6, which is not prime, because 8+6=14 and 1+8+6 =15 (neither of which is prime).
Thus the sequence begins: 0, 1, 8, 6.

Mathematicians believe that in this sequence there are no odd numbers aside from 1, and that all even numbers greater than 2 appear. According to Sloane, "there is no proof yet for either of these conjectures and this may be a problem that's too hard for twenty-first-century mathematics to handle." Hasler's sequence is like a new version of Fermat's Last Theorem, something that is very simple to state but requires deep excursions into the foundations of mathematics to prove. Like Fermat's theorem, this problem belongs to the domain of number theory, one of most difficult branches of mathematics. In an age when physicists have mapped the edges of the cosmos and created Higgs bosons, it is sobering to learn that mathematicians are still finding such richly confounding material in basic numerical games.

CABINET: So the fax numbers of the beast aren't in?

SLOANE: I don't think so. Let me look this up while we're talking. I can check them by name. Actually, the fax numbers of the beast *are* in. I sent in the sequence myself.

CABINET: Your standards have risen since then?

SLOANE: They go up and down. I get so many sequences. Until about 2009, I had to process everything myself. I processed the first 180,000 sequences. Since then, it's been a wiki and the editors do most of the work. I get called in to resolve disputes and have the final say.

CABINET: You now get about 20,000 new sequences submitted each year—that's an extraordinary amount.

SLOANE: Yes. It would be nice if you could mention in your article that we are overwhelmed with submissions and could use more editors. Editors don't get paid, but they get first crack at interesting sequences.

CABINET: Is it the articulation of a problem that makes a sequence interesting?

SLOANE: It could be that the problem is interesting and the person who sends it in doesn't realize quite how interesting it is. Or the proposer realizes it's an interesting question but doesn't have the mathematical skills to deal with it, in which case he or she will be grateful for help. That's resulted in a lot of joint papers, when one of our editors has collaborated with some submitter to study a problem formally. This is one of the reasons for submitting a sequence: somebody may see it who might be able to help you work out the formula or algorithm for producing it.

CABINET: Let's talk about a sequence recently submitted by Chai Wah Wu that is very enigmatic. It's about prime numbers and it has a kind of elegance that made me think it might be one the great mathematician Leonard Euler would have come up with in the eighteenth century. Who is Chai Wah Wu?

SLOANE: He's an engineer at IBM and a Fellow of the IEEE (Institute of Electrical and Electronics Engineers). He's submitted, and edited, a lot of sequences, and he's added programs for computing terms of many sequences, which is very useful. If I see a submission by him, I have a high degree of confidence it will be worthwhile.

CABINET: His prime number sequence seems like something that should have been known to mathematicians before, but I suppose the OEIS is showing us that there are still many basic unsolved questions in mathematics.

SLOANE: Absolutely. Mathematics is always expanding. There are more powerful techniques, we look at more complicated problems, and this kind of question about sequences of primes with certain properties is of continuing interest. You are right, Euler would have been interested in this. Some of the most recent developments in mathematics have to do with sequences of prime numbers. It's a very hot topic.

CABINET: Can you give an example of a sequence that's really odd or unusual?

SLOANE: Actually, I collect them. I keep notebooks where I jot them down and they now fill a bookcase. There's one by Douglas Hofstadter, who wrote *Gödel, Escher, Bach*; he's created quite a lot of interesting sequences. This one is called "Hofstadter's Q Sequence." It's got a very simple rule. It's a bit like the Fibonacci numbers, slightly different but similar in flavor. Someone has computed the first 10^{10} terms of this sequence, which is a lot! But there is no proof the sequence is infinite, so maybe at some point the computation ends and the sequence just stops. We don't know. From a mathematical perspective, that's remarkable.

CABINET: Aside from being a lovely curiosity, is this likely to have any application in the world?

SLOANE: Oh, I shouldn't think so.

THE HOLY FIRE AND THE LONELY SAINT
Matthew Spellberg

What the modern world calls ergotism was known in Europe for a thousand years by many names, identical in their ferocity but varied in their symbolism, like the banners of a barbarian army. *Ignis sacer*, read one heraldic device, the holy fire. *Ignis gehennae*, read another, the fire of Gehenna, the fire of hell. *Le mal des ardents*, the sickness of the ardent, of the burning ones. St. Martial's fire, after the saint whose relics dispatched the *miracle des ardents* of 994 CE in the Limousin. And eventually, above all, St. Anthony's fire, named for the saint who could heal it and also induce it. *Nemo impune peccat in Antonium*, read the inscription above the main portal of the abbey that housed his relics—no one sins against Anthony with impunity. *Nemo invanum currit ad Antonium*, read the second line. No one runs to Anthony in vain.

Ergotism takes its modern name from ergot, the hard, dormant stage, known scientifically as the sclerotium, in the lifecycle of the fungus *Claviceps purpurea*. It manifests as a conical structure colored purple, gray, or black, and it grows parasitically among the grains of certain cereals, especially rye. The livid prisms, called ergot because they look like *argot*, a cock's spur in Old French, flourish when a cold winter is followed by a wet spring, periods when in primitive agricultural societies harvests are poor, and farmers can't afford to discard blemished crops. Ergot contains a number of potent alkaloids, including lysergic acid, the key ingredient of LSD. Midwives have for centuries known that it can be used to induce uterine contractions.

It was not widely known until the seventeenth century, however, that when baked into bread and consumed in sufficient quantities, the ergot of rye is the cause of St. Anthony's fire, a terrible series of symptoms leading to permanent injury and, frequently, death. Modern outbreaks have shown that ergot-infected flour is slightly discolored and somewhat oily in texture, but it gives off no distinct odor, and in medieval Europe it probably seemed well within the wide boundaries of the edible, boundaries delineated not so much by ignorance as by a self-reproducing cycle of famine and warfare.[1] In years with a high yield of ergot, tens of thousands were affected.

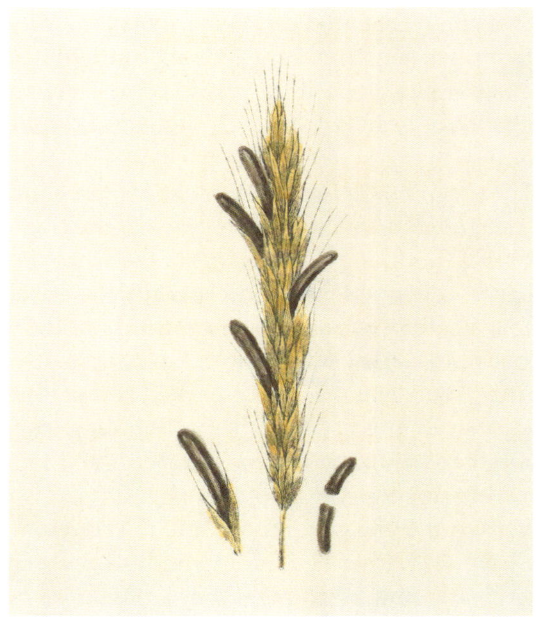

Ear of rye infected with ergot fungus. Illustration from Adam Neale, *Researches Respecting the Natural History, Chemical Analysis, and Medicinal Virtues, of the Spur, or Ergot of Rye, When Administered as a Remedy in Certain States of the Uterus*, 1828. Courtesy Edinburgh University Library.

A person who eats ergotic bread first suffers symptoms of an indistinct illness: a fever and an itching over his body. He may begin to feel an intermittent burning sensation in his limbs. He may plunge them into cold water for relief, and he may not think himself anything more than fatigued by hard work or, if he's a pilgrim on the way to Santiago de Compostela, by the long walk across southern France in the summer. The first distinctive sign of the ardent sickness, however, comes next. The itching becomes something subtler and more terrible, a light epidermal pattering, the feeling of ants crawling over the skin.

At this point the illness reaches a juncture, developing along two different paths. The first route sees the extremities turn pink, then yellow, and finally, as the skin peels off, black. There is acute ischemia—the reduction of blood flow—and motion becomes hard and painful. Sores begin to appear across the body, and the stomach swells. Lactating mothers

lose their milk, and pregnant women abort. There is a burning pain, and eventually gangrene sets in. The limbs—sometimes one, sometimes several—shrivel away, seem to char, and die. Sometimes they fall off on their own, sometimes they must be amputated. If the gangrenous limbs are removed completely, there is a chance of recovery. If they linger, death is almost certain.

The second path the disease takes is more insidious. It engenders involuntary spasms of the fingers and wrists, and soon convulsions of the whole body similar to epileptic seizures. Eventually the effects become as grotesque as they are painful, for the episodes can cause the body to collapse in on itself, and the patient contorts into a packed ball of limbs or a displaced gnarl of branches, resembling less a human than a human hacked into pieces and rebuilt with every appendage out of place.

Both forms, the gangrenous and the convulsive, were well described in the Middle Ages, and it was clearly understood that they were the same disease. The gangrenous tended to be more common in France, while the convulsive appeared more frequently east of the Rhine, a situation that physician Mervyn Eadie of the University of Queensland thinks might have been due to the effect of different soils on the exact chemical composition of ergot.[2]

There is, however, one possible, and perhaps important, difference between the modern clinical description of ergotism and the medieval clinical description of St. Anthony's fire. According to modern medical literature, mental disturbances, including confusion, dementia, and vivid hallucinations (effects of the lysergic acid), occur only in the convulsive variety. But the evidence for this is not definitive, as most of the cases of ergotism studied by science have been non-hallucinating gangrenous ones resulting from the excessive intake of ergot-based drugs, now used to treat migraines. Ergotamine drugs have not been known to cause the convulsive variety, and although doctors saw hallucinations paired with convulsions in the nineteenth and early twentieth centuries, ethical considerations make a modern study of this almost eradicated condition impossible. The most we can say for certain is that modern victims of gangrenous ergotism do not suffer hallucinations, and that victims of convulsive ergotism used to suffer them often.

Yet some circumstantial evidence suggests that for a thousand years in Europe, St. Anthony's fire caused hallucinations and mental terrors in sufferers *both* convulsive and gangrenous. For example, many artistic depictions of the disease by famous painters such as Hieronymus Bosch and Matthias Grünewald (the latter's painting commissioned for a hospital dedicated to treating *ignis sacer*) show someone with gangrenous physical symptoms who is surrounded, and in many cases totally upstaged, by a host of chimeras, by demons and angels pivoting between terror and ecstasy. There is also a striking closeness to metaphor in the otherwise literal descriptions of the French chronicles. It is written, over and over again, that the gangrenous disease arises from a fire that no water can quench and that no one can see, burning limbs from the inside out until they are black as coal. The chronicles suggest that people believed, and felt, and knew, that actual flames were burning in their stomachs and arms. This is borne out by the common depiction of St. Anthony stamping out a fire with his feet, and the fact that the walls of hospitals for ardents were painted all around with red flames.

This may seem a minor contention, but it has certain important implications. Something may have occurred during outbreaks of St. Anthony's fire that, were it to happen today, we would call a hallucination, but because it happened long ago, we don't. The history of St. Anthony's fire may therefore pose a question about the difference between a hallucination and a metaphor, a question that might have something to say about the effect of Christianity on the modern West, and on the role of culture in shaping consciousness.

Some further background is needed before we confront this boundary between the literal and the figurative. St. Anthony's fire is one of the most feared diseases in medieval Europe; it comes from nowhere and inflicts long-lasting horrors on its victims. They burn and blacken; they see demons; they convulse and seize; they jump from windows (as is also common during psychotic episodes triggered by consuming LSD). Medieval medicine is essentially helpless against it, though not for lack of trying. In fact, it is this disease that gives medieval medicine its distinctive character, that will impel it to make a major contribution to the history of healing. St. Anthony's fire—not the plague, not smallpox, not

syphilis—is the catalyst for the first pan-European network of hospitals, organized with a discipline unequaled in the West for many centuries.

At the close of the eleventh century, the holy fire breaks out in the Dauphiné, an ancient county of the Holy Roman Empire in present-day southeastern France. According to later sources, a nobleman named Gaston de La Valloire takes his son, afflicted with the disease, to pray at the relics of St. Anthony the Great, prince of hermits. Anthony's bones had been brought to the Dauphiné thirty years before by a Frankish knight named Jocelin, who received them from the Byzantine emperor Romanos IV Diogenes in thanks for his military service against the Saracens. The bones are said to have translated miraculously from the Egyptian desert to Alexandria and subsequently to Constantinople, where they rested in the Hagia Sophia before their departure for France. Gaston promises that if his son Gérin is healed, he will devote himself, in the name of St. Anthony, to the care of the ardents.

Whatever the true outcome of this story or its relation to reality, a group of noblemen forms a lay brotherhood named for St. Anthony in the last decade of the eleventh century. They build a hospital for holy fire in the town of Saint-Antoine-en-Viennois, where the relics are kept in the care of a Benedictine priory. True to its etymology, the hospital is also a hostel for pilgrims coming to pray to St. Anthony, or continuing on to Santiago.[3] The brotherhood and its patron flourish. Anthony will join Roch and Sebastian as one of the great protectors against illness in the Catholic pantheon. The lay organization will become by papal bull a monastic order using the Rule of St. Augustine, fitting because the story of Anthony's life had profoundly affected Augustine on the eve of his conversion to Christianity. The Antonites will eventually unseat the Benedictines in Saint-Antoine and take control of the relics; in the little town they build their mother abbey. They build commanderies and adjoining hospitals along the pilgrim routes, in Freiburg, Isenheim, Memmingen, Basel, Cologne, Paris, Avignon, Montpellier, Carcassonne, Toulouse, Turin, Rome, Naples, Castrojeriz, and León. At the order's height in the fourteenth century, there will be 369 such satellites in Europe, including in England and Hungary. In 1253, the Antonites are mentioned in papal documents as the official nurses to the Roman Curia, and they are the only order accorded this privilege until 1300.

The hospitals in the town of Saint-Antoine are a wonder. During times of epidemic, they house as many as two thousand patients. (On the other hand, in 1589, when a season of bubonic plague and religious war disrupts travel throughout France, only seven ardents remain in the abbey.) Everything is strictly and efficiently ordered. Upon entering, patients are carefully examined to make certain they actually suffer from St. Anthony's fire. Those who have another disease are put in separate wards and sometimes even sent away.[4] The true ardents, meanwhile, are ushered into a world of incredible spiritual and social strictness. They must pledge to be loyal to the faith and the order while in its care. They must live morally and chastely while in the hospital. If a male and female patient wish to be married, it can only be with explicit permission of the order. One of their number must serve as night watchman. If they are able, they must pray the canonical hours in the church, observing the matins and lauds and nones and vespers with the monks. Those who can't are taken care of by the pragmatic hospital architecture, which consists of a huge rectangular room with a rounded chapel at the end. The doors of the chapel can swing wide open, and suddenly the whole space with its hundreds of crowded beds (sometimes three or four amputees share a mattress) is an ark for prayer.

The order makes promises in return. First and foremost, the sick are fed every day, and given meat three times a week. On holidays, they get a small donation and a feast. At Easter, to each a lamb. At Christmas, white bread the size of four rolls and a full pitcher of undiluted wine, beef, pork, and a cup of wine with honey.[5] Although the cause of ergotism is unknown, the order somehow senses that fresh and healthy food is essential to recovery, perhaps the intuition of a society that knows intimately the many insidious effects of hunger. But possibly more than that, since the provision of food is also bound to the structures and symbols of the liturgical calendar. This is most clear when it comes to the main instruments of healing, which are, first, the *saint vinage*, wine mixed with herbs that has been poured over Anthony's bones, and second, Anthony's balsam, a closely guarded secret mixture of herbs

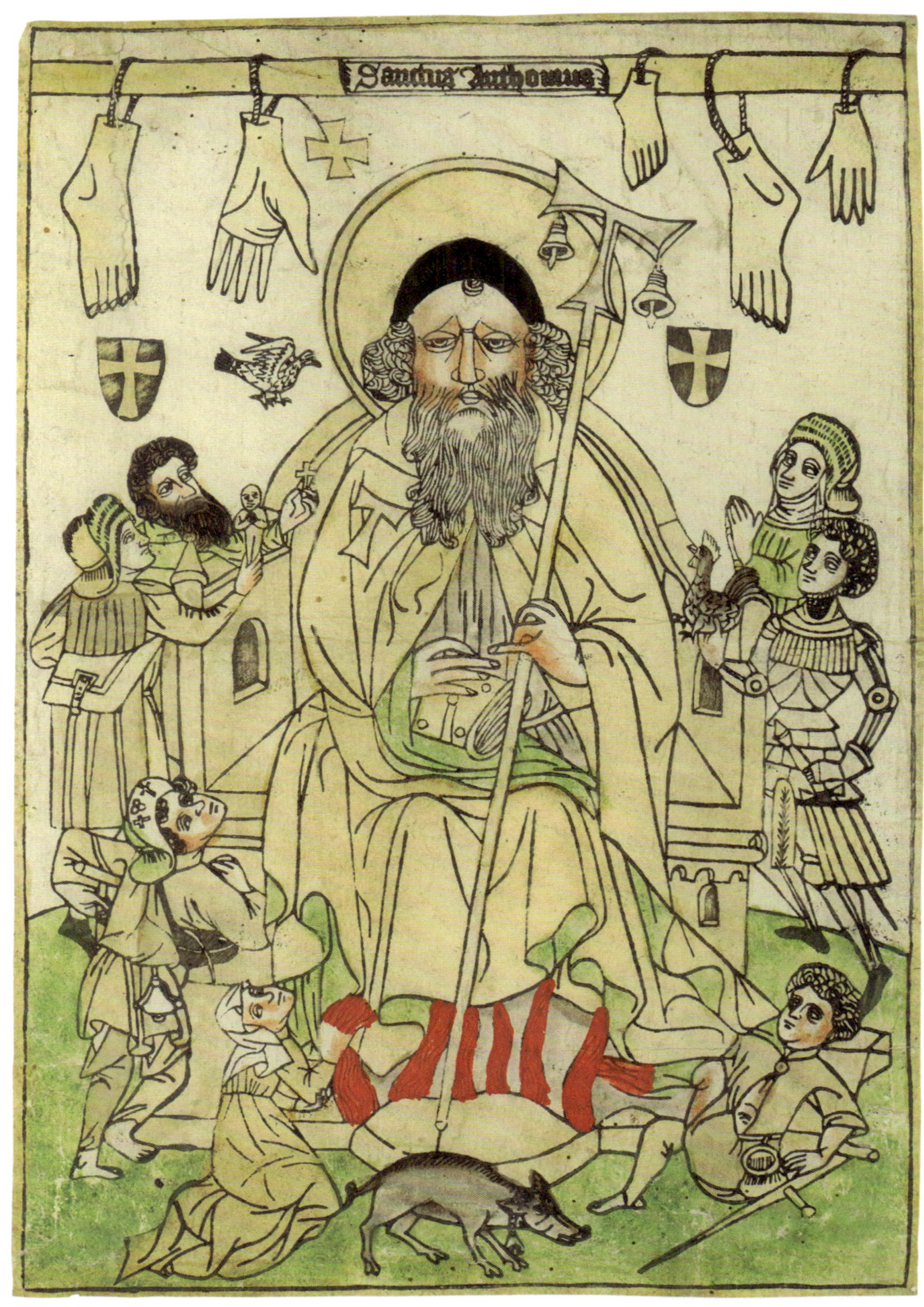

German woodcut by unknown artist depicting St. Anthony,
ca. 1440–1450. The saint, shown with his various symbols,
is surrounded by victims of the holy fire. Courtesy Staatliche
Graphische Sammlung, Munich.

(maybe the same as in the *saint vinage*) rubbed on the extremities to soothe the burning.[6] The main medicines—bread, wine, oil—are respectful parodies of the Eucharist and the chrism, modeled on the central spiritual performance of Christianity. Eating and drinking—essential to healing, and maybe the main reason for the order's successes—are a by-product of the Antonites' love of symbolic order, for the lamb at Easter is foremost the Lamb of God, and only second a lamb to eat.

Giorgio Agamben has written eloquently of what was variously called in European monasticism the *regula vitae*, the rule of life; the *regula et vita*, the rule and life; and the *regula vel vita*, the rule or life. He argues in his book *The Highest Poverty* that the interchangeability of these formulations (the rule *of* life is also rule *and* life) indicates that the governing of monastic life and the living of monastic life were thought by the monks to be completely coincident. The hours and rituals of the monastery did not compel behavior; behavior did not govern the hours and rituals. Rather, behavior and rules were meant to replicate each other exactly and organically, without any punishment or direct exercise of authority needed to make them cohere. Agamben considers this an unprecedented and unique form of non-authoritarian political organization.

The Antonites used something akin to this coincidence of rule and life as a template for healing. The sick needed continuous structure, communal protections, and, above all, a common set of symbols, like compass points indicating the way to health, in order to live. But this armature for living had to be actively embraced, not passively accepted, an axiom made explicit by the fact that the patients had to serve as their own watchmen and swear oaths of fealty, like temporary monks. An important effect of order is to invest the mutability of human experience, governed by the whim of subjective time, with a symbolic fixity. The wretchedness of illness rejects structure; it erases habit and makes time impossible to measure. Hours stretch into days, a week can seem to pass in a night. Even a minor fever without the disruptions of lysergic acid can cause confusion, delirium, dreams more vivid than reality. Aby Warburg, who went on to devote his life to studying the aliveness of images, remembered that during a bout of typhoid fever at the age of six, in 1873, the little devils and carriages from an illustrated edition of Balzac's *Les petites misères de la vie conjugale* started to dance across his bed, becoming ever more daring and capricious.

St. Anthony's fire, we know, can cause vivid hallucinations. A probable outbreak of convulsive ergotism in southern France in the 1950s (probable because there are some who allege it was mercury poisoning) afflicted hundreds of villagers with visions of snakes, soldiers, and heavenly lights ordering them to leap from windows.[7] And although gangrenous ergotism does not generally produce hallucinations of this sort, it seems reasonable, even obvious, that even for gangrenous patients in the medieval period, facing a disease they did not understand and could not effectively cure, their overwhelming physical pain would have been augmented by a mercenary parade of psychic fears capitalizing on each and every consequence of the disease —the body's betrayal, the mind's impotence, the approach of death. It is entirely conceivable that the manifestations of this fear took on the weight of physical reality, and began to resemble what we in the modern world would call hallucination.[8] For the afflicted would have tried desperately to describe in whatever vocabulary was available to them—that of fire, or demons, or curses, or just retribution for sins—what it was that was happening to their bodies. My own experience with the harrowing effects of hypochondria, especially hypochondria manifested on top of actual illness, leaves me in no doubt of the many avenues that a fire-addled mind might take, into self-pity or terror, toward delusion and paranoia.

The Antonites, helpless against most of the physical effects, could at least discipline the spiritual ones. The shifting fears of illness were straitjacketed in a series of ritualized, symbolic actions, actions borrowed from religious practice and made into a kind of therapy, an elaborate and theatrical placebo, healing by mimesis, by performance. For those who survived, the performance ended in a decisive valediction to illness, maybe intended to prevent lingering psychic trauma: the healed victims hung their blackened limbs in the abbey church as ex-votos to St. Anthony. In Lourdes or Santiago, the healed now leave little brass models of their legs or arms, or perhaps a crutch they once used, but in Antonite churches, it was the leg itself, the very limb, that was left behind, turned from a leg into the symbol

of a leg. What looks from afar to be a gruesome
practice is up close, by its own logic, a sanitizing act,
the transformation of the unpredictable vagaries of
bodily sensation into clean and ordered signs.

The planet around which all the symbols of healing orbit is Anthony himself. By the late Middle Ages,
he is rich in iconography. He has the flames at his feet,
a bell, a book, a pig, blackened hands and arms hanging above, and on his habit and his staff the order's
insignia, the Greek letter *tau*, which appropriately
resembles a crutch.[9] But why exactly is the prince of
hermits the patron of these monks, and of this illness?
Surprisingly, the question has been rarely asked with
the thoroughness it deserves. Many scholars have
written about Anthony, his life in late antiquity, and
his biography by Athanasius, which is among the
most famous and influential of hagiographies. Others
have written about his association with the holy fire.
But no one, so far as I know, has attempted rigorously to explain the connection between the historical
Anthony and the symbolic one, except to suggest that
medieval pictures showing the saint's temptation as a
psychedelic feast of demons might owe something to
the hallucinations of Anthony's fire.

A still less explored question is what he meant
to the Antonites and their ingenious system of symbolic caregiving. Adalbert Mischlewski, the foremost
modern historian of the Antonites, concludes that
it was all chance.[10] Anthony was just another local
saint invoked against a scourge, and circumstances
worked in such a way that his followers in the
Dauphiné became the founders of an international
brotherhood. The situation is admittedly curious,
at least on the surface. Why would a hermit be
the patron of hospitals, where the sick are packed
together in conditions of dependence? But this is
related to a larger question. How did a man living
alone in the desert serve as the model for European
monasticism, one of the most intense experiments in
communal living ever attempted?

For Anthony, in addition to patronizing this illness, is the key hermit of the Middle Ages. Not the
first, but the one whose influence, thanks to his biographer Athanasius, becomes most widespread and
accepted as a model for the holy life. His withdrawal
into the desert in fourth-century Egypt does as
much as any other action to destroy the foundations
of the ancient world, for he turns his back on *civitas*

and *virtus*, the foundational classical notions that a
person is constituted by the duties and privileges that
accrue to him within his society. But the revolution is
still more radical, for Anthony is not merely a person
who turns his back on the community; he is a person
constitutionally incapable of accepting community, at
least as it exists in his own time.

A powerful detail in Athanasius, so distinctive that even after sixteen hundred years it retains
an aura of authenticity, is that as a boy Anthony
does not like to play, neither alone nor with other
children. We often hear of artists-to-be creating
extravagant realities in their nurseries, orchestrating
precocious displays of puppetry or painting, corral-
ling their friends into pageants, actions which we
interpret as the necessary outpouring of the inner
life. There is a certain kind of person about whom
we think they *must* pour their life force into the
world. Anthony is not that kind of person, or does
not want to be, anyway. He keeps his life force hidden within him, pent up.

Anthony's story is about a refusal, or rather an
innate inability, to externalize the experience within.
His continued retreat from humanity, first into a
hut, then a tomb, then the desert, then a far, arid
mountain, is an attempt to reach a place where his
aliveness cannot escape, for there is no vessel into
which it can be poured, no piece of property, no
article of clothing, no object, no person. He is afraid
or unwilling to let his mind push beyond his body's
boundary, to make any mark on the earth.
The temptations of St. Anthony, and the holiness
he builds from them, become the blueprint for a
medieval hydraulics of spirit. What happens when
the pressure of the inner reservoir, kept clean and
undrunk so that it might one day quench the thirst
of God, builds to an unknown strength? The self
vacillates between exultation and despair, borne
aloft by images of other beings. Athanasius writes
that in solitude, Anthony faces a "great dustcloud
of thoughts" sent from the devil. They include a
lascivious woman; a terrifying small black boy (this
black boy will become a common apparition among
monks who read Athanasius too often); a dragon;
uncounted species of twisted reptile; invisible agents
who beat the hermit black and blue. The farther
Anthony retreats into himself and the more isolated he becomes, the more his thoughts take on the

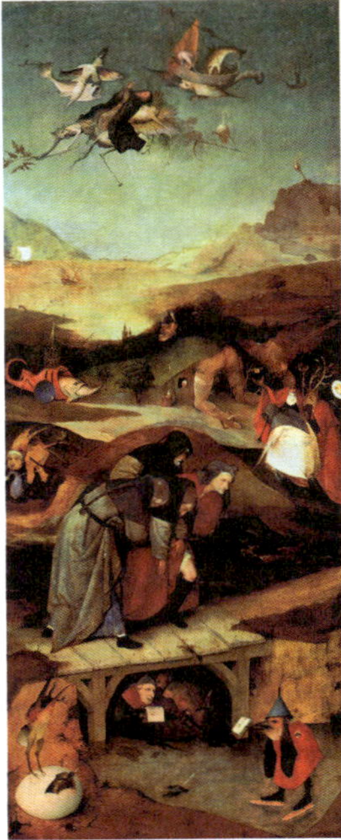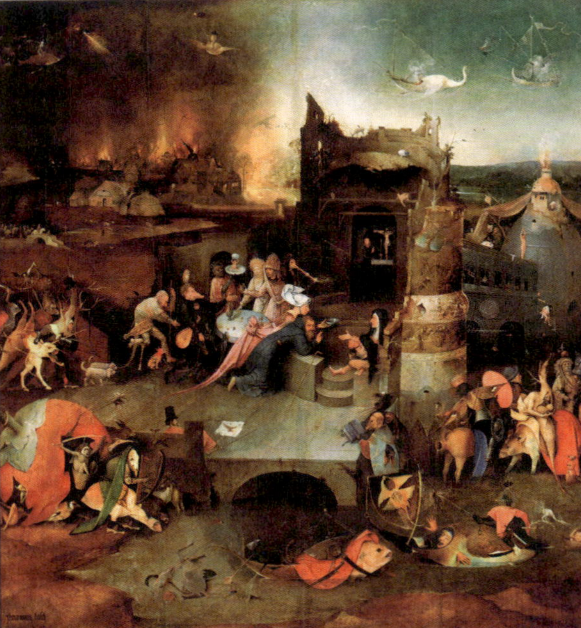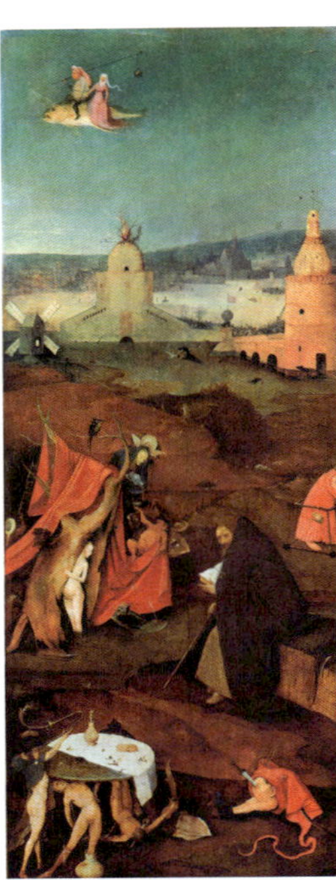

Hieronymus Bosch, *The Temptation of Saint Anthony*, ca. 1500.

weight of reality, and the more his existence comes to resemble a kingdom, crowded and oppressed, in a state of continuous insurrection.

Anthony represents a spectacular insight of the Christian worldview, foreshadowed in the Gospels by the Temptation of Christ. In solitude, whether geographical, spiritual, or the physical solitude of sickness, a person becomes a society. And a person unprepared for that solitude becomes a society in a state of extreme precariousness. At one moment, his empire exceeds that of all earthly realms; it grasps at eternity in the baroque splendor of its architecture, in the glitter of its jewels, in the desirability of the slaves in its harems, in the perfection of its awards, punishments, and perversions. In the next, it is in a state of utter catastrophe, buildings aflame and in ruin, the citizens and slaves deformed into factions savaging one another while wearing the masks of beasts. The more distant a person grows from the world of other people, the more complete this private universe becomes, the more real, and if unprepared, the more volatile. It begins to approximate that paradigmatic private universe, the dream, where the productions of mind *are* the floor and sky and windows and wall, not to mention every inhabitant malignant and benign.

But the Antonine solution, which becomes the monastic solution, and maybe the modern solution, is not simply to ignore this private world, to run from it back to the social one. Instead, the private world must be tamed from the inside before the social world can be rejoined. Communal life can be an armature for private life, providing a vocabulary of actions and images through which the solitary kingdom can be brought to order. But it can't actually do the ordering, it cannot simply impose beliefs in the way that self-righteous schoolteachers will later debase the Antonine impulse into ideology. Nor can it be a substitute. A person must pass through the rise and fall and restoration of the kingdom of solitude in order to become, to the core, part of the new society of humans.

Hieronymus Bosch's Lisbon triptych of the Temptation of St. Anthony, from the early sixteenth century, articulates this worldview very directly. In the left panel, St. Anthony, who wears the *tau* of an Antonite, is shown being carried by three friends after he has been dropped from the sky by a pack of flying monsters. In the other two panels, in contrast, Anthony is shown without any companions, surrounded only by a huge host of demons. If the panels are meant to be viewed from left to right (as

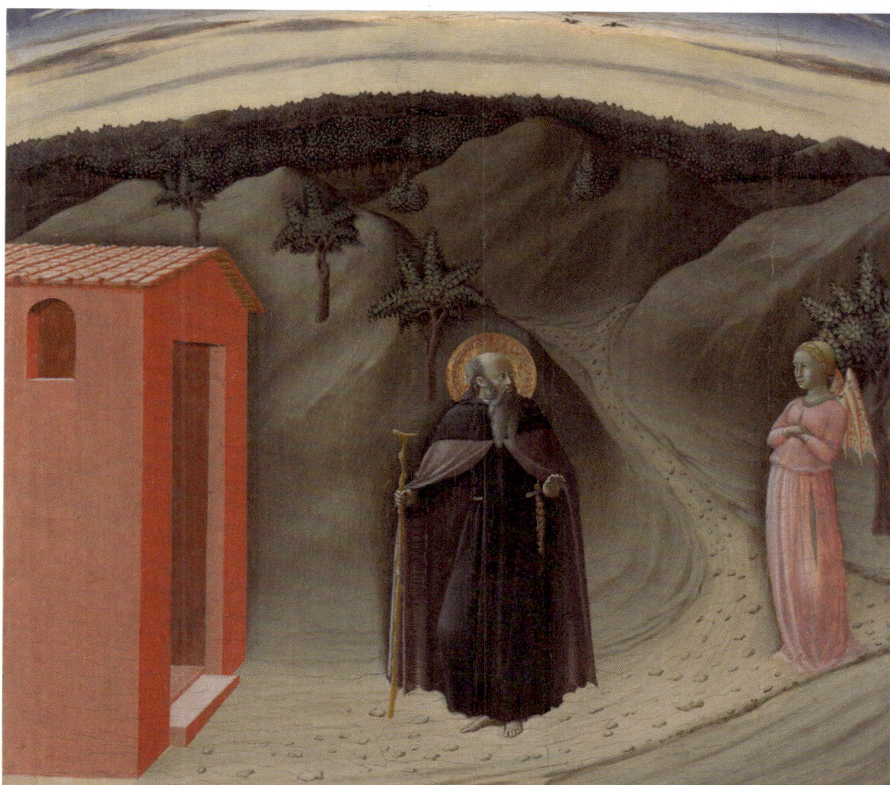

Master of the Osservanza, *Saint Anthony Tempted by the Devil in the Guise of a Woman*, ca. 1435.

many of Bosch's other triptychs very clearly are), then Anthony's friends in the left panel are carrying him into his isolation in the central panel, not away from it. This point doesn't require any great stretch of interpretation, because they are walking him along a path that points directly toward the middle of the work. It is the duty of Anthony's helpers to lead him to solitude, to prepare him for the battle over his private kingdom (perhaps they have offered to take the bruised saint back to their village and he has said to them, *no dear friends, no, carry me deeper into the wilderness*). One of these helpers carries a crucifix tied to his belt. In the next panel, a crucifix, or a *tau* almost transformed into a crucifix, dangles in the same position from Anthony's garment, as if the talisman has been passed from one to the other: *here, keep this, remember there are others in the world.*

The absolute ineffectiveness of medieval medicine meant, essentially, that the Antonite monks could do little more than exactly what Anthony's friends are doing. They could carry the sufferer into the solitude of his sickness, and leave some talisman of their common faith in his hand. Physical pain,

Elaine Scarry has eloquently explained, cuts off its perceiver from the rest of the world. Bosch's St. Anthony triptych shows the terrifying reality that can arise to fill the void, the apparitions that flood the mind which stubbornly persists to work while in isolation, whether that isolation is born from geographical distance or closeness to death. In such a situation, as the bridges fall away, the mind's own figurations become its reality, and what might be a simple metaphor or symbol in some other context becomes what we would call a hallucination and is, to the perceiver, the very stuff of being.

To plant a stable and reassuring set of metaphors into the overly fertile ground of mental isolation was the project of Antonite healing. The hours, the shrines, the flames, the votaries, the wine, the *tau*, and the white bread were an attempt to influence the shape of the world that each victim would inevitably be forced to construct and then suffer through. Bosch understood this exceptionally well, as he understood the logical conflation of Anthony and Antonite healing. In the central panel of his triptych, the major symbolic devices of the Antonite order

appear amid the devil's mercenaries. In the middle ground, there is a severed foot upon a white cloth, an ex-voto offering, still bleeding, in front of the living saint. Behind Anthony, partially hidden in a dark room, Jesus stands at an altar right next to a crucifix and imparts a blessing; the symbol of the Savior has become the Savior, alive and incarnate. Still more astonishing is a burning building in the distant background being looted by a pillaging army. This rectangular structure with a curved chapel on the shorter side is none other than an Antonite hospital, its falling tower mounted by the *tau*.[11] The painted flames that decorated the walls of the Antonite hospital have burst into actual fire, so that the dread of dying in fire might at least have a consistent and sympathetic continuity with the external world, as powerless as the victim.

The Antonites practiced what might now be called palliative care for the mental confusions and terrors of St. Anthony's fire, wherever those terrors fell on the spectrum between chemical hallucination and psychic disturbance. It was perhaps their special insight, born as much from ignorance as wisdom, to understand how extreme suffering, and not just suffering but many forms of extreme isolation, collapse the distinction between hallucination and imagination. In fact, the compassion of the Antonite project is the direct result of its minimal impact, as Bosch depicts with sobering clarity. In his painting, the symbols of healing are miniscule compared with everything that is not a symbol, or is a perversion of symbols (is that the *saint vinage* in the hands of a demon?), or an unformed matrix of meaning, a Eucharist and a theologian and a merchant and a fish and a devil and a monk and a chamber-pot all at once and never at all. The monks, following Anthony's example, were resigned to the fact that dreams are hostile to the influence of waking life, even though they plunder its stones to build their palaces. The Antonites mastered a discipline that we, thankfully, have been able to let lapse, although there is no guarantee that it won't be needed again soon. This discipline might be called understanding not-understanding, or helping when you are helpless, and it is a quixotic midwife to inner life, witness to the birth of attitudes that make a certain notion of selfhood possible.

1 In medieval Germany, the ergot spur was called *Hungerkorn*, the hunger grain.

2 See Mervyn J. Eadie, "Convulsive Ergotism: Epidemics of the Serotonin Syndrome?" *The Lancet Neurology*, vol. 2, no. 7 (July 2003).

3 The treatment of the holy fire was always related to the care of pilgrims on the roads to Santiago. This may be because many victims of *ignis sacer* set out for Santiago in the hope of being healed; it may also simply be because pilgrims, like all travelers, were vulnerable and in need of special care. I wonder if it might also be because pilgrims, many dependent on alms, were often given the bread no one else wanted, and so were more frequently exposed to ergot.

4 In Memmingen, the patients themselves were called on to judge whether or not a newly admitted person had their disease.

5 White bread, though less nutritious than dark bread, was highly valued in the Middle Ages. When founding his hospital, the Hôtel-Dieu in Beaune, the Burgundian chancellor Nicolas Rolin set aside funds for *white bread* to be regularly distributed to the poor, a gesture of unheard-of largesse.

6 The recipe of the balsam was a closely guarded secret, so closely guarded, in fact, that the Order itself forgot it. Adalbert Mischlewski reports that a 1601 letter from the head of the Antonite hospital in Isenheim to the Archduke Ferdinand of Austria says that the recipe has regrettably already been lost. Some art historians have thought that a clue to its composition might be found in the herbs depicted in Grünewald's *Isenheim Altarpiece*, a spectacular late medieval polyptych commissioned by the Isenheim monks. Under the panel showing St. Anthony meeting the hermit Paul, there are about a dozen herbs (by Lottelise Behling's count), including delicate tendrils of corn poppy, sage, ribwort, verbena, gentian, and ranunculus. The balsam may have had vasodilatory or disinfecting properties.

7 The poisonings at Pont-Saint-Esprit in 1951 have attracted many theories, including speculation that the CIA poured LSD into the water supply as an experiment in psychotropic warfare. John Fuller makes a case for the ergotism hypothesis in *The Day of St. Anthony's Fire* (New York: The Macmillan Company, 1968). Albert Hoffman, who first synthesized LSD from ergot, disputes the ergotism explanation in his book *LSD: Mein Sorgenkind* (Stuttgart: Klett-Cotta, 1979).

8 This argument owes a debt to an extraordinary observation in Elaine Scarry's book *The Body in Pain* (Oxford & New York: Oxford University Press, 1985). Scarry writes that pain and suffering so completely obliterate the normal parameters of experience that they appear to be without object: they just *are*, almost without cause. And yet, there is a deep need in the suffering mind to generate an objective cause for that pain: if we suffer from a terrible and mysterious pain in the spine, we say, as if to dilute the mystery, *It feels as if there is a hammer pounding on my spine*. What begins to be complicated, however, is when we begin to say, *There is a hammer pounding on my spine*, and we continue saying that until, before long, the hammer becomes enormous and alive and full of a malicious agency.

9 The pig was the famous "cochon d'Antoine," an extension of the order's communitarian principles into the lay world. Poor farmers could promise a piglet to the order, which would then feed on trash in the streets until it was fat enough to be sent to the monastery to be slaughtered and fed to the sick. It was an elegant solution, for it meant that everyone and no one was responsible for the care of the pig, and so it diminished the burden of the tithe.

10 Mischlewski's major work is *Grundzüge der Geschichte des Antoniterordens bis zum Ausgang des 15. Jahrhunderts* (Cologne and Vienna: Böhlau, 1976).

11 This, at least, is the convincing conclusion of the medical anthropologist Veit Harold Bauer in *Das Antonius-Feuer in Kunst und Medizin* (Berlin and Heidelberg; Springer Verlag, 1973). He notes that Bosch depicts another Antonite hospital in a drawing of the Temptation of Anthony now in the Kupferstich-Kabinett in Berlin.

RED STAR THEATER
William Firebrace

THREE

In the skies over Moscow, in the years before the collapse of the socialist state, stood three symbols of the space program: the rocket, the cosmonaut, and the red star. The rocket remains on the Monument to the Conquerors of Space (1964), a 110-meter-high titanium sculpture beside Mira Prospekt with the Alley of the Cosmonauts leading to its base. The Yuri Gargarin monument (1980)—featuring a statue of the cosmonaut on a 30-meter-high column with his arms pulled back in the style of a Marvel superhero, as though about to leap into the stratosphere—continues to overlook Leninsky Prospekt. These two landmarks at once look back to the period of Soviet space exploration and forward to the time of planetary probes and space stations. But the red star—symbol both of astronomy and of communism—is gone. Preceding the epic period of space flights, it once crowned the dome of the Moscow planetarium (1929), on Sadovaya-Kudrinskaya Ulitsa.

PATTERNS

Some buildings derive from tangled threads of different influences, which unexpectedly intertwine at the moment of their creation and which continue to exert an influence for many years. Some of these influences are tangential, some central; some are clearly defined, some discerned only through the traces they leave. Together, they indicate a pattern of movement rather than a simple object. The Moscow planetarium, a comparatively simple building, stands at the intersection of influences created by engineering, style, theater, astronomy, religion, and politics, each of which affects all the others.

PROJECTION

The Moscow planetarium is a variation on the original projection planetarium, invented by the German mechanical engineer Walther Bauersfeld and built in 1923 on the roof of the Zeiss factory in Jena. This experimental planetarium was the first to feature the Zeiss projector, whose complex sets of individual lamps, each moving on their own course, could project up onto a hemispherical screen the paths of the planets, the movement of comets, and

the relative brightness of the distant stars and galaxies. It was also the first building to feature a thin shell dome, designed by Bauersfeld and the engineer Franz Dischinger, based on a geodesic structure of thin metal rods sprayed with cement. Planetariums immediately became a craze in Germany and then in Europe, a must-have item for cities on the make, with the Moscow planetarium being the thirteenth to be constructed.

David Ryazanov—a former comrade in exile of Leon Trotsky and director of the Marx-Engels Institute, an organization devoted to Soviet philosophy and history—proposed the construction of the planetarium in 1926. The building was originally intended to be part of a large science complex—including a zoo, a museum, and a library—which would exemplify the rising power of pure science. Evolutionary time would be presented in the zoo and cosmic time in the planetarium, both set against the traditional religious time of the discredited Russian Orthodox Church. Ryazanov traveled to Germany to visit various planetariums and to persuade Bauersfeld and Dischinger to construct a planetarium for Moscow. At the time, the Weimar and the Soviet republics were on good terms, with considerable architectural interchange between the two. Bauersfeld and Dischinger possessed skills lacking in the USSR : the technology to construct the projector and the engineering expertise to put up the ferro-cement dome, lightweight construction and the projection of light thus combining to produce a building reduced to the minimum use of material. The new planetarium was to be on an ambitious scale, with an internal diameter of twenty-seven meters, and seating for 1,440 spectators. The Zeiss dumbbell projector provided by Bauersfeld was the latest model, able to project an astonishing 8,956 stars and to switch the projection point to various latitudes.

There had been considerable discussion in Germany as to what form the exterior of a planetarium should take. As a new building type, should it

Opposite: Moscow's Monument to the Conquerors of Space in 2009. Photo Jaime Silva.

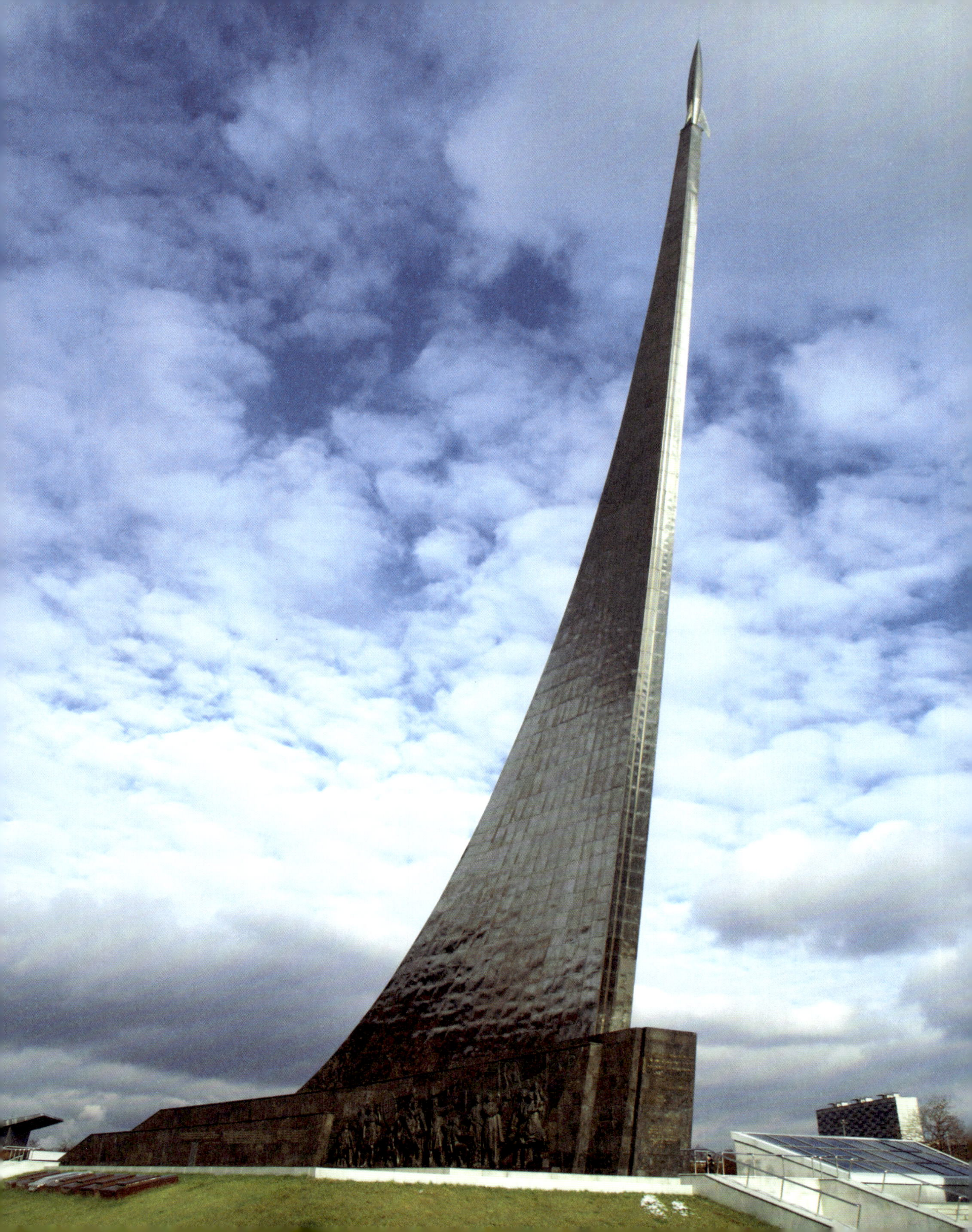

reflect the scientific nature of the interior? Should it be clearly part of the new age of modernism? Should it belong to the neoclassical tradition, a small temple featuring a formal entrance with columns and a portico? The discussion concerning the Moscow Planetarium, which took place within the confused cultural conditions of the Soviet Union of the late 1920s, went one stage further. The design is credited to two young Russian architects, Mikhail Barshch and Mikhail Sinyavsky, and is usually referred to as constructivist—though constructivism included any number of different approaches, and often implied little more than modernism. While both architects had emerged from the VKhUTEMAS school of architecture, established in 1920 by Lenin, they were also conversant in the eclectic mix of styles left over from the prerevolutionary period. This was the first, and only, building by this pair of architects. A photo from the time, taken in what looks like late evening, shows the architectural team climbing up the maintenance ladder attached to the outside of the dome with Barshch in front, as though leading his colleagues into the skies. Asked later how they had come to be awarded this prestigious design, Barshch commented that nobody in Moscow knew what a planetarium was—it was presumed to be some kind of toy for children, and therefore more experienced architects had not been interested in the project.[1]

The planetarium was thus a mix of German optical and engineering technology, which determined the basic layout of the building, and Soviet modernist architecture, which supplied a specific external appearance. It was built at a time when the experimental culture of the revolutionary period was coming to an end and a mix of modernist and traditional forms had become the official style. In fact, the various designs for the planetarium flickered between modern and traditional; an intermediate design by Barshch and Sinyavsky proposed a large neoclassical porch with Greek columns, at once looking back to prerevolutionary architecture and forward to the Stalinist period. This concept was abandoned for the clean simple form actually constructed, but hovers around it as an unconstructed phantom project.

Much of the design of the Moscow planetarium is determined by the technical requirements of the projection system. The building has three stories:

a basement, an entrance and foyer at ground level with a set of radial portal frames to support the floor above, and a main projection hall for the fourteen-hundred-odd visitors on the first floor. The internal hemispherical projection screen indicates a circular plan. There is requirement for additional service spaces that need to be added to the circular form, so four elements project from the central circle—the entrance, a box for storing the projector to the side when it is not in use, another box with an elegant spiral stair for services, and offices for the staff. But intertwined with this pragmatism are other influences, derived from the specifically Russian background, that move the building away from its German origins.

PARABOLA

The planetarium has two domes: the inner hemispherical projection screen and an outer ferro-cement shell whose parabolic form was a decision of the German engineers as much as the architects. The design is highly unusual, in fact the only parabolic dome ever built over a planetarium. A parabola is more efficient than a circle in distributing structural forces, and thus can save material. This outer dome is, astonishingly, only eight centimeters thick at the top and twelve at the bottom, giving it a ratio of shell thickness to internal volume of 1:280, less than that of an eggshell to an egg. This shell was constructed from a framework of steel rods laid according to a timber formwork and onto which was sprayed concrete. Due to a shortage of materials in Moscow, a cement substitute was created from ground-up clamshells, which have roughly the same chemical composition as cement—and which for some reason were available in landlocked Moscow. The insulation was a layer of moss. The materials of the sea and of the land were used to create a shell for the artificial sky, which was then covered externally with aluminum sheeting imported from Germany.

However, alongside the structural explanation there are other sources of influence—pragmatic, stylistic, intellectual. Mikhail Barshch had been on a tour of Soviet Asia and had become interested in the diverse forms of mosque domes. The planetarium's appearance, but not its material, is similar to the dome of the 1914 Glass Pavilion of Bruno Taut, constructed in Cologne, of which the German

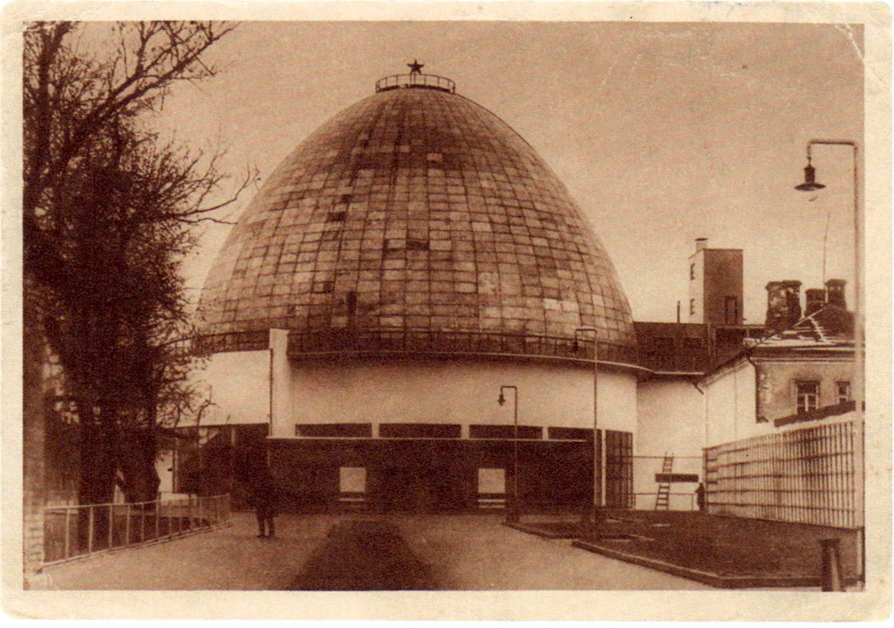

Postcard depicting the Moscow Planetarium, topped with its red star, 1930. Courtesy of Jeremy Storey.

writer Paul Scheerbart wrote that it would allow contemplation of the light of the moon and stars. Parabolic domes were perhaps becoming fashionable in Moscow, appearing in Ivan Leonodov's visionary project for Club of a New Social Type and also Moisei Ginzburg's unbuilt Palace of the Soviets. Pragmatically, the parabola provides more space between the dome and the hemispherical projection screen, in that strange zone between projected sky and real sky, allowing workers to assemble the screen more easily from above. From the exterior, the planetarium resembles a cylindrical eggcup cradling a great egg, which is particularly significant to the Russian celebration of Easter, the time of rebirth and resurrection. The red star at the summit of the dome inevitably evokes the stars on traditional Russian onion domes. It is not necessary to say that one of these influences was decisive; a building can be indebted to diverse, even contradictory sources.

INTERNAL MOVEMENTS

One of the themes of certain early Soviet artists, such as Kazimir Malevich, had been the elimination of the object and its replacement by abstract shapes and lines of movement. The planetarium can be seen as constructed of various movements. In section, the parabola of the exterior dome rises above the semicircle of the interior projection screen—the parabola

outlining the elliptical path of planetary motion, and the semicircle the more ancient notion of the perfect sphere of the heavens. The curves within the radial portal frames on the ground floor and the partial parabola of the entrance canopy echo these lines, so that the entire section consists of curved lines of potential movement. Meanwhile, the circular plan of the planetarium is based on both circumferential and centrifugal movement, as the circular lines of the great circular hall are balanced by the four forms flung outward, such as the elegant spiral stair descending in a glass cylinder. The architectural dynamic determines the movement of the spectators, who enter axially through the curved entrance, circulate among the portal frames which radiate out from the center of the foyer, and move up along the steps running around the circumference of the building to take their places in the projection hall. To these can be added the lines of movement created by the ingenious and complex Zeiss projector. Standing in the center of the domed hall, surrounded by the seated spectators and describing with its lights the paths of the celestial bodies, the projector produces not a geocentric but a heliocentric view of the solar system. The spectatorial illusion that the dome of the building has vanished and that there is only a night sky above results in the planetarium's final dematerialization.

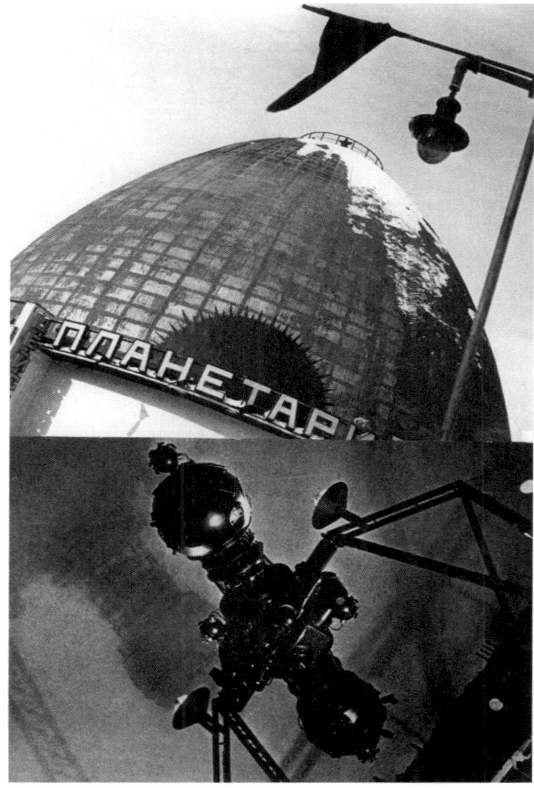

Alexander Rodchenko, *Planetarium Building. Projector Made by Zeiss*, 1932.

SKY THEATER

In 1927, Aleksei Gan, artistic editor of the architectural magazine *Sovremennaya Arkhitektura* and theorist of constructivism, published drawings of the first version of the planetarium and proclaimed it to be successor to both traditional theater and church:

The theater has been up until now nothing but a building dedicated to the service of cult. How this service has been performed, to which cult it is dedicated, plays no role. … Our theater must be different; it should draw the spectator to a love of science. The planetarium—a theater of optical science—is also one of the forms of our theater. In it, people do not act, but manage a complex technical apparatus. In this theater, all is mechanized. … So the theater at the service of cult passes to the service of science. In this theater, Man, equipped with machinery, extends his sense of perception, sees the most complicated mechanics of the movement of celestial bodies. This will help him forge a scientific understanding of the world and free himself from

both the fetishism and prejudice of savage priests and the pseudoscience of European civilization. For this theater, we need to build a new building.[2]

For Gan, traditional, prerevolutionary theater was little more than a kind of church service, whereas the planetarium would produce the most refined version of the theater performances proposed by Vsevolod Meyerhold and Lyubov Popova, in which narrative was abandoned, actors moved in precise patterns, and sets became large machines to accommodate these movements. By 1927, these performances were already part of the past, as the original impetus for a new theater had faded. For those like Gan, still hoping for a revival of the earlier enthusiasm, the planetarium offered a new opportunity. Its form resembles a temple, within which the audience sits reverently as the mysteries of the heavens are revealed on the interior of the dome, the traditional location in orthodox churches for a large painting of God staring back down. But this was a new kind of church. In one of his last poems, written in his highly individual style, Vladimir Mayakovsky declared: "Proletarian woman, proletarian man, come to the planetarium / Will come in, will hear the lively buzz / in the lecture hall / Spectators sit awaiting the sky to be shown / The director-of-the-skies came, the expert in sky matters / He came, pushed and twirled the million celestial bodies."[3] The director-of-the-skies—the poet's invented term for the lecturer who also controlled the projector—becomes in Mayakovsky's words part scientist, part priest, part shaman, part theater director. As is often the case with Mayakovsky, his support for the new socialist world has an undertone of mysticism. The projector could speed up time, summon up the vastness of the cosmos, and place the viewer in an alternate location within it. It was an appropriate mechanism to revive a declining revolutionary impulse.

COSMISM

Constructing a planetarium in Moscow was never going to be only about an educational display of the movements of the planets and the stars. Russia had had a long and diverse attitude to the cosmos, mixing science, esotericism, gnosticism, a belief in a world beyond the purely physical, and a feeling

that the nation was specially destined to explore the planets and beyond. The nineteenth-century writer Nikolai Fyodorov, founder of what is known as Cosmism, had proposed both that the atoms of the deceased were scattered throughout the universe and also that steps should be taken to resurrect the dead, who would then live on various planets since there would not be enough room for them to inhabit the earth. This resurrection theme would later filter into Soviet science fiction, for instance in Andrey Tarkovsky's film *Solaris* (1972), where the dead reappear on a spaceship above an aquatic planet. However, Fyodorov also inspired early Russian ideas about planetary travel. Konstantin Tsiolkovsky, the first Russian rocket designer—who in Czarist times had already worked out the basic formulas for the thrust required by engines intending to escape the earth's atmosphere—had been a follower of Fyodorov. Tsiolkovsky lived in the small town of Kaluga, just south of Moscow, where he constructed models of rockets and dirigibles,

indulged in complex and semi-mystical theories as to the makeup of the universe, and also wrote science fiction novels about Russian space explorers encountering aliens on other planets.[4] He was deeply eccentric—photos show him with long flowing locks, surrounded by his rockets and airships as he holds up his ear trumpet as though to detect distant sounds.

Other early Russian science fiction writers described the coming age of interplanetary flight. In *Red Star* (1908), Alexander Bogorov described Mars, the definitive red planet, as inhabited by a benign race keen to associate with the Russians. And in Aleksey Tolstoy's novella *Aelita* (1923), written at a time where the color red had acquired a political significance, two Soviet cosmonauts visit Mars, discover that its population is a slave race dominated by corrupt rulers, and assist in a 1917-style revolution, made slightly more complicated by the lead cosmonaut falling for the Martian queen. A year after its publication, *Aelita* was made into a spectacular and

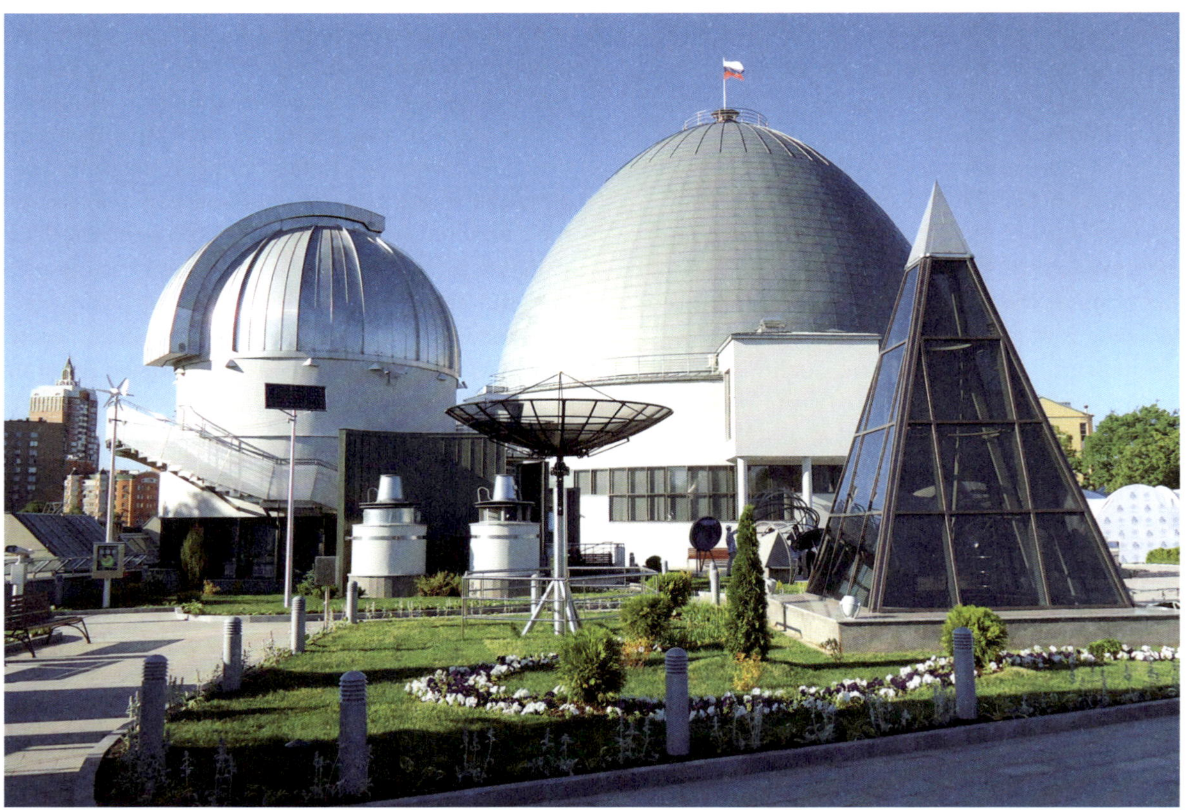

The Moscow Planetarium today.

very popular, if also what looks today absurdly antiquated and theatrical, film by Yakov Frotazanov.

By the late 1920s, popular societies were being
set up in Moscow to build on the enthusiasm for
space travel, with large-scale meetings and exhibitions on the subject. As a counterpart to this wave
of unscientific amateur enthusiasm, there was
also official interest in a more pragmatic, technological approach to space exploration. The Central
Bureau for the Study of the Problems of Rockets was
established in 1924 under the leadership of Yakov
Perelman, whose ultimate aim was the development of interplanetary travel.[5] "Onward to Mars,"
a phrase coined by the Soviet rocket designer
Friedrich Zander, later became one of the slogans of
the engineers working on the probes sent to Mars
and Venus by the country in the 1970s and 1980s.

This early Soviet enthusiasm for space travel,
mixing sci-fi and pragmatism, was reflected in the
planetarium, which provided a link between the
popular interest in space travel and the official, more
scientific approach. The large crowds that came to
the planetarium to see the scientific display of the
paths of the planets and stars understood that the
shows were also intended as an inspiration for the
future expansion of the Soviet people. Tsiolkovsky's
model rockets, accompanied by images of Soviet colonization of other planets, were shown prominently
in the lobby, and model rockets, imitating columns, were also placed by the entrance, as though
architecture and rocketry could be combined. In
the early 1940s, the planetarium hosted shows by
the Moscow Fantastic Theater about Copernicus,
Giordano Bruno, and Galileo, and during the early
1960s, Soviet spacecraft such as the spherical *Vostok
3KA-2*, launched with space dog Zvezdochka shortly
before the Gagarin mission, were displayed in the
lobby. The planetarium was used in the early 1960s
to show the workings of the solar system to prospective cosmonauts, some of whom, such as Gagarin,
returned to lecture to large audiences on their experiences. The planetarium was thus linked with the
early achievements of the Soviet space program—the
visible sign within Moscow of the success of Soviet
technology in comparison to its Western rivals—
and the venue was intended to inspire visitors to
imagine the gradual expansion of the Soviet program beyond the earth's atmosphere.

LATER MOVEMENTS

The later story of the Moscow planetarium mirrors
that of the Soviet Union. It had been brought to life
at a moment when Soviet society was rapidly changing, when the great hopes of the revolution were
fading before a political system moving towards the
Stalinist dictatorship of the 1930s. Built like other
constructivist projects during a period marked of
poor-quality materials, the building followed an
unsteady path. Soon after it was completed, the
Stalinist government added the red star—it did not
feature in the original design—so as to link the planetarium to the regime. At some point, the exterior
walls were painted bright blue, as though to deny its
links with the white modernism of the 1920s, and
the building's curving entrance porch was removed.
A photo from the early 1940s shows the building
already in a decayed state, surrounded by anti-
aircraft batteries dug into the rubble around it, ready
to fire up into, rather than investigate, the heavens.
After the war, the Soviet space program provided
a new sense of purpose for the planetarium; it was
renovated, received a new state-of-the-art Zeiss
projector in 1970, and once again became a popular
feature of Moscow society. By 1987, it was listed
as a monument, but with the collapse of the Soviet
Union, the building soon fell prey to the uncertain-
ties of the times. With the change in the political
system, the red star was removed and replaced by
the Russian flag, and the institution privatized. The
valuable property was situated in an affluent residen-
tial area, and rival property developers struggled for
ownership through legal and illegal means. Armed
thugs raided the building and threatened the staff,
some of the objects in the foyer were stolen and still
remain missing; others were hidden by the loyal staff.
Finally the site was sold to a development company.

The building remained closed between 1994 and
2011, during a period of political struggles, corrupt
judges, and bankruptcy. The revival in the fortunes
of the Russian state, however, coupled with the
public enthusiasm for the new age of Russian space
exploration shown by Mir and the International
Space Station, eventually led to redevelopment of
the site. The new plan called for the construction of a
large-scale, four-story astronomy museum designed
to accommodate not just a planetarium, but also
a cinema, lecture rooms, museum exhibits, and

educational displays. Most of the old planetarium building was controversially destroyed. Only the cupola, the portal frames, and some other minor elements were preserved; the rest of the original structure was rebuilt, and when the reconstructed planetarium was finally placed on top of the new museum building, it occupied a position six meters higher in the Moscow sky that it had previously. What stands there now looks something like the old building, but without its atmosphere.[6] In 2011, the new planetarium, equipped with the latest Zeiss digital projector, opened to the public.

Today, the building is part of a complex that includes a small park containing a selection of astronomy-related objects, two small observatories, models of Stonehenge and Jaipur, and glass pyramids and spheres: a broad version of astronomy mostly shorn of its specifically Russian themes. The hopes of Russian space exploration, kept alive by the existence of the International Space Station, have recently shown signs of revival, with declarations by Vladimir Putin that the colonization of space is once again the destiny of the Russian nation.

UPWARD

At the beginning of Aleksey Tolstoy's novel *Aelita*, the egg-like spaceship raises itself a few meters above the city before beginning its surprisingly rapid journey to Mars. The Moscow Planetarium, in a state somewhere between reconstruction and resurrection, both ghost and portent, has also now been elevated, as though it too were about to begin a long flight. Once again, it takes its place alongside Yuri Gagarin on his column and the rocket on its vast plume, all three in a state of barely restrained stasis, awaiting their next skyward move.

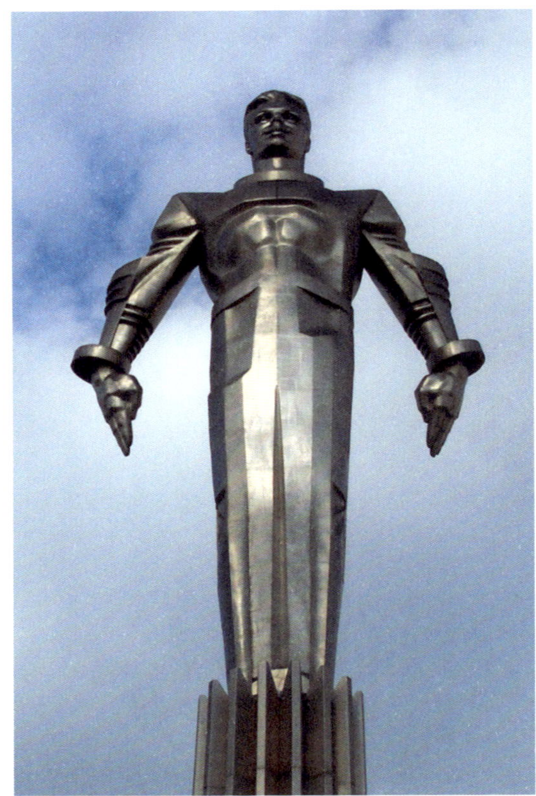

Yuri Gagarin, ready for takeoff from the top of his monument on Leninsky Prospekt, Moscow.

1 Selim Khan-Magomedov, *Michael Barshch* (Moscow: Russian Avant-garde Foundation, 2009).
2 Aleksei Gan, "Novye tipy mass-ovykh zrelyshch," *Sovremennaya Arkhitektura*, no. 3 (1927). Thanks to Nadezda Gobova for translation.
3 The entire untitled poem, written by Mayakovsky in 1929, is available in Vladimir Mayakovsky, *Polnoe sobranie sochinenii v dvenadtsati tomakh*, ed. Vasily Katanyan, vol. 10 (Moscow: Khudozhestvennaia literatura, 1941), p. 126. Thanks to Nadezda Gobova for translation.
4 Richard Stites, *Revolutionary Dreams: Utopian Vision and Experimental Life in the Russian Revolution* (Oxford & New York: Oxford University Press, 1989).
5 Asif A. Siddiqi, *The Red Rockets' Glare: Spaceflight and the Russian Imagination 1857–1957* (Cambridge and New York: Cambridge University Press, 2010).
6 See Anke Zalivako, "A Critique of the Preservation of Moscow's Planetarium," *Future Anterior*, vol. 5, no. 1 (Summer 2008), pp. 38–50.

CATASTROPHE

CATASTROPHE

THE BONDS OF CATASTROPHE
D. Graham Burnett

It is perhaps not widely understood (outside the specialized domains of risk modeling and property insurance) that the last twenty years have seen the relatively rapid growth of a new kind of financial instrument: the catastrophe bond. I aim in what follows to offer the reader a brief introduction to these innovative money-things, which sit at the precarious nexus of mathematical modeling, environmental instability, and vast sums of capital. Techno-legal creations of considerable complexity (and some genuine elegance), "cat bonds" circulate in the Olympian air of global high finance, where they afford investors an opportunity to place large bets on the occurrence and (non-occurrence) of various mass disasters: earthquakes, hurricanes, plagues, suitcase nukes. The lengthy, turgid, and highly confidential specifications that make up the prospectuses of these investments might be said to represent a special and entirely overlooked subgenre of science fiction: what we discover, turning the pages of such deals, are fanatically extensive metrical descriptions of countless doomsday scenarios, each story told in lovingly legalistic and scientific detail. Unlike most dystopian fantasizing, however, the worst-case scenarios played out in the appendices of cat bond issues come with very real-world prospective

———————

Below: Image from risk appendix to the offering prospective for the MultiCat Mexico Ltd. cat bond, series 2012-I. This $315-million issue has a double trigger structure, covering both hurricanes and earthquakes. The parametrics for the two kinds of natural disaster are different, but both make use of specific geographical "boxes" where a trigger event must occur. This graphic depicts the tracks of all of the historically recorded named storms to pass through the hurricane boxes. On the basis of the parametric model in the bond (which makes use of central pressure conditions in a given storm, as reported by NOAA), hurricanes Anita, Allen, Gilbert, and Dean would all have triggered a total loss for holders of MultiCat Mexico Ltd. bonds.

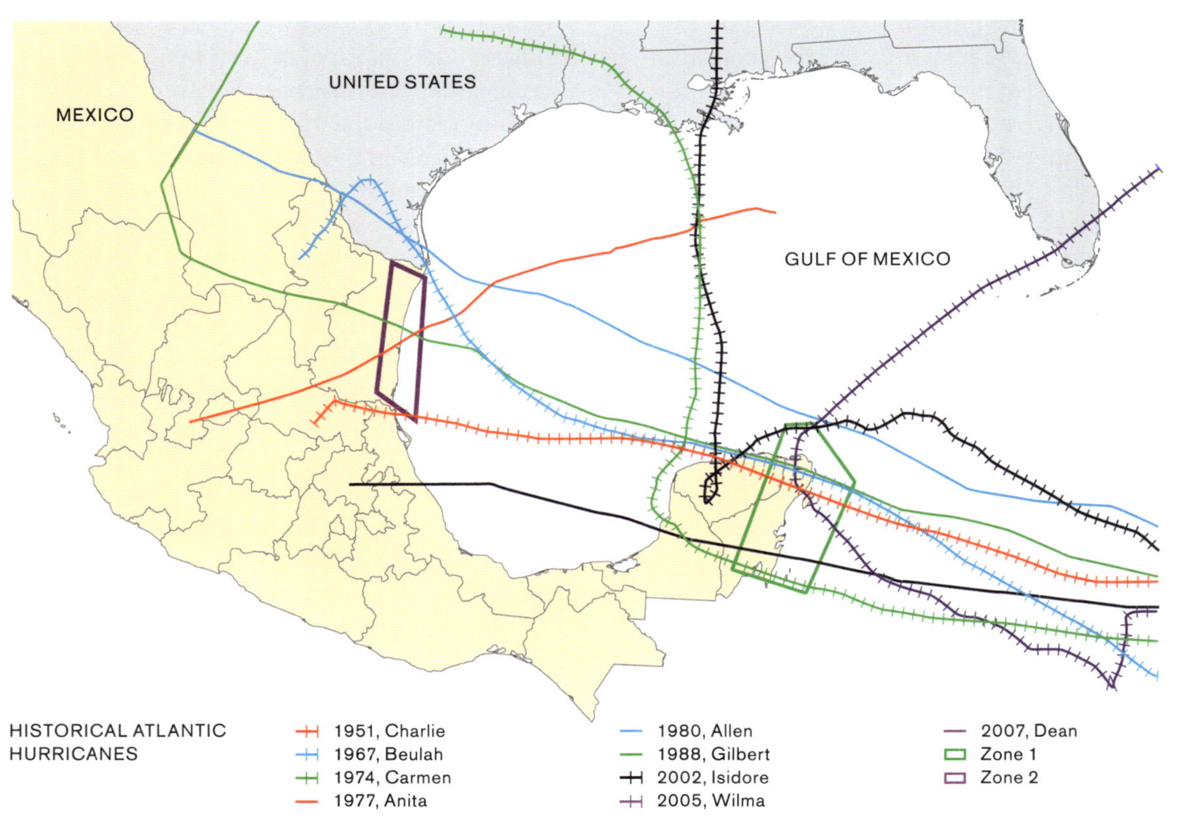

paydays, precisely priced and proper to the consideration of an imaginative portfolio manager looking to diversify her investments.

Put your paranoia aside (at least temporarily). It is quite possible that cat bonds are basically a good thing, creating mechanisms as they do for hedging against the tremendously disruptive costs of low-probability, high-negative-impact natural and/or social events. It is also possible, of course, that they are simply another sophisticated exercise in plutocratic self-dealing. We will bracket that thorny problem for now, and focus here on conveying (1) a general understanding of how these instruments work, and (2) a specific appreciation of the way that they constitute perhaps the most elaborate and powerful social technology currently available for articulating just what we mean when we say "catastrophe."

. . .

So what's a cat bond? A cat bond is, first of all, a bond—meaning a kind of debt arrangement. The holder of any bond has conveyed a sum of money to the bond issuer for a fixed term (say, a year or two) in return for the promise of some sort of interest payment: You hold my hundred thousand dollars this year, but you promise that at the end of the year you are going to give me back, not a hundred thousand dollars, but *a hundred and ten thousand dollars*—netting me a 10% return on my investment. With an ordinary high-quality corporate or municipal bond, my odds of getting my principal back are pretty close to 100%, and my rate of return (given the near-negligible risk of loss) is generally pretty low. US Treasury bonds are about as minimal-risk an investment as the earth seems to afford at present (since they are backed by the American government, which, despite its problems, looks unlikely to evaporate anytime soon), and so whatever they are paying in a given year basically sets the baseline for investors everywhere: it's a small rate of return but, for all intents and purposes, it's guaranteed. By contrast, if I am buying a "junk" bond—issued by some business guys with wild eyes and big ideas—I am promised considerably bigger interest payments than I would get on a "T-bill" (a short-term US Treasury bond), but I have to weigh the non-zero probability of a default on the part of

my debtors, who may in fact not only not pay me my nice premium, but could even lose some or all of my principal (though this is pretty rare in normal financial climates). That, in a nutshell, is the bond market: lend money to different folks, who have to promise to pay you more or less for the privilege of the loan, depending on how shady they look.

Catastrophe bonds have this basic structure. The holder of such a bond has indeed conveyed a sum of money to the bond issuer for a fixed term, in return for the promise of a downstream percentage premium. What makes a cat bond a cat bond, however, is that—unlike most ordinary bonds, which are issued by people/governments/institutions needing ready-to-hand money to build a building or a bridge or expand a business—a cat bond has been issued by somebody who is worried about some kind of possible disaster, somebody who is looking for protection from the financial effects of a catastrophe.

Think like a gigantic insurance corporation for a moment. If you've been writing property insurance for a large number of homeowners in southern Florida, you get pretty nervous every hurricane season. Yes, you've socked away everybody's premiums for years and years, so you are sitting on a mountain of cash, but you still have to reckon with the fear that, in your competitive drive to underbid the other insurance companies writing policies in the Sunshine State, you may have left yourself inadequately capitalized in the event that a massive storm flattens the region. You would do well to hedge against that whopper, by basically buying some insurance yourself. And indeed, the "reinsurance" market—insurance for insurers—has been around for a long time, and amounts to a circa $500 billion business, whereby the financial risks of different large-scale insurable events are carved up and spread out among a sizable (but relatively cozy) community of mutually re-insuring insurers. This is all good old-fashioned insurance. Meaning, basically, contracts with the following form: "If you lose *this* under *these* conditions, I will pay you back for it." It's a big deal to take on that sort of obligation. You had better be sure you can do what you say you are going to do—or else you go bankrupt (and your clients get screwed).

In the wake of Hurricane Andrew in 1992 (to that point the costliest such storm in US history,

tallying damages above $25 billion), the insurance and reinsurance industries were obliged to reckon with the fact that there might not actually be enough resources floating around in the entirety of the insurance universe to handle a *really* big storm. This was a scary thought, and it produced a good deal of hand-wringing, some soul-searching, various governmental committees and inquiries, and also some developments. Cat bonds can be understood as part of the resulting effort to bring more money (from new sources) into the quite private and arguably even arcane world of the big insurers.

The new source at issue in this case was the US capital market—meaning the $40 trillion or so that sloshes around in the liquid world of stocks and bonds under the jurisdiction of the US Security and Exchange Commission (SEC). There is no larger pool of money on the globe. Tapping it requires designing an instrument you can sell in that marketplace. And this is what the early cat bond innovators did: they designed relatively simple bonds that could be sold directly to (large, institutional) investors—bonds that permitted insurance companies to "rent" their risk to the market.

Here is an example of how such a bond works. Istanbul is a very large city that lies near a seismic fault. Big earthquakes have hit the place before, including one in 1509 that took down one of the towers of the Hagia Sophia and killed upwards of ten thousand people (contemporaries called it "The Little Day of Judgment"). There is currently Turkish legislation that mandates earthquake insurance for a large class of property holders in the city, and a kind of public-private entity (the "Turkish Catastrophe Insurance Pool," or TCIP) that manages those policies. The TCIP is on the hook for a lot of money if the North Anatolian Fault takes another big slip, as it has a few times over the last five hundred years. So the TCIP goes to Munich Re (a large German reinsurance firm) and some other dealmakers, and together they design, market, and sell a cat bond. The bond promises to pay 2.5 percent per year (which, when bank-to-bank interest rates are below 1 percent, doesn't look too bad), and investors can choose to leave their money with TCIP for one, two, or three years.[1] TCIP promises to take all the money they get for the bonds (and they end up getting $400 million for them, since this paper sells like

hotcakes in New York), and stick it in a dollar-denominated bank account in Germany, where it will just sit safely until the maturation date. There is only one kicker: if there is a big earthquake in Istanbul while your money is in that account, you can probably forget about your tidy 2.5 percent annual interest payment. In fact, you can probably forget about your million-plus principal investment too, because there's a good chance TCIP is going to get to keep all your cash—and use it (at least in theory) to help pay off all the claimants they are about to see.

How big an earthquake? That is where things get interesting. Cat bonds are built with what are called "triggers"—meaning specific criteria under which the "cedant" (the party seeking to hedge their potential losses, in this case TCIP) gets to keep some or all of the value of the bond. There are several different kinds of triggers: some are keyed to specific financial losses on the part of the cedant (e.g., "if, for whatever reason, we have to pay out more than $100 million in claims in a given year, we get to keep the money you invested in our bond"); others are keyed to the industry as a whole, or some subsection of it (e.g., "if earthquake insurers in Western Europe face an event that requires total payouts above $10 billion across the sector, we get to keep your money"). But the most interesting triggers are those that that *are keyed to the specific metrical parameters of a prospective disaster*. These are called "parametric" triggers, and they constitute a remarkable convergence of geophysical and financial modeling. In such trigger systems, the mathematics of meteorological, seismographic, and even epidemiological analysis is used to create spreadsheet disaster projections that are at the same time odds tables in a kind of high-stakes pari-mutuel pool. Think of it as something like off-track betting on global catastrophes.

What do parametric triggers look like? The figure on page 77, which has been taken from the prospectus for TCIP's actual cat bond prospectus (Bosphorus 1 Re Ltd.), depicts a schematic map of the Bosphorus, speckled with small, multicolored dots in and around the major urban areas of Istanbul.[2] Those dots represent seventy seismographic monitoring stations that are part of a global network of strong motion seismometers in urban

areas. The colors here represent a weighting code, by which each station is given more or less significance in the following summation:

$$15942.48 \times \sum_{j=1}^{J} w_j \left(\max\left(\min(S_j, 1.0) - 0.1, 0\right)\right)^{1.6}$$

Here, "j" is the number of a specific monitoring station ($J=70$), "w_j" is the weighting factor for a given station j (the range of these values is given in the key at the bottom of the figure), and "S_j" is the reported "spectral acceleration" for a given earthquake event at station j (spectral acceleration is a standard unit for measuring the effect of an earthquake at a given point).

The earth suddenly trembles, and then slips precipitously out in the lovely Princes' Islands off the southern coast of Istanbul. Calamity. You are a hedge fund manager in Westport, Connecticut, who holds a lot of Bosphorus 1 Re Ltd. cat bonds. You turn down the sound on CNN, and log onto the GIS website address given in your bond prospectus to pull down the reported quake numbers. You plug them into the formula above and do the arithmetic. If the resulting number is larger than 2,412, you just lost everything.[3]

. . .

Why such a complicated formula? Why not a nice simple trigger, like, "If there is an earthquake bigger than 7.4 on the Richter Scale, the epicenter of which is within the city limits of Istanbul, then TCIP gets your money"? There have indeed been much simpler parametric triggers than the multi-input, weighted model at the heart of Bosphorus 1 Re Ltd. For instance, one of the earliest large cat bonds, called Concentric Ltd., was issued by Tokyo Disneyland in 1999, and it spelled out a straightforward set of three concentric rings around the Magic Kingdom: a quake of 6.5 (measured in the Japanese seismic units) in the inner circle, or 7.1 in the middle ring, or 7.6 in the outer one tripped the switch—conveying the escrowed $100 million to Mickey's keepers. But the evolution of the cat bond industry has tended in the direction of increasingly complex parametric triggers.[4] This can be understood to reflect the increasing complexity of the modeling

systems that are used to structure these deals. On the one hand, there are a number of different hurricane and seismological models that can be used (largely on the basis of data about historical storms and earthquakes) to project conceivable atmospheric and geotectonic cataclysms, and to assess (at least notionally) associated risks and probabilities. On the other hand, there are various portfolio models that insurers and investors use to analyze their liquidity under different economic and market conditions. Intricate parametric triggers for cat bonds sit at the hinge of these two worlds.[5] For instance, the weighting of the different seismological monitoring stations in Bosphorus 1 Re Ltd. reflects, one must presume, the relative magnitude of TCIP's financial exposure in each zone: higher weightings in the formula would appear to correlate with a higher-density of higher-value insurance obligations (though without access to TCIP's books, it is difficult to assert this with certainty).

In this sense, the formula at the heart of Bosphorus 1 Re Ltd. reflects a meticulously crafted mathematical description of a very specific natural-social event: an expensive earthquake. An earthquake is an earthquake, but an expensive earthquake is a catastrophe. Hence,

$$15942.48 \times \sum_{j=1}^{J} w_j \left(\max\left(\min(S_j, 1.0) - 0.1, 0\right)\right)^{1.6}$$

should be understood as the way you say, in the computational patois of late capitalism, "a catastrophe in Istanbul."

. . .

What about the *human* dimension of the catastrophic? Yes, you may also wager on mass death (and not merely on catastrophic property loss). For instance, the spring of 2015 saw the rapid sale of 285 million euros' worth of mortality cat bonds issued by Benu Capital Ltd., a shell company incorporated in Ireland (the cedant is AXA Global Life, a Paris-based banking and insurance conglomerate). This bond is triggered by "excess mortality" in France, Japan, and/or the US over a five-year period ending in 2019. The exact details of the trigger model are not public, but the placement and

structuring agents for the instrument have reported that the "Class A notes will trigger at a mortality index level of 116% for France, 116% for Japan and 108% in the US," and that the Class B notes (the riskier tranche) "will trigger at a mortality index level of 108.1% for France, 108.2% for Japan and 104.1% in the US" Without being able to examine the underlying model, however, it is difficult to say exactly how these modestly elevated mortality rates would need to "manifest" in the relevant populations in order to trigger the bond, since the mortality index in use in the instrument is apparently weighted by age and gender in each covered region. The A Class notes pay 2.55%, and the B notes 3.35%.

Is this a good bet? In some sense, the market says it is, in that the offering was expanded from its initial prospectus, and even the larger issue promptly sold out. At the same time, it is perhaps worth pointing out that one of the rating agencies (Standard & Poor's) explicitly noted, in its rating report on the issue, the impossibility of meaningfully "modeling" all the potential events in a mortality transaction. For instance, a large tsunami, or terrorist attack, or pandemic, or the outbreak of a new Sino-Japanese war would all stand a very good chance of triggering the bond—and yet it is obviously very hard to put credible odds on such a basket of monstrous singularities.[6] What the successful sale of Benu Capital's bond can be said to "mean" however, is something like the following: a small coterie of the masters of the universe, sitting around tables in tall glass buildings, think they know (well enough) how likely it is that lots of us will suddenly die in the next few years. And they have backed up their wager with gigantic piles of money.

. . .

Let's return, in closing, to the paranoia—if just for a moment. On the one hand, there is something undeniably unsettling, I think, about cliques of billionaires placing large-stake bets on mass death. And there is something additionally troubling, perhaps, about many of the most sophisticated scientists of the earth and atmosphere taking on paid employment as bookies to a members-only numbers game played with global catastrophes. On the other hand,

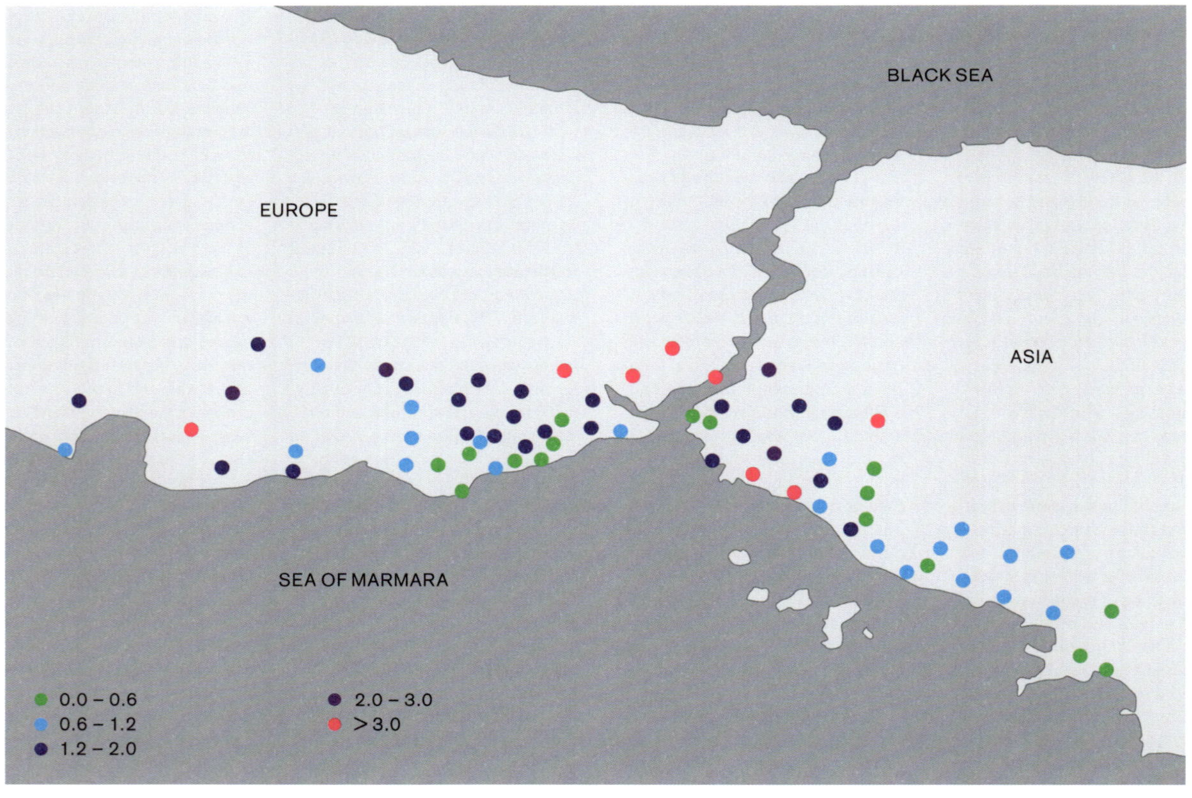

if there actually is, say, some horrible pandemic that sweeps across Japan, there are going to be a lot of ordinary people expecting to receive (and needing) payout from their life insurance policies. And if AXA Global Life goes bankrupt, many of them are likely never to see those payouts. Whereas if Benu Capital's cat bond triggers, AXA may be able to meet its obligations, and the impact of those sudden costs will be distributed across a broad pool of large-scale investors (who will simply have to write down some investment losses).

On the one hand, on the other hand. Perhaps it will have to suffice, in a short essay like this one, merely to state that the moral-cum-financial problem at issue in these instruments affords an interesting touchstone for any theory of wealth and social welfare. The problem is left to the reader.

Though that might be a bit too anodyne. After all, a dark and recursive specter haunts our topic: the vast aggregations of capital that are at play in the cat bond industry are themselves inextricable from the titanic, corporate-industrial refiguring of our planet—its external features, climatological dynamics, and even internal architecture. Which is to say, there is mounting evidence that the historical evolution of the "anthropocene" ought to be understood as a non-trivial component of what we still tend to think of, reflexively, as "natural" catastrophes. Or, to put it another way, it would seem that human beings—and specifically the wealthiest humans on earth—are in the process of creating a significant drift toward climatological and terrestrial changes that are increasing the frequency and intensity of disruptive natural-social calamities on our planet. Indeed, some specific corporate entities are large enough in themselves to be meaningful drivers of such changes. Upon which those same entities are now in a position, potentially, to capitalize, by means of well-placed cat bond bets. Which, looked at this way, amount to bets on a game in which they are actual players.

Outlandish? We will see.

---

1 Technically, the money is not left "with" TCIP, but with a "Special Purpose Vehicle" (SPV), a kind of shell company that exists exclusively for the purpose of holding the assets in question and discharging, across the term of the bond, the obligations occasioned by its prospectus. The actual structuring of these deals has much to do with the small print aspects of international tax law and corporate finance. The account given in the text here is schematic. For details, see Pauline Barrieu and Luca Albertini, eds., *The Handbook of Insurance-Linked Securities* (West Chichester, UK: John Wiley and Sons, 2009).

2 I was surprised, in doing this research, by the level of confidentiality that surrounds cat bond documentation. Most of the individuals who work with the actual offering circulars and prospectus materials have been obliged to sign non-disclosure agreements, and are therefore unwilling to share the specifics of these instruments, which are not subject to the obligatory public filing requirements of the SEC because they are not available to ordinary retail investors. The concern with secrecy is largely a function of a legal culture at banks and insurers—a culture that frets about liabilities and obsessively protects what could be construed as intellectual property. I was able to find several individuals in the industry who, on being assured anonymity, were willing to convey copies of some of the relevant documentation. This piece would not have been possible without their assistance, which is gratefully acknowledged here. Further thanks to Sophia Li and Aaron Hirsh.

3 For the record, only a very small number—roughly half a dozen—of the several hundred cat bonds issued since the mid-1990s have actually triggered (and not all triggering events occasion total loss of the principal invested in the bond, since some bonds are designed with different levels of loss pegged to different trigger levels).

4 Though it should be noted that the use of parametric triggers in cat bonds saw a brief hiatus in the period 2010–2014, for reasons that are debated among industry insiders. In general, cedants prefer "indemnity" triggers (triggers that are keyed to specific losses from an insurer's book), because they eliminate—at least in principle—what is called "basis risk," meaning the risk of differences between the insurer's obligations in an insurable event and the pay-in afforded by a triggered cat bond. It is ideal, for the cedant, if these match up dollar-for-dollar, but no parametric trigger, however precisely tuned, can insure a perfect fit with the particular losses an insurer will ultimately face in a given situation. (Basis risk can, of course, go both ways, and it is possible for a cedant to end up receiving more money from a triggered cat bond or other reinsurance relationship than the cedant is actually obliged to pay out to its policy holders in a given insurable event.) Parametric triggers, which appear to be back on the upswing in the last year, have always had an appeal for investors, in that they are arguably more transparent/objective than indemnity triggers (since the latter are contingent on the cedant's bookkeeping). It is perhaps worth adding that parametric triggers in insurance contracts predate the emergence of the cat bond industry itself, but information on how and where they were used is difficult to secure, given the even more private nature of the traditional insurance business.

5 A small number of companies specialize in the computer models that lie at the center of the cat bond industry, the most important of which are AIR Worldwide, RMS (Risk Management Solutions), and EQECAT (now part of CoreLogic, a large, global property information and analytics corporation). These firms employ considerable numbers of scientists and programmers who design, maintain, and retail the use of specialized risk-analyzing software (most of it derived from weather and seismographic models produced in academic settings). What is striking to an outsider is the extent to which these systems dominate the configuration and assessment of any given cat bond deal. Both buyers and sellers (and even the notionally independent rating agencies) tend to rely to a considerable degree on the same (or a very similar) model, and sometimes even on the same appendix of projected risk analysis. This seems quite remarkable, in view of how speculative much of this modeling is—historical data tends to be very limited, and the calculation of probabilities for unique, multi-variable events is a highly uncertain affair.

6 Details of the Benu Capital deal are courtesy of Steve Evans's Artemis website (www.artemis.bm), the primary clearinghouse for publicly available information about the cat bond industry.

THE LISBON EARTHQUAKE
Walter Benjamin

Between 1927 and 1933, Walter Benjamin wrote and presented some eighty programs on German radio, many designed, like this broadcast, for children. "The Lisbon Earthquake" aired on Berliner Rundfunk on 31 October 1931 and on Südwestdeutsche Rundfunk, Frankfurt, on 6 January 1932.

Have you ever had to wait at the pharmacy and noticed how the pharmacist fills a prescription? On a scale with very delicate weights, ounce by ounce, dram by dram, he weighs all the substances and specks that make up the final powder. That is how I feel when I tell you something over the radio. My weights are the minutes; very carefully I must weigh how much of this, how much of that, so the mixture is just right. You're probably saying, But why? If you want to tell us about the Lisbon earthquake, just start at the beginning. Then go ahead and tell us what happened next. But I don't think that would be much fun for you. House after house collapses, family after family is killed; the terror of the spreading fire, the terror of the water, the darkness and the looting, the wailing of the injured, and the cries of the people searching for loved ones—no one wants to hear just this and nothing more, and besides, these things are more or less the same in every natural catastrophe.

But the earthquake that destroyed Lisbon on November 1, 1755, was not a disaster like thousands of others. In many ways it was singular and strange, and this is what I'd like to talk to you about. To begin with, it was one of the greatest and most devastating earthquakes of all time. But it was not only for this reason that it moved and preoccupied the entire world in that century as few other things did. At the time, the destruction of Lisbon was comparable to the destruction of Chicago or London today. In the middle of the eighteenth century, Portugal was still at the height of its colonial power. Lisbon was one of the wealthiest commercial cities on Earth; at the mouth of the Tagus river, its harbor, full of ships year in and year out, was lined with trading houses belonging to merchants from England, France, and Germany, and above all from Hamburg. The city had thirty thousand dwellings and well over 250,000

inhabitants, roughly a quarter of whom died in the earthquake. The royal court was famed for both its austerity and its splendor. The many accounts of Lisbon published before the earthquake reveal the strangest details of the court's rigid formalities; how, for instance, on summer evenings courtiers and their families would rendezvous in the main square, the Rucio, where they chatted for a short spell without ever leaving their carriages. People had such an elevated notion of the king of Portugal that one of the many leaflets conveying detailed descriptions of the calamity all across Europe could not fathom that such a great king could also have been affected by it. "Just as the extent of a catastrophe can only be grasped once it has been overcome," writes this particular chronicler, "the dire ramifications of this frightful case can only be felt once one considers that the king and his wife, altogether abandoned, spent an entire day in a carriage under the most wretched conditions." Leaflets featuring such passages functioned as newspapers do for us today. Those with the capacity to do so collected detailed eyewitness accounts and had them printed and sold. Later on, I will read to you from another such report, one based on the experiences of an Englishman residing in Lisbon at the time.

Yet there's another, special reason that this event affected people so strongly, that it inspired countless leaflets to be passed from hand to hand, and that almost one hundred years later new accounts of the catastrophe were still being printed: the impact of this earthquake was greater than any ever heard of before. It was felt all over Europe and as far away as Africa, a colossal area calculated at two and a half million square kilometers if one includes the farthest reaches where it was detectable. The strongest tremors ranged from the coast of Morocco on one side to the coasts of Andalusia and France on the other. The cities of Cádiz, Jerez, and Algeciras were almost completely destroyed. According to one eyewitness, the cathedral towers in Seville trembled like reeds in the wind. But the most violent tremors traveled through the water. Massive groundswells were felt from Finland to the Dutch East Indies; it was calculated that ocean convulsions progressed from the

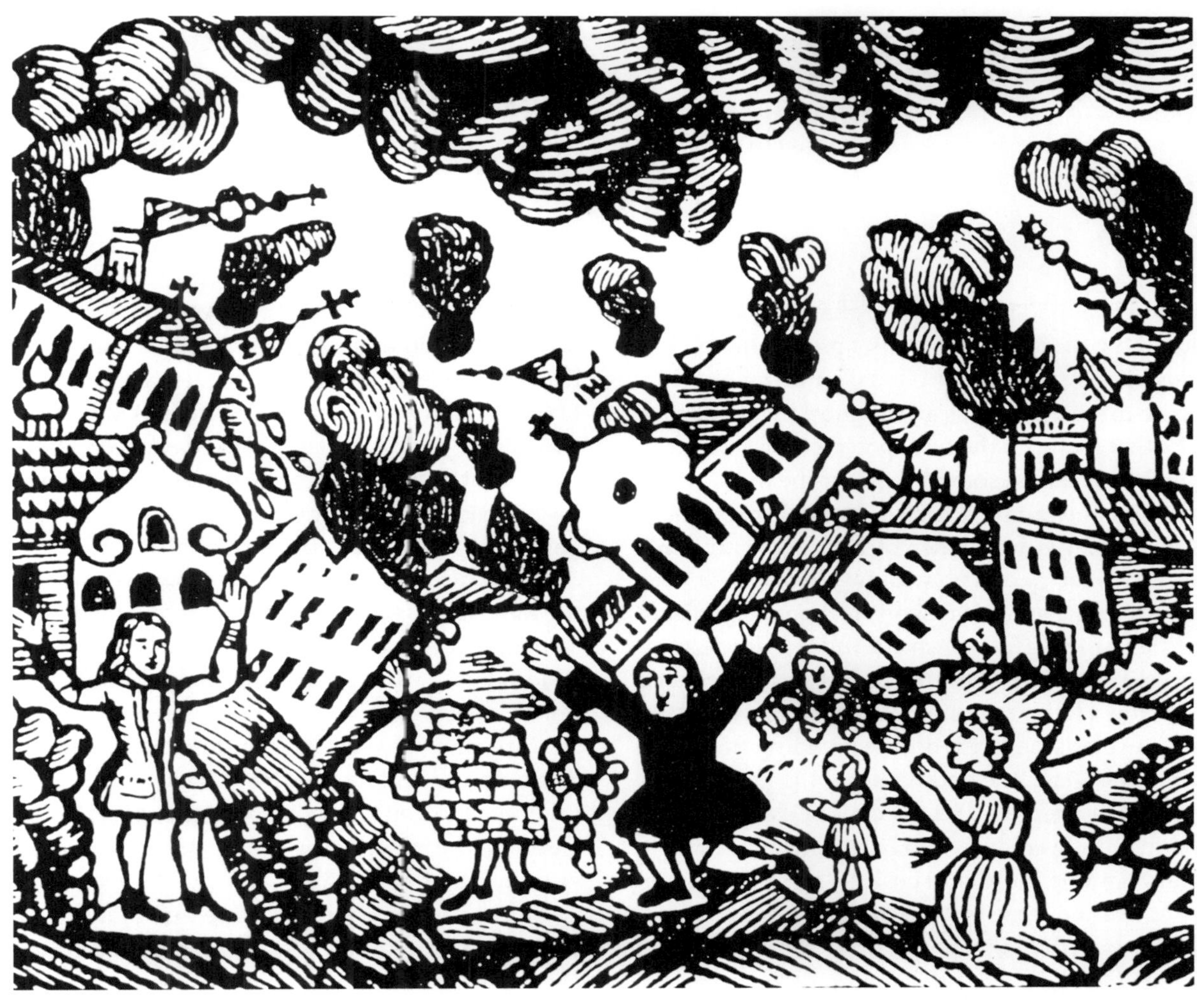

1755 woodcut from broadside printed in Litomysl, Bohemia, depicting the Lisbon earthquake. Note that the cityscape bears no resemblance to the Portuguese capital.

Portuguese coast to the mouth of the Elbe with tremendous speed, in only a quarter of an hour. But so much for what occurred at the moment of the calamity. The weeks leading up to it saw a series of strange natural phenomena that, after the fact and perhaps not wholly without reason, people looked back on as omens of the impending calamity. For example, in Locarno, in southern Switzerland, two weeks before the catastrophic day, vapor suddenly began rising from the ground. In two hours it had changed into a red mist, which around evening precipitated as purple rain. From then on frightful hurricanes, combined with cloudbursts and floods, were reported across western Europe. Eight days before the quake, the ground around Cádiz was covered with masses of worms emerging from the earth.

No one was more preoccupied with these strange events than Kant, the great German philosopher whose name some of you may already have heard. When the earthquake occurred, he was a man of twenty-four, and neither before nor after did he ever venture beyond his hometown of Königsberg; yet he collected all the accounts this earthquake he could find, with tremendous enthusiasm. The short works he published on the phenomenon constituted the beginnings of scientific geography in Germany.[1] The beginnings of seismology, at any rate. I'd like to tell you something about the path this discipline took from that portrayal of the 1755 earthquake up until today. But I must be careful that our Englishman, whose account of his experiences during the earthquake I would still like you to hear, does not get lost in the shuffle. He has been waiting impatiently; after 150 years of being ignored, he'd like once more to have his say, and has allowed me to share only a few words concerning what we now know about earthquakes. But one thing first: they are not what you think. If I could pause for a moment and ask how you would explain earthquakes, I bet the first thing you'd think of is volcanoes. It's true that volcanic eruptions are often linked to earthquakes, or at least heralded by them. So, for two thousand years, from the ancient Greeks through to Kant and on until about 1870, people believed that earthquakes were caused by fiery gases, steam from the earth's interior and suchlike. But once people began to use measuring instruments and to make calculations, whose subtlety and precision surpass anything you

might imagine—and that goes for me as well—in short, once people could verify the matter, they found something altogether different, at least for large earthquakes like the one in Lisbon. They do not originate from the deepest recesses of the earth—which we still think of as liquid, or more exactly muddy, like molten sludge—but rather from events in the earth's crust. The earth's crust is a layer roughly three thousand kilometers thick. This layer is in perpetual upheaval; the masses within it are constantly shifting in an ongoing attempt to find equilibrium. We know some of the factors that disturb this equilibrium, and ceaseless research is being conducted to discover others.

This much is certain: the most significant shifting is a result of the continuous cooling of the earth. This subjects the masses of rock to enormous tension, ultimately causing them to break apart and then to seek a new equilibrium by rearranging themselves, which we experience as an earthquake. Other shifting results from the erosion of mountains, which become lighter, and from alluvial deposits on the ocean floor, which becomes heavier. Storms, whirling about the earth, especially in autumn, do their bit to rattle the planet's surface; and finally, it remains to be determined just how the pull of celestial bodies exerts force on the earth's surface. But you might be thinking: if this is true, then the earth's crust is actually never at rest, so there must be earthquakes all the time. And you'd be right, there are. The incredible precision of the earthquake-monitoring instruments available today—in Germany alone we have thirteen seismological stations in various cities—is such that they are never completely still, which means that the earth is always quaking, only most of the time we don't feel it.

When, out of a clear blue sky, this quaking suddenly becomes noticeable, it's even worse. And literally out of a clear blue sky. "Because," writes our Englishman, who now finally gets his say,

the sun was shining in full splendor. The sky was impeccably clear, giving not the slightest sign of any natural phenomenon to come, when, between nine and ten in the

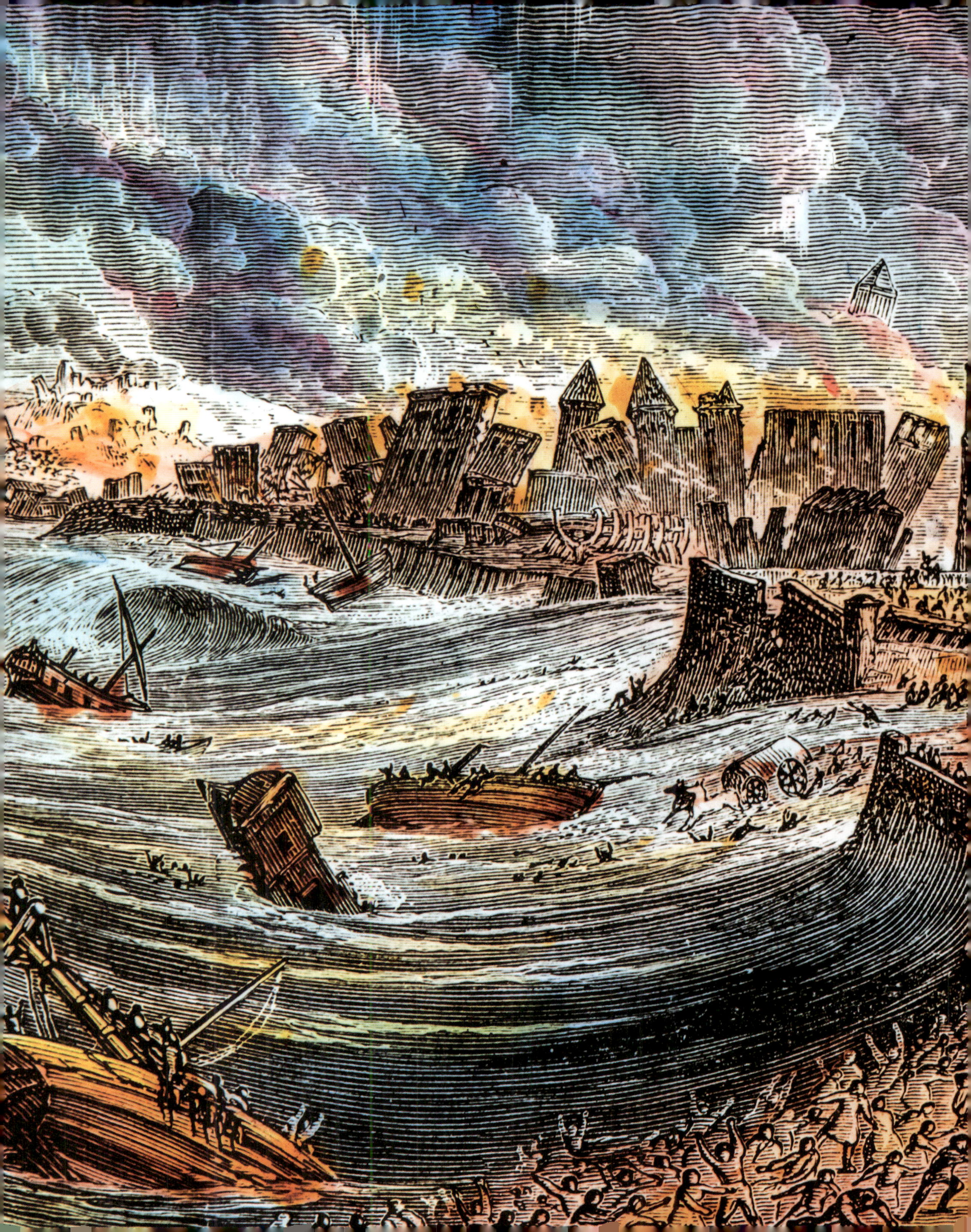

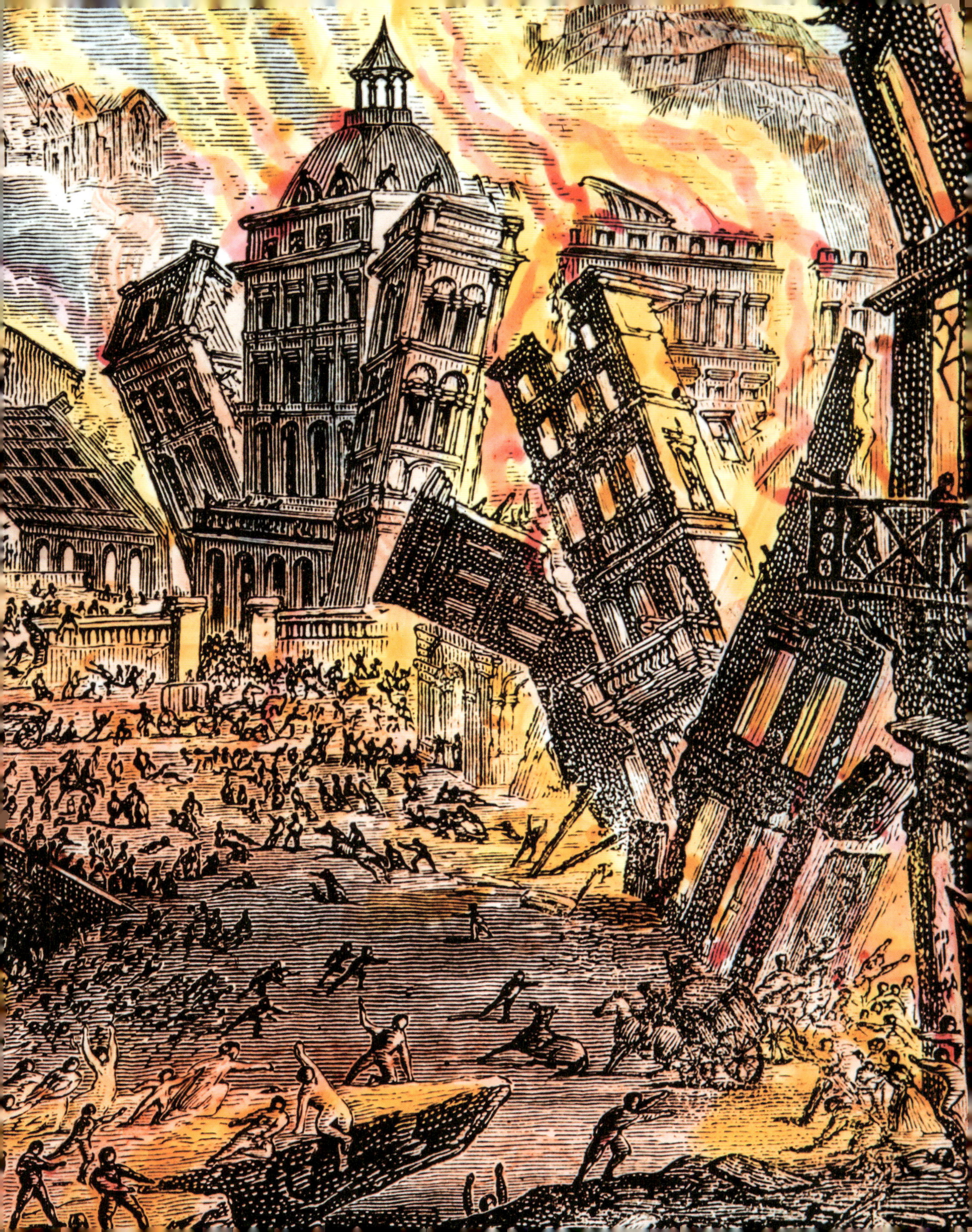

morning, I was sitting at my desk and the table began to move, which was rather surprising as there was no reason at all that it should have. While I was still pondering the cause of what had just happened, the house started to shake from top to bottom. From beneath the ground came a shuddering boom, as if a storm were raging in the distance. I quickly set down my pen and jumped to my feet. The danger was great but there was still hope that it would all pass without harm; the next moment, however, would erase any uncertainty. A horrible crackling noise was heard, as if all the buildings in the city were falling down at once. My building was so jolted that the upper floors caved in, and the rooms in which I resided swayed so much that everything was turned upside down. I expected to be struck dead at any moment; the walls were crumbling, large stones fell from their cracks, and the roof beams appeared to hover in midair. But at this time, the sky became so dark that people couldn't make out what was in front of them. Pitch dark prevailed, either as a result of the immense amount of dust caused by the collapsing houses, or because of the volumes of sulfurous vapor escaping from the earth. Finally the night brightened again, the violence of the shocks relented; I collected myself as best I could and had a look around. It became clear to me that I owed my survival thus far to a small bit of luck; that is, had I been dressed, I most certainly would have fled to the street and been struck dead by collapsing buildings. I quickly threw on some shoes and a coat, rushed outside and headed to St. Paul's cemetery, where I thought I would be safest given that it sits on a hill. People no longer recognized their own streets; most could not say what had happened; everything was destroyed and no one knew what had become of their loved ones and all that they owned. From the hill of the cemetery, I was then witness to a horrific spectacle: on the ocean, as far as the eye could see, countless ships surged with the waves, crashing into one another as if a massive storm were raging. All of a sudden the huge seaside pier sank, along with all the people who believed they would be safe there. The boats and vehicles so many people used to seek rescue fell equal prey to the sea.[2]

As we know from other accounts, it was about an hour after the second and most devastating seismic shock that the massive swell, twenty meters high, which the Englishman saw from afar, came tumbling over the city. When the tidal wave receded, the Tagus riverbed suddenly appeared completely dry; its recoil was so powerful that it took all the river's

water with it. "When evening lowered over the desolated city," the Englishman concludes, "it looked like a sea of fire: the light was so bright, you could read a letter by it. The flames soared from at least a hundred different points and raged for six days, consuming whatever the earthquake had spared. Petrified in anguish, thousands stood mesmerized before the city, as wives and children beseeched all saints and angels for help. All the while, the earth continued to quake with greater or lesser force, often for a quarter of an hour without cease."

So much for this fatal day, November 1, 1755. The disaster it brought is one of the very few before which mankind is as powerless today as it was 170 years ago. Here, too, technology will find a way out, albeit an indirect one: through prediction. For the time being, however, it seems that the sensory organs of some animals are still superior to our finest instruments. Dogs in particular will exhibit unmistakable agitation for days before the onset of earthquakes, which is why they are deployed to provide assistance to earthquake stations in vulnerable regions. And with that, my twenty minutes are up; I hope they didn't go by too slowly for you.

Translated by Jonathan Lutes. We are grateful to Verso for allowing us to publish this excerpt from Radio Benjamin, *their recent collection of Benjamin's writings for and on radio, edited by Lecia Rosenthal. We have made certain minor modifications in the text so that it is consistent with* Cabinet's *style sheet.*

1 In 1756, Kant wrote three essays on the subject of the earthquake, emphasizing the nature of its physical dynamics rather than theological justifications: "Von den Ursachen der Erderschütterungen bei Gelegenheit des Unglücks, welches die westliche Länder von Europa gegen das Ende des vorigen Jahres betroffen hat" ("On the Causes of Earthquakes, on the Occasion of the Calamity that Befell the Western Countries of Europe toward the End of Last Year"); "Geschichte und Naturbeschreibung der merkwürdigsten Vorfälle des Erdbebens, welches an dem Ende des 1755sten Jahres einen großen Teil der Erde erschüttert hat" ("History and Natural Description of the Most Noteworthy Occurrences of the Earthquake that Struck a Large Part of the Earth at the End of the Year 1755"); "Fortgesetzte Betrachtung der seit einiger Zeit wahrgenommenen Erderschütterungen" ("Continued Observations of the Terrestrial Convulsions that Have Been Perceived for Some Time"). See translations by Olaf Reinhardt in Kant, *Natural Science*, ed. Eric Watkins (Cambridge: Cambridge University Press, 2012).

2 Benjamin borrows from an account of the earthquake by Rev. Charles Davy. For Davy's text, see "The Earthquake at Lisbon," in Eva March Tappan, ed., *The World's Story: A History of the World in Story, Song and Art*, vol. 5 (Boston: Houghton Mifflin, 1914), pp. 618–628.

IN THE SHADOW OF CATASTROPHE:
AN INTERVIEW WITH ANSON RABINBACH
George Prochnik

In what way does writing about catastrophe, either predictively or retrospectively, risk kindling a new blaze? Conversely, is it possible to identify aspects of such texts that work against the drive to catastrophe? Conventional wisdom suggests that temporal distance from historical trauma increases the clarity of perspective, yet Central European intellectuals in the twentieth century had no opportunity to formulate their positions at a remove in space or time from the era's successive debacles. They careened from disaster to disaster, and the texts they composed under these conditions were porous to catastrophe at both ends. But unrelenting proximity to the apocalypse on the Continent, which negated any possibility of "ivory tower" sequestration from events, also gave their writing a uniquely instructive relationship to catastrophe. At once symptomatic, diagnostic, and—in theory, if not always in practice—therapeutic, these works betray a rare consanguinity with the events they analyze. For this reason, they make viscerally manifest questions of intellectual responsibility that continue to resonate. Written in the aftermath of the Cold War, Anson Rabinbach's *In the Shadow of Catastrophe: German Intellectuals Between Apocalypse and Enlightenment* (University of California Press, 1997), explores the interwoven life and works of seven influential thinkers in the age of world war. George Prochnik spoke with Rabinbach, professor of history at Princeton University, in May 2015.

———————

CABINET: Can you give us a sense of the basic premise and argument of the book?

ANSON RABINBACH: This book is a historian's meditation on how the catastrophic events of the twentieth century became the matrix of philosophical reflection in the periods immediately following the two world wars. It examines the aftershock of the apocalypse as it appeared in the writings of some of the central figures of twentieth-century German thought. Each of them recast the experience of catastrophe in his own unique philosophical idiom. After World War I, German-Jewish authors such as

Ernst Bloch and Walter Benjamin and the Dadaist Hugo Ball translated the cataclysm of the war into messianic images of redemption and revolutionary transfiguration. After World War II, the redemptive power of violence no longer figured in the works of Karl Jaspers, Martin Heidegger, or Max Horkheimer and Theodor Adorno; although politically these towering figures had little in common, all of them saw the apocalyptic event as symptomatic of what might be called the burdened traditions of modernity. For them, World War II dramatized the logic of catastrophe, as at once a deep rupture in the course of modernity and as the apotheosis of Western thought. In their bleak and dispirited mood, in their deep distrust of all redemptive schemes, the texts written in the shadow of World War II call to mind the first photographs documenting the vastness of ruin visited on European cities. In their backward glance at the ruined traditions of Central European thought, these texts are themselves events, the philosophical analogy to the panoramas of destruction. The book itself was also conceived in the shadow of a cataclysmic event—the collapse of Communism—and it seemed to me that we were living in a moment where there was another shadow cast by the end of this enormous period of time in which the Cold War dominated intellectual and cultural discourse in the West.

CABINET: I like very much your framing conceit, the notion that the figures you focus on were themselves so vitally enmeshed in the catastrophic events of the era that these disasters are legible in their writings not just as subtexts but as the organizing principle of their composition. You speak of the events as being almost embedded in the texts themselves.

RABINBACH: That was the central idea. What I was concerned with was thinking about how to write intellectual history without falling into two equally troubling traps: one was to avoid pure textualism, to write about these thinkers as if they were writing for the *Journal of Modern Philosophy* and completely separated from the world that they lived in. And the

other trap was to over-contextualize, to write as if the ideas were simply reflections of the events themselves. My goal was to talk about the way in which these ideas *were* events, the texts were themselves events—they had efficacy, permanence, and you might say they cast their own shadow. So I had these two notions of events: the event as part of the text, as a component of the text, and the text itself as event, and I tried to draw on both these alternatives.

CABINET: And that also brings to mind one of the central ways in which you're considering the shadow itself, which is through the suggestion that these individuals were themselves intellectually implicated in the catastrophe. It's not that you ever ascribe some direct causal link between a particular text and a particular event, but you suggest ways in which their critical/philosophical practices inscribed forms of explosive thought that had real world consequences.

RABINBACH: Yes, I think that the events themselves created a shock-effect in the text and for each of the authors, a shock-effect through which they were wedded to the events, and yet they had to create a certain amount of distance from them in order to write about them. Not all of them understand the catastrophe in the same way. Jaspers talks specifically about the Nuremberg trials and German guilt. He's the one who talks most specifically about an event. Heidegger's letter on humanism is over-determined by events, by his own personal and political circumstances and the political situation in Germany. For him, the signal event is the collapse of Germany, the site of Being's new beginning. But that is never explicitly mentioned in the text. For Horkheimer and Adorno, it was the Shoah, though they had no language to name it. So sometimes you have to think of the catastrophic event as being tattooed *into* the text, permanently there but not evident.

CABINET: This makes me think of your interesting reading of the work of Agnes Heller and the idea that she adopts from Hegel of reflective remembrance, a form of remembrance that is not concerned with integrating the event as much as preserving intact its shock. The passage you cite is from a 1995 essay and is worth quoting in full: "After the end of the catastrophic century, we look backwards, not from the plateau of the end of history, but from the flatland of the absolutely historical present. We could enter this absolute present with the empty consciousness of forgetting. Or we could instead practice a kind of remembering, which Hegel first called 'Andenken' (reflective remembrance). Remembrance is respect, the respect of thinking. If there is to be mourning, then the respect of thinking is a requiem. I am speaking of a requiem for a century."

RABINBACH: It's a way of thinking about the event without being nostalgic or sentimental or thinking about it as something we mourn or as traumatic. I think her word "Andenken" gives a very specific meaning to how we should contend with events: with respect but also with the capacity for criticism.

CABINET: And that idea resonates with another point you make, which partly informs your choice of these texts composed in such intense proximity to crisis: how it isn't necessarily the case, as psychoanalytic thought has it, that distance creates a useful perspective.

RABINBACH: It's the opposite, I think. The conventional psychoanalytic wisdom is that when a traumatic event occurs, it's a shock to the system, and so it is submerged into the unconscious, where it lives a kind of twilight existence, which is a period of latency. As a result of this period of latency, eventually the self comes to terms with the shock and works through it, and it becomes integrated into the personality. For the writers I discuss, this was not an option. They lived in a world of permanent catastrophe. Benjamin's famous Angel of History looking back at the rubble of progress is a perfect metaphor for this idea—that the past is a cataclysm so enormous that they can only think about it in the immediacy of the event, not after a long period of latency. That's why I chose texts that were written in the immediate aftermath of the events; two years at the most.

Opposite: The problem of death and the problem of evil. Machine guns and chemical warfare in World War I; the trains running to concentration camps in World War II.

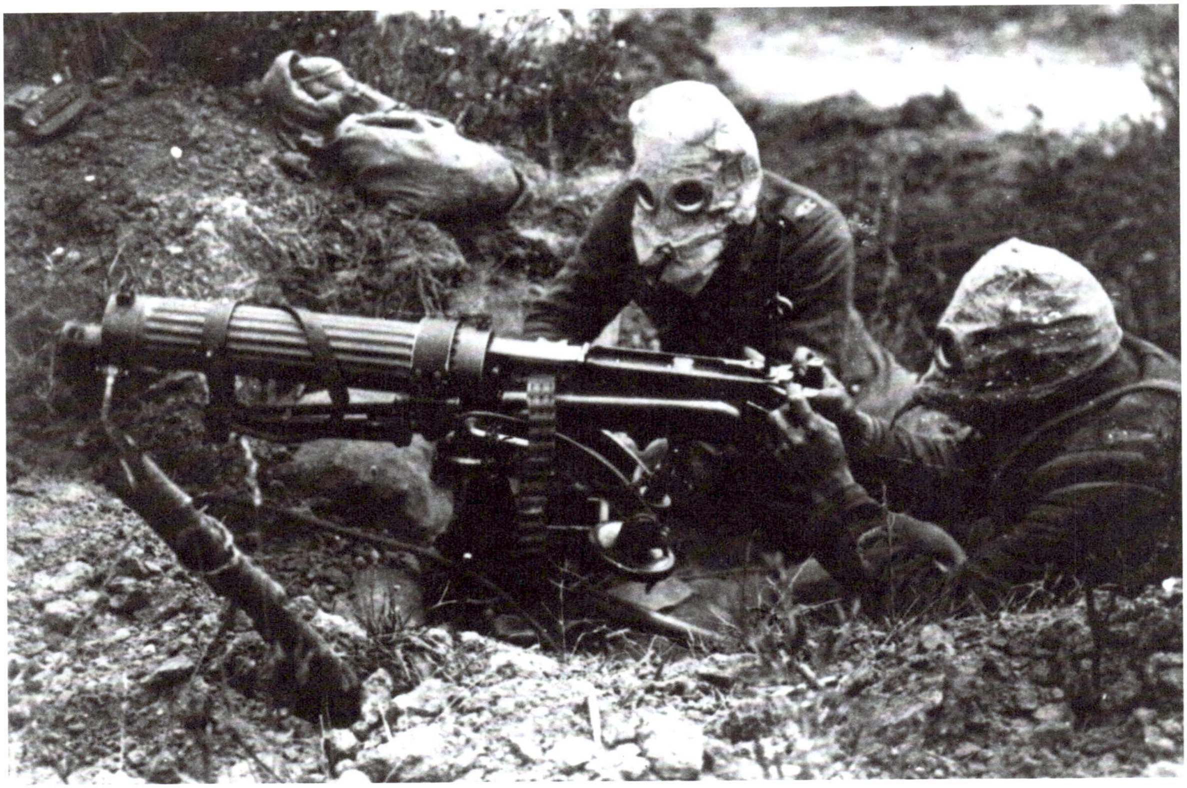

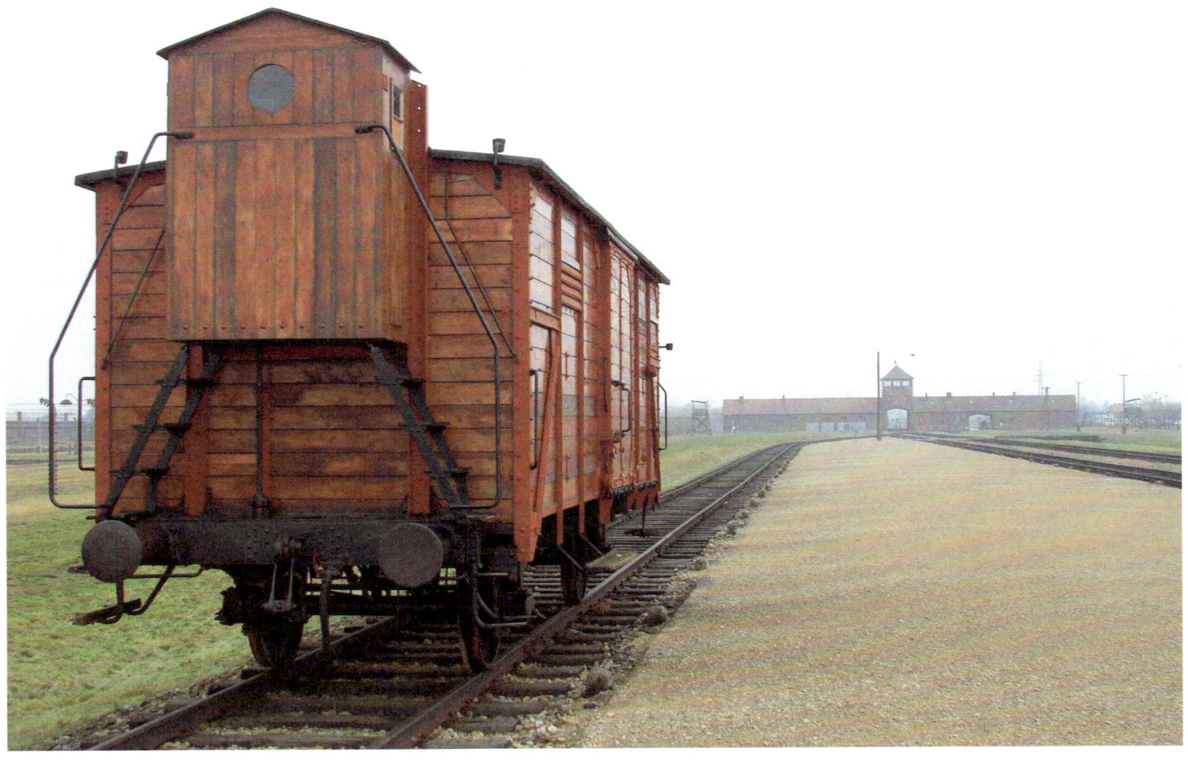

CABINET: And it's fitting that you were writing the book in the immediate aftermath of an event which was another twentieth-century cataclysm, the Eastern European catastrophe.

RABINBACH: I'm currently writing a book about three concepts— totalitarianism, genocide, and total war—invented in the twentieth century, and it's specifically about the Cold War and its end. But in *The Shadow of Catastrophe*, it was only in the Hugo Ball chapter that I was aware of the echoes between the historical experience of my subjects and the events I was living through in the late 1990s—in other words, the collapse of Communism. There, I discussed the ways that he represented a kind of inverted German nationalism that was all about German guilt and the failures of Germany, the malignancies of the German personality and of Prussianism. And Ball then inverted all of this into a kind of pride: "We are the worst and no one can best us for our worstness."

CABINET: A kind of negative exceptionalism. You cite Hannah Arendt's framing of the two postwar eras: "The reality is that 'the Nazis are men like ourselves'; the nightmare is that they have shown, have proven beyond doubt what man is capable of. In other words, the problem of evil will be the fundamental question of postwar intellectual life in Europe—as death became the fundamental problem after the last war." And I'm wondering if you can speak a little about how you understand this distinction, this transition from death to evil, and say whether in your own estimation this difference she's drawing is correct and whether we still live with evil as our predominant problem.

RABINBACH: Arendt was never more brilliant than when she wrote that sentence. Whether true or not, it's an extraordinary sentence. Obviously, you can find moments in the aftermath of World War I where people were talking about evil: about the evil of the Kaiser, whether or not to put him on trial, and about the right-wing militias that arose out of the war—the "trenchocracy," as Mussolini called them. There was plenty of evil to go around after the World War I. But she's basically right. The catastrophe of that war was seventeen million dead, twenty

million wounded; the magnitude of the cataclysm was enormous. People had never contended with that kind of mass death. Obviously in the Middle Ages, you had the Black Plague, but people had never contended with this level of seemingly purposeless mass death.

CABINET: Inflicted from person to person.

RABINBACH: And of course there was enormous mass death in World War II. How could you say that that war was not about death, with roughly fifty-five million people dead, including the Holocaust, which is a very small part of the overall death figures. But, nevertheless, I think she's right that people focused on a kind of evil that had never been manifested before. At no time previously had any group been singled out for absolute destruction by another group in the way that the Jews were. So for her, Auschwitz was a break with civilization. And I think she's right about that.

CABINET: And that rupture was something with which all the thinkers you consider had to engage.

RABINBACH: Yes. And that's why when I wrote the chapter on Adorno and Horkheimer's *Dialectic of Enlightenment*, I interpreted it as a book about the murder of the Jews. The book had not been read that way before, although there's plenty of evidence once you look at the book from that point of view.

CABINET: Let's talk about the first chapter where you're also focused on Jewish thought from a very different perspective; if not exactly a hopeful perspective, it is at least a perspective in which apocalypse might be turned into something more promising than what the intellectuals felt in the wake of World War II. You start by looking at the generation of Jews in the early twentieth century, a whole enormously varied group of intellectuals, who were thinking about messianism in a new way.

RABINBACH: There was an explosion of interest in things Jewish, in what it meant to be Jewish, although it's anachronistic to talk about identity because these people didn't think about identity. They invented the Judaism they needed.

CABINET: And what brought them to that?

RABINBACH: The immediate occasion were Martin Buber's *Three Speeches to the Jews* in, roughly, 1910. By 1912, there was this enormous interest in discussion about anti-Semitism, what it meant to be Jewish; people made jokes, they wanted to absorb Hasidism without becoming Hasidic. It was a kind of experimentation with what it meant to be Jewish, with the Jewish condition. It wasn't about identity; it was about what it meant to be Jewish in Europe.

CABINET: The marginality.

RABINBACH: Marginality and how they related to the assimilationists, to the diaspora, to the Zionists who dreamed of Palestine, and also to the cultural Zionists. There were all these manifestations and varieties of Jewish intellectualism; there was a famous case in Berlin where somebody named Moritz Goldstein wrote an article in which he said that Jews had to abandon assimilationism, that it had been a colossal failure and that liberalism had not worked out for the Jews. The young Walter Benjamin also participated in all this; he had an extensive correspondence with Buber's son-in-law, Ludwig Strauss, talking about what it meant to be Jewish. He says at one point that as far as Zionism goes, he wouldn't object to it for the Eastern European Jews because for them, it was the question of whether or not to leave a burning building.

CABINET: I was struck by his incredibly precocious evaluations. You quote a letter that Benjamin writes to Strauss in 1913, when he's all of twenty-one, where he talks about the idea of the "creative culture-Jew," and imagined Judaism as a kind of inverted Tower of Babel. The Jews, he writes, "handle ideas like quarry stones." But they "build from above without ever reaching the ground."

RABINBACH: The idea of not reaching the ground is a messianic idea of tremendous potential without any vehicle to bring it into realization or existence. So you live between potential or hope and the absence of any possibility of its realization.

CABINET: That goes to the question of Benjamin's

anti-political urge for radical change, and what it meant for him to feel that any sort of normative political behavior was doomed by definition.

RABINBACH: Benjamin's sensibility was to bring it so close to the skin that you understand that he has his finger on exactly what the situation is, and there is no exit from that situation. He considers various options—he toys with Communism with Brecht, and with Zionism with Gershom Scholem. But for him, there is no exit. It's a cliché that his suicide is symbolic, but it is a metaphor for the fact that he couldn't see himself exiting Europe.

CABINET: What, then, is he advocating? Somehow, it seems, in at least some of his writings, that he manages to still believe that there is a kind of sublime activism that can be galvanized in opposition to the status quo, while disavowing the potential for substantive political action.

RABINBACH: He has a wonderful affinity for these moments of activism, but he has absolutely no heart for engaging with it. He talks about surrealism, but in the past tense, when it's over. He talks about Dada in the same way. Communism is also not a possibility. He captures the core messianism of the Communist idea, but his philosophy of history is totally opposed to Communism. The idea of progress is inimical to him.

CABINET: And how do you align that idea with an essay like "The Critique of Violence" where Benjamin seems to imply that there are forms of general action—the proletarian strike, etc.—that can entertain violence without violating?

RABINBACH: It's exactly the same thing. He admires and invokes Sorel, but in the end, it's divine violence— not human violence—that is ultimately the final judgment.

CABINET: How do you contrast that with Ernst Bloch's approach to these messianic, redemptive ideals?

RABINBACH: Well, Bloch was engaged with the Communist Party. But it's important that, coming

back to what we were saying earlier about the Jewish ferment around 1912, when he wrote *The Spirit of Utopia* in 1918, it had a Jewish section, a couple of Jewish chapters. When he republished the book a few years later, he took them out.

CABINET: Why?

RABINBACH: I think that the ferment, the excitement, the electricity was over, and that his communism didn't allow it. It didn't fit with his new socialist utopianism.

CABINET: You had a great observation about how "the messianic idea implied the radical rejection of any sort of quotidian politics combined with a characteristically apocalyptic attitude, which often incorporated antipolitics *in extremis*."

RABINBACH: That's about Benjamin, but Bloch too had it. During World War I, they were all part of an anti-Prussian, anti-German exile group in Switzerland. Scholem was also part of it: Hugo Ball was the central figure in that movement.

CABINET: Let's turn to Ball. First of all, who was he, and how did he come to this group of people?

RABINBACH: He was a young Catholic intellectual who had two simultaneous careers: one was as an anti-war activist and a philosopher, and the other was as the founder of Zurich Dada, as a Dada poet and performer. And he was the editor of the anti-war newspaper *Die Freie Zeitung* in Bern. Bloch was part of his staff at that newspaper; they all krew each other. His book *Flight Out of Time*, a diary, is a central text of the Dada movement and is still read widely. Later in his career, he became very religious and recommitted himself to Catholicism, and became a close associate of Carl Schmitt and an admirer of his conservative political theology.

CABINET: What happened between Bloch and Ball at *Die Freie Zeitung*?

RABINBACH: It emerged that Ball was, among many things, also an anti-Semite. His book *Critique of the German Intelligentsia*, written in 1919, is not an anti-Semitic book, *except* when you restore the parts that were deleted after World War II to make the book more palatable for post-World War II generations.

His view was that the central feature of German militarism and authoritarianism was German Protestantism. Luther's idea that you can be a good Christian, and at the same time, you must obey secular authority, was for Ball the crux of the problem with German nationalism. He identified more with French Catholicism and Russian anarchism, but he also said that the Protestant Junkers and materialistic Jews were responsible for Germany's descent into war and apocalypse. After the war, he accused the Weimar Republic of being a Jewish republic, the marriage of Marx and Walther Rathenau, the foreign minister who was assassinated in 1922. Why were the Jews responsible? Because they were manipulative, they held the purse strings of the Prussian government, the usual litany of complaints. He was a conventional anti-Semite, but the expurgation of the egregious passages meant that this was completely undiscovered until recently. Bloch eventually got totally fed up with Ball and left Basel.

CABINET: We had spoken before but let's return to that idea of the possibility that anti-Semitism was in fact so pervasive that it was imagined to be a force unlikely to ever effloresce in physically toxic ways.

RABINBACH: Before World War II, anti-Semitism was completely normal in polite and impolite discourse. It was only after World War II and the Holocaust that it became taboo, and so, that's why Ball's anti-Semitic pages were excised from the book. Because you couldn't have this sophisticated, intellectual artist be thought of as an anti-Semite in the new, Western-oriented, and contrite Federal Republic of Germany.

CABINET: In some way, there may have even been something anesthetizing about the omnipresence of anit-Semitism. But let's turn to Heidegger and his "Letter on Humanism." You have a wonderful line about how the letter exemplifies Heidegger's characteristic ability to assume a position that pretends to the highest philosophical rigor while positioning himself in the most opportune political light.

RABINBACH: I think that characterizes Heidegger very well. He had an ability to think himself through his astute philosophical lens and at the same time he had an absolute inability to think of himself apart from his most banal and mundane circumstances. In "Taking Philosophy Seriously," Richard Rorty said that Heidegger was a "redneck," "a good old boy from the Black Forest."

CABINET: What were the circumstances of the composition of Heidegger's letter?

RABINBACH: Well, the situation was that Heidegger was in dire straits in 1945. His house had been confiscated by the French occupation authorities and the university had established a commission to discuss whether he would be allowed to teach in the future, which did not look like it would turn out very well. But there was one bright spot in all this darkness and that was that a number of French intellectuals visited Heidegger at this time. One of the visitors was a young man called Jean Beaufret, who arranged to ask him a series of questions to which Heidegger would respond. They would be published in French; French authorities would not allow him to publish in German. The "Letter on Humanism," which was written in the fall of 1946 and published in 1947, came out of this exchange with Beaufret.

It gets more complicated because the other figure who played an enormous role in the partial rehabilitation of Heidegger was Jean-Paul Sartre, who was influenced by Heidegger and never made any bones about it. As the very powerful editor of *Les Temps modernes*, he devoted three issues to the Heidegger case in the first few years after the war. In the end, Sartre's verdict was that Heidegger was no more culpable for Nazism than Hegel was for the Prussian state. Heidegger repaid Sartre by attacking him in the letter as an example of humanism and existentialism, which he rejected because all humanism, all self-assertion—whether it be intellectual self-assertion, technology, science, knowledge—represented metaphysics, the false beginning of putting man at the center of the universe, whereas the center has to be Being, with man relegated to the humble position of shepherd of Being.

CABINET: I like the idea of humility being invoked

as the ultimate value by someone who at the same time is positioning himself as the ultimate victim of Nazism.

RABINBACH: He's only the victim of Nazism to the extent that Nazism is itself a manifestation of the arrogance and metaphysical hubris of humanism. Nazism is a humanism—he doesn't say that, but the implication is there—because the idea of race is the self-assertion of the human. Heidegger argued that he himself was only culpable to the extent that he was culpable for all of Western civilization, from the Greeks to the moderns, which represented this false road of metaphysics. Heidegger claimed that he himself, through error or misjudgment, had taken that road too.

CABINET: How do you fathom his charisma and his influence over the next generation of French intellectuals, such as Derrida?

RABINBACH: I don't understand it. Even without the anti-Semitism, what do we learn from him? Pure, unsullied Heideggerianism is the idea that we have to pay attention to thinking, to poetry, to nature, to immerse ourselves in the Being of nature and the Being of language, and not to engage in political adventures.

CABINET: That's a good transition point to your treatment of Adorno and Horkheimer's *Dialectic of Enlightenment*, which opposes the Heideggerian glorification of rootedness and the idea that "dwelling" rules supreme. Their book starts with the figure of Odysseus, but you've conjured something subtler than just the archetype of the wanderer through that connection.

RABINBACH: Adorno once said that he went back to Germany to finish off Heidegger; the Frankfurt School saw him for who he really was. I think *Dialectic of Enlightenment* is a very anti-Heideggerian book in the sense that, although it is intensely critical of not just *the* Enlightenment but of enlightenment—in the sense of the domination of nature by concepts as the most fundamental source of reification and domination—they refuse to posit an alternative in the sense that Heidegger posited an alternative: his

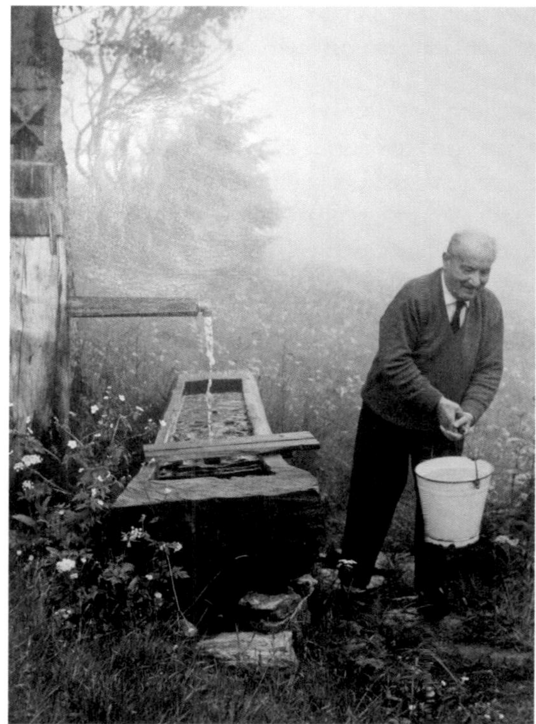

Undated photograph of Heidegger outside his hut in the Black Forest.

idea of the truth of Being. For them, the idea of this alternative is anathema, and in this they stayed faithful to Benjamin's legacy. I think it's not unimportant that *Dialectic of the Enlightenment* was written just after the time that Benjamin's manuscripts arrived in New York.

CABINET: So they were thinking about his "Theses on the Philosophy of History"?

RABINBACH: And the Jewish dimension was paramount.

CABINET: What do make of the way they take the idea of anti-Semitism and almost extend it into a philosophical principle affecting all the ways in which civilization failed?

RABINBACH: The more I immersed myself in their correspondence and in the texts, the more I became convinced that this was a book about anti-Semitism, and that *Dialectic of Enlightenment* is not just about how Odysseus, escaping myth and nature, becomes

the source of enlightenment and domination. There was a second thesis, maybe even more important, namely that that the Jews were sacrificed—this is the word they use—because they represented the taboo on mimesis, the taboo on art and representation. The austerity of the Jews, in a way, revealed through negative example, the mythical, pre-modern, pre-enlightenment character of Christianity, and anti-Semitism, and by extension the Holocaust, was a revolt of this mythicized, image-bound, Christianity against the Jewish taboo on mimesis.

CABINET: Do they position it as a repetition of the fundamental Christian revolt against Judaism?

RABINBACH: Exactly; the mythicized, image-bound Christianity was always present latently. Protestantism was one attempt to rebel against, or to remove, this magical quality of Christianity. But, ultimately—and here Adorno and Horkheimer followed Freud—only Jews manifested the abstract non-sensual character that they identified as *Bilderverbot*, the proscription on images. Christianity revolted against the "demagified" world, and the Jews represent "demagification." You can't even translate the word that Adorno and Horkheimer use.

CABINET: I think you use "disenchantment" at one point.

RABINBACH: That's not so good. But it is true that their idea was that Christianity represented a kind of revolt against disenchantment, and the Jews were identified with a disenchanted world.

CABINET: And do Adorno and Horkheimer advocate for disenchantment?

RABINBACH: It's not that they advocate it; it is just the nature of the human condition, and they were convinced that Max Weber was right and that this is our fate.

CABINET: You speak about living with that as something distinct from solace, but still a position— a kind of composure in the face of disenchantment. They saw themselves as permanent exiles, but

their lives were not entirely without enchantment. You write about the names that they had for each other.

RABINBACH: The animal names. That's very important; you can't do work on them unless you know the names, because you wouldn't know who the characters are in the correspondence. Adorno was "the hippopotamus," his wife Gretel "the giraffe," and Horkheimer "the wooly mammoth."

CABINET: How did you come to see the importance of these names, apart from being able to recognize who they were talking about?

RABINBACH: Eventually, I began to think it was important, that there was something about staying in this childhood world that made life worth living for them.

CABINET: And there is something beautiful in your suggestion that this form of childhood fantasy is very distinct from the re-mythification that they are indicting in Heidegger.

RABINBACH: It's a better alternative than re-mythification.

CABINET: I wonder if you can expand a bit on the figure of the shadow and the way you use it in relation to catastrophe. It seems to me one of the many merits of the book is how you complicate the idea of the shadow, giving us something of a taxonomy of its multifarious nature, as manifested through the works of the thinkers you focus on. A shadow can be retrospective in this sense, but it can be foreshadowing as well; it's a figure operating temporally and spatially as the signal of a new beginning or of a final collapse. And you suggest that the shadow lingers but the shadow is not uniform.

RABINBACH: The conceit of the shadow was initially employed to try to indicate the different ways in which events were both perpetuated and elongated, as you say, but also short-circuited in a variety of intellectual contexts. And it seemed to me that the shadow was a good metaphor for thinking about the ways in which the two different catastrophes of the twentieth century impacted the intellectual engagement that occurred as a result of those events.

There is a huge field concerned with the history of concepts, but it's almost entirely devoted to concepts invented between 1750 and 1850. Historians have even given a name to that period: the "saddle time," the period in which modernity became established in science, politics, and philosophy. So where are the twentieth-century concepts? Where is the shadow? Is it latency? People have said that the shadow is another word for latency; the concepts invented in the twentieth century are too traumatic, and so they have been driven underground. So, that is one argument, the trauma argument. I understand the shadow of catastrophe in two dimensions; first, the one cast by the cataclysmic events of the twentieth century, and second, the shadow cast by the texts I examine, the protracted impact of catastrophe in what have become iconic works, in part because they are themselves the incarnation of those events.

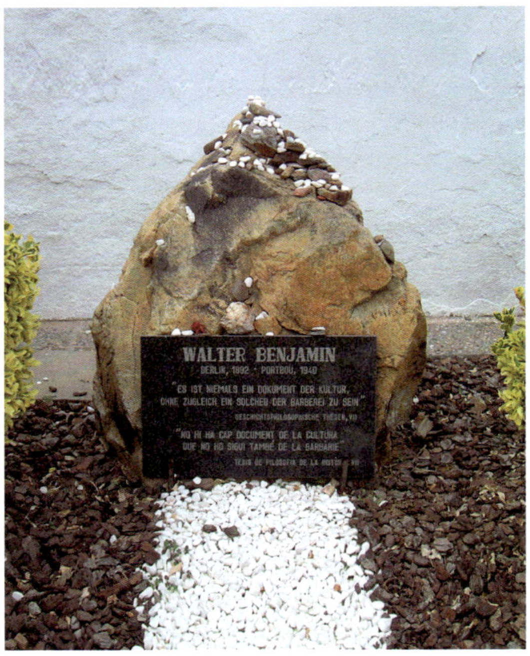

Walter Benjamin's grave in Portbou, Catalonia, where he committed suicide in September 1940. The epitaph, in German and in Catalan, is from Benjamin's "Theses on the Philosophy of History": "There is no document of civilization which is not at the same time a document of barbarism."

IT CAME FROM OUTER SPACE
Maria Golia

The solar system has filled up a lot since the dawn of the science of meteoritics in the late eighteenth century; Jupiter, which had four known moons, now has fifty.[1] Four asteroids were known by 1807; as of 2013, over six hundred thousand were catalogued—some little more than flying rocks, the biggest a third the size of the moon—but by some estimates they number in the millions.[2] Typically depicted as orbiting the sun within a thickly peppered belt between Mars and Jupiter some two hundred million kilometers from Earth, asteroids are in fact at immense distances from one another, though they are not as far apart as the planets. Agoraphobics are advised not to contemplate what the solar system looks like drawn to scale. Reduce Earth to the size of a pea and Jupiter would be three hundred meters away, Pluto two kilometers away "and about the size of a bacterium." The closest star, Proxima Centauri, would be sixteen thousand kilometers away from the pea-sized Earth.[3] Having calculated the possible number of planets that may exist beyond our solar system, Carl Sagan noted that the emptiness between them is so great "that if you were randomly inserted into the universe" the chances of landing on or near one would be less than one in a billion trillion.[4] Advances in astronomy suggest that stars and galaxies comprise only four to five percent of a universe composed largely of invisible "dark matter" and the "dark energies" that drive its expansion.[5] Science may sketch the contours of this reality, but the intellect, even aided by intuition, can neither grasp nor convey the spaciousness of space.

That Earth should regularly encounter asteroidal, cometary, and planetary debris may seem extraordinary, but our planet whizzes through the quasi-void around the sun at a speed of thirty kilometers per second, in constant collision with such objects. An impact event with the energy of the Hiroshima nuclear bomb occurs around once a year, while a megaton event is expected at least once a century. No one would be around to calculate these probabilities, however, were it not for Earth's superbly protective atmosphere; most bodies break up when they encounter it and are fragmented and dispersed by aerodynamic stresses before they reach its lower realms. More discrete is the microscopic powdering of interplanetary and interstellar dust that Earth receives annually by the tens of thousands of tons. This dust contains enough micrometeorites (a.k.a. magnetic spherules, average size 0.2 millimeters) for at least one to fall on each meter of the planet's surface per year. Every mundane stretch of highway hosts some tiny relic of the early solar system.[6]

The flux of meteorites is not constant. In its youth and at various points in its 4.5-billion-year history, our planet was severely battered, which is why geologist Derek Ager has compared Earth's life to that of a soldier: "long periods of boredom and short periods of terror."[7] But meteorite impacts and the terrific craters some caused were not always recognized as external forces acting on Earth's geological development. It was only at the end of the nineteenth century that some geologists began to take a new interest in terrestrial craters, which had long been attributed to volcanic activity. Among them was Grove Karl Gilbert (1843–1918), chief geologist of the US Geological Survey, who had been present at the 1891 gathering of the American Association for the Advancement of Science when mineral merchant Albert E. Foote described the unusual meteorites he had found in the vicinity of Coon Butte, Arizona, which contained microscopic diamonds. Foote was so intent on announcing his exceptional find that he barely mentioned that Coon Butte was the rim of a gigantic crater, soon to become the first of its kind ever studied on Earth. An estimated two hundred million tons of rock was displaced to form its perfect bowl, measuring 1 kilometer across and 180 meters deep. In keeping with prevailing views, Foote thought the crater was volcanic and dismissed the small meteorites lying in its proximity as coincidence.[8]

Gilbert suspected that the crater had been made by an impact and the large mass that caused it

Opposite: Meteor Crater (formerly known as Coon Butte and now also called Barringer Meteorite Crater), attributed to the impact of a three-hundred-thousand-ton meteor some fifty thousand years ago. Photo Jonathan Blair. From *National Geographic*, September 1986.

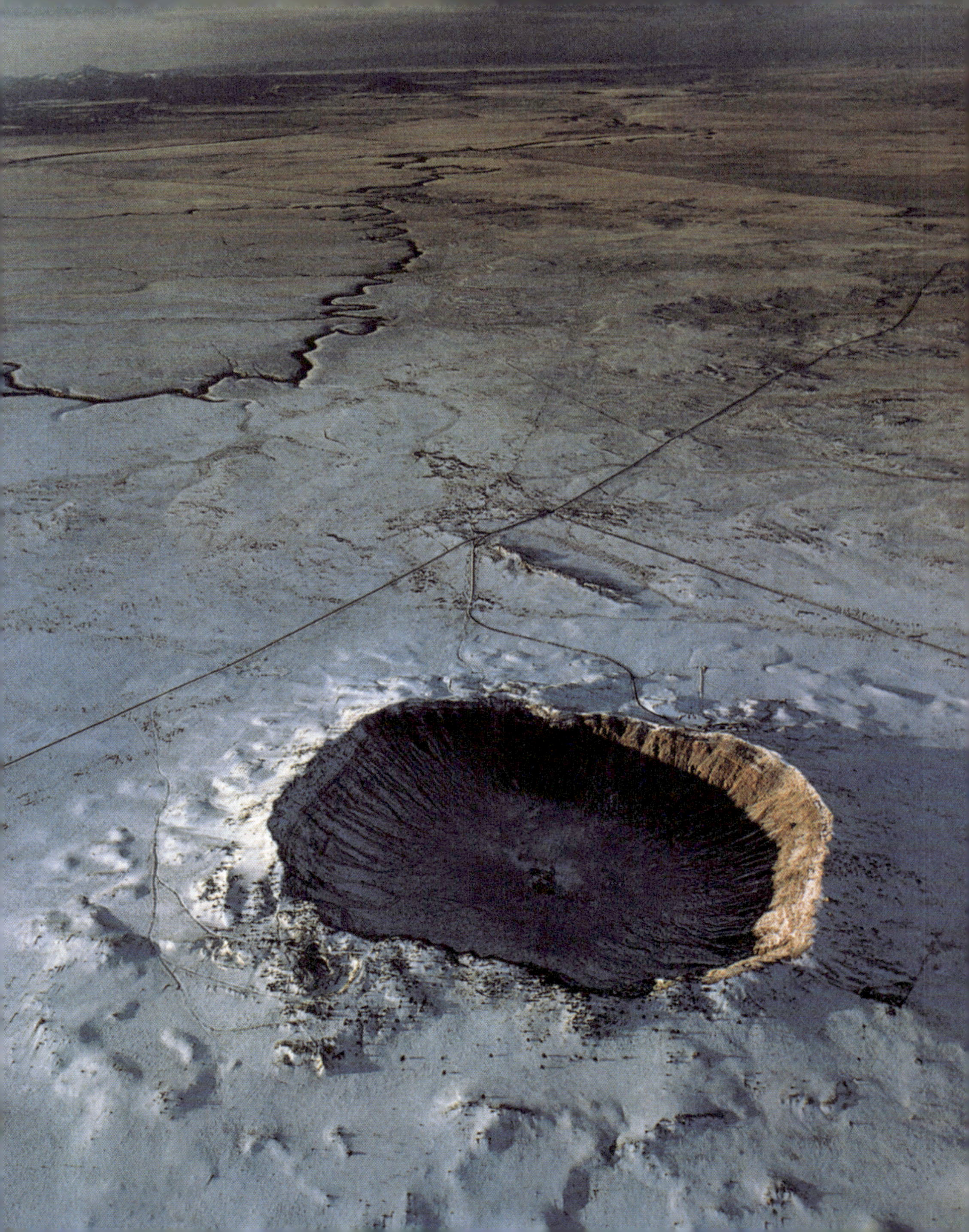

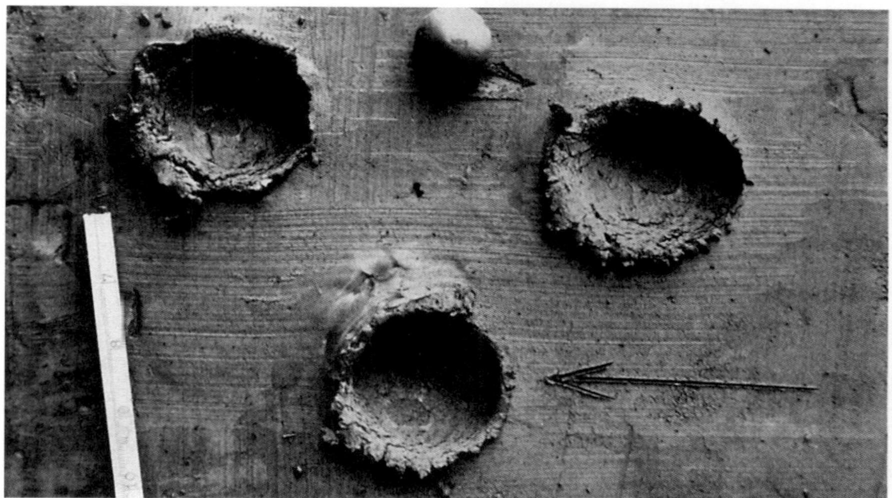

Grove Karl Gilbert's 1891 mudball experiment designed to prove that an object thrown obliquely will make a hole similar to that made by an object dropped vertically. Photo Grove Karl Gilbert. Courtesy US Geological Survey.

might still be buried there. He soon set out "to hunt a star," spending weeks examining the crater and hurling mud balls into mud surfaces to observe the cavities they made, which led him to conclude that an impact object that arrived obliquely could still leave a round, rather than elliptical, crater.[9] Gilbert's measurements—involving the probable size of the impact object, the volume of the crater, and the amount of material thrown up to form its rim—were compromised by his failure to take into account fifty thousand years of erosion and resulted in a calculation that could not account for the mass of any meteorite that might have landed there. Nor did he find the magnetic anomalies that a large iron-rich body would have produced. Remaining faithful to science, Gilbert reluctantly concluded that the crater could not have resulted from an impact and that the meteorites around it were coincidental.[10] (Soon, however, he would turn his attention to lunar craters, and in 1892 delivered a paper in which he rightly asserted that they had been formed not by volcanic activity, as was widely believed at the time, but by impacts.)

To Daniel Moreau Barringer (1860–1929), a quintessential American entrepreneur, this was "highfalutin" nonsense. Born in Raleigh, North Carolina, his father was a US congressman who shared an office with Abraham Lincoln. At military school, Barringer's disrespect for authority won him an early dismissal. At fifteen, he enrolled at the College of New Jersey (later Princeton University) where he befriended classmates who would influence his own and America's destinies, including future US president Woodrow Wilson. Although he received a law degree from the University of Pennsylvania, Moreau, as he now called himself, opted out of a legal career, partnered with a geologist, and spent several years prospecting for minerals in Spain, South America, Mexico, California, and the southwest United States. In 1897, he hit the jackpot, acquiring the mining rights for the Commonwealth Silver Mine in Pearce, Arizona. He married, and celebrated his newfound wealth with a yearlong honeymoon around the world.[11]

Moreau heard of the Arizona crater in 1902 through a chance encounter at the Tucson Opera with Samuel Holsinger, who had also stepped out for a smoke. A US Land Office agent who knew the territory, Holsinger said that according to local legend, the bowl was formed by a meteorite. Moreau was intrigued but incredulous because he knew that the crater had, as he later noted, been examined "by members of the United States Geological Survey while making topographic maps of the region, and in their report they evidently did not accept this theory." Holsinger sent Moreau samples of the meteorites from around the crater; analysis revealed 92 percent iron, 5 percent nickel, and trace amounts of iridium, platinum, and microdiamonds. The iron and nickel contained in the samples were valued at 125 dollars per ton at the time, and Moreau, riding a long lucky streak, figured there were at least tens of thousands of these meteorites.[12]

Unlike Gilbert, Moreau was convinced the impact meteorite still existed and was ready to dig to the antipodes to find it. Apart from the monetary benefits, he was compelled to prove academia wrong about the crater's origin, calling their volcanic, and later "steam explosion" theories, "blind" and "demented."[13] Moving in the circles of Theodore Roosevelt and the trustees of Princeton and MIT, Moreau found many enthusiastic investors, but they abandoned him as results failed to materialize. Moreau, who took his fortune from the earth, put it back where he found it, drilling unsuccessfully for twenty-six years to find the meteoritic mother lode. In the words of his grandson, he "was not just a man of strong opinions, he was a man of constant opinions." Moreau's stubborn prospecting eventually ruined him. He never imagined that the mass (later estimated at three hundred thousand tons) had vaporized in the bombastic energies of impact (equivalent to approximately nine megatons of TNT) and the small scattered meteorites were all that remained.[14]

A nine-page spread in the June 1928 issue of the *National Geographic Magazine*, entitled "The Mysterious Tomb of a Giant Meteorite," outlined mining operations at the site without mentioning Moreau or his quest. The article's urbane author described a "splash in stone" so deep "that [Lower Manhattan] could be dropped into the hole and only the Woolworth Tower would project prominent above the rim."[15] The article highlighted Gilbert's investigations, perhaps as a nod to the esteemed US Geological Survey, even though Gilbert had held firm to the crater's volcanic origin until his death. Moreau died in 1929, before the substantial evidence he had gathered would help prove the mandarins wrong.[16]

In the 1950s, geologist Eugene Shoemaker (1928–1997) brought a unique perspective to Meteor Crater (as it has become known) from his recent study of nuclear blast zones at a testing field in Nevada, where he saw parallel signs of destruction. With a colleague, he identified coesite, a quartz formed only under intense shock at high temperatures, in samples taken from both the blast zones

---

Below: Core sample taken from southern perimeter of Meteor Crater in 1966. The material in this box is from a drill depth of 102.5 to 122 feet, and was collected to provide examples of unshocked rock to serve as a baseline for investigating the effects of the impact at Meteor Crater. Courtesy United States Geological Survey.

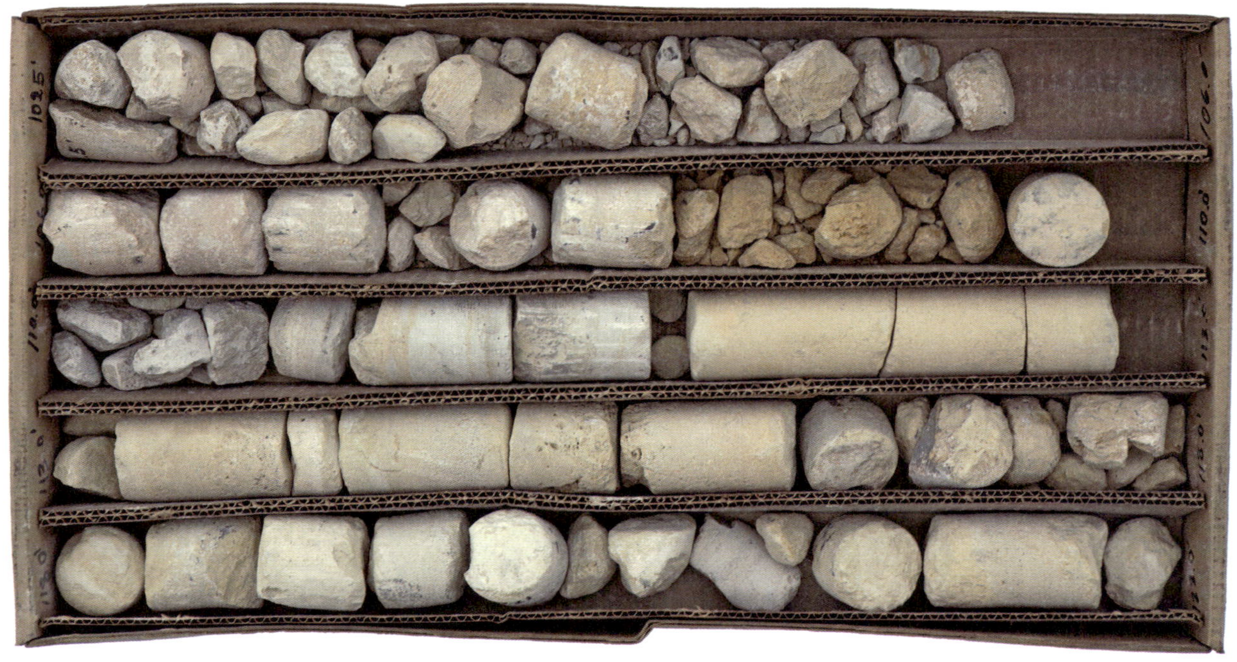

and Meteor Crater. Having proven the impact origin of the crater conclusively by 1963, Shoemaker's next move was not to seek out other craters, but to look to space for what caused them.[17] In the 1970s, with his wife Carolyn and other colleagues, Shoemaker conducted a systematic survey of the inner solar system, tracking asteroids. Only twelve had so far been discovered, not because science lacked the means, but the interest. "Astronomers in the twentieth century essentially abandoned the solar system." Shoemaker explained in an interview. "Their attention was turned to the stars, the galaxies." When Shoemaker's team focused the Palomar Observatory telescope closer to home, the findings were startling: asteroids and their detritus crossed Earth's path regularly.[18]

In his *Nature of the Stratigraphical Record* (1973), Derek Ager pointed out that what humans consider rare catastrophes are a routine aspect of Earth's geological process. "The hurricane, flood or the tsunami may do more in an hour or a day than the ordinary processes of nature have achieved in a thousand years," he wrote.[19] While Ager refrained from naming meteorite impacts as geological game-changers, he cited respected paleontologist Digby McClaren, who in 1970 had linked them to mass extinctions. At the time, impact-related topics were treated by the scientific community like some private indiscretion, admitted but rarely discussed. Geologists and paleontologists, among others, followed the maxim that "nature does not make jumps." Anything significant occurs not because of some anomalous "paroxysm," but as a result of well-observed, familiar processes. Since the simplest solution is always the best, the notion that extraterrestrial forces directed Earthbound processes "violated [scientists'] parsimonious instincts."[20]

Yet the idea kept cropping up. In the late 1600s, Edmond Halley had remarked to the Royal Society that the Bible's great flood was possibly caused by a comet. A century later, Pierre Simon Laplace (1749–1827), whose modified version of Kant's nebular hypothesis remains current, thought that a large meteorite could kill off whole species.[21] Examining the fossil record, naturalist George Cuvier (1769–1832) postulated "a world previous to ours, destroyed by some kind of catastrophe."[22] Over time, other scientists aired the possibility of mass extinction, and H. G. Wells (1866–1946), who

studied biology under T. H. Huxley and advocated Darwinian theory, essayed it for a wider audience in his two-volume nonfiction *Outline of History* (1920), an international best seller:

We do not know what jars and jolts the solar system may have suffered in the past. … Some huge dark projectile from outer space may have come hurtling through the planets and deflected or even struck our world and turned the whole course of evolution into a new direction … but this is a lapse into pure speculation.[23]

In the 1970s, Derek Ager effectively "rehabilitated" catastrophes by presenting them as relatively regular catalysts of the geological process, but to scientists from a variety of disciplines, mass extinction was still not worthy of speculation.

That impacts and their consequences were so reluctantly explored reflects the same adherence to accepted theories that prevented meteorites themselves from being readily embraced as significant phenomena.[24] To assess the effects of major impacts, it was necessary to overcome not only attachments to familiar concepts but also the territoriality separating members of different disciplines and their suspicion of findings not originating in their own fields. In the late 1960s, the Apollo missions produced the first photographs of Earth, inspiring pride and environmental awareness, on the one hand, and warnings about alien invasions and the forthcoming apocalypse from the "pseudoscientific popular fringe," on the other. Scientists may have wished to distance themselves from sentimentality or sensationalism, but the persistent denial of meteorites, first as extraterrestrial objects and then as forces of cataclysmic change, betrays an almost organic outrage that life on earth should be subject to such intrusions, as if it existed somehow on its own, suspended not in space but in cautious consideration.

The theory that the "age of the dinosaurs" ended as a result of cataclysmic impact sixty-five million years ago passed from heresy to orthodoxy over the next twenty years. Persuasive proof was found in a thin geological stratum encircling the earth between the layers corresponding to the Cretaceous and subsequent Tertiary periods, the so-called "K/T Boundary." Geologist Walter Alvarez gathered samples of the peculiar stratum in Umbria, and with

his father Luis Alvarez, a nuclear physicist, enlisted a colleague at Berkeley to analyze it. Unheard-of quantities of iridium were found, an element abundant in meteorites and space dust but rare on Earth. Samples gathered from the K/T Boundary at worldwide locations produced the same results. The Alvarezes' 1980 paper, announcing their belief that the dinosaur extinction was triggered by a massive asteroidal or cometary impact, was hotly contested, not least because its authors had trespassed paleontological territory.[25] Luis Alvarez further insulted the naysayers by calling them "stamp collectors." Habeas corpus was once more demanded, not in the form of the impact mass but of its crater. Eugene Shoemaker proposed a crater in Manson, Iowa, which was adjudged to have been formed nine million years too early. In 1990, Carlos Byars, a *Houston Chronicle* journalist, was attending the annual Lunar and Planetary Science conference in Houston when he heard graduate student Alan Hildebrand's paper on a possible impact site in the Caribbean Sea. Byars told Hildebrand about a paper given at a 1981 conference by Glen Penfield, a geophysicist working for the Mexican oil company Pemex, about a colossal circle of magnetic and gravitational anomalies in the Yucatan, a phenomenon first noted by Pemex scientists as early as 1950. These readings, Penfield had asserted, were the signature of a now-buried circular impact crater that extended from the Mexican mainland into the Gulf of Mexico.[26] Though Penfield's hypothesis had not originally found a receptive audience, he and Hildebrand, now working together, soon managed to gather sufficient geological evidence to prove that the crater—which they named Chicxulub—was the *memento mori* of a world-wrecking impact. We now know that object that made it weighed over a trillion tons and was at least ten kilometers wide, and the crater it made upon impact was briefly more than thirty kilometers deep before it began to collapse because of the inability of rock to support a hole of that size. Scientists estimate that the crater today is some 170 kilometers wide.

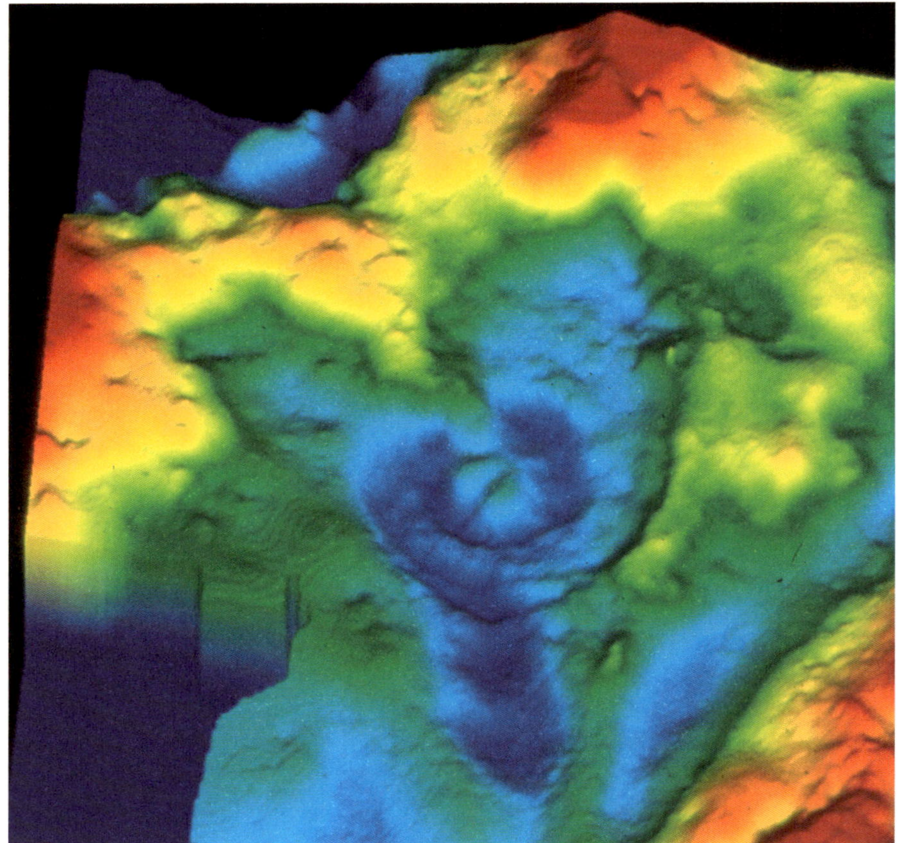

Three-dimensional Bouguer gravity anomaly map over the Chicxulub crater. The crater is represented by the near-circular low central to the figure (with contained concentric structure). This image does not show the shape of the crater; the negative gravity anomaly of the crater instead corresponds to the relatively low densities of the rocks within it (breccias and the melt sheet) and the Tertiary sediments filling it. Courtesy Mark Pilkington and the Geological Survey of Canada.

Nowadays, any schoolchild can tell you that an asteroid was behind the dinosaurs' demise.[27] But the controversy surrounding the K/T extinction is not over, with Princeton University researchers presenting evidence that extensive volcanic activity (in India's Deccan Traps) had already done most of the work of killing off 70 percent of Earth's species and claiming that the Chicxulub impact only delivered the *coup de grâce*.[28] Either way, it is now accepted that at random points in time, Earth experienced bombardments that altered planetary chemistries, presenting an evolutionary *cul de sac* for some types of life and favorable conditions for others, including us. Cosmochemists now speak of a "biology of revolutionary rather than evolutionary change."[29]

Investigations of the transformative power of large impacts indicate that even events much smaller than Chicxulub could produce enough dust and ash to block the sun and launch a global winter.[30] People living in desert cities know how a few gusts of wind can kick up a sandstorm so dense that visibility is reduced to almost zero. Witnesses of volcanic eruptions have likewise watched ash clouds towering into contused skies, blotting out the sun. Those who have survived bombings can attest to the deafening shockwaves and lung-searing heat. But there is nothing in human experience—including Hiroshima and Nagasaki—that remotely resembles the sheer power, many orders of magnitude greater than any man-made weapon, of a cosmic impact, for which death itself is but a puny metaphor.

The speed of an object the size of the one that created the Chicxulub crater would compress the air beneath it to such an extent that it would generate temperatures some ten times higher than the surface of the sun (60,000° C). One second after hitting the atmosphere, the meteorite would slam into the ground and vaporize, shattering nearly one million cubic kilometers of the surrounding rock and creating a glowing fireball of more than a thousand cubic kilometers of rock vapor that would incinerate everything within a 250-kilometer radius. Everyone within 1,500 kilometers of the epicenter would be hurled to the ground amid a blinding flash of light. Earthquakes and tsunamis would follow as showers of burning debris falling back into the Earth's upper atmosphere would set the world aflame. Survival would be possible but not necessarily preferable.

The first day's potential death toll has been projected to be 1.5 billion.[31] Scientists still debate the exact size of the asteroid that created the Chicxulub crater, and some have even proposed that it might in fact have been a smaller, faster-moving comet, but given the scale of the destruction, the point seems almost moot.

Imagining destruction of such scope remains essentially, perhaps mercifully, impossible but that hasn't stopped Hollywood from trying. Impact events have inspired a genre of popular film (and fiction) worthy of a book of its own.[32] That mass extinction should become a subject of mass entertainment is nonetheless suggestive, as are academia's jocularly titled contributions to the literature, works like "Killer Rocks from Outer Space," "Earth's Greatest Hits," and "Coming Attractions."[33] In US military and scientific circles, the idea of planetary defense systems designed to intercept meteorite attacks is likewise subject to "the giggle factor," according to Air Force Lieutenant Colonel Martin E. B. France:

Even the most ardent supporters of defending the earth from cataclysmic asteroidal and cometary impacts share occasional public or private chuckles with colleagues and skeptics—behavior considered unthinkable when discussing means to avert or mitigate [terrestrial catastrophes].[34]

If laughter, as has been said, is the confusion between "yes" and "no," then the "GF," as Lt. Col. France calls it, may be owed to the paradox of a threat so seemingly remote yet ever present. "Ours is indeed an age of extremity," wrote Susan Sontag in her 1965 essay "The Imagination of Disaster," "for we live under the continual threat of two equally fearful but seemingly opposed destinies: unremitting banality and inconceivable terror."[35]

In the last two hundred years, it is not the probability of impact-related catastrophe that has increased, only our awareness of it. Dismissing the danger of falling stones in 1803, a contributor to the *Journal des Débats* confidently wrote that "one should not worry; we are not at war with the moon."[36] A century later, the author of *Astronomy for Amateurs* assured his readers that "there is little to fear of the destruction of humanity by these balls of wind [comets]," based on the fact that two comets had been observed the previous century without incident.[37]

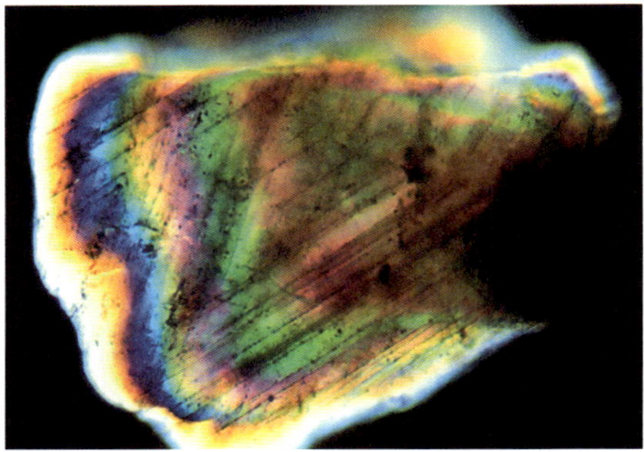

Shocked quartz grain produced by the impact at Chicxulub. In quartz, the passage of a strong shock wave can cause dislocation of the grain's crystal structure along preferred crystallographic orientations. This grain shows at least eight sets of planar deformation features when rotated. Courtesy Alan Hildebrand.

In light of recent space surveys, we are now informed that earth exists in "a sort of cosmic shooting gallery" and the threat has been far from fully assessed.[38] Since NASA began monitoring Near-Earth Objects (NEOs) in 1984, the danger of mass extinction has been taken with greater seriousness. The "Spacewatch" program was expanded in the 1990s and renamed "Spaceguard" in response to a catastrophic event on Jupiter, the first of its kind ever predicted and observed from Earth.[39] In July 1994, fifteen fragments of the comet Shoemaker-Levy 9 (named for its discoverers Eugene and Carolyn Shoemaker and David Levy), several of them over a kilometer wide, struck Jupiter with a devastating force equal to three hundred gigatons of TNT, underscoring the threat of a similar event to our planet.[40]

Earth has in fact experienced several near misses. On 15 February 2013, a NEO passed, as predicted, within 17,200 kilometers of the earth, darting gracefully through a flock of orbiting telecommunications satellites without grazing so much as an antenna. But that same day, an unobserved asteroid exploded above Chelyabinsk, Russia, causing considerable mayhem and prompting the US House Science Committee to convene a meeting to discuss threats from space. In June 2013 NASA, which claims to have found 95 percent of all large asteroids near Earth's orbit, launched its "asteroid grand challenge," aimed at identifying the rest in

cooperation with the private sector, academia, and ordinary citizens. As of 27 February 2015, 12,328 NEOs have been discovered. Some 866 of these are asteroids with a diameter of approximately 1 kilometer or larger and 1,558 have been classified as Potentially Hazardous Asteroids.

Many scientists are now convinced that Earth has been subject to impacts "100 times more energetic [than Chicxulub] … with effects dwarfing that of the K/T," partially and perhaps fully vaporizing oceans.[41] Our earliest ancestors were life forms capable of taking refuge in the murkiest mulch at the bottom of the sea, places that coincidentally have yet to be as well mapped as the surfaces of the Moon and Mars. That *homo sapiens* has overcome the cosmic odds to not only exist but to examine its place in the universe must give pause, especially considering that the process was randomly detoured by flying rocks. The brilliant and eccentric cosmologist Sir Fred Hoyle (1915–2001) compared the chances of natural selection producing results like us to a hurricane blowing through a junkyard and assembling a Boeing 747.[42] Whether or not evolution was aiming in our direction, its mind-bending trajectory demonstrates the relentlessly creative force that V. I. Vernadsky, author of *The Biosphere*, called "the pressure of life."

Humanity seems rather less enthralled with creation than destruction, predicting apocalypses throughout history, producing them repeatedly through war and greed, and watching filmic enactments of them in its spare time. In portrayals of planetary destruction, the most familiar narrative involves a last-minute human intervention that saves Earth, allowing us to enjoy the frisson of imagined catastrophe safe in the expectation that the crisis will ultimately be averted. In February 2013, one potentially city-smashing asteroid went relatively softly into the night and the impact of yet another in Russia caused injuries but no loss of life, but there was no global elation, no music and handholding, no peace treaties or amnesties to celebrate not one but two miraculously narrow escapes. Instead, we save our cheers for Hollywood heroes who save Earth from sinister asteroids, even though such deliverance is in fact frequent enough and quite real.

1 NASA also lists seventeen "provisional" moons. See <solarsystem.nasa.gov/planets/profile.cfm?Object=Jupiter>.

2 See <solarsystem.nasa.gov/planets/profile.cfm?Object=Asteroids&Display=OverviewLong>.

3 The scale analogy is from Bill Bryson, *A Short History of Nearly Everything* (London: Black Swan, 2004), p. 45.

4 Ibid, p. 49. These cosmic odds are reminiscent of the Tibetan notion that the consciousness released at a person's death would have about the same chance of finding a new body as a turtle surfacing in one of several rings floating randomly atop an ocean.

5 Author's conversation with astrophysicist Amr Zant, 24 January 2014.

6 Jon Larsen, "A Hunt for Micrometeorites," *Meteorite: International Quarterly Magazine for Meteorites and Meteorite Science*, vol. 18, no. 2 (May 2012), pp. 31–36.

7 Ted Nield, *Incoming* (London: Granta Books, 2011) p. 95. A student and, later, colleague of Derek Ager, Nield speaks affectionately of his mentor's independent thinking and achievements.

8 Ibid, p. 100. The microdiamonds, an example of shock metamorphism, were formed from carbon in the meteorite under the pressures of impact. In Foote's day, it was theorized that the meteorite was a fragment of a body large enough to form diamonds in its core.

9 Ibid, p. 102.

10 Ted Nield, *Incoming*, p. 104.

11 Drew N. Barringer, "A Grand Obsession—Daniel Moreau Barringer and Meteor Crater," *Meteorite: International Quarterly Magazine for Meteorites and Meteorite Science*, vol. 16, no. 4 (November 2010), pp. 8–9.

12 Ibid, p. 9.

13 Ted Nield, *Incoming*, p. 106.

14 Drew N. Barringer, "A Grand Obsession," p. 12.

15 William D. Boutwell, "The Mysterious Tomb of a Giant Meteorite," *The National Geographic Magazine*, vol. 53, no. 6 (June 1928), p. 722.

16 Drew N. Barringer, "A Grand Obsession," pp. 11–12. Aside from two mining-related books that became standard references in mining and engineering schools, Daniel Moreau Barringer authored two scientific papers supporting Meteor Crater's impact origin, noting that the finely pulverized silica found within it (later understood as formed by shock metamorphosis) and large quantities of magnetic iron oxide (abundant in meteorites) around its rim were inconsistent with known volcanic materials, none of which were found in the vicinity.

17 Recognizable impact craters were rare in Shoemaker's day; as of 2012, 180 had been identified worldwide, mostly by satellite imagery. The oldest, at three billion years, was discovered in Greenland in 2012 and is nearly one hundred kilometers wide. The largest is the three-hundred-kilometer-wide Vredefort crater in South Africa.

18 Bill Bryson, *A Short History of Nearly Everything*, p. 240.

19 Ted Nield, *Incoming*, pp. 96–98.

20 Ibid., p. 98.

21 Ibid., p. 117.

22 Cuvier cited in translator's footnotes to Vladimir I. Vernadsky, "Evolution of Species and Living Matter," trans. Meghan Rouillard, *21st Century Science & Technology* (Spring–Summer 2012), p. 36.

23 H. G. Wells, *The Outline of History* (New York: The Macmillan Company, 1956), vol. 1, p. 41.

24 "Falling stones" were observed throughout history but claims that they originated in space were largely refuted until the mid-nineteenth century owing to Aristotle and Newton, whose theories essentially held that the heavenly bodies were well-ordered in space, and there were no odd, unaccounted-for bits flying about.

25 Luis Alvarez, Walter Alvarez, Frank Asaro, and Helen V. Michel, "Extraterrestrial Cause for the Cretaceous–Tertiary Extinction," *Science*, vol. 208, no. 4448 (6 June 1980), pp. 1095–1108.

26 The author and *Cabinet* wish to thank Professor Alan Hildebrand for his generous assistance in clarifying the details of the events surrounding the discovery of the role played by the Chicxulub impact in the mass extinctions at the end of the Cretaceous period.

27 An online computer game called Dinosaurs and Meteors offers the former a chance to resist their extinction. "When meteors threaten to destroy all of the life on Earth, the dinosaurs ... evolved into having laser beams in their eyes, as well as missile launchers!" See <arcadeprehacks.com/game/17461/Dinosaurs-and-Meteors.html>.

28 Stuart Mason Dambrot, "Not by Asteroid Alone: Rethinking the Cretaceous Mass Extinction," (19 January 2012). Available at <phys.org/news/2012-01-asteroid-rethinking-cretaceous-mass-extinction.html>.

29 Kevin Zahnle and Norman H. Sleep, "Impacts and the Early Evolution of Life," in Paul J. Thomas, Roland D. Hicks, Christopher F. Chyba, and Christopher P. McKay, eds., *Comets and the Origin and Evolution of Life* (Berlin: Springer, 2006), p. 243.

30 A drop of several degrees Celsius would be enough to drastically reduce crop yields. See David Morrison, "The Contemporary Hazard of Comet Impacts," in Paul J. Thomas, Roland D. Hicks, Christopher F. Chyba, and Christopher P. McKay, eds., *Comets and the Origin and Evolution of Life*, p. 291.

31 Much of this scenario is borrowed from Bill Bryson, *A Short History of Nearly Everything*, pp. 253–255. The author and *Cabinet* are grateful to Professor H. Jay Melosh for reviewing this paragraph and correcting some inaccuracies in Bryson's account.

32 Impact-related films became a genre in the 1950s. A short list includes *When Worlds Collide* (1951), *The Day the Sky Exploded* (1958), *The Green Slime* (1968), *Meteor* (1979), *Deep Impact* (1998), and, the author's personal favorite, *Armageddon* (1998). The impending release of the latter two prompted a US Congressional hearing on space defense in anticipation of the spike in public concern. See Martin E. B. France, "Planetary Defense: Eliminating the Giggle Factor," p. 10. Available at <www.dtic.mil/dtic/tr/fulltext/u2/a430995.pdf>.

33 From an ebscohost.com search for papers on "mass extinction events."

34 See Martin E. B. France, "Planetary Defense," for a synopsis of US-initiated planetary defense efforts.

35 Susan Sontag, "The Imagination of Disaster," in *Against Interpretation and Other Essays* (New York: Picador, 1966), p. 224.

36 Matthieu Gounelle, "The Meteorite Fall at L'Aigle and the Biot Report," in Gerald Joseph Home McCall, Alan J. Bowden, and Richard J. Howarth, eds., *The History of Meteoritics and Key Meteorite Collections: Fireballs, Falls and Finds* (London: Geological Society, 2006), p. 77.

37 Camille Flammarion, *Astronomy for Amateurs*, trans. Francis A. Welby (London: Thomas Nelson & Sons, 1903), p. 203.

38 The oft-quoted phrase "cosmic shooting gallery" seems to have been coined by William J. Broad, "Earth Is Target for Space Rocks at Higher Rate than Thought," *The New York Times*, 7 January 1997.

39 NASA's early warning system was named after the one envisaged by Arthur C. Clarke in his 1972 *Rendezvous with Rama*.

40 D. A. Crawford, "Comet Shoemaker-Levy 9 Fragment Size and Mass Estimates from Light Flux Observations," paper given at the 28th Lunar and Planetary Science Conference, Houston (1997). Available at <www.lpi.usra.edu/meetings/lpsc97/pdf/1351.PDF>. Eugene Shoemaker led the first NEO Study Working Group and collaborated with the Spaceguard Foundation until his death in 1997.

41 Kevin Zahnle and Norman H. Sleep, "Impacts and the Early Evolution of Life," p. 243.

42 Ted Nield, *Incoming*, p. 180.

BUNKER CORRESPONDENCE
Patrick Lyons

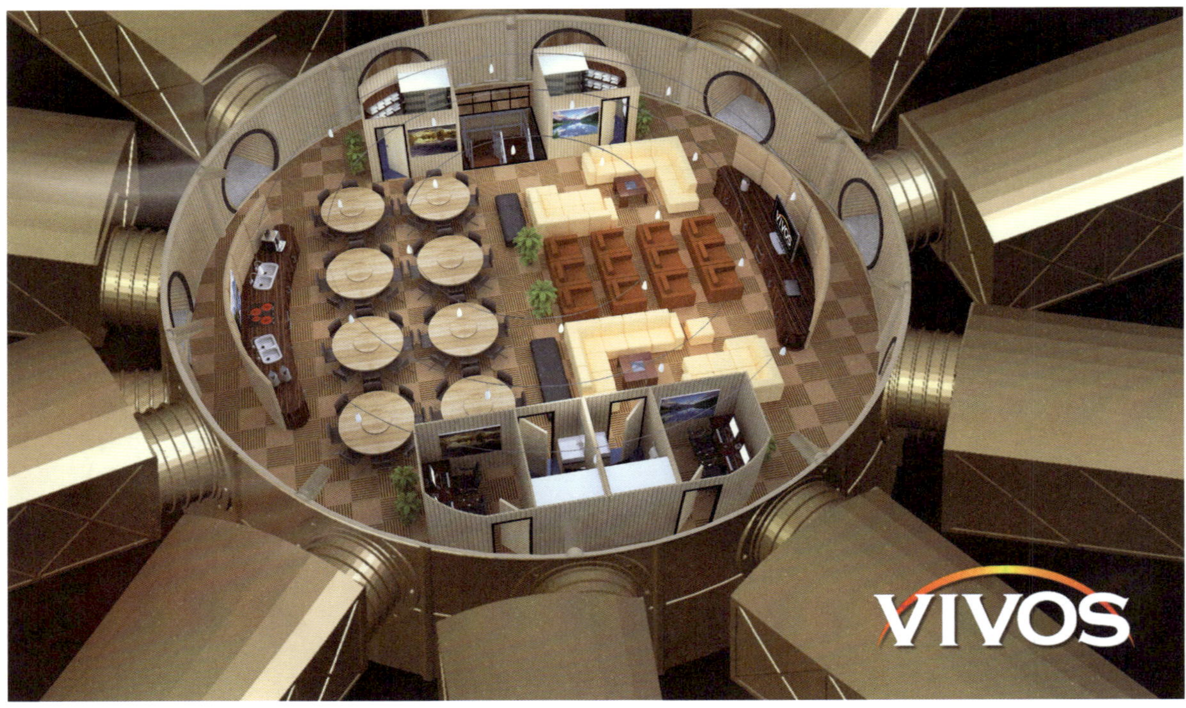

There's nothing out of the ordinary about insuring against the unknown. A vast insurance industry exists so that buyers can experience relative calm in the present by casting a virtual safety net over the unknown future—all at a price. Insurance allows one to tame the future and pick it apart into tangible outcomes. But what are its limits? What does insurance for the end of times look like?

Consider Robert Vicino, founder of the Vivos Group (and a former inflatables entrepreneur), which owns a luxury underground bunker in Indiana that can house eighty individuals, as well as a second in the "heart of Europe" that offers more than 225,000 square feet of blastproof living area. His company, whose motto is "Life Assurance for a Dangerous World," sells off spots in these facilities to anyone who (1) passes the screening process, and (2) is willing to spend somewhere around $35,000 (children under sixteen are offered a $10,000 discount). The bunkers are "fully stocked with food, toiletries, linens, medical supplies, a one-year supply of fuel, a deep water well, NBC filtration systems, geothermal heating and cooling,

bedroom suites, full-size showers and bathrooms, a theater area, dining area, lounge area, exercise equipment, kennels, a garden area for fresh vegetables, laundry area, abundant storage areas, ATVs, bicycles, tools, a workshop, security devices; and, just about everything else that may be needed to ride out virtually any catastrophic event." Each is built to withstand nuclear terrorism, social anarchy, electromagnetic pulses, solar flares—the list goes on and on.

The application process is relatively straightforward. Applicants plug in their basic personal information and check off boxes concerning personal skills and professional background. I went through the process, but, lacking any of the requisite expertise, was unable to check anything off. No military background, no carpentry or medical skills— basically no potential as a survivalist. For my personal statement, I provided an honest assessment of my worth, fluffed with the best "prepper" ideological stance I could muster:

———————

Above: A communal space in a Vivos shelter.

Given the current state of widespread political, economic, and social disrepair in our nation today, it seems to me that the only direction left to go is down. Down, that is, in one of two ways: For the unprepared, down leads to disaster, destruction, and chaos. For those granted the precious gift of foresight, however, down leads simply underground, to safety, towards the future. After extensive research, I've come to conclude that Vivos, among all other shelter complexes, holds the most promise for the protection and preservation of future generations in the face of the unimaginable crises that bear down upon us. In the interest of forward movement for humanity, I wish to apply for placement in your Indiana compound.

From your emails I understand that you are no longer accepting applicants without significant medical, military, or survivalist expertise. While I cannot claim to have any of the above, I have many skills to offer your community. In filling out the Skills and Expertise section of my application, I was struck by the absence of interest in culture and the humanities. As a scholar of French and German Literature and philosophy, I believe that my critical perspective and engagement with the humanities would be of great use to your society, and serve an integral role in the ethical and intellectual cultivation of future generations.

If my perspective appeals to you, I will be happy to discuss in further detail my potential contributions to your project, and my potential candidacy as a member of your movement.

Surprisingly, my application was advanced to the next round of scrutiny: a phone interview. I put off the interview for several months, and in the meantime received regular emails detailing the slashing of bunker prices, further options for me and my party of hopeful survivors, and even a stock email from Vicino himself urging me and my family (never mentioned in my application) to continue our application:

Dear Patrick,

Are you still looking for a survival shelter for your family? I have just reviewed your application for membership in Vivos and noted the size of your group. We have limited space remaining in our completed Indiana shelter and are looking to fill it with one or two more like-minded families that can benefit the existing shelter community, before potential shelter lockdown.

This would be a very significant discount from our listed pricing to make Vivos as affordable as possible for you.

Please let me know if this interests you and when would be a good time to receive my call to discuss the details.

Sincerely,
Robert Vicino
Founder and CEO, *The Vivos Group*

Most striking among the many e-promotions was something called the "Ark of Humanity," with a link to an Indiegogo page crowdsourcing funds for the scheme. While an actual seat in Vicino's bunker costs more than most can afford, the Ark project was quite reasonably priced, at only thirty dollars per kit (with discounts for bulk orders, naturally). The catch was that the Ark only houses a sample of your DNA, which you provide Vivos by mailing in "5 droplets of whole blood" on a special "donor card." It's up to you to survive the apocalypse, but once you have, you can count on your DNA being stored in the company's Genome Vault, just in case old you needs some of young you's DNA.

Curious, I rekindled contact with a Vivos representative and finally scheduled my phone interview. When the time came, I spoke with a woman for about twenty minutes, posing questions about the educational structure in the bunker for post-fallout generations and about the preservation of the humanities. Her blanket answer to both inquiries was that whoever bought space would be responsible for education and the preservation of culture. When I asked about the Ark, she said that they were backordered on DNA sample kits, which I found strange because at the time the Indiegogo campaign had raised only $261 of its $100,000 goal. Given the uncertain state of the arts and humanities in this new world order, the editors at *Cabinet* and I decided to pitch in and so, despite the chronic shortage, we dished out eighty dollars for a "Four Early Bird Donor Kits" package. Then, on June 22nd, the end did come—not for humanity, the humanities, or even for us, but for the Ark itself. Still stuck on $261 at the conclusion of its month-long campaign, the fundraiser was terminated. Our kits were not coming, our credit card was not going to be charged, and our blood stayed in our veins. The floods might be on their way, but the Ark was not ready.

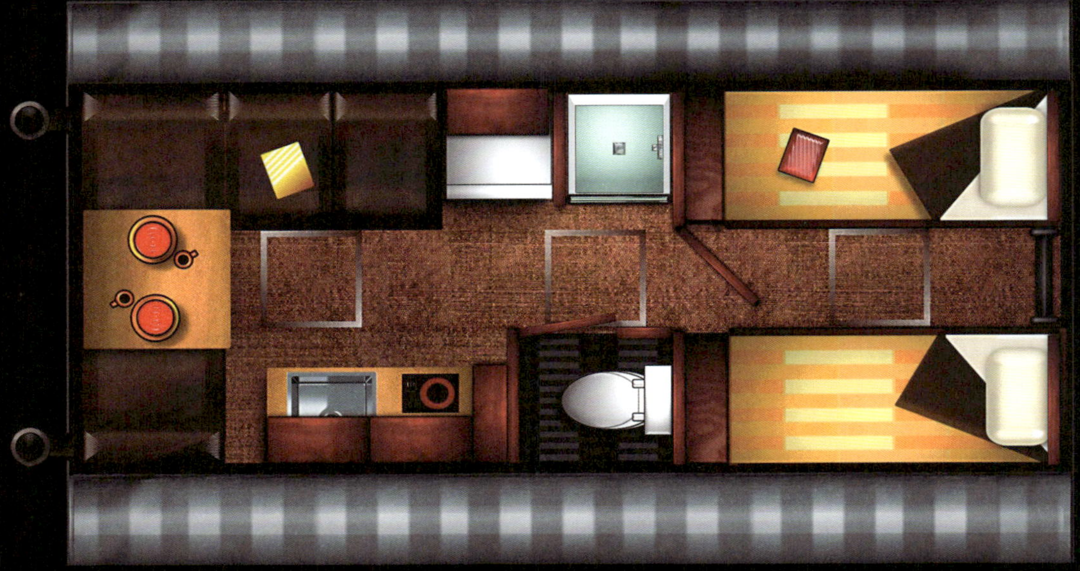

"Just add food, fuel, water and your loved ones!,"
is how Vivos promotes its line of family-sized
turnkey shelters that can be installed underground
on private property. Here, a room from the four-
person Luna model.

Some awards are harder to get than others. Take the Dickin Medal, for instance, which honors animals' service during war (see George Pendle's article in this issue). Dozens of dogs and pigeons, and a handful of horses, have won the award but only one cat—the mighty Simon—has been recognized in the seventy-odd years that the medal has been given. This makes a certain sense, given that dogs, pigeons, and horses can be trained to carry out duties crucial to the war effort. But this downplays the vital role of morale, which is where the cat really comes into its own. During the darkest days of war, the cat offers comfort by sitting in soldiers' laps, purring in the right way, and turning over to have its belly rubbed vigorously. This may seem like a small service, one that does not merit official recognition, but it is worth noting that the cat alone behaves as it does entirely of its own volition. Knowing that an animal has been trained to perform a certain duty effectively turns that animal into another soldier, but the cat, in its utter indifference to any form of instruction, is the only one that can raise morale, precisely because the soldier knows that the cat is keeping him company because that's what it really wants to do. Perhaps the bestowers of the Dickin Medal should consider this when making their selections in the future, though it is of course highly unlikely that any cat would deign to attend a ceremony that imagines humans to be in a position to be handing out medals.

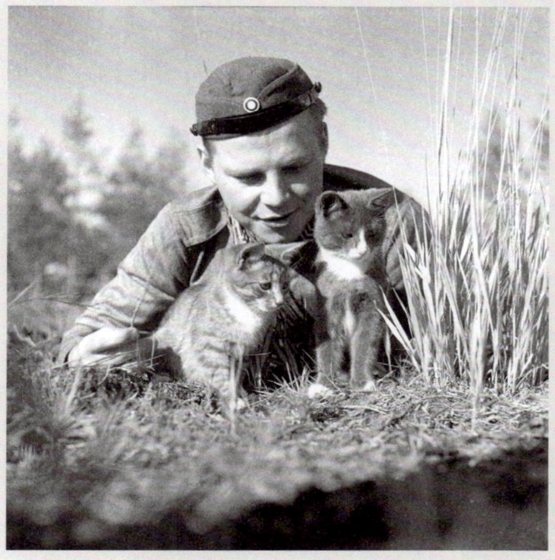

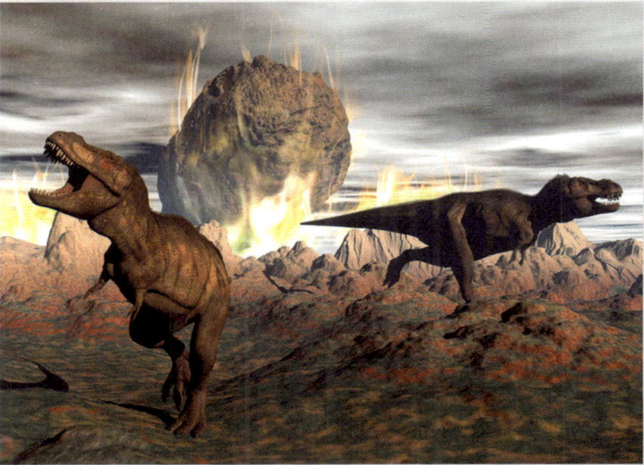

Author Bill Bryon, on the other hand, has attended numerous prize ceremonies. His bestselling *A Short History of Nearly Everything*, which sold millions of copies worldwide, won the 2004 Royal Society Aventis Prize and the European Union's 2005 Descartes Prize. In researching the Chicxulub meteorite (see Maria Golia's text in this issue), we came across some data in Bryson's book that made our eyes pop. Did you know, for instance, that the shockwave produced by such an object striking Earth would travel at "nearly the speed of light"? We hope not, because this figure is massively wrong. In fact, if an error this large were to hit Earth, there would be no crater; it would simply rip through the planet and keep going on its merry way. That is because this figure is fifty thousand times too high. When we called H. Jay Melosh, University Distinguished Professor of Earth Atmospheric and Planetary Sciences at Purdue University and author of many articles modeling meteor impacts, to ask him about this extraordinary number, he informed us that the shockwave would travel at roughly six kilometers per second. He was also generous enough with his time to correct a number of other assertions in Bryson's account of the Chicxulub impact event. Some awards are easier to get than others, it would seem.

Speaking of large objects in outer space, when does a satellite become large enough to effectively function as a building? This question came up when we were editing William Firebrace's essay in this issue. In print, the names of satellites—like all vessels'—should be italicized, per *The Chicago Manual of Style*. But the International Space Station looked very awkward to our eyes when it was rendered as the *International Space Station*, so we turned to the Arbiters of Style in Chicago. We are reproducing here our correspondence with them:

```
From: Cabinet <info@cabinetmagazine.org>
Date: Monday, 22 June 2015
To: The Chicago Manual of Style
```

```
We are currently editing a text that includes a
number of satellite names. We have italicized Vostok,
etc., per Chicago section 8.115. But we now have a
sentence that refers to the space stations Mir and
International Space Station. Our feeling is that Mir
should be italicized and International Space Station
should not, but we can't defend this since they are
both proper names referring to the same exact kind
of object (i.e.; a satellite, albeit one that is very
large and can have multiple people living on it).
Are these two to be treated the same as regular
satellite names (e.g., Sputnik) and italicized?
The fact that International Space Station is also
functioning as a descriptor of the object makes it
especially awkward-looking in italics. Any help
would be greatly appreciated.
```

```
From: The Chicago Manual of Style <chicagomanual@
press.uchicago.edu>
Date: Tuesday, 23 Jun 2015
To: Cabinet
```

```
Since Mir and ISS are the same kind of object, they
should be treated in the same way. It's an editorial
decision, but they seem more like the names of
buildings or communities or even projects than ships
or vessels, and can therefore justifiably remain in
caps only without further treatment.
```

```
All the best,
Staff
```

We appreciate the clarification but now live in dread of receiving an excellent text on, say, the history of the USS *Intrepid* and its transition from being an active ship in the US Navy to becoming the Intrepid Sea, Air & Space Museum. Here is the kind of nightmarish italics scenario that such a text might put on our plate: "When the *Intrepid* was originally commissioned, no one imagined that it would one day become the Intrepid, a museum docked on the west side of Manhattan showcasing, among other things, the history of the *Intrepid*'s war service and its transformation into the Intrepid."

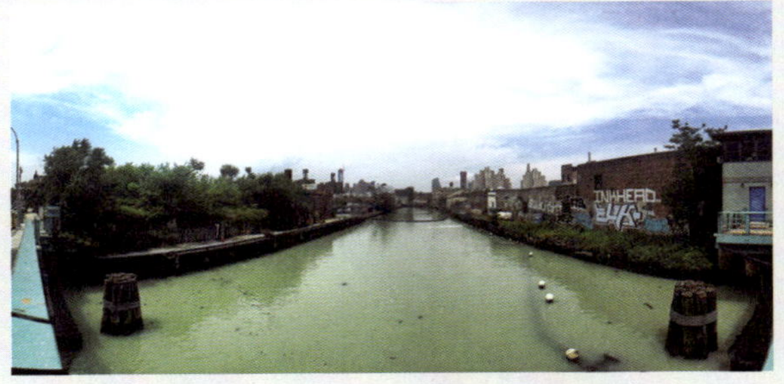

We've always loved scratch-and-sniff films, where cinemagoers are given cards impregnated with various scents and asked during the film to release the appropriate odor for a given scene. The characters are eating pizza, say, and the cinema can be made to smell like a pizza parlor. While editing Stassa Edwards's essay on the Great Stink of 1858, when the funk of London's Thames finally overwhelmed the population, we were greatly helped by the matching olfactory ambience of our office, courtesy of a summer-warmed Gowanus Canal.

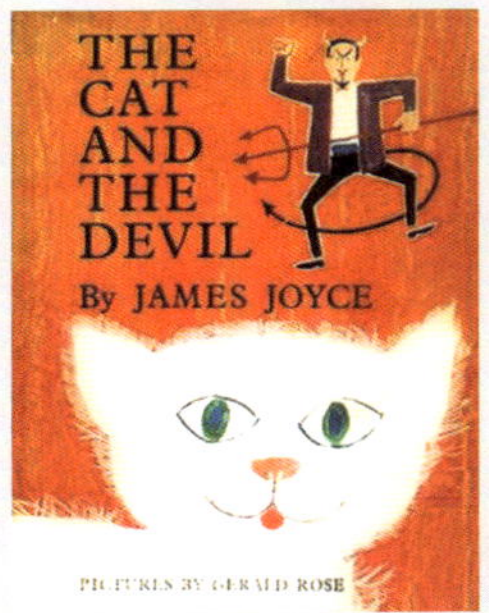

The Walter Benjamin text in this issue was hard to choose. He created many excellent radio broadcasts for children, and so many of them focused on terrible disasters! But reading Benjamin also reminded us of a time when intellectual giants did not think it beneath them to write books for children—Oscar Wilde, Daniil Kharms, Gertrude Stein, James Joyce, Langston Hughes, T. S. Eliot, Leo Tolstoy, and Ludwig Wittgenstein are only a few of the names to be added to Benjamin's. We can't vouch that all of them wrote great books, but it would be wonderful if someone revived the tradition, or at least sent us an essay on why it withered.

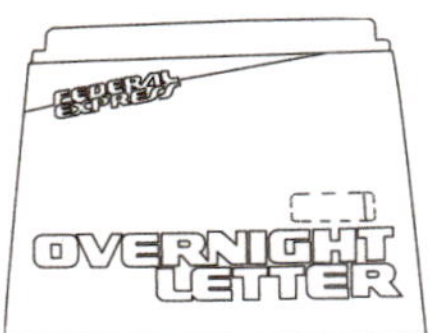

ARCHAEOLOGY OF THE DIGITAL
01

PETER EISENMAN: BIOZENTRUM

< >

cca.qc.ca/epub

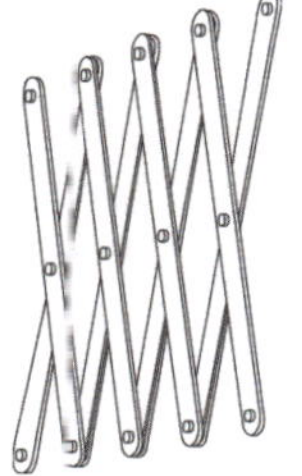

ARCHAEOLOGY OF THE DIGITAL
02

CHUCK HOBERMAN: EXPANDING SPHERE / IRIS DOME

◀ ▶

cca.qc.ca/epub

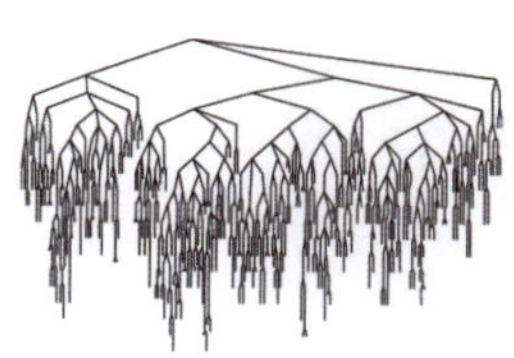

ARCHAEOLOGY OF THE DIGITAL
03

SHOEI YOH: SPORTS COMPLEX, GALAXY TOYAMA / ODAWARA GYMNASIUM

◁ ▷

cca.qc.ca/epub

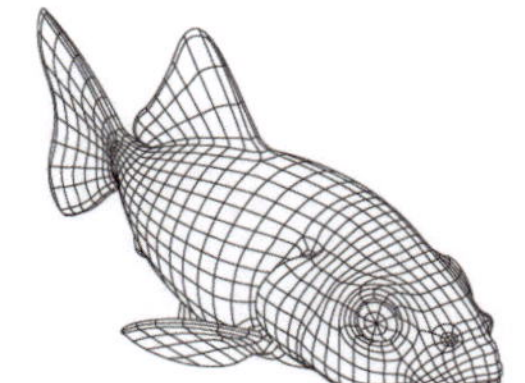

ARCHAEOLOGY OF THE DIGITAL
04

FRANK GEHRY: LEWIS RESIDENCE

< >

cca.qc.ca/epub

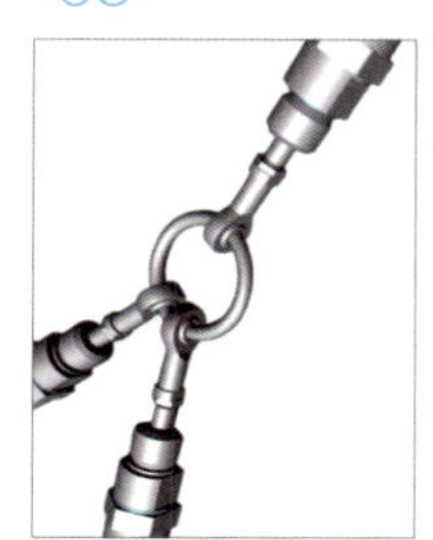

ARCHAEOLOGY OF THE DIGITAL
05

KAS OOSTERHUIS: NSA MUSCLE

← →

cca.qc.ca/epub

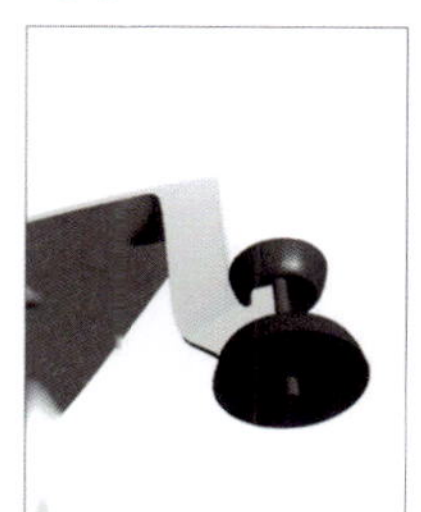

ARCHAEOLOGY OF THE DIGITAL
06

MARK GOULTHORPE: HYPOSURFACE

⟵ ⟶

cca.qc.ca/epub

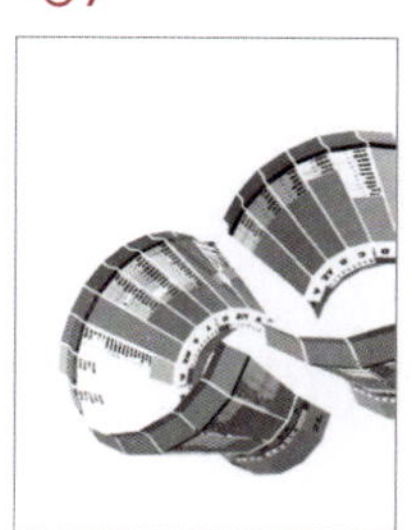

ARCHAEOLOGY OF THE DIGITAL
07

ASYMPTOTE ARCHITECTURE: NYSE VIRTUAL TRADING FLOOR

◁ ▷

cca.qc.ca/epub

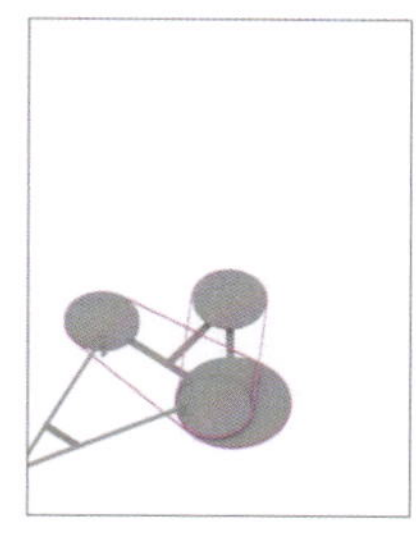

ARCHAEOLOGY OF THE DIGITAL
08

KARL CHU: X PHYLUM / CATASTROPHE MACHINE

← →

cca.qc.ca/epub

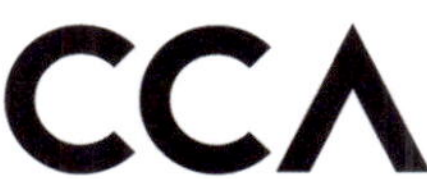

Centre Canadien d'Architecture
Canadian Centre for Architecture

Archaeology of the Digital is an ongoing research project at the Canadian Centre for Architecture that investigates early uses of computers in architecture. This project has raised many questions about the mpact of these tools on the conceptualization, visualization, and production of architecture. It has also led to questions about the output of the CCA itself, in particular the publications that accompany this project. The series of reflowable, dynamic digital publications – edited by Greg Lynn and designed by New York studio Linked by Air, provides new ways of reading architectural processes. These bookmarks are physical links to our latest phase of digital production. Please cut and mark.

e-flux

CONTEMPORARY ART

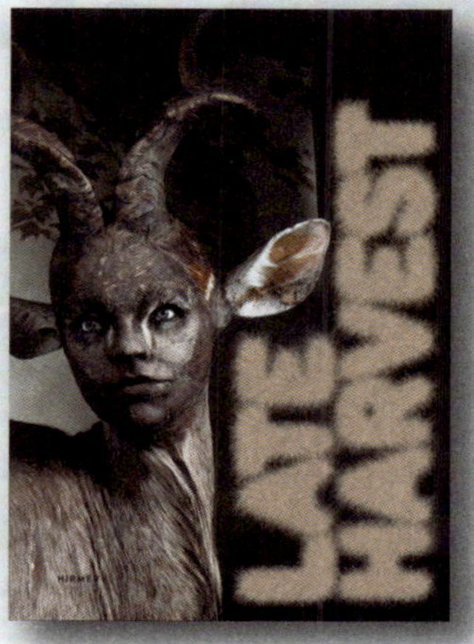

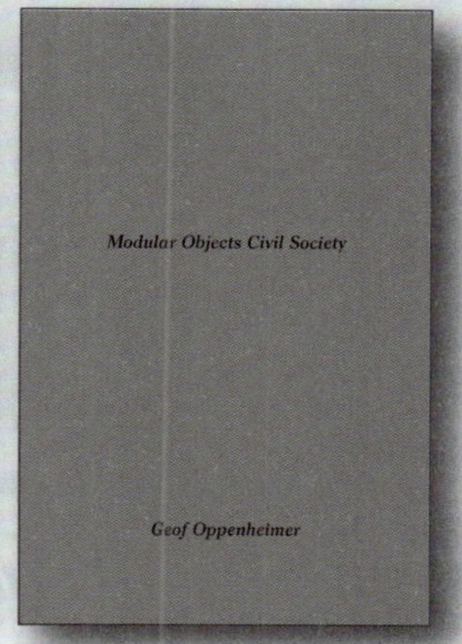

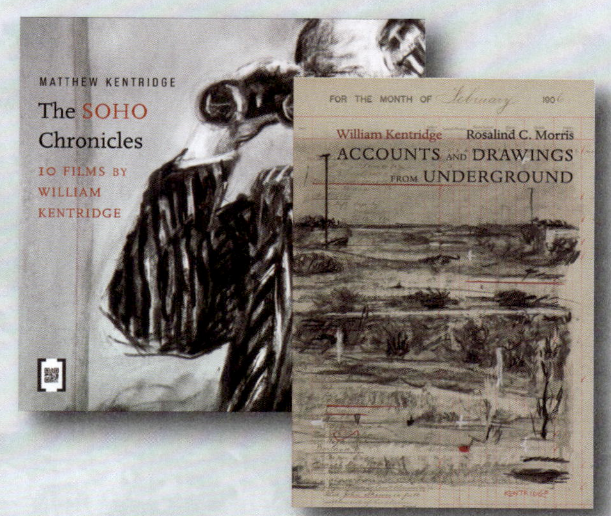

From Hirmer Publishers
LATE HARVEST

HIRMER

Edited by JoAnne Northrup

Late Harvest juxtaposes contemporary art created with taxidermy with historically significant wildlife paintings. The result highlights intriguing parallels and startling aesthetic contrasts while simultaneously confirming and subverting viewers' preconception of the place of animals in culture.

192 p., 107 color plates
Cloth $45.00

From WhiteWalls

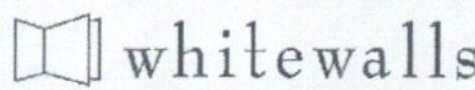 whitewalls

MODULAR OBJECTS CIVIL SOCIETY

Geof Oppenheimer

At its heart, *Modular Objects Civil Society* is a reflection on the performance of living, asking how we move, act, and create meaning within a world of objects—and how those objects accrue value in relation to one another.

152 p., 143 halftones
Cloth $25.00

WILLIAM KENTRIDGE

From Seagull Books
THE SOHO CHRONICLES

Seagull BOOKS

10 Films by William Kentridge

Matthew Kentridge

The Soho Chronicles tells the story of artist William Kentridge's alter ego, Soho Eckstein, through stories and illustrations. Throughout, Matthew Kentridge reflects on his brother's artistic process and his life.

438 p., illustrated in color throughout
Cloth $150.00

ACCOUNTS AND DRAWINGS FROM UNDERGROUND

The East Rand Proprietary Mines Cash Book, 1906

William Kentridge and Rosalind C. Morris

This collaboration between William Kentridge and Rosalind C. Morris uses the 1906 Cash Book of the East Rand Proprietary Mines Corporation to create art reflecting on labor, capital, and environmental devastation.

196 p., 61 color plates
Cloth $100.00

DISTRIBUTED BY THE UNIVERSITY OF CHICAGO PRESS   www.press.uchicago.edu

HOW TO ORDER

1. Mail a check to Cabinet, 181 Wyckoff Street, Brooklyn, NY 11217, USA.
2. Shop online at <cabinetmagazine.org/shop>.
3. Call +1 718 222 8434.
4. Fax +1 718 222 3700.

Checks, made out to "Cabinet," must be in USD and drawn on a US bank. We also accept Visa, MC, AmEx, Discover, and Paypal (paypal@cabinetmagazine.org). Prices valid till 1 December 2015. Visit <cabinetmagazine.org> to view our limited and unlimited editions, posters, and other tchotchkes.

CABINET BOOKS
Prices include postage.

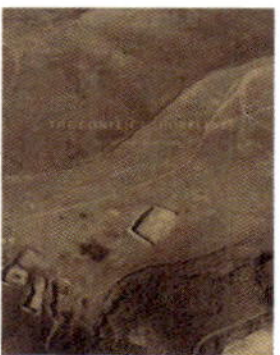

The Conflict Shoreline:
Colonialism as Climate Change
Eyal Weizman's analysis of climate change as a political tool used to displace the Bedouins in the Negev Desert.
US $33
Elsewhere $40
(Subscriber discount: -$7)

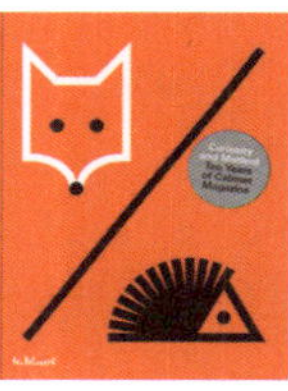

Curiosity and Method:
Ten Years of Cabinet Magazine
An encyclopedia with entries culled from the first ten years of Cabinet.

US $41
Canada & Europe $57
Elsewhere $63
(Subscriber discount: -$5)

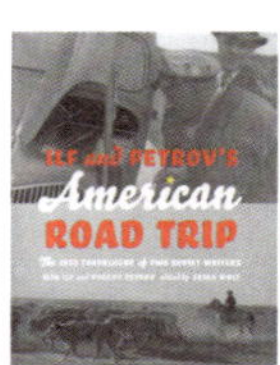

Ilf and Petrov's American Road Trip
The 1935 travelogue of two Soviet writers journeying through America.

US $24
Elsewhere $30
(Subscriber discount: -$7)

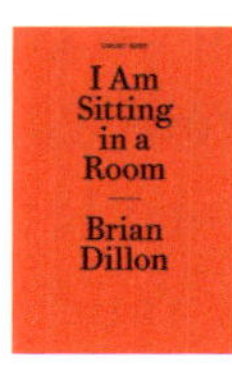

I Am Sitting in a Room
Inaugural volume, by Brian Dillon, in Cabinet's "24-Hour Book" series.

US $15
Canada $16
Elsewhere $20
(Subscriber discount: -$2)

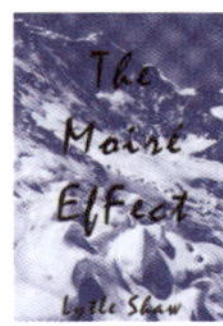

The Moiré Effect
Lytle Shaw tracks Ernst Moiré from his humble Alpine beginnings to his fateful founding of a Zurich photography studio.

US $15
Canada $16
Elsewhere $19
(Subscriber discount: -$2)

CABINET BACK ISSUES

Available back issues (pictured below) are $10 each plus postage. Postage rates: US $2 per issue; Elsewhere $7 per issue, $17 for 3 issues.

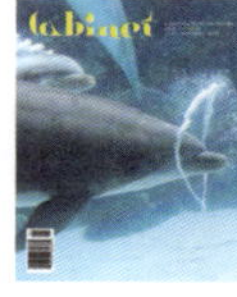
Issue 37
Bubbles

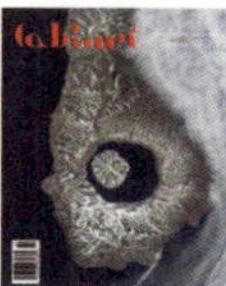
Issue 38
Islands

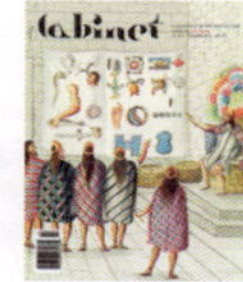
Issue 39
Learning

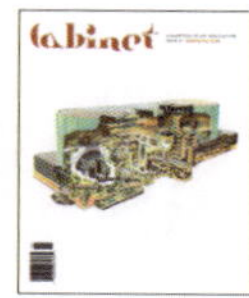
Issue 41
Infrastructure

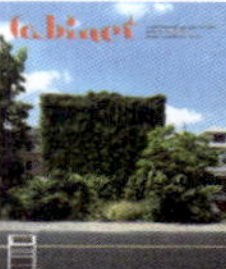
Issue 42
Forgetting

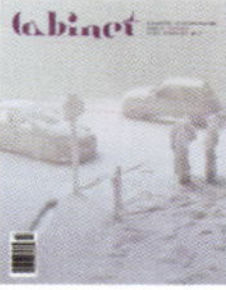
Issue 43
Forensics

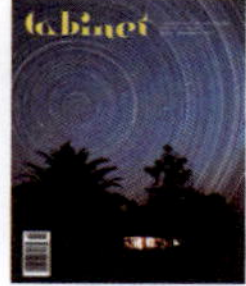
Issue 44
24 Hours

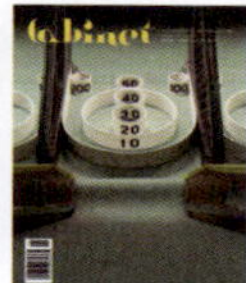
Issue 45
Games

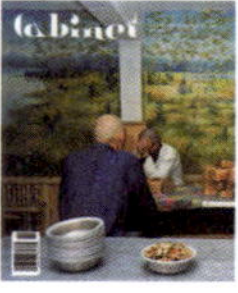
Issue 46
Punishment

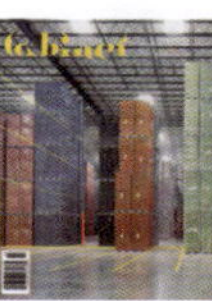
Issue 47
Logistics

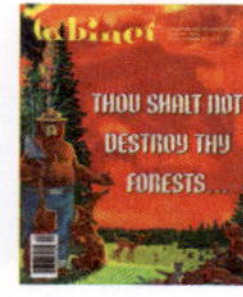
Issue 48
Trees

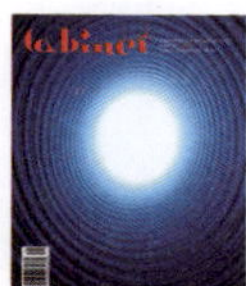
Issue 49
Death

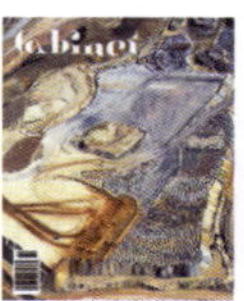
Issue 50
Money

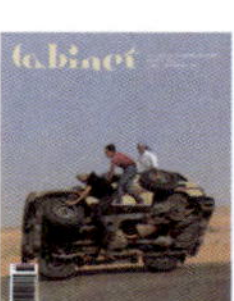
Issue 51
Wheels

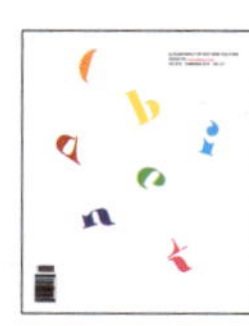
Issue 52
Celebration

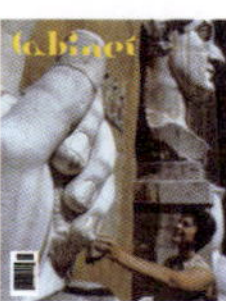
Issue 53
Stones

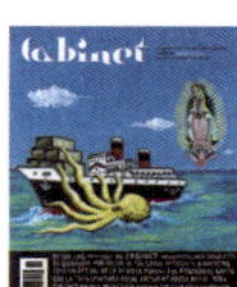
Issue 54
The Accident

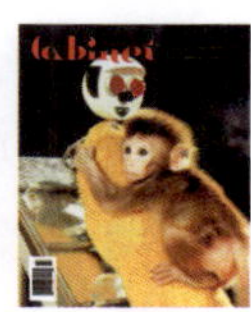
Issue 55
Love

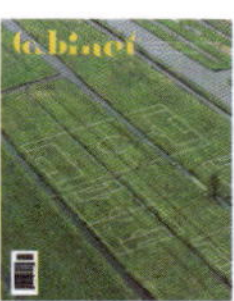
Issue 56
Sports

CABINET
300 Nevins Street
Brooklyn, NY 11217 USA
phone + 1 718 222-8434
fax + 1 718 222-3700
info@cabinetmagazine.org
www.cabinetmagazine.org

Issue 62, Fall 2016–Winter 2017

Cover: Still from Jeremy Everett, *Floy*, 2015.

Cabinet (ISSN 1531-1430, USPS # 020-348) is a quarterly magazine published by Immaterial Incorporated, 181 Wyckoff Street, Brooklyn, NY 11217. Periodicals Postage paid at Brooklyn, NY, and additional mailing offices.

POSTMASTER: Please send address changes to Cabinet, 300 Nevins Street, Brooklyn, NY 11217.

Printed in Belgium by Die Keure, who are the *crème de la crème*.

ADVERTISING
phone + 1 718 222-8434
advertising@cabinetmagazine.org

DISTRIBUTION
Cabinet is available in the US and Canada through Disticor, which distributes both using its own network and through Ingram, Ubiquity, Small Changes, Cowley Distribution, Kent News, MSolutions, the News Group, Chris Stadler, and Don Olson Distribution.

To carry Cabinet through one of these distributors, contact Melanie Raucci at Disticor: phone + 1 631 587-1160, mraucci@disticor.com

Cabinet is available in Europe and elsewhere through Central Books, London: orders@centralbooks.com

Cabinet is available worldwide as a book, with an ISBN, through DAP: phone + 1 212 627-1999, dap@dapinc.com

For further information, contact: circulation@cabinetmagazine.org

INDIVIDUAL SUBSCRIPTIONS

1 year (4 issues):	2 years (8 issues):
US $32	US $60
Canada $38	Canada $72
Western Europe $40	Western Europe $76
Elsewhere $50	Elsewhere $96

Please send a check in US dollars made out to "Cabinet," or mail, fax, or email us your Visa/MC/AmEx/Discover info to:

300 Nevins Street
Brooklyn, NY 11217 USA
phone + 1 718 222-8434
fax + 1 718 222-3700
subscriptions@cabinetmagazine.org
www.cabinetmagazine.org/subscribe

INSTITUTIONAL SUBSCRIPTIONS
Institutional subscriptions are available through library agencies such as EBSCO, or directly from Cabinet:
www.cabinetmagazine.org/subscribe

SUBMISSIONS
We only accept submissions via email. Guidelines available at:
www.cabinetmagazine.org/information/submissions.php

Editor-in-chief
Sina Najafi

Senior editor
Jeffrey Kastner

Editors
D. Graham Burnett, Christopher Turner

UK editor
Brian Dillon

Associate director
Kelley Deane McKinney

Art director
Everything Studio

Associate editor
Julian Lucas

Editorial assistant
Evdoxia Ragkou

Website directors
Ryan O'Toole, Luke Murphy

Editors-at-large
Saul Anton, Sasha Archibald, Mats Bigert, Brian Conley, Christoph Cox, Jeff Dolven, Leland de la Durantaye, Jesse Lerner, Jennifer Liese, Ryo Manabe, Alexander Nagel, Sally O'Reilly, George Prochnik, Frances Richard, Daniel Rosenberg, Aaron Schuster, David Serlin, Debra Singer, Justin E. H. Smith, Margaret Sundell, Allen S. Weiss, Eyal Weizman, Margaret Wertheim, Gregory Williams, Jay Worthington, Tirdad Zolghadr

Contributing editors
Molly Blieden, Eric Bunge, Pip Day, Charles Green, Adam Jasper, Srdjan Jovanovic Weiss, Lytle Shaw, Cecilia Sjöholm, Carl Michael von Hausswolff, Sven-Olov Wallenstein

Events
Bryony Quinn (London)

Cabinet national librarian
Matthew Passmore

Cabinet is a non-profit 501(c)(3) magazine published by Immaterial Incorporated. Our survival depends on support from generous foundations and individuals. Please consider supporting us at whatever level you can. Donations are tax-deductible for those who deal with Uncle Sam. All gifts are acknowledged online. Contributions of $25 or more will be acknowledged in the next possible issue; those above $100 will be noted in four issues. Checks to "Cabinet" can be sent to our office; please write "Say cheese" on the envelope.

Cabinet wishes to thank the following visionary foundations and individuals for their support of our activities during 2017. Additionally, we will forever be indebted to the extraordinary contribution of the Flora Family Foundation from 1999 to 2004; without their support, this publication would not exist. We would also like to extend our enormous gratitude to the Orphiflamme Foundation and the Opaline Fund for their generous support.

$100,000
The Lambent Foundation

$50,000
The Warhol Foundation for Visual Arts

$15,000
The New York City Department of Cultural Affairs

$10,000
The National Endowment for the Arts

$8,000
The New York State Council on the Arts

$6,000
Margaret Sundell & Reinaldo Laddaga

$3,000
The Danielson Foundation

$1,500–$2,500
Stina & Herant Katchadourian, Steven Rand & Nancy Wender, Terry Winters

$501–$1,000
Anonymous, Martha & Thomas G. Armstrong, Sara Clugage, Spencer Finch, Christian Scheidemann, Sandy Tait & Hal Foster, Edward C. Wilson and Hesu Coue Wilson Family Fund

$500 or under
Pamela Cederquist, David Hariton & Tod Lippy, Steven Igou, Lenore & Richard Niles, Debra Singer & Jay Worthington

$250 or under
Tauba Auerbach, Jeff Beall, Mia Enell & Nicholas Fries, George Ganat, Alex Goodfriend, Cynthia Hansen, Peter Hapstak, Peter Jaszi, Craig Kalpakjian, James Katzenberger, Carin Kuoni & John Oakes, Scott LeBouef, Deborah Lovely, Meredith Martin & Joshua Siegel, Paul McConnell, Helen Mirra, Jason Olin, Andrew Pederson, Jocelyn Price & Christopher Leone, John Sargent, Eric Schmid, Pooja Shah & Rebecca Ward, John Sherburne, James Siena, Jude Tallichet & Matt Freedman, Volker Welter, Margaret Wertheim

$100 or under
David Brynan, Peter Cohen, Avril Danczak, Øyvind Osmo Eriksen, Elizabeth Esch, Samuel Gaty, Cat Ingrams, Jen Knuth & Greg Tucker, Aden Kumler, Rupert Maitland, Jim Martin, Lewis Nicholson, Paul Cameron Opperman, Amy Jean Porter, Kaye Reeves, Hanneline Rogeberg, Sarah Rudledge, David Sckrabulis, Rick Skibinski, Jeannie Weissglass, Lucas van der Velden

CONTRIBUTORS

Mats Bigert is one half of Bigert & Bergström, an artist and filmmaker duo based in Stockholm. On the occasion of the thirtieth anniversary of their collaboration, Art & Theory Publishing is releasing a book about their work later in 2017. They are currently the subject of a survey exhibition at the Shanghai Minsheng Art Museum that will travel later this year to Artipelag, Stockholm.

D. Graham Burnett is an editor of *Cabinet* and teaches at Princeton University. Recent collaborative work includes "The Oannes Scrap," presented by TBA21 at the Kochi Biennial in December 2016. He is affiliated with the collective ESTAR(SER). For more information, visit <estarser.net>.

Alice Butler is a writer based in London. Her work has been published widely in art and culture magazines, including *Frieze*, *Art Monthly*, and *Cabinet*, and in June 2016, she contributed a chapbook project to the Whitstable Biennale in Kent, UK. She is currently working toward a PhD in the department of Art History and Visual Studies at the University of Manchester, with a thesis provisionally titled "Close Writing: The Personal Performances of Kathy Acker and Cookie Mueller."

Eduardo Cadava teaches at Princeton University. He is the author of *Words of Light: Theses on the Photography of History* (Princeton University Press, 1997) and *Emerson and the Climates of History* (Stanford University Press, 1997). He has also coedited *Who Comes After the Subject?* (Routledge, 1991); *Cities Without Citizens* (Slought Foundation, 2003); a special 2004 issue of *South Atlantic Quarterly* entitled "And Justice for All?: The Claims of Human Rights"; and *The Itinerant Languages of Photography* (Yale University Press, 2013). His book *Paper Graveyards: Essays on Art and Photography* is forthcoming from Princeton University Press.

Brian Dillon is UK editor of *Cabinet*, and teaches critical writing at the Royal College of Art, London. His books include *The Great Explosion* (Penguin Books, 2015), *Objects in This Mirror: Essays* (Sternberg Press, 2014), *I Am Sitting in a Room* (Cabinet Books, 2012), and *The Hypochondriacs* (Faber & Faber, 2010). He writes regularly for *Artforum*, *Frieze*, the *Guardian*, and the *London Review of Books*. He is working on a book about essays and essayists.

Jeff Dolven teaches poetry and poetics, especially of the English Renaissance, at Princeton University. A new book of criticism, *Senses of Style*, is forthcoming in late 2017 from the University of Chicago Press.

Jeremy Everett is an American artist based in Paris and Los Angeles. He received his MA from the Institute without Boundaries in 2009. For his work *Floy* (2014), a still from which is featured on the cover of this issue, he arranged for a truck full of milk to flip over on a US highway. His new book, as yet untitled, will be released later this year by Idea.

Marta Figlerowicz teaches literature, film, and critical theory at Yale University. She is the author of *Flat Protagonists* (Oxford University Press, 2016) and *Spaces of Feeling* (Cornell University Press, 2017, forthcoming), and is currently working on a new project about myth and fantasy in the digital age.

Allen Ginsberg (1926–1997) was an American poet and author.

Melanie Jackson is an artist working with writing, moving image, and sculpture. She is based in London and represented by Matt's Gallery. Recent solo exhibitions in London include "The Urpflanze (Part 1)" and "The Urpflanze (Part 2)" at Drawing Room and Flat Time House, respectively. This article is part of a collaboration with Esther Leslie, and is an extract from their forthcoming book *Deeper in the Pyramid*, which will be launched at their exhibition of the same name at Grand Union, Birmingham, in spring 2018.

Esther Leslie is professor of political aesthetics at Birkbeck, University of London. Her books include *Hollywood Flatlands: Animation, Critical Theory and the Avant-Garde* (Verso, 2002); *Synthetic Worlds: Nature, Art and the Chemical Industry* (Reaktion Books, 2005); *Derelicts: Thought Worms from the Wreckage* (Unkant, 2014); and *Liquid Crystals: The Science and Art of a Fluid Form* (Reaktion Books, 2016).

S. Billie Mandle is an artist living in western Massachusetts, where she is an assistant professor at Hampshire College.

Sally O'Reilly is a UK-based writer. Her recent projects include the novel *Crude* (Eros Press, 2016), and the libretto for the opera *The Virtues of Things* (co-commissioned by the Royal Opera, Aldeburgh Music, and Opera North, 2015). In 2016, she had a year-long writing residency at Modern Art Oxford.

George Prochnik is a Brooklyn-based author. His most recent book is *Stranger in a Strange Land: Searching for Gershom Scholem and Jerusalem* (Other Press, 2017). He has written for the *New York Times*, the *New Yorker*, *Bookforum*, and the *Los Angeles Review of Books*.

Xenia Vytuleva is an art historian, theorist, and curator. Her scholarship focuses on new modes of preservation and on the intersection of architecture and politics. Until recently, she taught at the Graduate School of Architecture, Planning and Preservation at Columbia University.

Will Wiles is an architecture and design journalist based in London. He is the author two novels: *Care of Wooden Floors* (Little A/New Harvest, 2012) and *The Way Inn* (Harper Perennial, 2014). A third novel is forthcoming from Fourth Estate.

Annie Julia Wyman is a screenwriter, essayist, and doctoral candidate at Harvard University. She is the co-translator of Giorgio Agamben's *Unspeakable Girl* (Seagull Books, 2012) and the editor of *Book Stories* (McSweeney's, 2014). Her most recent academic work was presented at a 2017 conference in Dehradun, India, titled "Materialities: Objects, Matter, Things" and co-organized by the Forum on Contemporary Theory in Baroda and the Department of English at Doon University.

AF328623

COLUMNS

COLUMNS

COLORS / MOUNTBATTEN PINK
Annie Julia Wyman

"Colors" is a column in which a writer responds to a specific color assigned by the editors of Cabinet.

———

All stories, even stranger ones, must begin with a unifying thread. The camera must focus; one must establish some central fact or tone. Say, for instance, that the man whom this story treats lived and died in an effervescence of letters that might strike the ordinary mortal as absurd. He was Louis Francis Albert Victor Nicholas Mountbatten, born Seine Durchlaucht Prinz Ludwig von Battenberg: His Serene Highness Prince Louis of B. And he was further called, once he was done growing up—and once World War I had convinced his mostly German family to alter that "Battenberg" slightly, so that they came off as more convincingly English—he was further called Admiral of the Fleet The Right Honourable The Earl Mountbatten of Burma, KG, PC, GCB, OM, GCSI, GCIE, GCVO, DSO. In that order.

Visualize, if you will, all these letters scrolling over black while the voice-over informs us that "The Earl of Mountbatten went by *Dickie*." Zoom in on one of his official portraits—the blush in a cheek so narrow, next to a nose so low and long—and you know you are dealing with the very pink of inbreeding. To be called Dickie, we might feel, would be below the dignity of a person otherwise knit into every royal family, not just in England but on the Continent.

Nonetheless "Dickie" was what you called this dazzlingly be-monikered person if, like him, you had a certain number of ruffles in your collar and pins on your lapels and kinks in your DNA and baffling acronyms

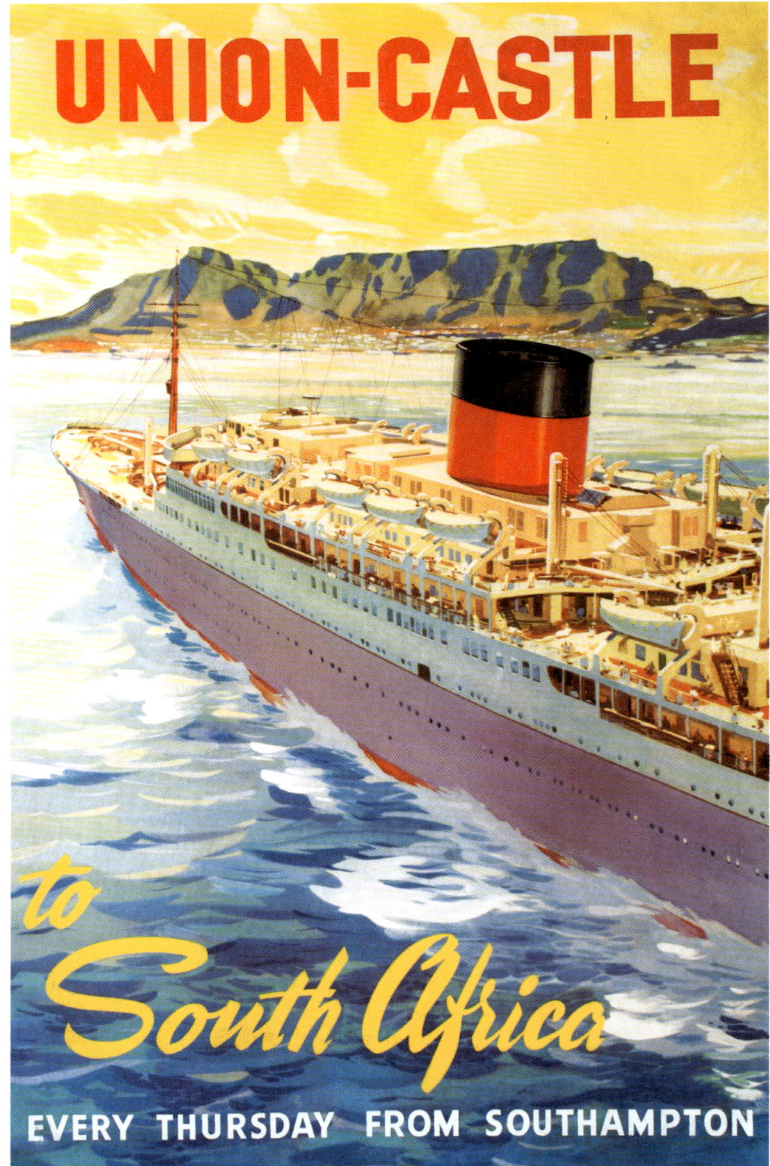

Louis Mountbatten's inspiration. Poster for Union-Castle Line, ca. 1948.

bringing up your nomenclatural train—that is, if you could get close enough to address an actual Mountbatten. Dickie's nephew, Philip, Prince of Greece and Denmark, married Queen Elizabeth II, if that tells you anything about what a Mountbatten is. Dickie's own maternal great-grandmother was Queen Victoria, she who was called Empress of India.

And indeed it was Victoria who had first suggested "Nicky" for this the umpteenth of her many great-grand-progeny. (She had nine children, forty grandchildren, and eighty-three great-grandchildren; "Grandmother of Europe" was one of her own unofficial identifiers.) But there were already too many Nickys in her clan, Czar Nicholas II of Russia among them. So: "Dickie," so as not to confound the Ruskies.

Dickie attended a fancy school: slow pan across rows of boys in

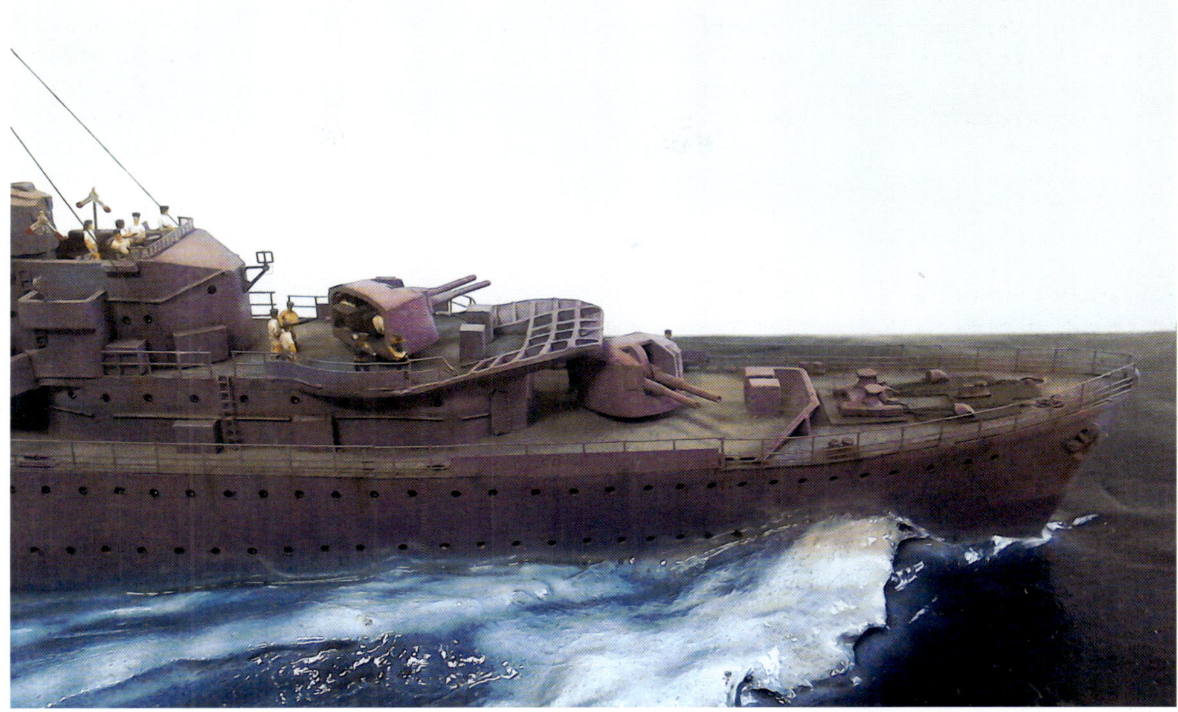

Model of *HMS Kelly*, a World War II Royal Navy "⟨" class destroyer that was painted the strategic shade of pink when under Mountbatten's command. The ship is shown here as it appeared in May 1941. Model and photo Ian Ruscoe.

chapel, poking each other, whispering, sneaking cookies out of their pockets. They head out into the yard, scraps of paper on which they've doodled "DICKIE MOUNTBATTEN IS A TOSSER" blowing around their ankles. At fourteen, he was sent to a fancy naval academy. And soon afterward, War. And then another War after that. For various forms of derring-do, Dickie was covered in decorations and put in charge of the entire British fleet. For this, he was given his most important and most evocative title: First Sea Lord.

Pause, then. And introduce a certain amount of retrospective explication. Put the slight brakes on our barreling narrative. Perhaps a professor, in a tweed coat, poses artfully in front of a PowerPoint. Are we surprised that a man of this titular magnitude, from a family of Germans disguised to seem English, would be interested in detection, and in camouflage, in acts of distinguishing

and the panic of being distinguished? War came, and with it more questions about who fits in, and who doesn't. Along what lines of language and violence and fantasy were these deceptions undertaken?

Well, Dickie had a whole lot of ideas. He got himself a patent for a sensor system allowing ships to remain stationary relative to one another. He supported plans for an enormous aircraft carrier made of ice (never built; cost far too much money). But it was ship camouflage that drew his most intent interest. Not the striped dazzle patterns that turned ships into eye-baffling arrays of cubism. In 1940, the 5th Destroyer Flotilla, under Dickie's command, was escorting a group of civilian ships that had been pressed into service as naval vessels when he apparently saw one of them, a Union-Castle ocean liner—*Travel the Big Ship Way! 14 Days to South Africa!*—still painted in the firm's characteristic

pink tones disappear into the dusk. And so he had all of the boats under his command painted what came to be called Mountbatten Pink, which was in fact a dusky rose. The protected lent its cloak to its protectors, you might say.

Dickie must have watched his first pink ship disappear against the horizon and felt some exhilaration. Though someone less credulous might have seen the pink persist against the sky and felt bad for Dickie. Someone might have said, without meaning it, "Well done, sah." Close on the face of another sailor, less of a bootlicker, standing behind the first one and rolling his eyes. And maybe we see the same two chatter over tinned fish or cocoa or bangers in the mess.

"It's called the Purkinje Effect."
"The what?"
"The Purkinje Effect."
Sarcastically: "Oh, to be sure."
"Something to do with reds and

pinks being less visible at night than some other colors. Never mind that in daylight, reddish colors appear brighter than any other kind of color."

"Well, as long he's happy."

And both men sigh.

A fantastical person, Dickie Mountbatten, and fantastically convinced that his undertaking was based on scientific fact. What a Victorian, says the professor, smiling with delight, and cites the *OED* entry for *pink*. A flower, in fact, much older than Victoria: dianthus. And bounteous in namesakes: the flower gives us the color. And for its tattery petals, *pink* also means a series of perforations or cuts, a zigzag, a path of escape. Pink, a color for little girls, originally a color for little boys, a color for Christ, specifically—see, in Raphael's *Madonna of the Pinks*, the Christ-child offer the viewer the little dianthus in his fat baby hand. See two museum-goers in the National Gallery stroll away from the *Madonna of the Pinks*. One mutters: "Raphael was better at blues." Imagine Raphael, rolling in his grave.

There is a city in India painted pink. Jaipur, in Rajasthan, has nothing to do with Dickie Mountbatten, but then again one story, widespread but apocryphal, claims that it does. According to the legend, Maharaja Ram Singh II, ruler of Jaipur, did up the whole burg in the color because he wanted to impress Dickie's great-uncle, the Prince of Wales, on his 1876 visit. Pink, the color of terracotta, the color of Hindu wedding turbans, the color of hospitality. One hopes Dickie saw it, since when he went to India in 1947, the Indians were on the verge of kicking the British out.

Some called him the Man who Gave Away India, as if it were a substance. Churchill was pissed. But as India's last viceroy and first governor-general, Dickie oversaw the hand-off to Gandhi and Jinnah, that was all, and he may have prevented civil war—though he certainly bears

some responsibility for the tens of thousands of people who have been killed in Kashmir. A trifle unclear, really, how history works (except that those to whom evil is done, as the poet wrote, sometimes do evil in return). Dickie brought along his wife, Edwina, who was by no means as noble as he but just as fun. Her long affair with Jawaharlal Nehru passed many a bright New Delhi hour. Pink was the color of the exotic, and of seduction, though mainly for whiter kinds of people—pink, the color of parts unseen.

Meanwhile, the world spun on. Empires fell. Victory in those two Wars—but at the same time, Britain was mastering the art of losing generally; reality was beginning to shiver, to edge away. The Heisenberg Principle; Schrödinger's animal. The liquidation of a hundred thousand people at Hiroshima. Atomic energy, the space race: cue a supercut montage of every stupid public safety video the baby boomers were shown in school. By the 1970s, it was hard to say whether that cat had ever been in the box, much less whether it was alive or dead. In the 1940s, the Philadelphia Experiment had purportedly made a ship invisible, sailors and all, though the experience of being made see-through had made them all seasick upon the ship's re-coalescence. One is said to have lost his hand, since it was reconstituted stuck inside the ship's hull. But this was a price that had to be paid (if it was paid at all). Postmodern forms of deception would have been unrecognizable to a man like Lord Mountbatten. The invention of radar had made all ship's camouflage short of phase change, or maybe interdimensional slippage, irrelevant.

In the meantime, Dickie served as admiral of this, and admiral of that. Admiral for NATO in the Mediterranean, perhaps most importantly. Dickie went to America, and tried to get Nixon to encourage Francisco Franco to hand over

power to his distant royal cousin Juan Carlos. Dickie went to the Soviet Union, and made an ass of himself by telling Stalin stories about his relatives in the Russian aristocracy (perhaps he related the "Nicky" anecdote). There are late photographs of Lord Mountbatten so covered in medals you can't see anything but his long horsey face. A public person now, thoroughly—and the subject of a rather tepid television miniseries—but did his public self conceal some other identity? There were rumors he was bisexual. There were rumors he was homosexual. Imagine, if you will, on or off camera, another sort of photograph, less public: Edward, Prince of Wales, squinting from a short distance at his longtime consort, the light bouncing up off the deckside pool he and Dickie swim in right into the prince's pale eyes.

No way to know, most unfortunately. But if there is not a thread, there is at least a quality: a color, a set of themes. If words are too much, and if stories fail—well. Even that is a predicament each of us will finally escape. In 1979, Lord Mountbatten, his grandson Nicholas, and two others were killed by the Irish Republican Army, which had placed a bomb in his fishing boat, *Shadow V*, in the waters off Mullaghmore, County Sligo, in Ireland. Gone—to put it briefly—in a flash. Oh, who knows how history works, and where we go, to what undiscovered country we retire when our mortal coils get blown off? We can say that the sun will surely rise again, after it sets on each one of us. We can say, in lieu of any sense of destination or ending, that Dickie Mountbatten was survived by that selfsame lady who will survive us all, the child of the morning, she whom the Greeks called Rosy-Fingered Dawn.

SENTENCES / HOW HOW HOW WHAT WHAT WHAT HOW—WHEN
Brian Dillon

"Sentences" is a column by Brian Dillon each installment of which examines the mechanics and style of a single sentence chosen by the author.

———

"Considering how common illness is, how tremendous the spiritual change that it brings, how astonishing, when the lights of health go down, the undiscovered countries that are then disclosed, what wastes and deserts of the soul a slight attack of influenza brings to light, what precipices and lawns sprinkled with bright flowers a little rise of temperature reveals, what ancient and obdurate oaks are uprooted in us in the act of sickness, how we go down into the pit of death and feel the waters of annihilation close above our heads and wake thinking to find ourselves in the presence of the angels and the harpers when we have a tooth out and come to the surface in the dentist's arm chair and confuse his 'Rinse the mouth—rinse the mouth' with the greeting of the Deity stooping from the floor of Heaven to welcome us—when we think of this and infinitely more, as we are so frequently forced to think of it, it becomes strange indeed that illness has not taken its place with love, battle, and jealousy among the prime themes of literature."
—Virginia Woolf

It may well be the sentence that for diverse reasons—because thinking about Woolf, or sickness, or essays, because trying to emulate a certain rhythm in my own writing—I've copied out by hand more than any other. Each time, I've marveled at the logic and ease and length (181 words) of the sentence, the hard clausal steps that slowly mount (or is it descend?) to a grammatically wrong-footing conclusion—the dash's flat fall where we might have expected a "then…" or "so.…" I have wondered about the oddity of Woolf's metaphors—the sentence is mostly made of metaphors—and their unabashed mixture: the lights go up, the lights go down, the patient rises and falls as though in a rickety old elevator, till at last the cage clatters open, slightly missing the floor one wanted. This is the first sentence of Woolf's 1926 essay "On Being Ill," and it's hard to think of a verbal array whose structure better mimics both its subject and the larger text of which it's part: precisely because, despite its exquisitely shaped adventure, the sentence finally fails to hold itself together.

Everything that rises must converge, or not. Seven times—four *hows* and three *whats*—the sentence invites us to anticipate a logically and artistically satisfying terminus. With the final *how* we may reasonably expect that the grammatical, argumentative, and symbolic denouement is just around the comma-swiveling corner. Instead, we embark on a mysterious paratactic excursion, with no punctuation and no hint, for what seems an age, that our destination is the dentist's chair: "we go down … and feel … and wake … and come to the surface … and confuse.…" Everything tends toward the sentence's second and final dash—the first dash, the dentist's, may as well be any instrument at all—and an abrupt meta-swerve: "—when we think of this.…" Do we, does even Woolf, really think of this? The sentence has allured us a long way, but I'm not certain I follow, not even sure what "this" consists of, never mind the "infinitely more."

Woolf was complexly unwell in the autumn of 1925, when T. S. Eliot asked if he might publish a piece of hers in the literary magazine *The Criterion*, which he had founded in 1922. (By the time Woolf's essay appeared, the journal had relaunched as *The New Criterion*.) The novelist was trying to start work on *To the Lighthouse*, but had been laid low by flu, headaches, and a vulturous pecking at the spine: this last, in a letter to her friend and lover Vita Sackville-West, is Woolf's way of describing her most recent mental and emotional breakdown. When she speaks in "On Being Ill" about "the act of illness" (how odd, to think of it as an act) and "the great experience," when she imagines the moment when "we cease to be soldiers in the army of the upright," one may assume she has more vicious symptoms in mind than feebling coughs and sniffles. The essay is a lurid reflection on the uses of melancholy, the limits of sympathy, and the triumph of death.

You can hear in the delaying rhythms of the opening sentence the influence of Marcel Proust and the digressive, paid-by-the-word style of Thomas De Quincey, whose essays Woolf had lately looked into for the first time. The asthmatic novelist and the opium-eating essayist are among the very few writers in whom, she tells us on the first page, we will find the subject of illness authoritatively or even adequately treated—"literature does its best to maintain that its concern is with the mind; that the body is a sheet of plain glass through which the soul looks straight and clear, and, save for one or two passions such as desire and greed, is null, negligible and nonexistent." We lack a language to capture "this monster, the body, this miracle, its pain," and if we tried to coin new words for the shiver and the headache, taking "pain in one hand and a lump of sound in the other," the result would likely be laughable. Only poets come close. So what would a prose literature devoted to illness sound

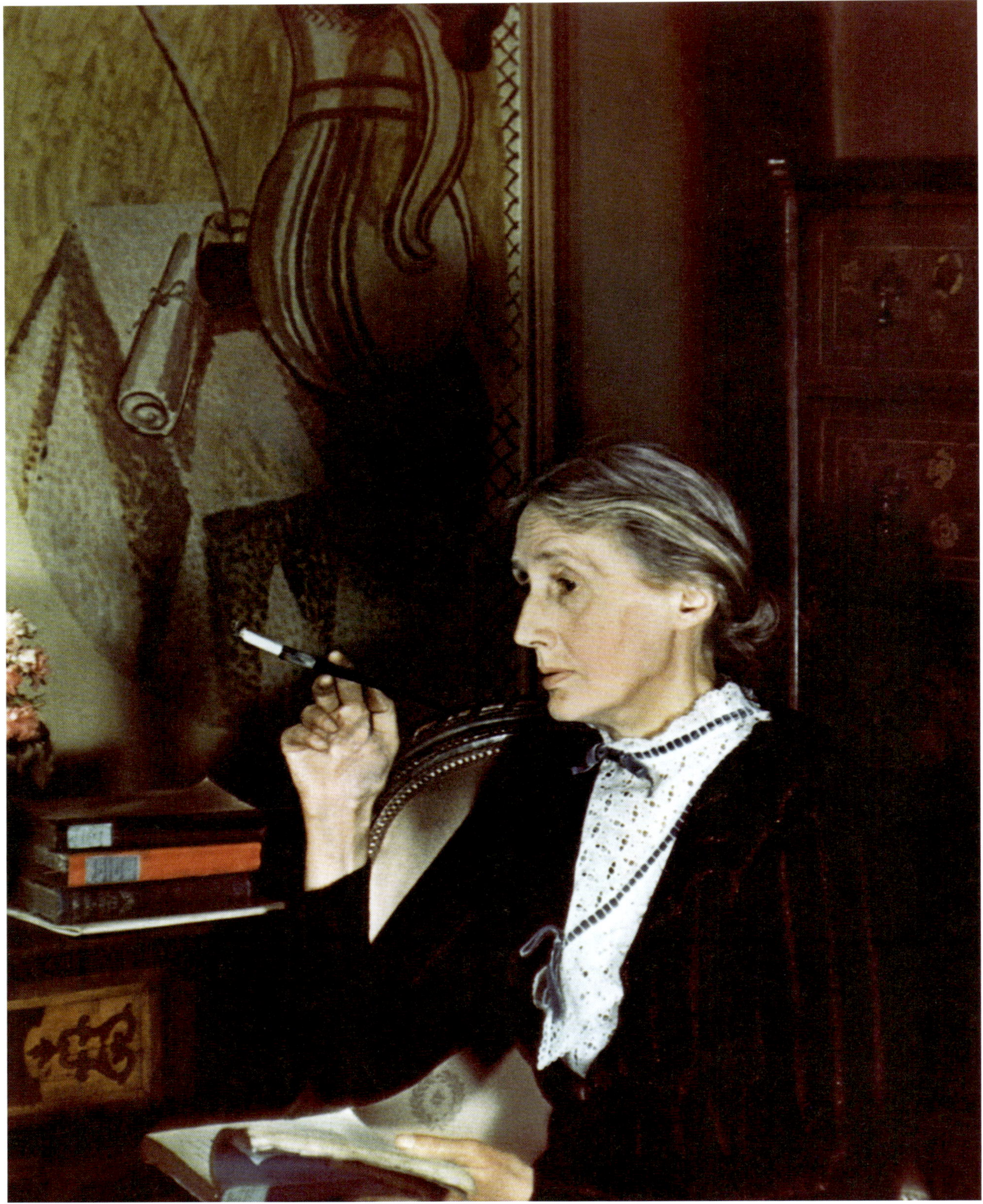

Virginia Woolf in 1939. Photo Gisèle Freund.

like? Perhaps it could only exist in the form of the essay, of which genre Woolf's opening sentence is both an elegant part-for-whole and a less than obvious parody.

Woolf herself was ambivalent about "On Being Ill," and about its opening sentence. At first she and her husband Leonard Woolf thought the essay one of her best: it is funny, learned, vagrant, strange, and quite aware of the Montaigne-mimicking cliché of its titular "On...." Woolf was late sending it to Eliot, informing him, as the deadline passed, that the manuscript was imminent but she had been "working under difficulties." Eliot was willing to publish, but had reservations. His postcard to that effect has not survived; instead we have Woolf's letters and diaries, in which she laments that she may have overwritten. Returning to the text in light of Eliot's note, she "saw wordiness, feebleness, and all the vices in it." She had composed the essay from her sickbed, and it seemed that one of the main arguments of the piece—that the hiatus and the solitude of illness encourage a febrile sort of reading, and writing—had proved correct: Woolf had simply used too many words.

Four years after it first appeared, Woolf reprinted "On Being Ill" as part of a series of essay-length books for the Hogarth Press, which she had set up with Leonard. She took the opportunity to rein in what must have seemed syntactic and figural excesses in the work. In a passage about the invalid's attitude to poetry, the 1930 version states: "We rifle the poets of their flowers. We break off a line or two and let them open in the depths of the mind." But in 1926, Woolf had let the second prose flower bloom: "We break off a line or two and let them open in the depths of the mind, spread their bright wings, swim like coloured fish in green waters." Time and again in 1930, she strips away such decor: images disappear, adjectives vanish, and

sentences quite as long as the opening one are pruned at their extremities as if they were rangy roses in her Sussex garden. The excess clauses are sometimes replanted or grafted nearby, not disposed of entirely.

There's a contradiction, not quite buried, in the way the essay characterizes the sick person's experience of language. On the one hand: "Illness makes us disinclined for the long campaigns that prose exacts." The works of Edward Gibbon, Gustave Flaubert, and Henry James are beyond the powers of the bedridden, whose memory, judgment, and attention are apt to stray "while chapter swings on top of chapter." On the other hand, illness makes us adventurers, in language and imagination; we are pleased to abandon concision and coherence. Above all, so it seems as "On Being Ill" starts to mimic the shape of its own beginning, illness frees us to fall back on the pillows and give up pretending to the logical progression of our thoughts.

Here is what happens in 1930 to the first sentence of 1926: very little, almost nothing. There are some small changes to punctuation, as when "arm chair" acquires a hyphen. In a sentence that is governed in its opening lines by the (somewhat confusing) play of light and dark, Woolf avoids a minor repetition when she writes "what wastes and deserts of the soul a slight attack of influenza brings to view" instead of "... brings to light." Perhaps that change diverts the metaphoric force of the sentence a touch, but we are, after all, still in the territory of the visible, inside a reverie that with its field of flowers and "Deity stooping from the floor of Heaven" could be straight out of a medieval dream poem. The real alteration from the version of the sentence in *The New Criterion* comes a little way after the dash, when "and infinitely more" is quietly forgotten. It's hard not to conclude that Woolf's "infinitely more" is just this: the swelling perplex of metaphors, which

she is doing her best to soothe and shrink.

What remains? Most of the sentence, and of course the crucial dash, which is the sveltest emblem possible of the license afforded to the sick, to the essayist, and to the sentence itself. "On Being Ill" contains one of Woolf's boldest essayistic deviations. She has been thinking about *Hamlet*, and the way rashness, "one of the properties of illness," allows at last a proper, because "outlaw," reading of the play's illogic and excess. And then, without warning: "But enough of Shakespeare—let us turn to Augustus Hare." Hare was a mediocre nineteenth-century biographer: his 1893 book *The Story of Two Noble Lives* (on Countess Canning and the Marchioness of Waterford) is the sort of thing one might have read in bed with flu in 1925. But it gives Woolf her last, long paragraph, on the eruption of violent death into poised, aristocratic Victorian lives. The essay ends in a kind of dream— with the image of a plush red curtain clasped and crushed in grief. And we're happy to follow Woolf there, in part, because of that dash in her opening sentence, which denotes a passage from the dream-fugue of sickness, depression, and undirected reading into the dirigible madness of writing.

INGESTION / HOW TO BOIL AN EGG
Mats Bigert

"Ingestion" is a column that explores its topic within a framework informed by history, aesthetics, and philosophy.

———

In 1995, when fifty-year-old Malcolm Eccles was diagnosed with terminal bowel cancer, he decided that he would leave his wife Brenda a memento she would never forget. There was one thing she couldn't cook and that was eggs. Always mistimed, hers would come out either too hard or too soft. Malcolm engaged a specialist glassblower in south London to make a foot-tall hourglass in which a portion of his ashes would be encased. Interviewed by the *Independent* in 1997, just after Malcolm had passed away, Brenda commented: "It's just what he wanted. I can see him now laughing his head off at me. He said he had worked so hard all his life and enjoyed it, so he couldn't see why he should stop working when he was dead. … He said: 'At least when you turn me over it will make you smile rather than make you cry.'"

The art of boiling an egg doesn't have to be a story about life and death, but for many of us it is a serious business that needs some practice to perfect. When I was growing up, my mother boiled our eggs until they were hard as stones, with a sulfuric green aura around their yellow innards. It was Sweden in the 1970s, and in my world, eggs were eaten that way. Often presented as part of a smorgasbord, they were halved and then topped with even smaller eggs squeezed out from fish behinds. But when I had to begin feeding myself, my awareness of the diversity of how eggs could be ingested increased. The first time I

ever ate soft egg yolk, however, was a deeply traumatic experience. It wasn't a boiled egg but a fried one—sunny-side up—presented on a slice of rye bread. After munching into the white corners of the egg, I approached the yellow center. I made a bold decision and took the whole yolk in one ravenous bite. As the sandwich, which I had bought at a canteen, had probably spent most of the day in a covered plastic container awaiting its eater, it had developed a thin coating and its convex geometry adhered perfectly to my concave upper palate, like glue. I had to scrape it out of my mouth with a spoon.

But this experience somehow cracked the *ovum philosophicum*—the alchemist's "philosophical egg." A mystical, gooey substance, which I had only ever encountered in a solid form hermetically sealed in its oval container, was now leaking out from its vessel. It was death, and rebirth. My mother's hard-boiled egg-stone had metamorphosed into the philosopher's stone, changing any substance it came into contact with, including my upper palate.

I soon developed a soft spot for soft-boiled eggs and my first serious girlfriend taught me how to do them right. She put them in cold water with a pinch of salt, and when the water came to a boil, the egg timer was set to four minutes. The egg timer was also shaped like an egg, ticking away counterclockwise until a buzzing noise signaled that the eggs should be taken off the stove and given a cold shower. It was best if they were not too fresh—the shell of an egg that is a week old, preferably two, can be peeled more successfully, without any of the white stuck to it. As an egg ages, it gradually loses moisture through the pores in its shell and the air pocket at its tip expands. The pH of the egg white also changes, going from a low pH to a relatively high one, which makes it adhere less strongly to the shell. For decades this

method provided me with perfectly boiled eggs, until one morning in Brooklyn, in the kitchen of *Cabinet*'s editor-in-chief, my long-held conviction about how to boil the perfect egg was challenged by what my colleague called the "Turner Method." This protocol had been demonstrated by Christopher Turner, a *Cabinet* colleague from London who also frequently stays at the same house in Brooklyn. Turner's way with eggs was different than mine, and, according to the editor-in-chief, more precise. My world was shaken.

In the Turner Method, the eggs are placed in a pan full of cold water, which is brought to a full, rolling boil and then removed from the heat. Now the timing begins, with the help of a digital device (egg timers R.I.P.) set to exactly five minutes. Eggs thus cooked yield perfect, soft yolks with the same consistency all the way through. My debunked method generated eggs whose yolks exhibited a gradient of solidity, ranging from very hard on the outskirts to softer at the center. And as with any paradigm shift overturning one's worldview, I strongly objected to this abhorrent method. How could half of the process of boiling eggs involve not boiling them?

But looking deeper into the mysteries of not-boiling pots revealed a host of new methods devised by molecular gastronomists for cooking the humble egg. There is, for instance, the method that recommends dropping the egg into water heated to between sixty-four and sixty-five degrees Celsius (though some suggest going as high as sixty-nine degrees), which warms it to a temperature where the white coagulates but the yolk still has a smooth, custardy texture. Using this method, your egg cannot overcook no matter how long it remains in the bath, which means you can have preheated soft-boiled eggs always ready to go. But is this really cooking eggs, or merely heating eggs? We

might call it poaching eggs, only with their shells on.

A more radical development in the world of eggs—conceptual in its twist and apparently revolutionary in its scientific benefits—is the recent discovery of how to "uncook" an already cooked egg. Let's say your egg timer breaks down while you're perfecting your breakfast ovum; then what? Well, you could always call Gregory Weiss, a biochemist at the University of California, Irvine, who has been developing a device for pulling apart tangled proteins and allowing them to fold back into their original states. This breakthrough might be used in the future to treat cancer, but it also means that the impossibly entangled proteins of my mother's 1970s eggs could be returned to their pristine fluid form. Unfortunately, the "vortex fluid device" Weiss uses for this regenerative process requires that urea, one of the main components of urine, be added to the cooked egg white. Even molecular chefs, who like to refer to their kitchens as laboratories, would have a hard time defending this recipe.

But let's leave aside the dissonance of mixing bodily fluids and look at the other end of our oval-shaped spectrum. Here, we find classical music fans who time their eggs using the overture of Mozart's *Marriage of Figaro*, the length of which is said to be ideal for producing the perfect soft-boiled egg. This is a favorite story told by conductors before concerts, but a quick search reveals that the ninety-five different versions currently available on Spotify range in length from three minutes and fifty seconds to five minutes and fourteen seconds, which to my mind renders this method too imprecise. But who knows, maybe the music enveloping the egg can soothe it into a perfect consistency—after all, the composition's purported salutary effects have even led to it being included in compilations such as *Kids Love Mozart!* and *Baby Mozart*.

Eggs contain the promise of life, and chickens support the population of the world by laying some 1.3 trillion eggs each year, according to data from 2014. Given that eggs actually contain everything we need in terms of protein, minerals, and vitamins—except vitamin C, for which you'll need an additional squeeze of fresh orange juice—one can understand the alchemists' use of the egg as a symbol of eternal life. When Emma Morano, the oldest woman in the world when she died last year at the age of 116, was asked about the secret to her extravagant longevity, she answered that she had been eating three raw eggs every day for the last hundred years. I hope that the one boiled egg I eat for breakfast every day will do instead, since the idea of gulping raw eggs, like some Rocky Balboa, fills me with disgust. Leaving aside the morality of eating animals, or even potential animals, the idea of ingesting an egg in its primordial form puts me too much in mind of the sort of primal act our ancestors engaged in, long before their descendants invented induction stoves and molecular gastronomy. I would rather end up in that hourglass a little prematurely, my ashes gently flowing through the funnel, particle by particle, clocking time for future generations of perfectly boiled eggs.

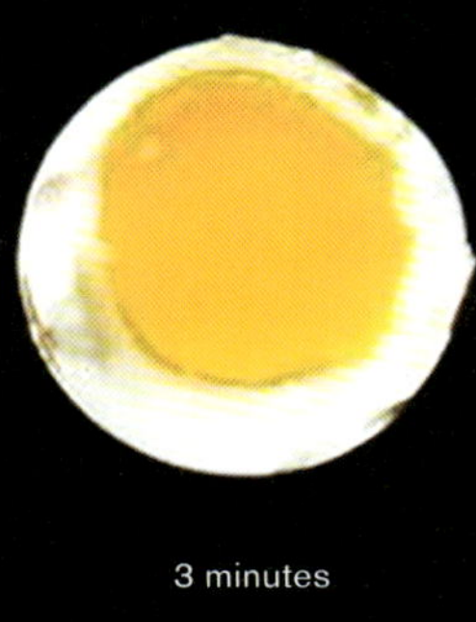

3 minutes

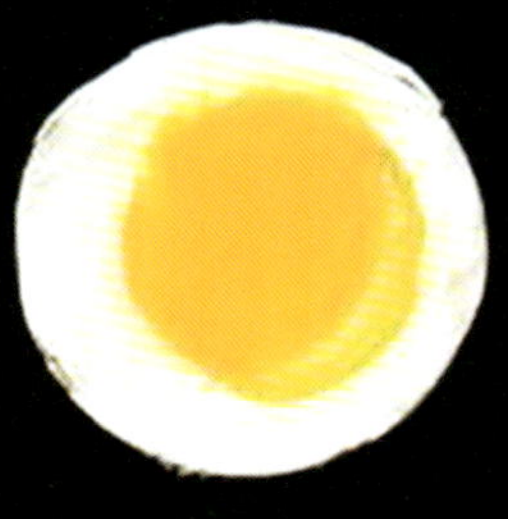

5 minutes

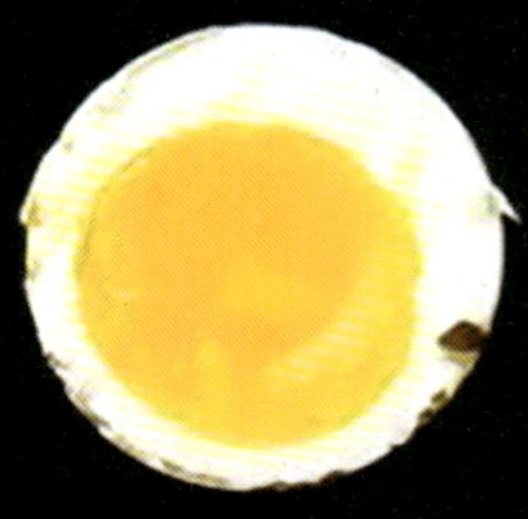

6 minutes

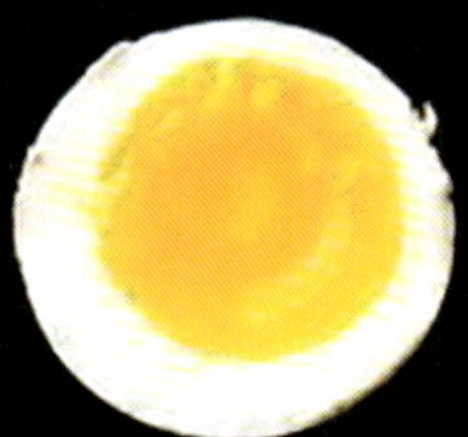

7 minutes

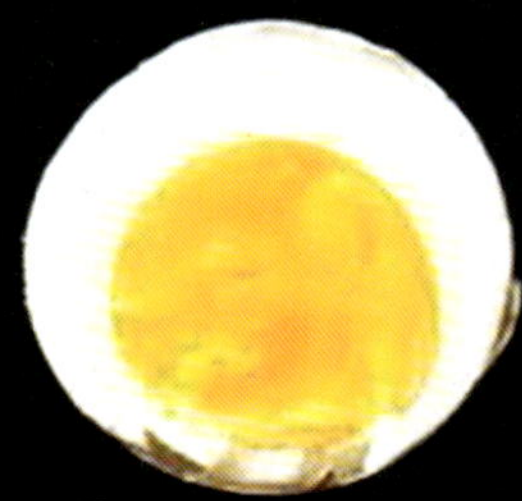

8 minutes

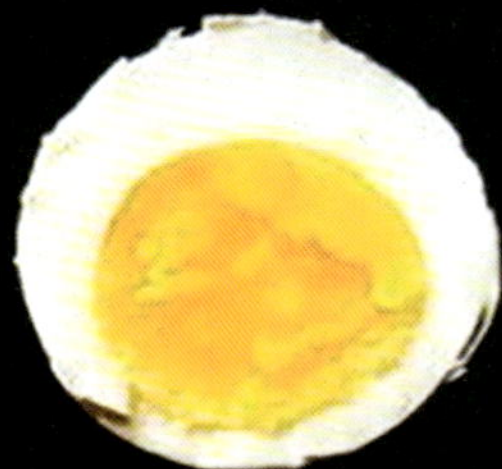

9 minutes

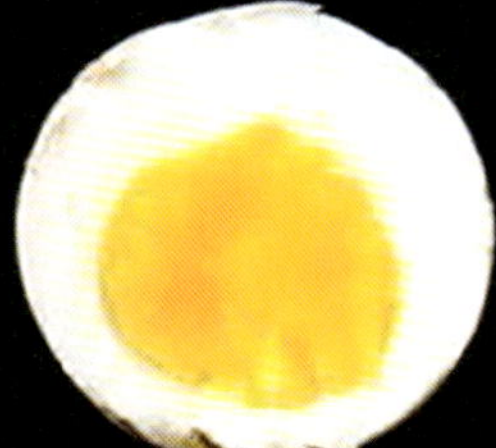

11 minutes

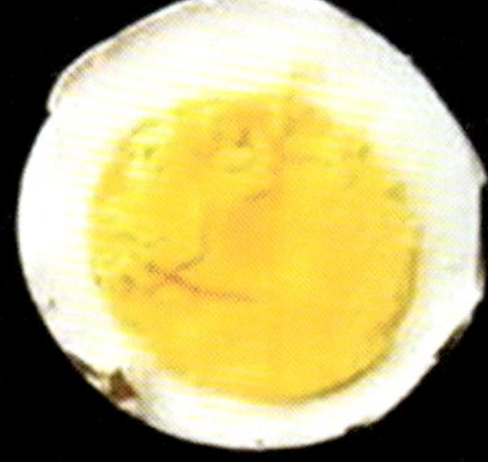

12 minutes

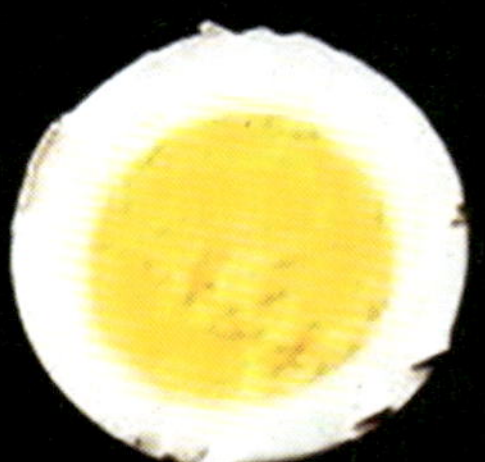

13 minutes

A good yolk is a matter of timing.

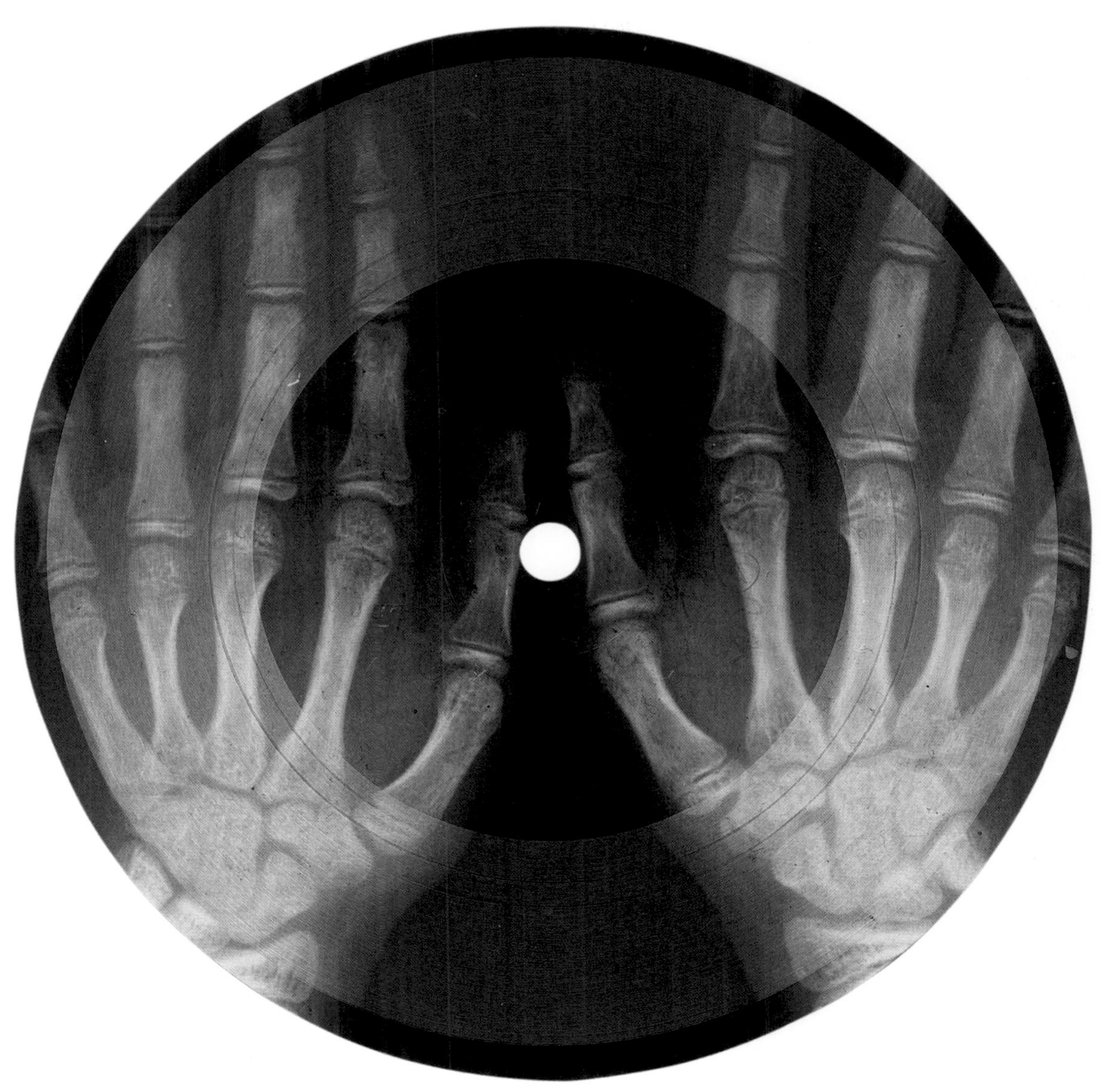

Ars longa, vita brevis. X-ray record, mid-twentieth century. Records courtesy Rudolf Fuks.
Photos Xenia Vytuleva and Francesco Benelli.

LEFTOVERS / PLAYING THE X-RECORD
Eduardo Cadava and Xenia Vytuleva

"Leftovers" investigates the cultural significance of detritus.

———

Look around, the world is shimmering.
Alexander Vvedensky, *The Gray Notebook*, ca. 1932

In recent years, globalization and transnational processes have destabilized conventional ways of reading culture, locality, and place. Although the mechanics of the visual and auditory aspects of dissident culture have been exhaustively mapped in the course of recent decades, its shadow narratives and improbable pasts are less well known. Dissident, material dispatches moving across borders bear the traces of variegated processes of diffusion within asymmetrical contexts. Among early attempts to transmit global ideals, a wonderfully rich case involves the Soviet dissident practice of illegally producing records on exposed X-ray films.[1]

"Music on bones"—as the practice, which began in the mid-1940s and lasted through the 1960s, was referred to in KGB documents and so-called anti-propaganda movies circulated by the government—was the only way to gain access to Western hits and, indeed, to some kinds of globalized cultural exchange. A master disc was pressed onto already-exposed, heated X-ray film— taken from hospital trashcans and medical archives—in order to make a crude phonographic recording whose barely visible grooves were etched on skulls, chest cavities, and spinal cords. No longer regarded as a medical document, no longer serving as a record of human physical identity, these exposed X-rays became the foundation of a new form of media, the abstract techno-basis of a new layer of "secret" and "precious" information. The Rolling Stones, the Beatles, and Elvis Presley, as well as jazz and foxtrot, were recorded on images of the interiors of Soviet bodies. Remarkably, the first examples served primarily as a means of personal escape, an "inner emigration," by multiplying the forbidden copies of banned songs by the so-called white immigrants, such as Alexander Vertinsky, Leonid Utesov, and Pjotr Leschenko. Crossing both physical and political borders, this hybrid, mediatic form provided an opportunity for a parallel narrative—a kind of sidewalk or by-product—which became the means for accessing a different kind of cognitum and even for survival vis-à-vis the official regime.[2]

The technology itself, embodying and demonstrating a logic of material reuse and repurposing, activated a memory of others' lives and invoked the progression from birth to death. With the postwar state program for fighting tuberculosis, fluorography became a routine, mandatory, nationwide procedure that produced a massive amount of X-ray waste that could now serve as a surface on which music could be "printed on ribs." Whether damaged or in perfect condition, the grayscale translucent celluloid was no longer associated with lethal maladies, but rather with the everyday medical routines of Soviet citizens. Because of the extreme photochemical deterioration built into the medium, the exposed X-rays had to be stored in the dark and, indeed, they were to be found in the cellars of most medical institutions. The silvery black-and-white images were exceptionally vulnerable to heat, moisture, and harmful gases such as sulfur dioxide and nitrogen oxide—a common chemical mix in the air of modernized urban environments. At the same time, organic compounds such as gelatin, which contained the photographic emulsion, were susceptible to fungal growth in sealed storage areas. The physical impossibility of managing X-ray films in federal archives condemned them to be only short-term or "transit" documents. The recycling of the film provided a happy opportunity for hospitals and health institutions, which had been asked to eliminate chemically treated plates because they were so extremely fragile and flammable. Similarly, the active life of the newly constructed X-record was also locked into a particular temporality—the discs could really only be played five to ten times.

The key laboratory for these homemade X-ray records was established at the end of 1946 in Leningrad—today's St. Petersburg— under the label Zolotaya Sobaka, the "Golden Dog."[3] To differentiate its agenda from other underground entities, the group issued a stamp featuring a cozy, domestic, even bourgeois image of a dog attentively listening to a gramophone. In reality, however, the origins of the technology were far from intimate and romantic. The basic equipment—called the "Bogoslovsky Machine"—was constructed from the remains of the Telefunken 45-rpm and 78-rpm models with adjustments made with military tools. Roughly cut out with manicure scissors, and with pencil titles scratched on their surfaces, each "record on bones" could cost up to five rubles, at a time when the average salary was eighty rubles a month. To own such an unusual record was a matter of social privilege and prestige. Its possession also signaled participation in certain underground, cluster cultures, regardless of one's education or social status. One of the cofounders of the Golden Dog, Boris Taigin, was a tram driver, a poet, and the publisher of *Be-Ta*, a magazine

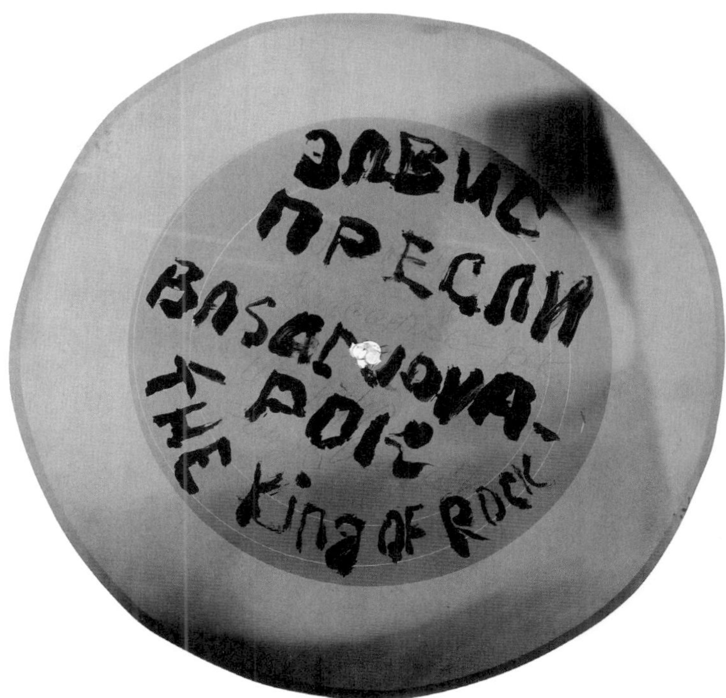

Elvis Presley, *From Elvis in Memphis*, 1969.

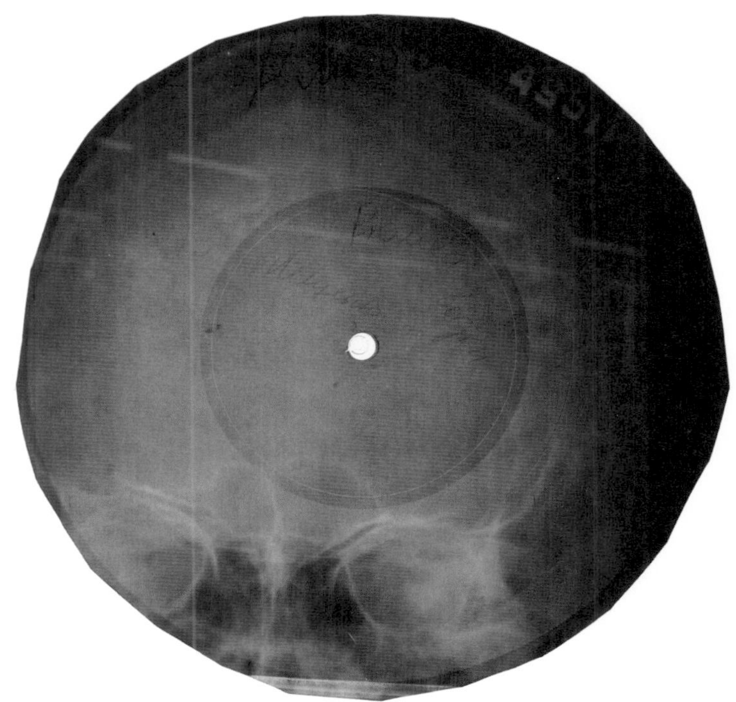

Steve Lawrence, *Lawrence Goes Latin*, 1961.

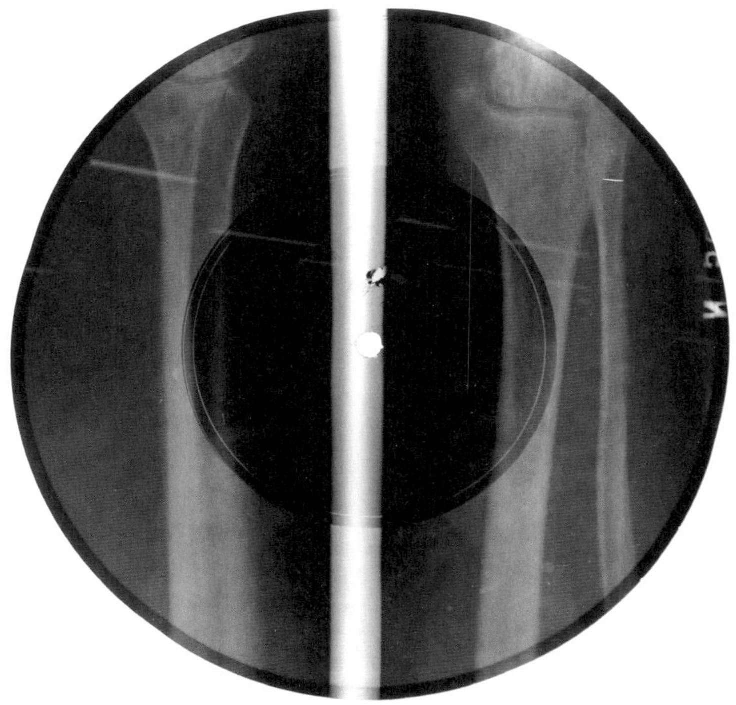

Louis Armstrong, *The Best of Satchmo*, 1974.

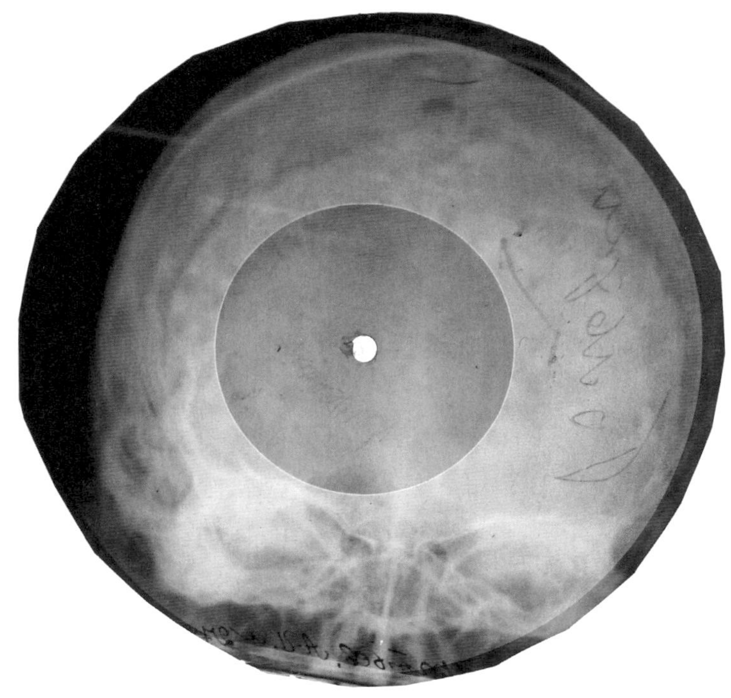

Lou Klayman and His Orchestra, *Twistin the Freilach
(To Make Every Party a Ball!)*, 1962.

whose average print run was ten copies.[4] Engineers, doctors, workers, artists, janitors, and students were all interested in the records, signaling a massive obsession that soon permeated Soviet society. Particularly popular in the resort areas of the Caucuses and Crimea, "music on bones" became a transnational phenomenon that took advantage of the dense and well-articulated network between the various Soviet republics. The Golden Dog was not only an ideological danger, but also an extremely influential, economic intervention against the very grain of Marxist-Leninist doctrine, especially given its non-socialist, private mode of production. "Music on bones" was a business.

The circulation of so-called *roentgenizdat* was hard to control; it was rather unpredictable and could emerge on the critical edge of various cultural zones. In the words of human rights activist and historian Lyudmila Alexeyeva, "its appearance was more rhizomatic and spontaneous than the underground mediums, it was like mushroom spores."[5] Mirroring samizdat, a backbone of Soviet dissidence, the name *roentgenizdat* literally means "publishing on X-rays." Samizdat was a particular, textual "mode of existence"—one that was similar to print, and even dependent on it, but not print. Following Alexeyeva, it should be considered a medium, a genre, even a corpus of texts. The *Oxford English Dictionary* defines samizdat as "the clandestine or illegal copying and distribution of literature," mainly a parody of an official print run, recalling the abbreviated names for official publishing houses: Gosizdat (the Soviet State Publishing House), Voenizdat (the Military Publishing House), and Detizdat (the Children's Literature Publishing House). Despite its bitter humor and playful references, *roentgenizdat* was viewed as a highly anti-Soviet activity and those involved faced sentences of three to seven

years in prison. From 1946 to 1957, "music on bones" was registered as a general anti-Soviet activity. In 1958, the influence of the practice had reached such a point that the authorities issued a special law declaring the home-production of recordings "a criminally hooligan trend."[6] A year later, however, the establishment of the official "music patrol," soon followed by the new availability of the tape recorder, signaled the end for "music on bones," and, by the early 1960s, production began to decrease rapidly.

The signature of this practice was not necessarily the quality of the sound that resulted from the reproduction, which was relatively poor. Rather, it was the way it discreetly, and in a way that mostly went unrecognized, organized several motifs and modes of reproduction—music, technology, photography, radiography, phonography, history, writing, memory, repetition, the senses—around the experience of death and mourning, but also around recycling and the promise of another life. To put it another way: this singular form of recycling transcribed music onto a shadowy representation of our mortality and finitude that also indicated a strange kind of survival.[7] If we are to believe André Malraux, however, music has always only been "music on bones." As he writes in *Man's Fate*, his 1933 account of the early days of the Chinese Revolution, "music alone speaks of death." If he suggests that, of all the arts, only music can speak of death, for him it is also the case that music can *only* speak of death, can speak of nothing else but death. What makes music music is that, in our experience of it, we encounter death, we encounter what is always about to vanish. Indeed, music is, as it were, the least incorporated matter. It remains, even after we hear it, even after we incorporate its trace, somewhere outside us, resonating in an exteriority that we experience as the opening

of a world. Music dispossesses us; it takes us away from ourselves. To say that music always has been "music on bones," then, is to say that music always has signaled our departure from ourselves, our imminent death.

As the material support for this clandestine practice, the X-ray film itself evokes a process of loss and disappearance, a *damnatio memoriae*, a kind of anti-memory, as the rays that produce the image also produce death in the process of its production. By illuminating bones and chests, by making flesh disappear and revealing an image of death beneath it, the X-ray enters the body and fixes an image of its passage. Translucency, shadows, and dissolution are more than a dominant aesthetic. Announcing the death-bringing age of radiation, they offer a view of the remains that all bodies are destined to become. In the first paper published on the subject, Wilhelm Röntgen designated his discovery the "X-ray," a name that, for him, suggested its mysterious nature—a kind of "twilight," a total enigma. The X-ray's high-energy, high-speed vibrations allow them to penetrate almost anything; when the film is illuminated, surface appearances disappear to reveal the death beneath the surface of life. Its inscriptional force is perhaps best registered in the consequences of its development in the field of nuclear physics: the lightning flash of Hiroshima and Nagasaki. Lasting one fifteen-millionth of a second, the X-ray flash penetrated every building, leaving its imprint on stone walls, tattooing kimono patterns on the victims' bodies, and, in this way, preserving the traces of the very things and persons it erased.

The diverse historical and ideological implications of the X-ray in the context of *roentgenizdat* should not be overlooked. Paradoxically, the same metanarratives, traumatic scenarios, and references to death, mourning, and disappearance would be actively displayed by the

"anti-propaganda" movies created against this dissident practice. *Shadows on the Sidewalks*, issued by the State Central Documentary Committee in 1960, was the first of these films to evoke shadowy, virtual bodies, and to reiterate the metaphorical corpus of the translucent medium.[8] Despite the expectation that a film against "music on bones" would be about music, its dominant focus and rhetoric are directed to the limitations and pathologies of the visual regime of the X-ray. Obsessively referencing the dark side of the roentgen—the blurred, distorted, grayscale image—the almost magical power of transformation through which an image could be turned into memory was negated. The act of "judgment" was translated into a solid visual formula, dividing society into "shadowy" illegal dissidents and the government's music patrol.

There is another dimension to the "new evil," at least as it is represented in the film: the staged "newsreel" is totally urban. It starts with an uncanny scene on the sidewalks in the center of Moscow: the black-market distribution of these X-ray records next to the enormous GUM department store on Red Square. The camera moves slowly from the cracks of the asphalt to rotating X-ray records, superimposing the bones onto the face of the evil main smuggler. "Hey, Zhenya Gorkun," says the voiceover, "how does the world look through the narrow groove of X-ray rock and roll?" The camera zooms in on the translucency of the X-ray and suddenly jumps out to the dancing shadows on the sidewalks. Both human and nonhuman are locked in an embrace in the optical logic of the X-ray. But the cityscape is much more than simply the indifferent backdrop to these scenes. Also under attack are certain patterns of modernity and urban existence, ones in which the smugglers and the victims of globalized culture coexist on sidewalks, in

traffic, and in clubs and restaurants. This coexistence is staged in the tension between the film's depiction of urban modernity and views of endless rural landscapes and the making of bread, which suggest different modes of living and prosperity. Indeed, Soviet propaganda movies excelled in the application of romantic motifs, redirecting them across the terrain of sacral and secular cults, and exploiting the total reversibility of the metaphors. (The relationship among materials, collective memory, and globalization is not a trivial one, especially since the practice of "music on bones" transgressed international copyright law.)

Looking back at the genealogies of dissidence and of the transnational connections that were often entangled with them, we see more paradoxical mergers: between different technologies, several modes of reproduction, material culture, and artistic practices. The radical cross-temporal and cross-disciplinary phenomenon of "music on bones" allows us, in Walter Benjamin's words, to "brush history against the grain," and to redefine the boundaries of the "transnational object"— the object that bears the traces of an entire network of historical relations, technological developments, and heterogeneous, but shared, desires and motivations. "Music on bones" is an extreme example of an almost clandestine form of globalization. Through a weird coincidence, and in a wildly absurd political context, the X-record, in its particular form of "recycling," transcribed music onto an obscured representation of our mortality, blurred the borders of the personal and the impersonal, introduced intimacy into cross-national and global cultures, and marked the fatal displacement of radiation onto music.

The authors are grateful to Rudolf Fuks for his assistance.

1 This article is based on research conducted for the exhibition "Re-cycle; Strategies for Architecture, the City, and the Planet" at MAXXI, Rome, in 2011. See the catalogue of the same name, edited by Pippo Ciorra and Sara Marini (Milan and Rome: Electa and MAXXI, 2012).

2 The preferred term for Soviet dissidents was *inakomysliashchie*, which literally means "those who think differently." See Yuri M. Lotman and Boris A. Uspensky, "On the Semiotic Mechanism of Culture," *New Literary History*, vol. 9, no. 2 (Winter 1978).

3 According to Boris Taigin, one of the cofounders of the Golden Dog, the first laboratory was established by the Leningrad engineer Stanislav Kazimirovich Fillon and was to be found at 75 Nevsky Prospekt under the innocent name Photography and Sound Letters, where one could record a personal voice message on a record and send it in the mail. At night, however, the studio was transformed into an illicit workshop.

4 For more on *Be-Ta*, see Emily Lygo, *Leningrad Poetry, 1953–1975: The Thaw Generation* (Berne: Peter Lang, 2010).

5 Lyudmila Alexeyeva described samizdat as the "backbone," the "core," of dissidence. See Lyudmilla Alexeyeva, *Soviet Dissent: Contemporary Movements for National, Religious, and Human Rights*, trans. Carol Pearce and John Glad (Middletown, CT: Wesleyan University Press, 1985), p. 284.

6 See Alexei Yurchak, "Gagarin and the Rave Kids: Transforming Power, Identity, and Aesthetics in Post-Soviet Nightlife," in *Consuming Russia: Popular Culture, Sex, and Society Since Gorbachev*, ed. Adele Marie Barker (Durham, NC: Duke University Press, 1999), p. 82.

7 Much has been written on the paradoxical nature of dissident practices. See, for example, Chantal Mouffe, *The Democratic Paradox* (London: Verso, 2000) or *Architecture and the Paradox of Dissidence*, ed. Ines Weizman (Abingdon, UK: Routledge, 2014).

8 *Shadows on the Sidewalks* was the debut film of Vladimir Krasnopolsky and Valeriy Uskov, two young progressive moviemakers. Responsibility for its script was given to Galina Shergova, an established propaganda writer.

WITH LOVE, A LETTER TO COOKIE, AND HER STORIES
Alice Butler

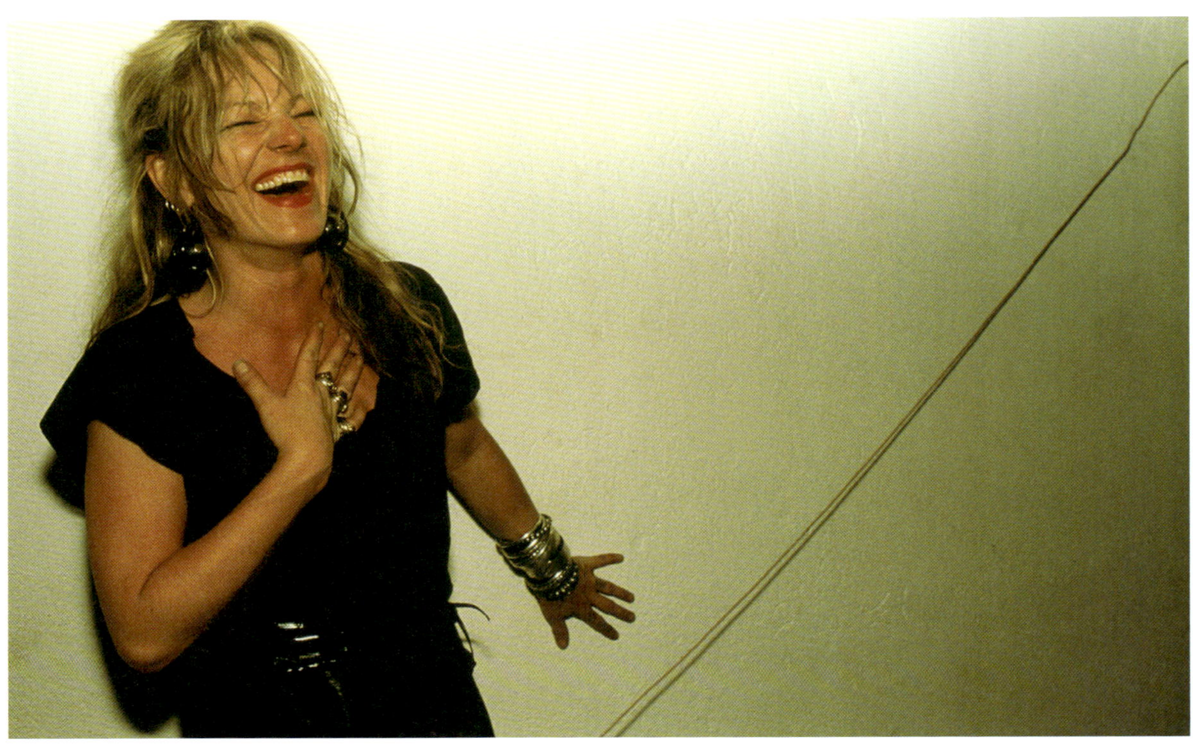

Dear Cookie,

I knew your face from the pictures first.

No one looks as ravishing in red at 4 a.m. on a toilet seat, lacy red knickers stretched down to your knees, with triangles of skin peeping through the folds of red fabric you probably fashioned together a few hours before the party.

No one looks as "alive" dead as you do in your casket, with bangles stacked up to your elbow like a glistening, gold Cleopatra.

I knew your face from the pictures first, but then I found your books and came to your writing. It is this body that I long for, the body of your stories.

I long to touch those eyes, that skin, that face, that fabric, but instead it's my writing you that touches, a second skin.

It is a skin that scratches, to find the other you.

Cookie Mueller and Nan Goldin became friends while staying in Provincetown in the summer of 1976, a wild and windy outpost for two young women breaking from their past. Nan had broken from the name Nancy, and Dorothy Karen somehow "got the name Cookie," before she "could walk."[1]

Cookie was having a yard sale, and Nan, a photographer from Boston's School of the Museum of Fine Arts, was enamored by her image: "a cross between a Tobacco Road outlaw and a Hollywood B-Girl, the most fabulous woman I'd ever seen."[2] After their first meeting, Nan shot Cookie in various settings, dressed in disorderly silks, always *fabulous*. And so they became closer with each click of the shutter, as they traveled from Provincetown to Baltimore to New York to the Amalfi coast in Italy, in unpredictable zigzags.

Many of the photographs are part of Nan's 35 mm, soundtracked slideshow *The Ballad of Sexual Dependency*, while others are to be found in *The Cookie Portfolio*, a collection of fifteen images later made into a book. The portfolio's pictures begin in Provincetown, with a sun-kissed Cookie locking her arms around her son Max in one picture, and her girlfriend Sharon in another, before moving through the New York party

---

Above: Nan Goldin, *Cookie laughing, NYC*, 1985. All Goldin images copyright Nan Goldin and courtesy Matthew Marks Gallery.

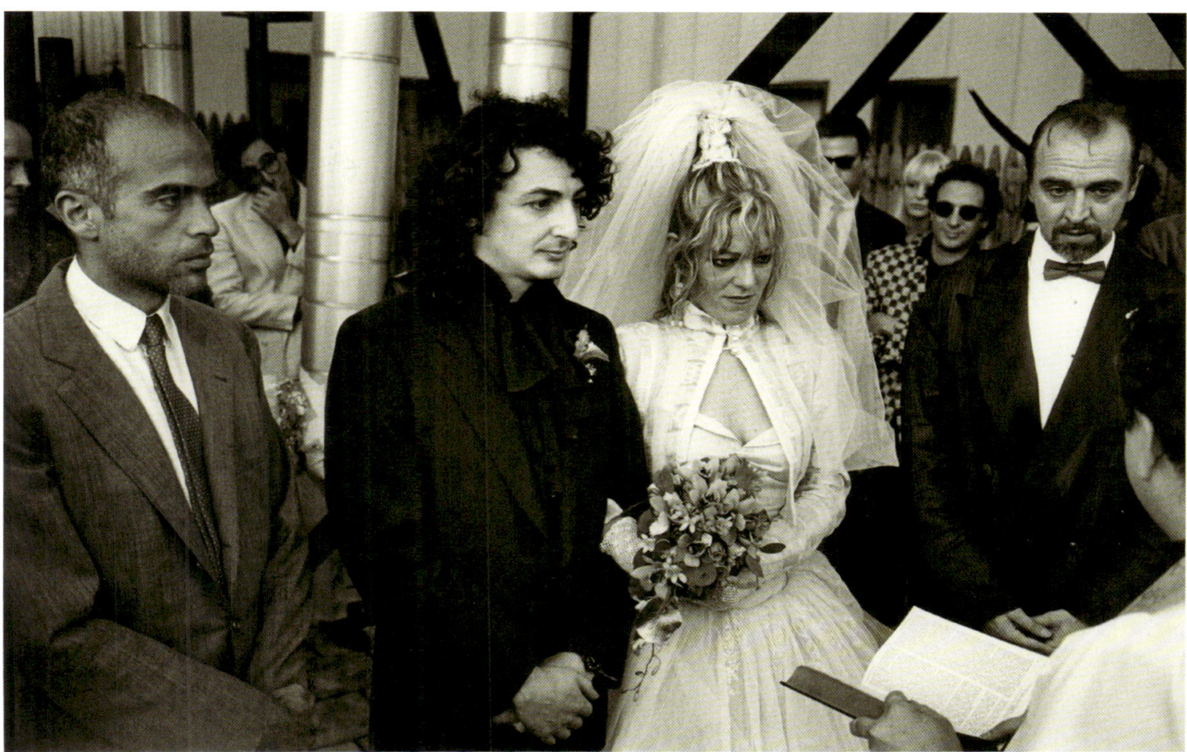

days, her mouth wide open in more than one picture; then her wedding to the artist Vittorio Scarpati, and the fairly sudden arrival of the symptoms of the disease that would kill her. Her face becomes less clear, as the carefree cackle fades with stroke-induced pain. In many of the later photographs, we see her only in profile, in shadow, or abstracted by the scans of an X-ray machine. Nan's final picture of "Cookie" is of her empty apartment on New York's Bleecker Street: with no body present, it is the striped sofa that remains, framed by framed portraits, and the pointless stuff of the living.

Aged just forty, Cookie died from AIDS-related illness on November 10, 1989, a few weeks before Nan took the picture of her apartment, and only eight weeks after her husband, Vittorio. She missed the opening of Nan's "Witnesses: Against Our Vanishing" exhibition at Artists Space in New York, featuring Vittorio's drawings, as well as works by artists including David Wojnarowicz, Mark Morrisroe, and Philip-Lorca diCorcia. The catalogue reprinted Cookie's text "A Last Letter," published a year earlier in the second issue of *City Lights Review*. As Nan Goldin writes in her introduction: "One of the writers for this catalogue has become too sick to write,"[3] and so, the title of Cookie's

text became more prophetic, more painful, with time, as her death mirrored the fate of those to whom she was writing.

In it, she writes *in memoriam* to her friends, now dead as a result of the epidemic, and the pitiful care from the state:

Each friend I've lost was an extraordinary person, not just to me, but to hundreds of people who knew their work and their fight. These were the kind of people who lifted the quality of all our lives, their war was against ignorance, the bankruptcy of beauty, and the truancy of culture. These were people who hated and scorned pettiness, intolerance, bigotry, mediocrity, ugliness, and spiritual myopia; the blindness that makes life hollow and insipid was unacceptable. They tried to make us see.[4]

Cookie has helped me see; she has helped me *write* through seeing. For so long she has been historicized by the image, either as the blond and beehived Cookie

Above: Peter Hujar, *Cookie Mueller's wedding to Vittorio*, 1986. Courtesy Peter Hujar Archive, Ira Silverberg, and the Fales Library and Special Collections, New York University.

of John Waters's early films (including *Multiple Maniacs*, *Pink Flamingos*, and *Female Trouble*) or as the Cookie in Nan's photographs: the girl laughing, or the girl clutching a cane, unable to walk because the disease was wasting her.

Born into the suburban enclaves of Baltimore in 1949, Cookie left home while still a teenager. As she writes in "Alien": "I was always leaving. Every time I left I had a different hair color and I would be standing on the porch saying goodbye to the older couple in the living room."[5] Dressed in colorful, thrift-shop chaos, her grimy glamour was a perfect match for the oddball love of John Waters's Baltimore Dreamlanders, whose alien arms she fell into when she "accidentally broke into show bizz."[6] An underground film career, together with all kinds of part-time jobs, from dealing drugs to working in a fish factory to designing clothes, saw her through the heady days of the 1970s.[7]

When she moved to New York in 1976, Cookie jumped into the downtown art world, what Robert Siegle has called "an alternative community but not an alternative state," in which painting, performance, film, sculpture, and writing became a permeable mesh of activity.[8] Cookie wrote candidly about the artists she loved for Annie Flanders's *Details* magazine, writing about her friends, the artists Keith Haring, Robert Mapplethorpe, and Jean-Michel Basquiat, whose death became the subject of Cookie's November 1988 "Art and About" column-cum-memorial. "The host of the party looked sad," she wrote. "He was sitting in the corner on the gray wall-to-wall industrial carpeting watching his shimmering, gilded, celebrated guests with his sloe eyes full of apathy and his oft-kissed lips frozen into a disingenuous smile."[9]

For the artists and writers of Cookie's scene, dwelling in the murky "abyss of the Lower East Side tunnel of tenements," downtown New York in the 1980s was its venues—ABC No Rio and Area, the Mudd Club and Saint Mark's Church—and Cookie, in a sense, was New York.[10] She came out of the clubs at 7 a.m., and then went back to read in them twelve hours later, with figures such as Eileen Myles, Joe Brainard, Kathy Acker, and Gary Indiana. Billy Sullivan's photograph of her pissing outside a club with her back turned—wearing a full-length black coat, feet slid into white stilettos—is suggestive of this history, and a suggestion of what was to come: the stigmatized fear of bodily fluids that would leave sick communities

neglected and maltreated. The "AIDS Coalition to Unleash Power," also known as ACT UP, was a direct action group established in the spring of 1987 to fight for improved legislation, education, medical research, and treatment for AIDS patients. Protesting the government's treatment of the infected as a harmful and deviant "object of scrutiny," ACT UP staged public demonstrations and politicized the funerals of those who had died of AIDS.[11] Artist and ACT UP activist David Wojnarowicz writes in his contribution to the "Witnesses" catalogue: "I imagine what it would be like if friends had a demonstration each time a lover or friend or stranger died of AIDS."[12]

The scrutiny I bestow on Cookie is written from love. With Nan's pictures of her showing a life in discontinuous fragments, I turn to Cookie's writing: let us focus on the life-writing performances she enacted in words while alive, rather than the prologue of death that these photographs tantalize.

When I look at the photograph of Cookie's empty apartment, I try to imagine the ephemera of writing strewn across the floor, *outside* the camera's frame. The scattered fragments of plays, poems, stories, and novels. I picture her hands moving feverishly across the typewriter, after making loose, intimate scribbles in her notebooks. I picture her body *writing*, as the seduced, and the seducer.

Writing to the author in Cookie is a way of letting her touching texts speak anew. It is a way of saying that her words touch me in a way that no other writer's words have before, an embodied relationship that has only one cause: the loving mesh of correspondence. It is a protest of sorts, an activist scream at the society of hate that, to borrow the words of Eve Kosofsky Sedgwick (speaking of the art critic Craig Owens, dead from AIDS in 1990, and whose memorial was held at Artists Space), "finally found it (to put it no more strongly than this) so possible, so little painful to let" her die.[13]

I don't wish to simply ignore the photographs, and the laughter and loss they document, but I want to know how Cookie performed those narratives in her own writing when alive, before she was robbed of her future by the epidemic. I am the reparative reader, writing from love. As Sedgwick writes: "Hope, often a fracturing, even a traumatic thing to experience, is among the energies by which the reparatively positioned reader tries to organize the fragments and

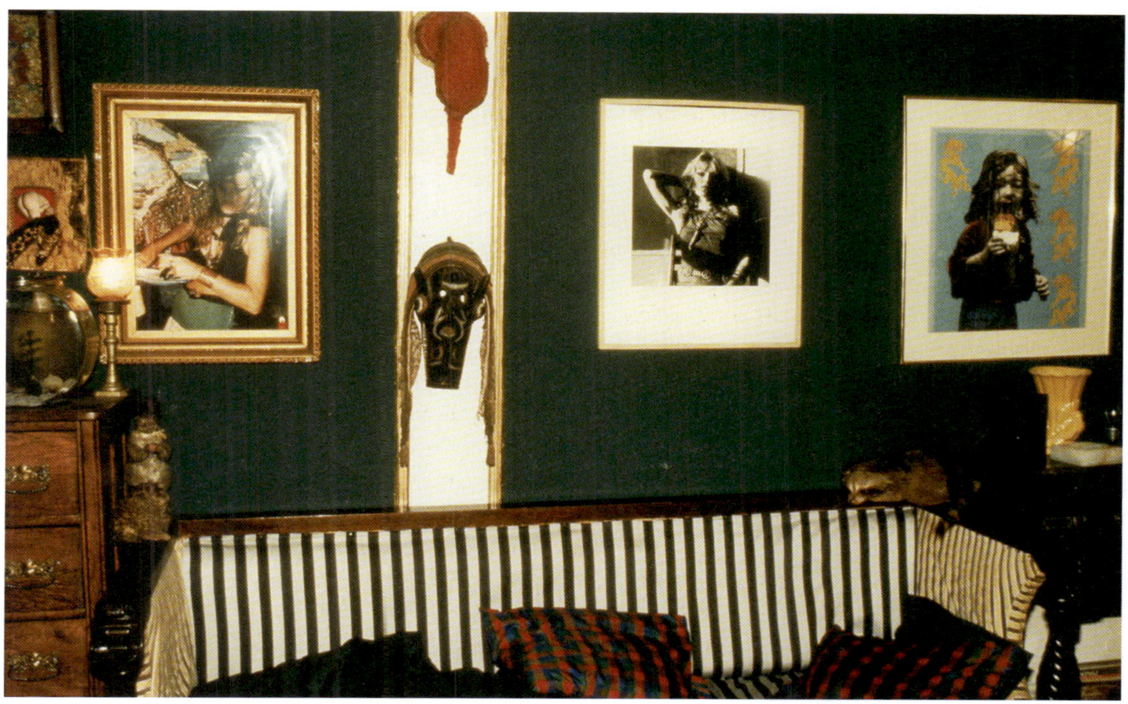

Nan Goldin, *Cookie and Vittorio's living room, NYC, Christmas 1989*, 1989.

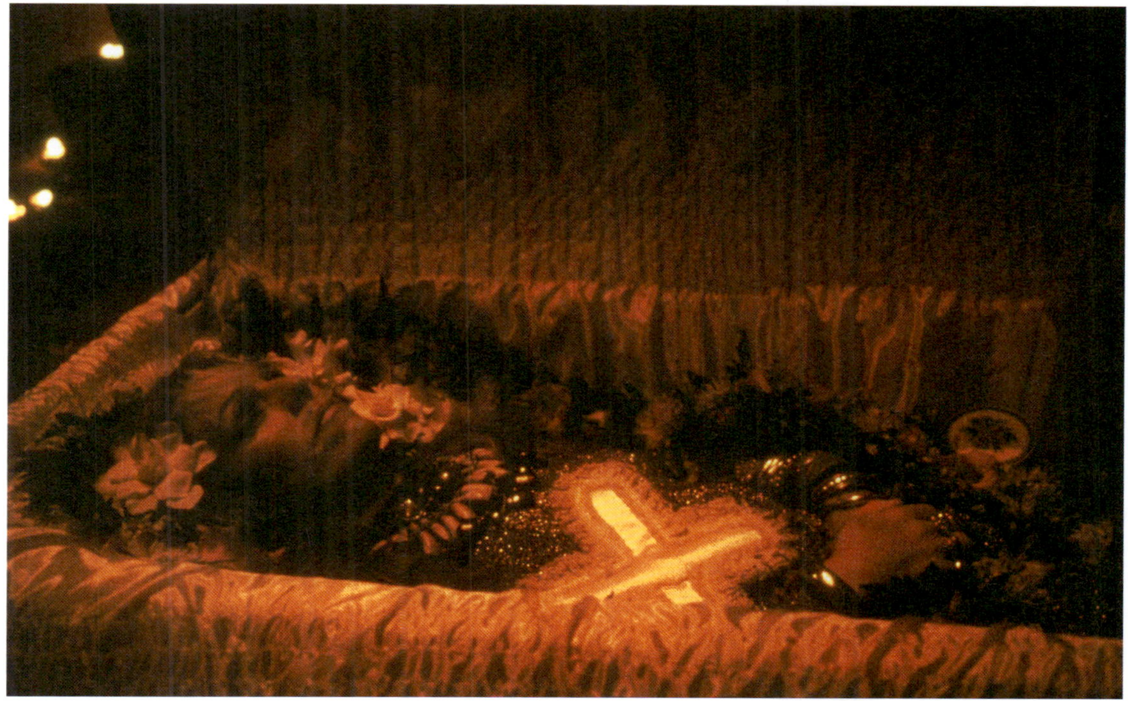

Nan Goldin, *Cookie in her casket, NYC, November 15, 1989*, 1989.

part-objects she encounters or creates."[14] As I feel for Cookie's body in writing fragments, hers and mine, I claim her in correspondence in order to enable a reclaiming of her work that might begin to understand her writing alongside (not after, or not without) her life cut short.

Walking through Clear Water in a Pool Painted Black was the first major collection of Cookie's stories to be published, when Chris Kraus picked it up, after no one else would, as the first in her Native Agents series for Semiotext(e).[15] Alongside Ann Rower's *If You're a Girl*, Cookie's book would launch in spring 1990, and so she missed it, with Richard Hell and Sharon Niesp reading in her place at the New York venue Quick! (formerly the club Area) on March 21, 1990.

Arranged chronologically, *Walking through Clear Water in a Pool Painted Black* comprises life stories from 1964 to 1989 that flirt with what once occurred: from Baltimore high school lust and a San Francisco peyote ceremony to an attempted rape in Maryland and a house fire in British Columbia. It is not so much the craziness of her tales that I find seductive, as the language and laughter with which she chooses to relay them. A lover of metaphor, her figurative sentences waver from haunting image ("There was no moon. The sky was like black cotton batting that felt like walking through clear water in a pool painted black.") to hilarious comparison, as when she raucously writes of the trauma of the attempted rape with affective young-girl innocence: "I felt very proud that I had melted so well into the underbrush, just like Bambi."[16]

If we take Cookie for her (written) word, she came to writing as a child ("I started writing when I was six and then never stopped completely."), later experimenting with a self-published novel around the time she hit puberty. She describes this stealthy act in cataloguing: "I wrote a novel when I was twelve and put it in cardboard and Saran Wrap, took it to the library and put it on the shelves in the correct alphabetical order."[17] It is possible Cookie's zine-like novel was the last long-form narrative she would piece together, in spite of her desire to write another one, and see it published. I "want to have a novel written in 2 months time," she wrote on a page in the back of her blue notebook, now in the Serpent's Tail/High Risk Archives at New York University's Fales Library and Special Collections, in which other fragmented attempts at this autobiographical novel, with allusive chapter subtitles, also appear.[18]

Cookie's novelistic desire belongs to an inventory of professional and personal longings, with other writing forms to conquer, and addictions to battle, filling out the numbered list. It is tempting to read Cookie's desire to write a novel as a craving intimately connected to her disease, which would later make writing difficult, eventually impossible. But instead of an autobiographical novel, the short stories piled up in ad hoc fragments, a *nearly novel*, amounting to a form she calls, in a note for the "Semiotext" [*sic*] book, "Quazi-Auto-Bio-Etc."[19] The many scribbled lists of stories found throughout the archive reveal the desire "to write" above all else, giving way to a life in textual pieces.

Or, as she wrote in a tiny text first published in the chapbook *Garden of Ashes*: "I believe that my short stories are novels for people with short attention spans."[20] It's from one of the little Hanuman Books that has Cookie's face printed on its cover (like her *Fan Mail, Frank Letters, and Crank Calls* of 1988), her yellow hair matched by a yellow border, and a red ribbon tied around her neck. Founded by editor Raymond Foye and painter Francesco Clemente, the press published tiny, colorful books (only three by four inches) that promoted avant-garde writing by authors and poets such as Bob Flanagan, Eileen Myles, and Gary Indiana.

Cookie's stories soar beyond their small scale, helping us to look and love closely, and to feel free and write freely. As Denise Duhamel wrote in a poem about Cookie: "Your rib cage lives on as a tree house for adolescent swallows / who, if they've never had a chance to rebel, do now."[21] Cookie's short stories, with narratives and forms that express adolescent tendencies, are like these adolescent swallows bursting forth, as rebellious now as they were in writing, helping *my* writing fly as I read her.

Published in downtown zines, artist periodicals, and Hanuman's chapbooks, or performed at live readings in venues such as the Mudd Club (where the toilet-scene photograph with which I started was taken), Cookie's autobiographical short stories might "fail" at the continuity of the novel, but they are illuminated by photographic detail, poetic lyricism, and feminist wit, as she turns the ephemeral autobiographical moment into ephemeral performative writing.[22] It is the passing of time that enables the writer in Cookie to pervert her own autobiography, as seen in the shameless way she writes shame, more specifically the vocation of go-go dancing: "I had decided to

Above: Mueller's handwritten list of short stories with page numbers, undated. Courtesy Ira Silverberg and the Fales Library and Special Collections, New York University.

Opposite: Note from Mueller to Richard Hell (recto and verso), ca. 1984. Courtesy Richard Hell and the Fales Library and Special Collections, New York University.

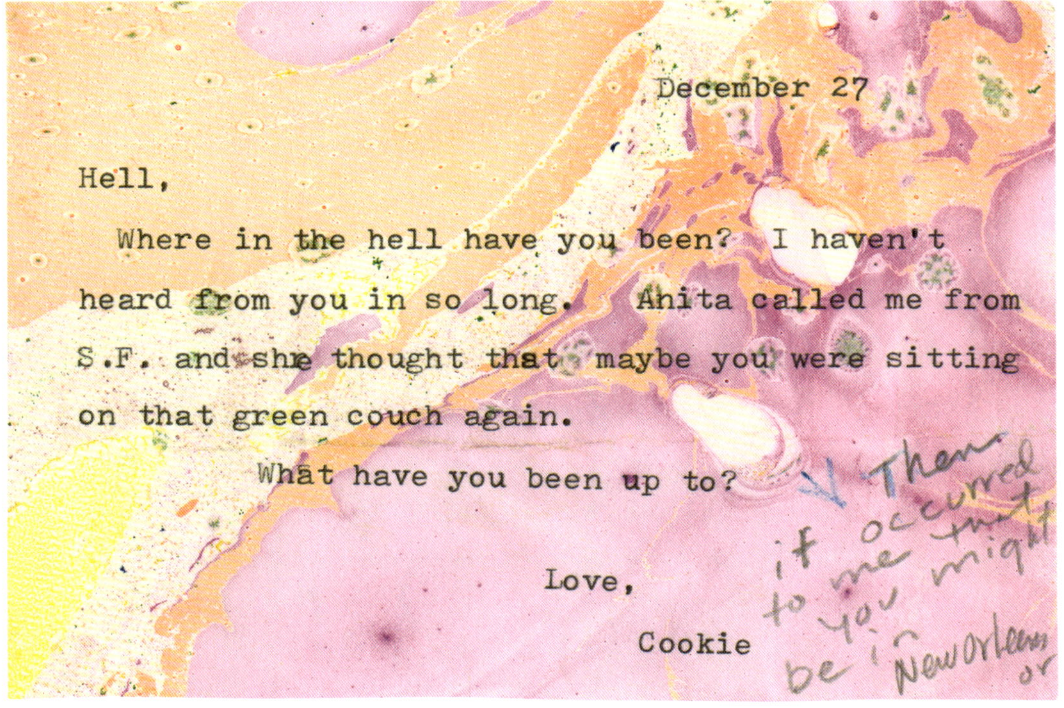
December 27

Hell,

    Where in the hell have you been? I haven't
heard from you in so long.   Ahita called me from
S.F. and she thought that maybe you were sitting
on that green couch again.

        What have you been up to?

                    Love,

                        Cookie

Then
it occurred
to me that
you might
be in
New orleans
or

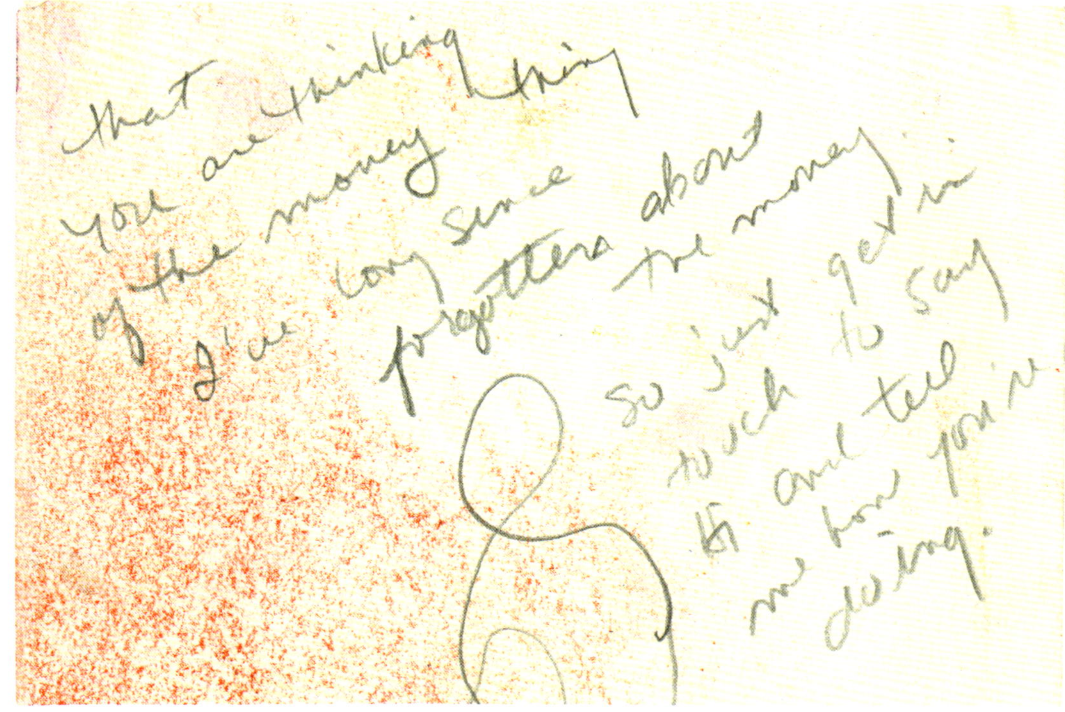
that are thinking thing
you are thinking thing
of the money
I've long since
forgotten about
the money
so just get in
touch to say
hi and tell
me how you're
doing.

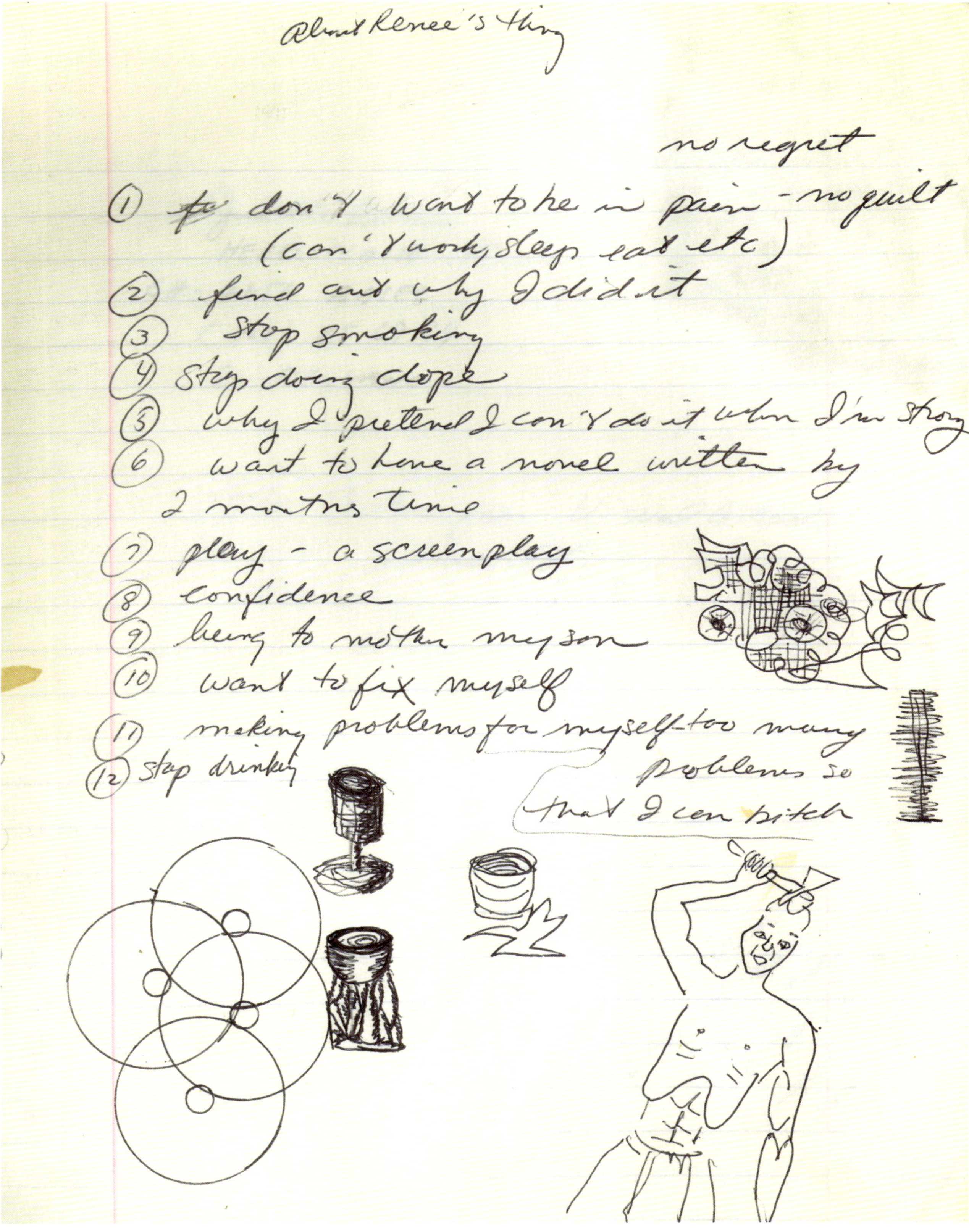
About Renee's thing

no regret

① you don't want to be in pain — no guilt
(can't work, sleep, eat etc)
② find out why I did it
③ stop smoking
④ stop doing dope
⑤ why I pretend I can't do it when I'm strong
⑥ want to have a novel written by
2 months time
⑦ play — a screenplay
⑧ confidence
⑨ being to mother my son
⑩ want to fix myself
⑪ making problems for myself — too many
problems so
⑫ stop drinking
that I can bitch

topless go-go dance when I first moved to New York from Provincetown. It wasn't something I especially wanted on my resume but I had been casting around, looking for work…something to pay the bills while I was making a start at designing clothes, searching film parts and writing."[23]

Cookie's "Go-Going—New York & New Jersey—1978–79" is stamped with a time and a place, making it into a kind of retrospective diary entry of performed first-person desire. As an ephemeral smattering of textual fragments, the diary—like the letter and the list—is a form favored by the adolescent discovering writing: rapid and unfinished, rebellious in confession. And so I also turn to these forms to find her, to discover the writer in Cookie through the stuff of adolescent writing. The amateur, adolescent writer appropriates these forms as ephemeral outlets for the precarious, perverse expression of desire and love. And Cookie appropriates them, too, as an adult-adolescent, working against the neat order of things, as it relates to gender, sexuality, sickness, and writing.

It is also possible to read the form of the short story itself, as it is owned and appropriated by Cookie, before her illness and during, as "adolescent." Many of her stories are rooted in her childhood and adolescence, and even those that focus on her later life, her twenties and thirties, remain adolescently charged, in their narratives and forms.

Indeed, when Carol Mavor writes in *Reading Boyishly* that "the adolescent wastes time," yet "when one is old, one panics at the thought of wasting time," the suggestion of a sickened temporality that touches death at the same time it touches youth comes to the fore.[24] With the pileup of stories that came thick and fast, Cookie's determination in her later writing to document teen anecdotes suggests a queer temporality that strives for both adolescent brevity and lasting posterity.

Cookie's short stories, with their diaries, lists, and letters, represent the "bit before" the novel, the in-between: the adolescent.

<h3 style="text-align:center">1. DIARY</h3>

Cookie's diary-stories are littered with raw attachments to personal information, which she subverts in writing with tricksy, feminist laughter. In "Haight-Ashbury—San Francisco—1967," for example, a story of her West Coast adventures and an LSD capping party gone

wrong, Cookie confesses to her adolescent sexual antics in candid storytelling. She remembers passing a "gathering of women" in which the "blond in the center of the group was extolling the virtues of Jimi Hendrix, after having fucked him the night before." "I walked on by," writes Cookie, adding casually, "I'd fucked him the night before she had."[25] The adult-adolescent writer in Cookie appropriates the conversational chatter of the young girl diary in the public, political space of the short story, teasing the reader with its languid, spoken confessions. This sex talk depicts a girl-adolescent in radical ownership of her own sexuality, but it also reveals a writer in ownership of her past, so that these confessions are not simply spoken, but written, too—in lasting, diary documents of first-person exhibitionism.

<h3 style="text-align:center">2. LETTER</h3>

Part of the reason why I have sought to get close to Cookie by writing a letter is because that's one of the ways she discovered closeness for herself, as when she prefaced a letter sent to her by her friend Gordon Stevenson (the "last letter" she received from him before he died) with a text that works like an epistolary memorial to him, and to the thousands of others dead from AIDS.[26]

Showing the affective pull of correspondence, Cookie's text becomes an open, public letter to Gordon's singular, private letter, when she writes:

"It's like wartime now," my aunt told me a few weeks ago. She lived in France during World War II. "You young people are losing friends and relatives just as if it were bullets taking them away." She's right, it's a war zone, but it's a different battlefield. It's not bullets that catch these soldiers, and there's no bombs and no gunfire. These people are dying in a whisper.[27]

As she thinks through the bodies of the dead through the living words of her aunt, Cookie's epistolary storytelling is her attempt to increase the volume of this whisper. She writes on behalf of her friends' sick bodies, aching to be remembered in their extended adolescence. She turns to the materiality of Gordon's letter and describes it, makes it a metaphor: "It was the

Opposite: Page from one of Mueller's notebooks, undated. Courtesy Ira Silverberg and the Fales Library and Special Collections, New York University.

last letter I received from him. He died the day I got it. I still have it, it's all frayed but the message is crisp."[28] The epistle is weathered and worn, but its message and meaning are fresh and alive with political energy, in spite of its age. And Cookie's reply sends this energy out into the world with a message just as crisp, just as close, driven by desire, perversity, grief, and love: we must write our deathly intimacies in public to make our sicknesses heard. My letter to Cookie is an imaginary chain in this vital correspondence; I reach for her in writing, to resurrect her whispers.

3. LIST

As a doodled indicator of desire, the adolescent's list (often located at the back of a notebook, much like Cookie's) is precarious in its permeability. And it is a form found in her stories, as well as her ephemera, as Cookie, with her artificial lists of clothes and objects, revels in its potential for riotous excess and infinite possibility. In "The Berlin Film Festival—1981," when Cookie is held at customs to be strip-searched ("carrying hashish, cocaine, MDA and opium, of course in small amounts, just tads really…"), she is specific in the details of what she was wearing, a cumbersome array of things to reduce the "bulk of my suitcase": "tights, leg warmers, over-the-knee boots, a dress, two sweaters, a vest, a leather jacket, various fur pieces and a long black coat."[29] Showing the jumbled chaos of her look, like the faulty, unfashionable adolescent, Cookie makes a joke out of her addiction to clothes with the unbounded form of the list.

In reading Cookie's work, it is possible to see the list as a queer form of multiplicity—an "open mesh," we might call it, to pilfer Sedgwick's phrase in her essay "Queer and Now." As she writes in full: "That's one of the things that 'queer' can refer to: the open mesh of possibilities, gaps, overlaps, dissonances and resonances, lapses and excesses of meaning when the constituent elements of anyone's gender, of anyone's sexuality aren't made (or *can't be* made) to signify monolithically."[30] The adolescent's list, as it is played with by Cookie in writing, is open like this mesh, allowing for radical multiplicities. (The relationship between queerness and adolescence is already evident early in Sedgwick's essay, with the much more melancholic recognition that: "I think everyone who does gay and lesbian studies is haunted by the suicides of adolescents.")[31]

The form of the list is aptly used by Cookie in a story about her bisexual adolescence that begins, "I had two lovers and I wasn't ashamed,"[32] one lover being Jack and the other being Gloria, whose hairstyles she catalogues like a hysterical archivist: "I watched her hair-dos from the back. Every day they were different: Beehives, Barrelcurls, Air-Lifts, Pixies, flips, French Twists, Bubbles, Doublebubbles."[33] Gloria is the teenage girl collector of hairsprayed images, queer in her awkward artificiality, her riotous multiplicity, her open mesh, which Cookie gives form to with enumerative words.

In 1997, eight years after Cookie's death, High Risk Books published the anthology *Ask Dr. Mueller*. Its epigraph, taken from Cookie's writings, reads:

Fortunately I am not the first person to tell you that you will never die. You simply lose your body. You will be the same except you won't have to worry about rent or mortgages or fashionable clothes. You will be released from sexual obsessions. You will not have drug addictions. You will not need alcohol. You will not have to worry about cellulite or cigarettes or cancer or AIDS or venereal disease. You will be free. [34]

Was this something she scribbled on one of the back pages of her notebook, feeling the destructive power of the disease? Another of Cookie's lists, it records her most toxic attachments, the things she loved and the things that made her sick, in her life as a writer and in her life *in* stories.

I go to her writing, to feel her fly.
With love.

1 Cookie Mueller, "My Bio—Notes on an American Childhood," in Cookie Mueller, *Walking through Clear Water in a Pool Painted Black* (New York: Semiotext(e), 1990), p. 137.

2 Nan Goldin, *I'll Be Your Mirror* (New York: Whitney Museum of American Art, 1996), p. 256.

3 Nan Goldin, "In the Valley of the Shadow," in *Witnesses: Against Our Vanishing* (New York: Artists Space, 1989), p. 5.

4 Cookie Mueller, "A Last Letter," in *City Lights Review*, no. 2 (1988), p. 51. Earlier versions of this text, of which there are manuscripts in the Serpent's Tail/High Risk Archives, were given the title "Gordon Stevenson," suggesting a much more direct form of obituary. Mueller's preface to Stevenson's letter is shorter, with the focus almost entirely on Stevenson, and Mueller's relationship with him (rather than the AIDS epidemic more widely). In its published versions, it is a text that has gone through many changes. In *City Lights Review*, it is set entirely in roman type; in the Artists Space catalogue, the preface remains in roman but Stevenson's letter has now been set in italics; in the version that was published posthumously in Semiotext(e)'s *Walking through Clear Water in a Pool Painted Black*, the entire text is in italics. A date has also been added to the title of this last version, "Last Letter—1989." The essay does not even appear in a proofreading copy of this book, perhaps suggesting that its late inclusion was a response to Mueller's death, with the different wording of the title placing greater emphasis on Mueller's authorship, her life and death. Its new title, "Last Letter—1989," leads us to think of it as Mueller's last letter, her last word.

5 Cookie Mueller, "Alien," in Cookie Mueller, *Ask Dr. Mueller: The Writings of Cookie Mueller*, ed. Amy Scholder (New York: High Risk Books, 1997), p. 201.

6 Cookie Mueller, "Breaking into Show Bizz," in Cookie Mueller, *Ask Dr. Mueller*, p. 203.

7 Other jobs on her list were "racehorse hot walker… go-go dancer… theater actress, playwright, theatre director, performance artist, house cleaner… credit clerk, barmaid, sailor, high seas cook, film script doctor, herbal therapist, unwed welfare mother, film extra, leg model, watercolorist, and briefly as a barmitzvah entertainer, although I'm not even Jewish." See the autobiographical text "Cookie Mueller, born 1949 Baltimore, Maryland," originally published in Cookie Mueller, *Garden of Ashes*, and reprinted in Cookie Mueller, *Ask Dr. Mueller*, p. 199.

8 Robert Siegle, *Suburban Ambush: Downtown Writing and the Fiction of Insurgency* (Baltimore: Johns Hopkins University Press, 1989), p. 3.

9 Cookie Mueller, "November 1988," in Cookie Mueller, *Ask Dr. Mueller*, p. 285.

10 The quotation is from Cookie Mueller, "Sam's Party—Lower East Side, NYC—1979," in Cookie Mueller, *Walking through Clear Water*, p. 115.

11 "Object of scrutiny" is a term from Cindy Patton, "Performativity and Spatial Distinction: The Ends of AIDS Epidemiology," in Andrew Parker and Eve Kosofsky Sedgwick, eds., *Performativity and Performance* (New York: Routledge, 1995), p. 188.

12 David Wojnarowicz, "Post Cards from America: X-Rays from Hell," in *Witnesses*, p. 11. With Wojnarowicz's essay criticizing Cardinal John O'Connor for keeping "safer-sex information off the local television stations … thereby helping thousands and thousands to their unnecessary deaths," and Senator Jesse Helms's attempt "to dismantle the NEA for supporting the work of Andres Serrano and Robert Mapplethorpe," it was the content of the exhibition catalogue, rather than the works on view, that caused the National Endowment for the Arts, under its chair John Frohnmayer, to rescind the grant given to Artists Space for the exhibition. Artists Space director Susan Wyatt challenged the decision with a great deal of support from the artistic community: the grant was partially restored, but to fund only the exhibition, not the catalogue.

13 Eve Kosofsky Sedgwick, "Memorial for Craig Owens," in Eve Kosofsky Sedgwick, *Tendencies* (Durham, NC: Duke University Press, 1993), p. 105.

14 Eve Kosofsky Sedgwick, "Paranoid Reading and Reparative Reading; or, You're So Paranoid, You Probably Think This Introduction Is about You," in Eve Kosofsky Sedgwick, ed., *Novel Gazing: Queer Readings in Fiction* (Durham, NC: Duke University Press, 1997), p. 24.

15 As Chris Kraus told me in a telephone call on 12 December 2016: "The first book was Cookie Mueller's *Walking through Clear Water in a Pool Painted Black*, and I didn't know Cookie personally, but I had heard her read at the Poetry Project, when she had already been diagnosed with AIDS. It was an amazing reading, and I'd heard through friends that she really wanted to publish this book, but despite her enormous popularity and her knowing everybody in the media and culture world in New York, nobody would publish it as it was. We went to her and said, 'We'll publish your book.'"

16 Cookie Mueller, "Route 95 South—Baltimore to Orlando," and "Abduction & Rape—Highway 31 Elkton, Maryland—1969," in Cookie Mueller, *Walking through Clear Water*, pages 34 and 51, respectively. The title of the latter story includes the city and state on the book's table of contents, but on the story's title page, it is given only as "Abduction & Rape—Highway 31—1969."

17 Cookie Mueller, "Cookie Mueller, born 1949 Baltimore, Maryland," originally published in Cookie Mueller, *Garden of Ashes*, and reprinted in Cookie Mueller, *Ask Dr. Mueller*, p. 199.

18 Cookie Mueller, notebook, undated, Serpent's Tail/High Risk Archives, MSS 86, Box V.II.1, Folder 17, Fales Library and Special Collections, New York University Libraries. Reproduced with the permission of Ira Silverberg.

19 Cookie Mueller, handwritten page, undated, Serpent's Tail/High Risk Archives, MSS 86, Box V.II.1, Folder 14, Fales Library and Special Collections, New York University Libraries. Reproduced with the permission of Ira Silverberg.

20 Cookie Mueller, "Cookie Mueller, born 1949 Baltimore, Maryland," originally published in Cookie Mueller, *Garden of Ashes*, and reprinted in Cookie Mueller, *Ask Dr. Mueller*, p. 199.

21 Denise Duhamel, "Beauties Who Live Only for an Afternoon," in Brandon Stosuy, ed., *Up Is Up, But So Is Down: New York's Downtown Literary Scene, 1974–1992* (New York: New York University Press, 2006), p. 305.

22 Among the periodicals that published Mueller's writing were the *East Village Eye*, *Avenue E*, *Verbal Abuse*, *Just Another Asshole*, *Bomb*, *Top Stories*, and *Wild History*.

23 Cookie Mueller, "Go-Going—New York & New Jersey—1978–79," in Cookie Mueller, *Walking through Clear Water*, pp. 100–101.

24 Carol Mavor, *Reading Boyishly: Roland Barthes, J. M. Barrie, Jacques Henri Lartigue, Marcel Proust, and D. W. Winnicott* (Durham, NC: Duke University Press, 2007), p. 339.

25 Cookie Mueller, "Haight-Ashbury—San Francisco, California—1967," in Cookie Mueller, *Walking through Clear Water*, p. 8. The title of the story is rendered in this way on the table of contents, but is given as "Haight Ashbury—San Francisco—1967" on the story's title page.

26 Cookie Mueller, "A Last Letter," *City Lights Review*, no. 2, p. 51.

27 Ibid.

28 Ibid.

29 Cookie Mueller, "The Berlin Film Festival—Berlin, West Germany—1981," in Cookie Mueller, *Walking through Clear Water*, pp. 126–127. The title of the story is rendered in this way on the table of contents, but is given simply as "The Berlin Film Festival—1981" on the story's title page.

30 Eve Kosofsky Sedgwick, "Queer and Now," in Eve Kosofsky Sedgwick, *Tendencies*, p. 8.

31 Ibid., p. 1.

32 Cookie Mueller, "Two People—Baltimore—1964," in Cookie Mueller, *Walking through Clear Water*, p. 1.

33 Ibid., p. 2.

34 Cookie Mueller, epigraph to Cookie Mueller, *Ask Dr. Mueller*, p. v.

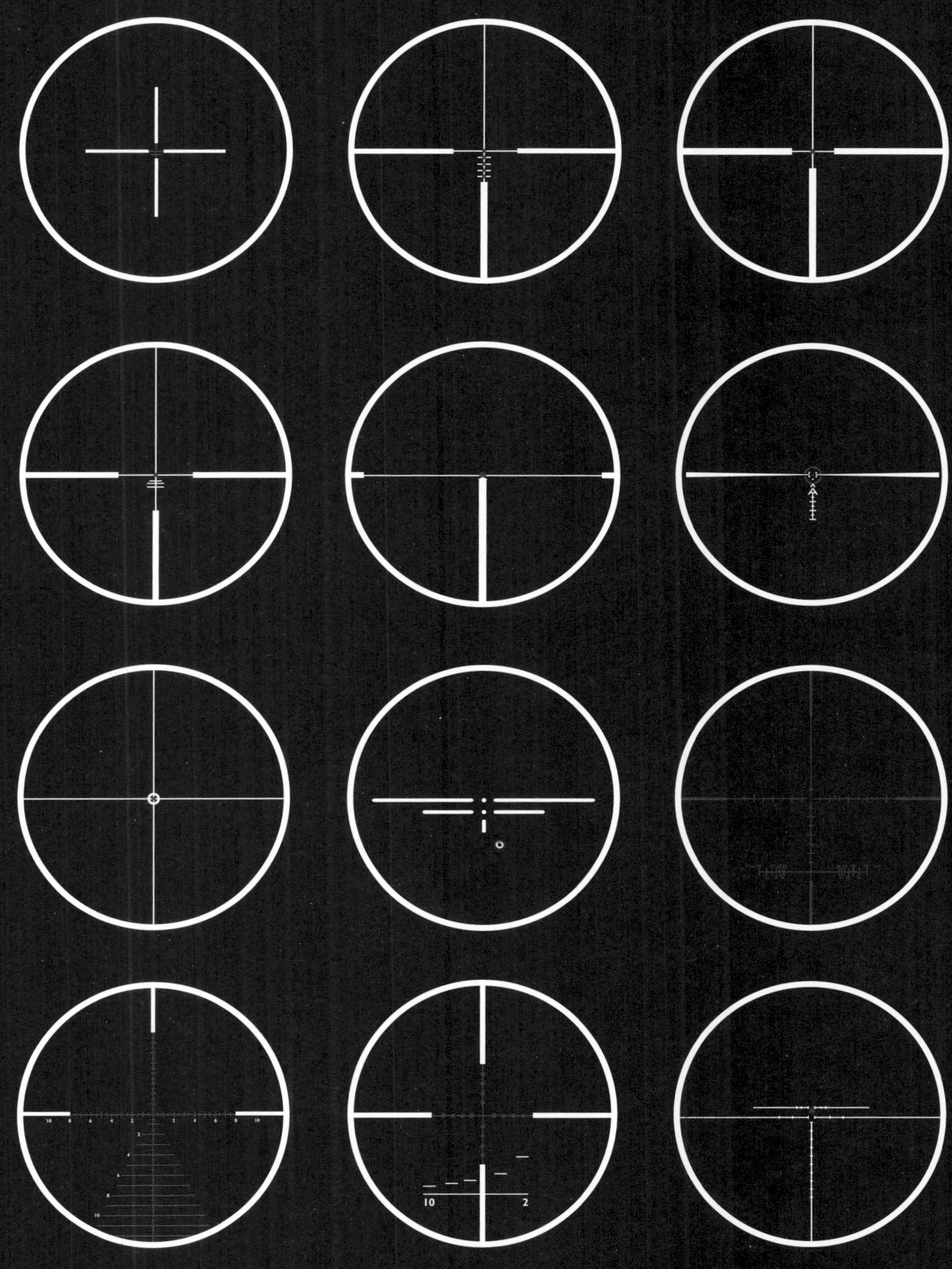

A selection of riflescope reticles available from Kahles,
an Austrian optical instruments manufacturer.

SPIDERS, STARS, AND DEATH
D. Graham Burnett

In the autumn of 2016, Colin Kaepernick, the African-American quarterback of the San Francisco–based American football team known as the "49ers," initiated a quiet protest in response to a series of well-publicized police shootings of black men under questionable circumstances: he ceased to stand for the singing of the national anthem. By early October, his gesture had drawn considerable attention, spawned emulation, and attracted virulent hostility. Perhaps the most notorious instance of the latter? The sale of T-shirts featuring his image under the superimposed conventional iconography of impending death: the plus-sign-within-a-ring figure knows as "crosshairs."

It will be worth taking a moment to recover a genealogy for this potent symbol—the universal modern index of imminent violent killing.

• • •

One morning in the late 1630s, in Yorkshire, not far from the town of Leeds, a gentleman by the name of William Gascoigne (he was then twenty-eight or so) rose and returned to his avocation: tinkering with one of the very new "viewing tubes" that had become the rage among learned persons across Europe and beyond in the wake of celebrated publications by Galileo and Descartes. Gascoigne enjoyed the company of a circle of provincial virtuosi in the Midlands, and he was justifiably proud of his success in securing and configuring the lenses necessary to make a reasonably powerful telescope, one that made use of the design advocated by Johannes Kepler—two biconvex lenses mounted in a cylinder of brass (or sometimes lacquered leather). Gascoigne's tube was not, however, hermetically sealed. For on this particular day, turning to his observations, he was startled to discern, in the visual field of his instrument, clearly delineated upon whatever he viewed, a thread-like filament. Further investigation revealed that a spider had, overnight, insinuated itself into his optical device, and had begun to spin a web therein. As fate would have it, the creature had undertaken this fruitless endeavor in the precise focal plane of the objective lens—producing an uncanny effect: a clear, distinct, and ultrafine line that seemed to hover over whatever Gascoigne observed though his telescope. He wrote of the discovery to his friend, the

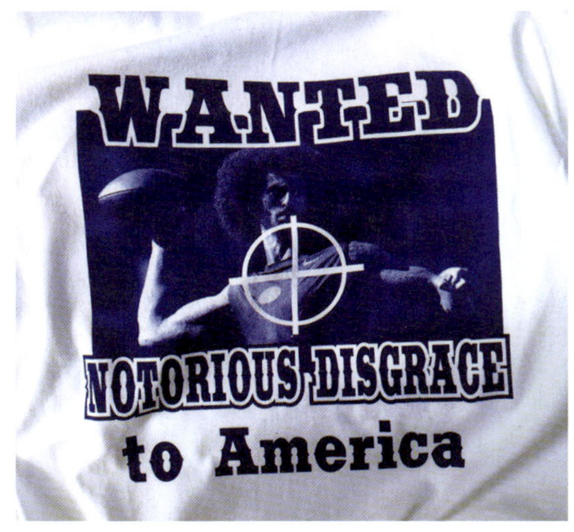

T-shirt targeting Colin Kaepernick for sale outside the Buffalo Bills' stadium when the team hosted the San Francisco 49ers on 16 October 2016.

mathematician William Oughtred, declaring it a providential gift from the "All Disposer" Himself.

Why? Because that serendipitous bit of silk immediately suggested a technique for introducing index lines into telescopic (and microscopic) instruments—lines that could be used to make metrical observations newly precise. Following the spider's principle, Gascoigne soon configured the world's first "micrometer," in effect a tiny ruler within the viewing tube, suitable for taking the measure of celestial bodies.

The whole episode marks the origin of what has come to be called (since the early eighteenth century) the reticle: "A grid or other pattern of fine threads, wires, lines, etc., in the focal plane or eyepiece of a telescope or other optical instrument in order to facilitate positioning, aiming, and measurement."

The crosshairs of our contemporary death-wishes are a species in the reticle genus: we could designate them *Reticulum trucidatorum*, the reticle of the assassins.

• • •

Importantly, then: for most of the history of crosshairs, these fine lines were trained on the heavens. The bulk labor of astronomers for several centuries consisted of the making and refining of star charts, necessary to navigation and cartography. The perfecting

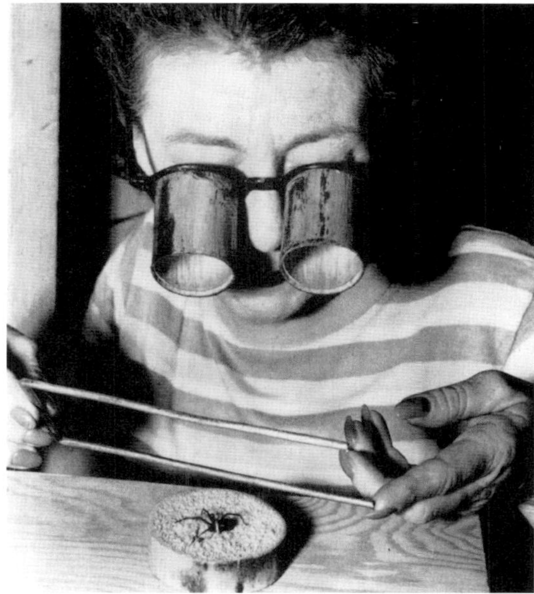

Nan Songer, who like Mary Pfeiffer supplied manufacturers with spider silk for crosshairs, extracting the material from one of her charges. Photo from *Natural History*, November 1955.

of such celestial maps hinged on the observation of stellar "transits," the passage of a given star across the "meridian"—which amounts to the measurement of the star's "noon," its apogee in the sky, its highest point on a given night from a given location.

Which is to say, for hundreds of years, we used crosshairs to take aim at rising stars. In dark observatories, peaceful, patient snipers waited, watching the bright specks walk slowly into their sights—which were often called "spider lines," no wire or thread or etching having proven as fine and resilient as the silk of the web weavers.

. . .

The unholy marriage of the gun and the telescope came late. Not until the middle of the nineteenth century were rifles sufficiently accurate that a marksman, taking aim squintingly down the barrel, could wish for preternatural sight—could want to see beyond the reach of his eyes, more clearly to direct the lead slug at his command. While there had been experiments with telescopic range finders for cannons, and while a few early suggestions of gunsights that made use of lenses can be found, it is really only with the publication of the English-born American engineer John Ratcliffe

Chapman's 1848 *Instructions to Young Marksmen* that we find wide dissemination of the design for an integrated telescope-rifle, suitable for improved death-dealing at long range. The idea caught on rapidly. The catalogues for the Crystal Palace exhibition of 1851 list a number of the novel systems, and by the US Civil War, carefully selected "sharpshooters" were training spider-silk crosshairs on human beings in combat.

This is the earliest account of the killing of a specific person by telescopic sight that I have been able to find. It reports a skirmish in Virginia in April of 1862: "Several times one bolder than the rest would take off his cap and wave it defiantly in the air, and upon one occasion, while doing this [sic], Colonel Berdan directed one of his men to wing him. Notwithstanding the distance, at least thirteen hundred (1,300) yards, the unerring telescopic rifle brought down the bold rebel."

In scenes like this, we turned an instrument for measuring the heavens into a new mechanism for effecting fatal action at a distance.

. . .

As late as 1941, in Hoboken, New Jersey, a woman named Mary Pfeiffer remained employed, as she had been since 1889, collecting some two thousand feet of spider silk every year for use in gunsights and optical instruments. During World War II, black widows were amassed at the military base of Fort Knox, and milked for their weapon-grade web-strands.

. . .

It amounts, perhaps, to this: our primary global icon of hate is a kind of re-fallen angel. Those nearly invisible threads by which the spider craftily seizes its prey became, for a time, nothing less than the rational yardstick of the infinitesimal and the infinite. But it did not last. Repurposed by the men-at-arms, those same micro-meticulous reticles once again snared victims, who danced with death on the head of a pin.

. . .

Genealogy cannot save us. But it offers options, queers conditions—e.g., every person upon whom the cross-hairs fall momentarily shares the subject position of a celestial body, cresting across its apogee in the night sky.

Strangely enough, the astronomers call this point in the transit of a star its *culmination*.

ARTIST PROJECT / RECONCILIATION
S. Billie Mandle

Saint Christopher, the enigmatic martyr and patron saint of travelers and children who bore the increasingly heavy Christ child across a deadly river before his own decapitation, bears brown water stains across his acoustical tiles. Light falls in displaced blades through his half-shut opening, across his little ledge, glaring the green cover of a volume lying there, angling down brown half-wall panels into the shadow realm. Saint Elizabeth—who vanishes from the Bible eight days after giving birth, when the men who are to circumcise her son arrive and try to name him Zechariah, whereupon she cries out, "No, he is to be called John!" for this is John the Baptist—is transformed, as in a Greek myth, into the black constellations of perforations in her soundproof paneling, then mantled with a jointed beam of light. And Saint Thomas More, intently principled, severe and merciless, who would not bow to kings, is a single, narrow ray plunging down a wooden wall, illuminating the grain in patterns reminiscent of a seizure patient's EKG.

For seven years, S. Billie Mandle traveled across the United States, photographing church confessionals, searching, she has written, "for what might be left behind in these private rooms." One recognition she came to—documented in her series *Reconciliation*, selections from which are presented here—is that the imprint of what these spaces not only witnessed but lived through was so palpably vivid that the rooms themselves assumed the character of the church's heroic intercessors. These chambers carried scars suggesting martyrdom and sacrifice—as well as lyric plays of light and color, attesting to the possibility of grace. In both their luminous composure and rank degradation, we sense the extreme experiences that once quivered the air here, reflected by and absorbed into the well-worn surfaces. This may help explain why the pictures share a kind of harrowing "afterlife" quality with early Nan Goldin hotel rooms, when Goldin was helping to develop the language of "confessional art."

Though the obligation and urge to confess may be among the primal religious responses to unsanctioned acts and wishes, it was at the Fourth Lateran Council in 1215 that the Roman Catholic Church first announced that church members must make at least one annual confession to avoid excommunication. This injunction was accompanied by the elimination of trial by ordeal, which some historians believe prompted legal courts to embrace confession, together with eyewitness testimony, as the core evidentiary props of secular law. The penitent, like the defendant, became "authenticated by the discourse of truth he was able or obliged to pronounce concerning himself," writes the philosopher Chloë Taylor. Michel Foucault understood the new emphasis on the individual, embodied in the act of confession, as a critical stage in a greater process of "individualization."[1]

It was at least 350 years after the council that private booths were introduced, with their visual cloaks and verbal apertures, consummating what's been described as the church's shift from "monstration to articulation."[2] Among the earliest allusions to the contrivance of a box with a grille on one side through which the kneeling penitent could "pour the story of his sins into the ghostly father's ears" occurs at Valencia in 1565.[3] A decade later, a reference to a rudimentary confessional in Milan crops up. Over the next ten years, boxes manifest in Aix and Toulouse. Throughout the seventeenth century, confessionals become increasingly ubiquitous.

Warnings about their susceptibility to abuse multiply in tandem with their spreading popularity, mostly as part of broader indictments of Popish doctrine and practices. As one early eighteenth-century Baptist sermon railed, the confessional presented "the utmost danger of violating all rules of modesty and decency, by putting questions, under pretence of searching sin to the bottom, which shall suggest wicked thoughts to the minds of young and inexperienced persons," along with being calculated "to put the poor penitent wholly in the priest's power with regard to estate, and reputation, and even life itself."[4] This twofold indictment of these archaic containers remained the principal line of attack for generations. Yet on the question of power, Foucault, exploring how spatial relations evolved in tandem with the demands of new discursive practices, saw the rooms both enhancing opportunities for surveillance and

facilitating the conferral of consolation. To Foucault, the confessional booth represented "the material crystallization of all the rules."[5] Indeed, notwithstanding the perils of sequestered anonymity pertaining to these spaces, there were always those in and outside the church who saw therapeutic possibilities attached to their lack of transparency. Voltaire, among the church's most vehement adversaries, characterized confession as an "excellent thing," a "curb to the greater crimes," and "the greatest curb on secret crimes."[6]

Misgivings about the vulnerabilities of these booths to exploitative confessors, combined with diminished faith in the efficacy of forgiveness that could be dispensed from them, culminated in the 1970s with a precipitous drop-off in confessions. Numbers never really recovered. Recently, churches have been eliminating confessionals altogether and replacing them with "reconciliation" spaces that embrace face-to-face dialogues with priests. Conversations less concerned with judging and prescribing penitential measures than with cultivating frank exchanges modeled on talk therapy. Confession is now everywhere in our culture, but has blurred with self-expression—as such, it has become a right more than a responsibility, with authority invested in one's own firsthand experience rather than any auditor, human or divine.

A twilit, elegiac atmosphere in many of Mandle's images resonates with the confessional's progressive disempowerment, and perhaps foreshadows their eventual total obsolescence. On balance, given their contributions to the bodily and spiritual afflictions of their occupants, this may be for the best. Yet, as Mandle's photographs reveal, these rooms are also richly layered repositories of passions spent and forever pent inside. We may feel grateful that such an archive exists. The smooth glass cages of our devices will preserve no physical relics of our psychic suffering. In a poignant twist of faith, Mandle has created images that allow us to begin achieving reconciliation with the confessionals themselves.

—George Prochnik

1 My overview of the history of the confessional is deeply indebted both to Chloë Taylor, *The Culture of Confession from Augustine to Foucault* (New York: Routledge, 2009) and to Alexander Freund, "'Confessing Animals': Toward a *Longue Durée* History of the Oral History Interview," *Oral History Review*, vol. 41, no. 1 (Winter–Spring 2014).

2 The genesis of this reading in relation to Foucault's history of the confessional is traced in Brian T. Kaylor, *Presidential Campaign Rhetoric in an Age of Confessional Politics* (Plymouth, UK: Lexington Books, 2011); see in particular p. 194.

3 Henry Charles Lea, *A History of Auricular Confession and Indulgences in the Latin Church* (Philadelphia: Lea Brothers & Co., 1896), pp. 394–396.

4 Joseph Burroughs, *The Popish Doctrine of Auricular Confession and Priestly Absolution Considered: A Sermon Preached at Salters-Hall, March 13, 1734* (London: Printed for J. Noon and J. Gray, 1735).

5 Cited by Sara Mills in "Geography, Gender and Power," in *Space, Knowledge and Power: Foucault and Geography*, ed. Jeremy W. Crampton and Stuart Elden (New York: Routledge, 2007), p. 50.

6 Raphael Melia, *A Treatise on Auricular Confession, Dogmatical, Historical, & Practical* (Dublin and London: James Duffy, 1865), p. 94.

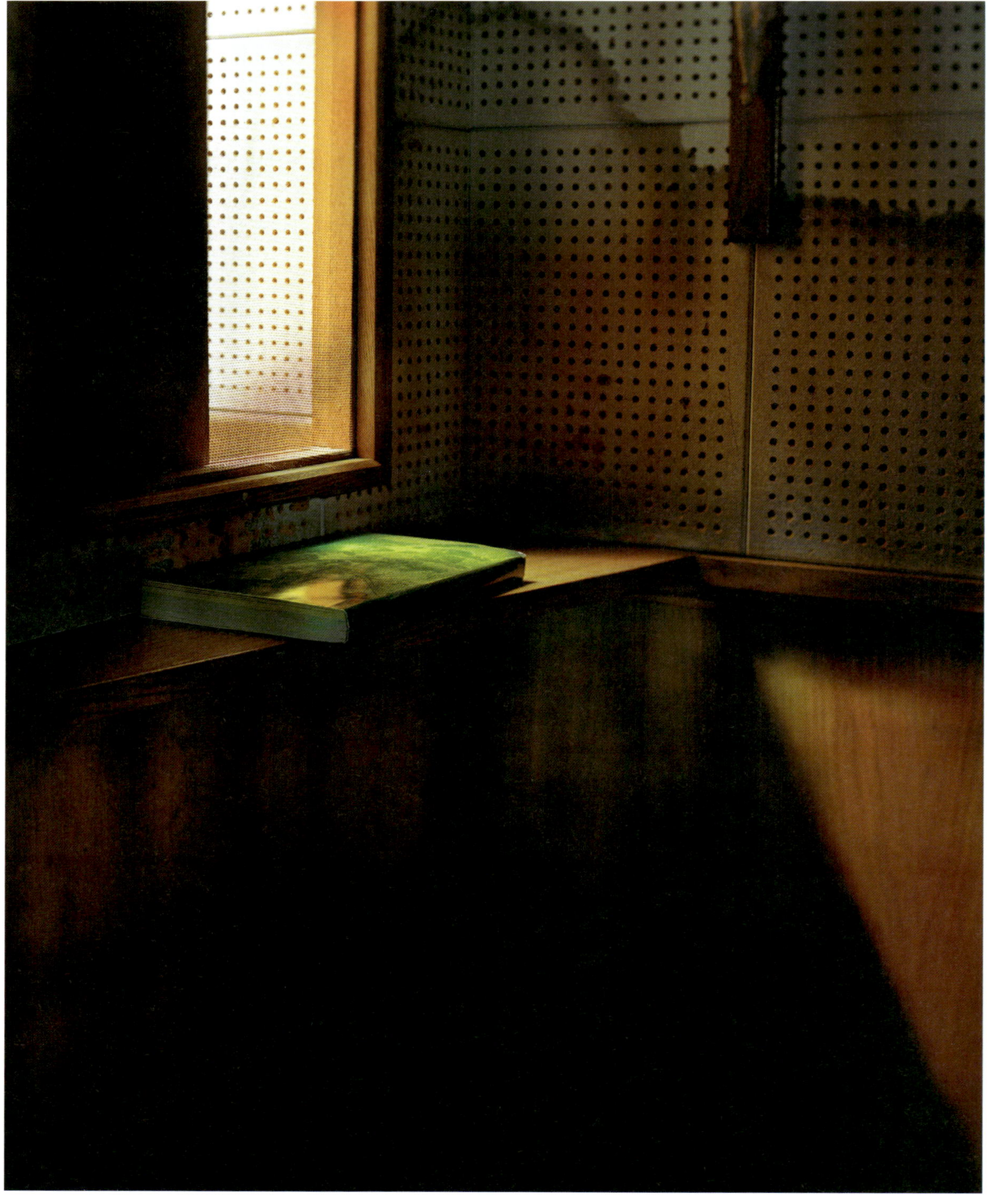

Saint Christopher.

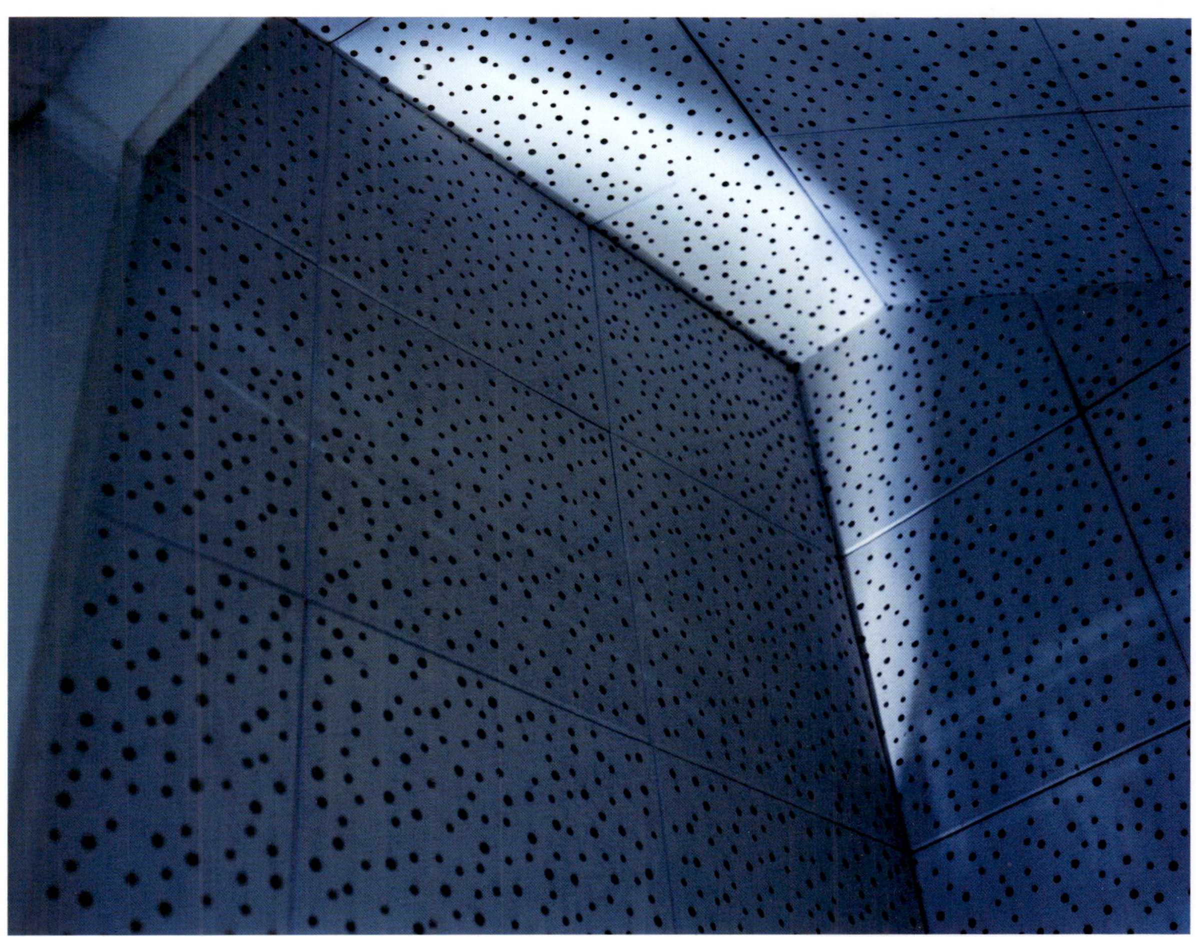

Saint Elizabeth.

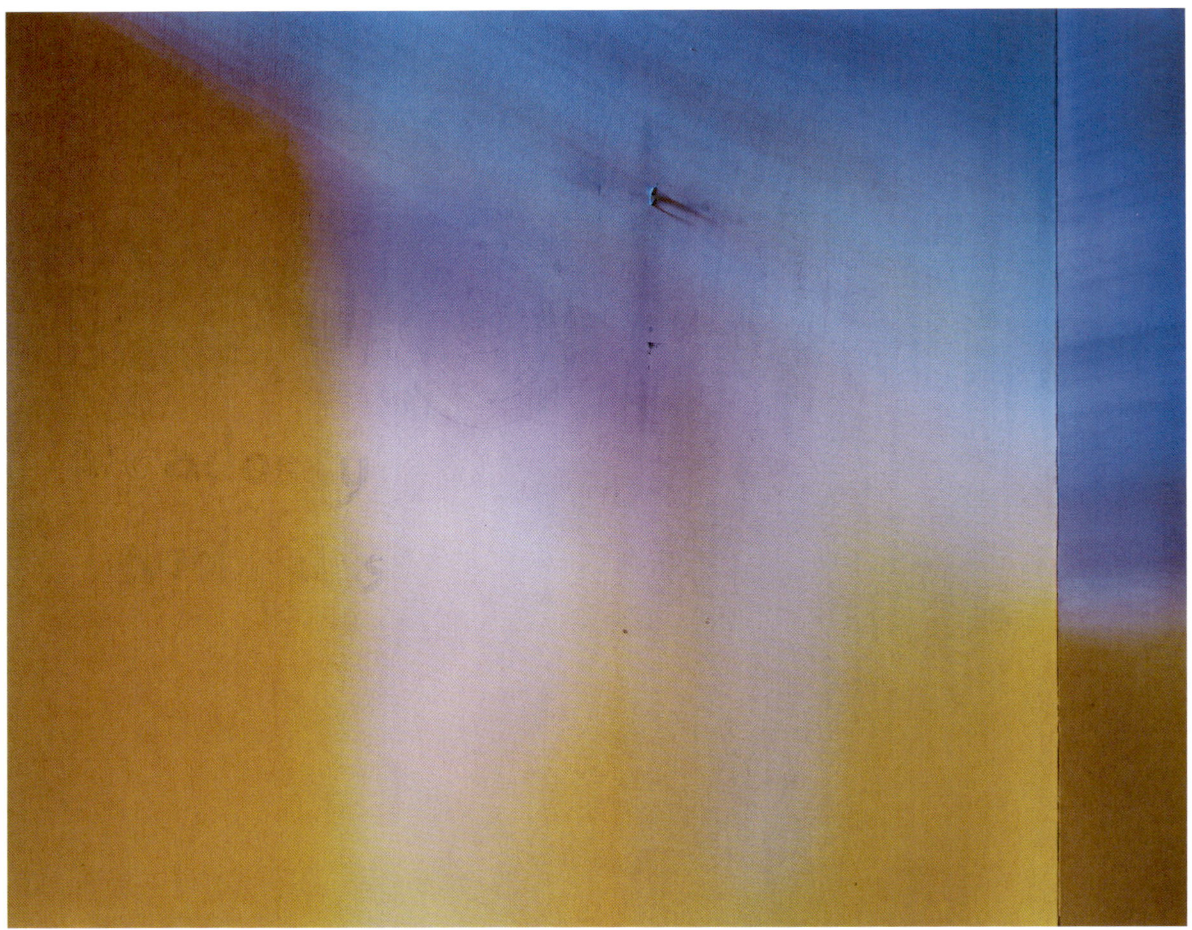

Saint Joseph.

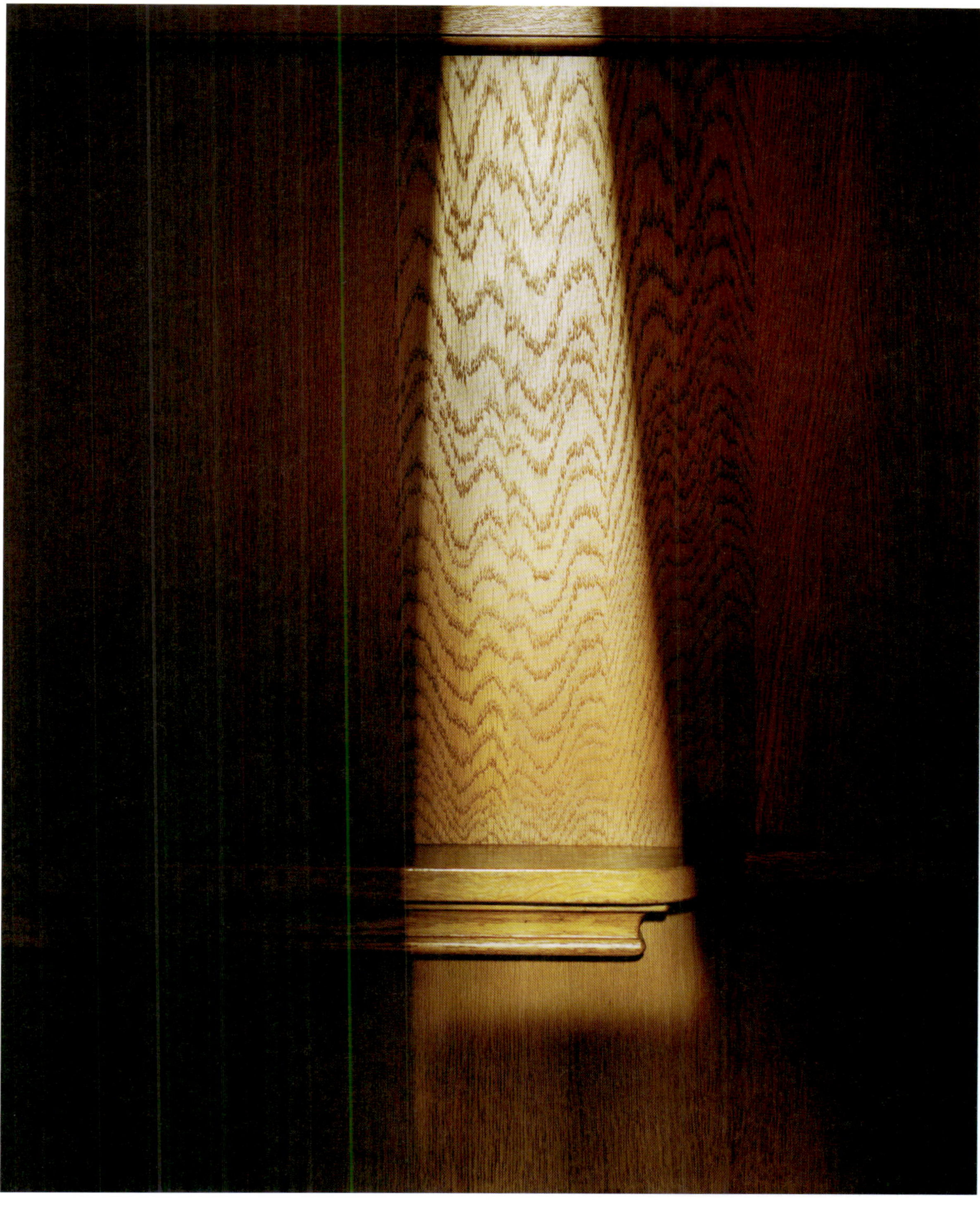

Saint Thomas More.

Saint Peter.

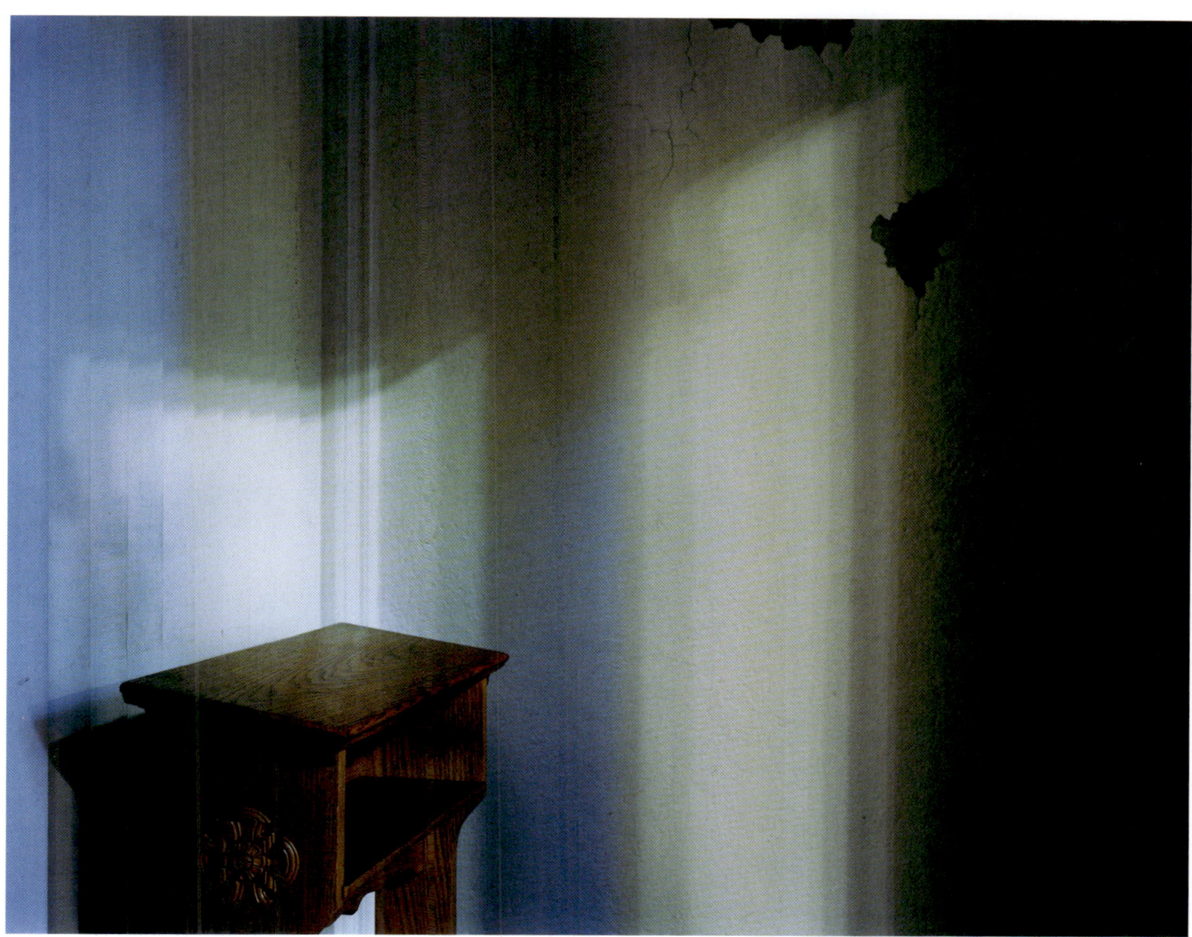

Saint Pancras.

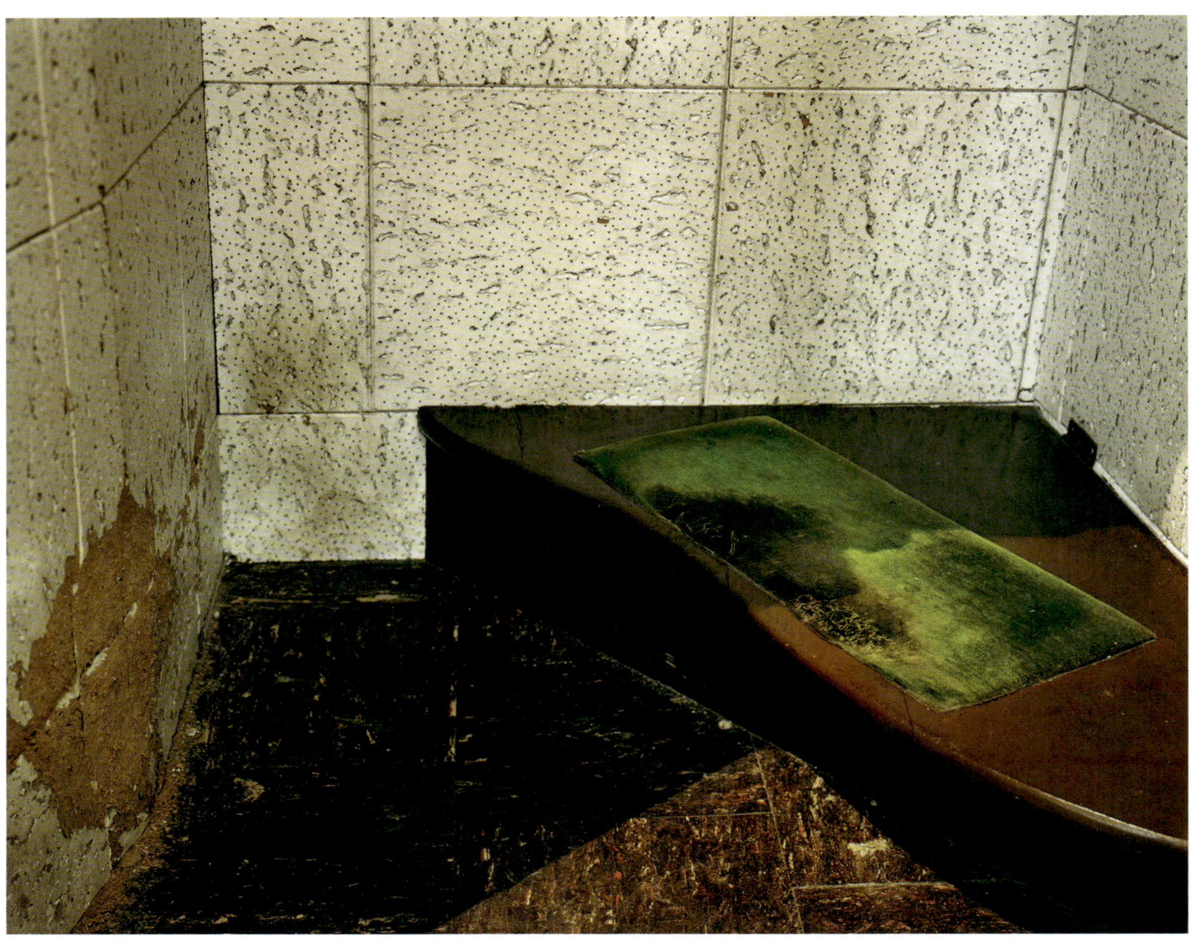

Our Lady of Perpetual Help.

CARDINAL DIRECTIONS
Marta Figlerowicz

"Your country's going to hell," said the immigration officer who checked my green card at JFK airport on my way back from Poland. It was October 2016, and Poland was reeling from a wave of conservative reforms instituted by our new, right-wing government. The officer—his name was Jeremy—knew a lot about politics, and we started talking, even though there was a line of impatient travelers behind me. Jeremy was reading a radical socialist pamphlet under his desk. He shoved it at me: it was a hastily stapled, crookedly xeroxed wad of papers. "I'm left of Bernie Sanders," he said. "I'm left of Karl Marx and even of Jesus." He finally stamped my passport. "America's going to hell, too," he declared as he handed it back to me. We both laughed; this still seemed like a sympathetic overstatement.

Back in the eighties and nineties, before my move from Poland to America, changes in time zone seemed equivalent to actual time travel. We would look out onto the West for models of the forward path we were hoping to take. Turning around, we would look east to shudder at the past we were leaving behind. We probably wouldn't catch up with Europe and the United States for a while, we assumed, but this delay also gave us a comforting sense of control over our future. If one had the money to drive over to Germany or France, or maybe even fly out to visit family in Chicago, one could get a sneak peek of what this glorious, capitalist future would look like. At the same time, the further we got from our own Soviet period, the more our neighbors to the east seemed stuck in that earlier era. East of Poland, the other Slavs were using our discarded train cars, and movies arrived in their theaters months after ours. Before long, we were making these comparisons with nostalgia rather than with fear. Indeed, taking a page out of *Goodbye, Lenin,* some older people I knew began to travel to Ukraine or Belarus to relive their twenties.

Poland was still catching up with the Western future, and fleeing the Russian-occupied past, even in 2010. That was when its centrist coalition government incurred the disaster that would ensure a right-wing takeover of both the executive and the legislative government six years later. Ninety-six passengers, most of them high-ranking politicians, died in a plane that crashed in the Russian city of Smoleńsk. They had been on their way to Katyń, a site where the Red Army shot thousands of Polish intelligentsia during World War II. The liberal left attributed the crash to human error and bad weather. But on the right, conspiracy theories blamed it on the Russian government and on the centrist Polish leaders who—it was said—had been their allies. Their view became increasingly popular, as national pride swelled over the notion that the Russians had gone to so much trouble to destroy our government. The incident also invited parallels to 9/11, which made Poland seem not only decisively non-Russian, but akin to the major Western powers whom countries east of us continued to oppose. Poles were vaguely proud that our national tragedy had involved aircraft; as official investigations of its causes prolonged themselves, many also began to take pleasure in their endlessness. Every Polish citizen of my generation has a story about where they were when they first heard of the crash, the way that most Americans know exactly where they were on 9/11. I, for one, found out about it in Cleveland, Ohio, around 5 am local time. I'd stepped out of my conference hotel to smoke and brace myself for my morning flight. As I lit up, a neon crawl on an adjacent building began announcing that half of my national government was dead.

But shortly after Smoleńsk, these narratives of catching up with the West became ever less appealing. The year 2010 was also when the great recession overtook Eastern Europe, leaving many Poles resentful of Western mirages of prosperity. As it became ever clearer that capitalism wasn't working for us as well as we'd expected, people began to suspect that perhaps it hadn't been an ideal goal for Poland all along. Instead, the European Union had merely colonized and indoctrinated our unknowing population.

And then, our national sense of time inverted even further: as I watched the neo-conservative consolidation of power in the United States, the events I had witnessed in Poland only weeks before the American election loomed before me like foreshadowings of what was to come. For once, it seemed as if Poland had gotten there first. The Polish government became right wing eight months before Trump won the presidential election. The first mass antigovernmental demonstrations in Warsaw occurred about three months before the Women's March. These former demonstrations

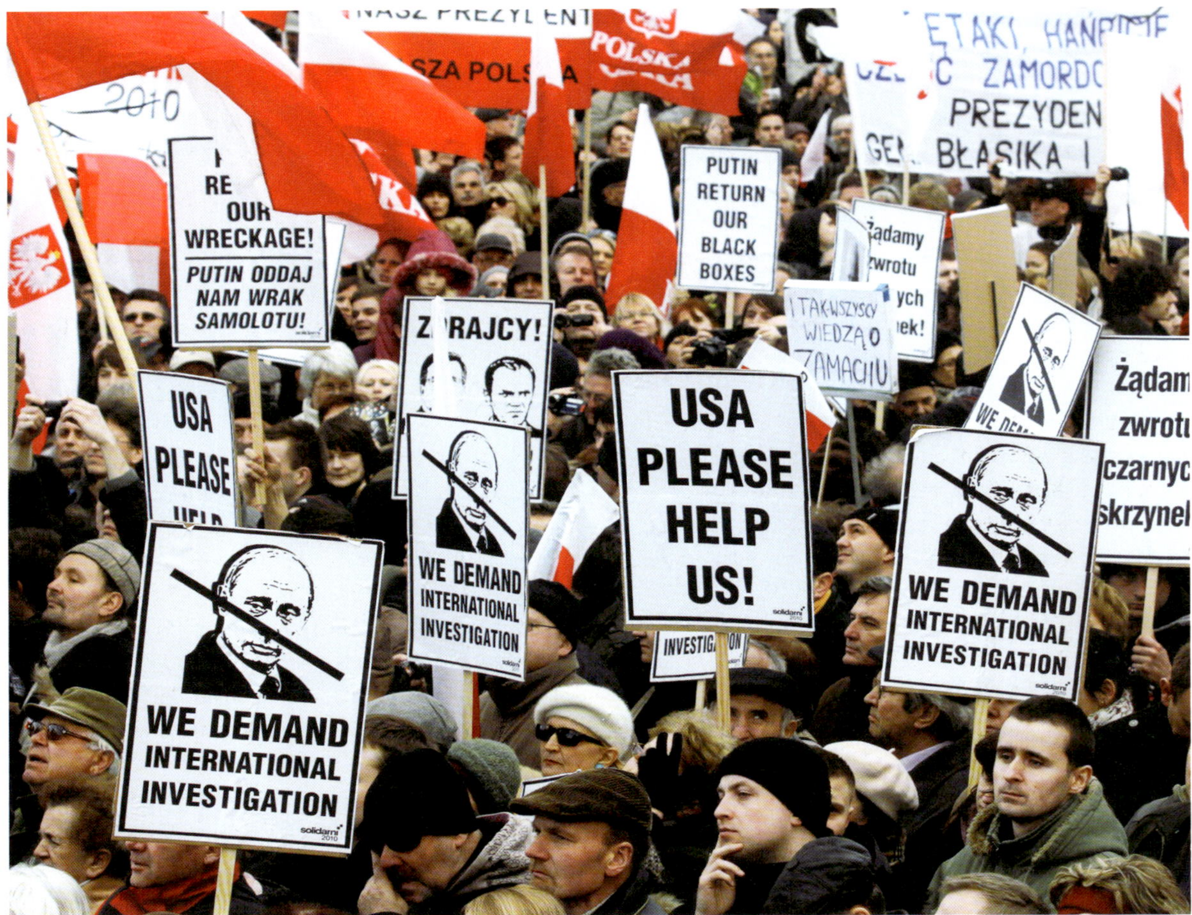

were women's marches, too—and indeed, their major (if not only) trigger had been a looming repeal of Poland's equivalent of *Roe v. Wade*. Back in fall 2016, the US press had covered the unrest in Poland with a certain condescension; little did anyone think that these same fundamental rights could come under fire in the West only a few months later.

Throughout February, the Polish press noted our tragicomic political precocity with triumphant, if somewhat masochistic, *Schadenfreude*. Writing for Anglophone audiences, Slawomir Sierakowski boldly proclaimed that the West now needed to look east to see what it is about to become, and prepare for it. As I marched down Fifth Avenue toward Trump Tower in the Women's March, while Louis Vuitton employees gazed down at us from their second-floor outlet and the bells of the nearby St. Patrick's Cathedral switched from the noon call to prayer to Lady Gaga's "Paparazzi," I similarly couldn't shake my sense of *déjà vu*.

But despite this *Groundhog Day* air of necromantic certainty, what I felt was mostly disorientation. These various local outbursts seemed additive, rather than repetitive, their prospects as indiscernible in New York as they were in Warsaw. The protests' broader triggers, as well as their human expressions, differed in ways that accidents of adjacent timing hid only from a vague aerial view. Whatever else I wanted to tell myself, I no longer knew where the future would come from. Indeed, I was not sure anymore why I had migrated to America in the first place. Back in the day, when I was leaving Poland, people saw my move as a bold, politically progressive choice; now, it seemed sadly quietist, like an attempt to live not in history, but in an idea of where history had already gone.

———

Above: Demonstration in Warsaw on 10 April 2011 marking the first anniversary of the plane crash in Smoleńsk, Russia.

MILK

JOURNEYS OF LACTIC ABSTRACTION
Melanie Jackson and Esther Leslie

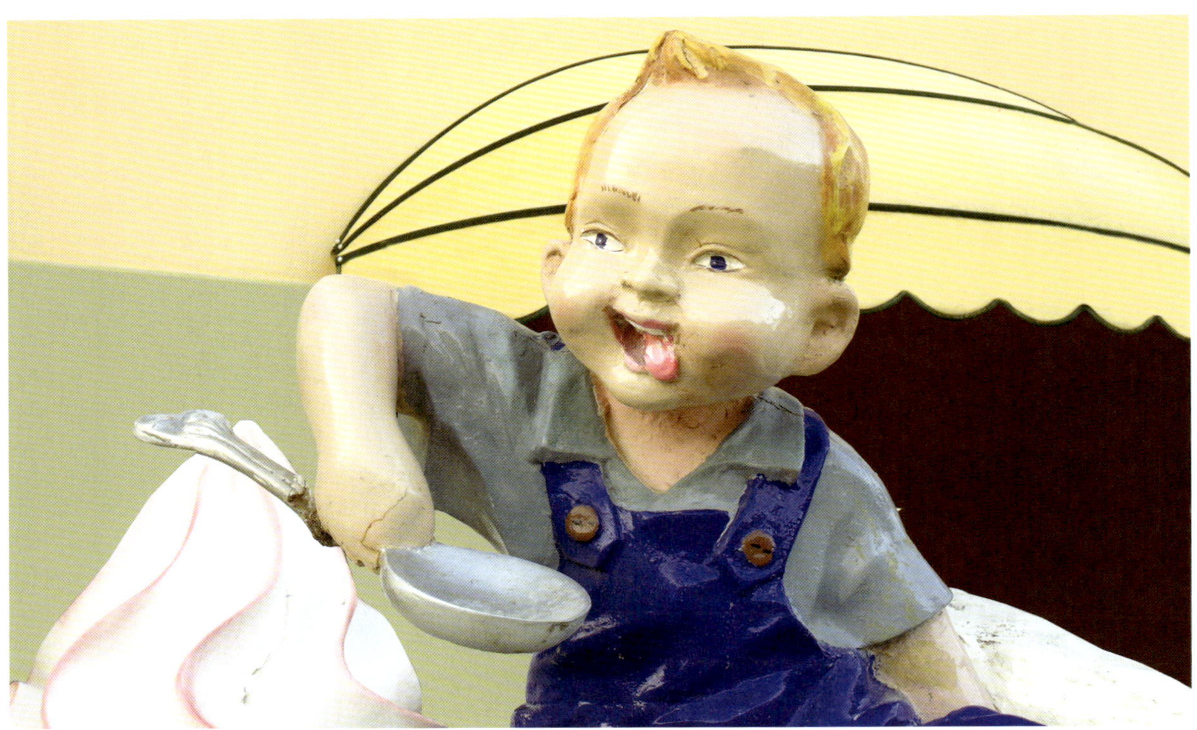

MILK AND BEGINNINGS

Milk is a primal substance. Milk is the first fluid to enter our mouths, to touch the tongue, to fill the belly. Our first words form around it and it flows into our language: in our thoughts and actions, we skim, condense, homogenize, express, churn, curdle, culture, sour, combine, separate. Milk, the milk of human kindness, is there with life from its beginnings and is essential for its continuation. For a premodern order, milk was life-giving and productive. Life, milk-sustained life, linked to fate and destiny. The land that flows with milk and honey was a specific reference to the homeland of a herder people—Canaan. This bountiful pasture became the model of a life sweet and fulfilled. Contemporary idiomatic speech is replete with spilt milk, milksops, milch cows, cash cows, sacred cows, the milk-hearted, the milk-livered, milk for free, milking it, milking it for all it's worth—all expressions of negativity, weakening, and exploitation. These phrases signal something of our contemporary dis-ease with anything that evokes dependency, an abject state in an age dominated by a form of capital that despises welfare, but thrives on precarity. There is, then, a milky language that speaks to our emotions, our socialization, and our hopes. If we disrupt milk's turbid body, it may be mobilized as a "filter" through which to explore the contradictions of the present.

Milk is primary, but also multiple. It is liquid, solid, powder, emulsion. It is poured, pressed, molded, cast, extruded. It is formless, but can take on any form, even indexing other things that press into it when solidified. It adopts shapes, of vessels or the shapes made of it or in it, when in solid form. Milk is a substance prone to mimesis and abstraction, a duality echoed in the ebullient packaging that places it before us as an industrial staple. For pats of butter or rich creamy milks, there are countless hand-drawn bucolic scenes, realistically formed, that essentialize the gift of nature, of the mother, Mother Nature. Equally, milk is prone to abstraction through technical processing into

Above: Melanie Jackson, *The Lick 2*, 2016. This fiberglass mascot from northern France was part of a larger display advertising ice cream.

powdered formulas or constituent parts. This abstraction is reflected in the aseptic geometries of plastic cartons, milk sticks, and Tetra Pak pyramids. The representations on the packaging and the forms of the container either reinforce sentimentalized versions of the chains that lead from cows to humans via commodification, or they bask in the alienation foregrounded by the technologies of production and the industrial triumph of invariant standardization.

Milk is a complicated liquid. It lends itself to reformulation and innovation, just as it reinforces existing social orders as natural. Milk articulates the rules of the nanny and the boss, as well as the technologist and the venture capitalist: it adapts to every kind of flow that the economy demands. Milk participates in a busy activity of human and bovine transformations. In solid, liquid, and powder forms, it is the matter of infinite innovation. Milk is refined, monetized, mechanized, and modernized. It is processed and recombined to extend its functionality.

Below: The Nesquik bunny hawking his wares.

The McFlurry, Mr. Whippy, Dairy Queen Blizzard, Cheese String, Dreaming Cow, Laughing Cow, Skinny Cow, Happy Cow, Crusha, Marvel—these dairy icons perform health and the abuse of health; an array of high-calorie, high-fat, low-calorie, low-fat, high-sugar, sugar-free, highly processed glimmer, with techno-scientific, multicolor, hedonistic, and eroticized appeal. These are the products of aggressive marketing, of low-margin, highly complex modes of manufacture. Dairy turns airy in ice creams that swell up with nothingness injected, and, as with microfoams in coffee, this airiness—or "overrun," as it is known in the industry—not only changes the texture, but also seems to stand as a symbol of milk's overinflated presence and excessive connotative ability in contemporary culture. Transgressive in relation to species origin, and in relation to the edicts of health, yet utterly pervasive, many of these hypernormative products are pitched at young people and children. They collaborate with a plethora of high-energy animated mascots in ecstatic reverie, weaning children from the breast and the bottle through a sugary lure.

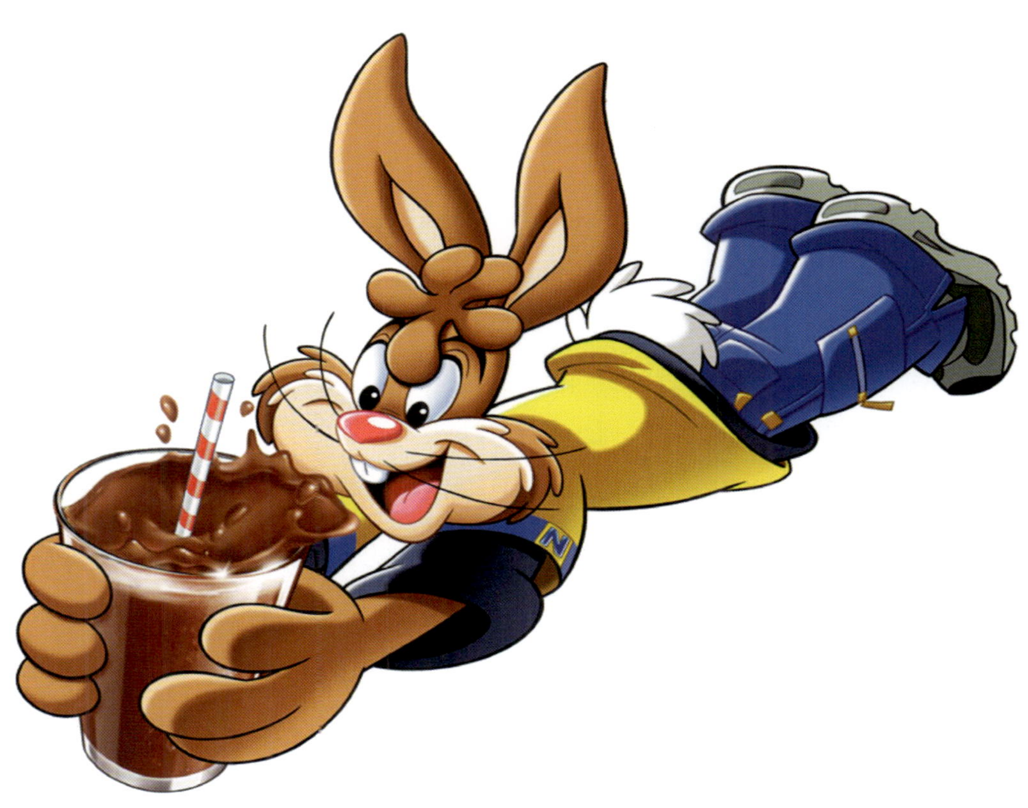

Milk's propensity for animation, for shape-shifting and transformation, teams it commercially with a bestiary of cartoon avatars and a dazzling spectrum of synthetic colors. Milk is frozen into colorful crystals with personality for a teeming frozen-treats market whose products bear ever less tangible relations to milk. In this format, milk adopts any and every shape, that of superheroes or cartoon villains, baroque architectonics or body parts. The cow, used frequently as a metaphor for the passive, dumb, and exploited, is replaced by wily, smart-talking animals and apocryphal consumers of its milk—cats, rabbits, mice—leaving only a vestigial hint of the originating animality. The ontologies of donor species collapse as milk re-forms into consumable biomass.

Though we associate milk with the nursery, a liquid of our childhood, and the childhood of human life, milk is now increasingly a substance for adults. One of the most technologized liquids on the planet, it appears in recombination not only as foodstuff—most visibly in the current proliferation of corporate froth in milky coffee microfoams—but also in fertilizers, deicers, bottle-labeling adhesives, antiwrinkle agents, shampoo, hand cream, floor-leveling compounds, leather finishes, paper coating, concrete, and cement. It can be used to produce ethanol (from whey), and is found in supplements and catalysts, emulsifiers and surfactants. Milk re-enters the human body surreptitiously, as concentrates and isolates. Advertising promotes the incorporation of whey isolates to expand the muscle mass of male bodybuilders, at the same time as it promotes their power to diminish the body mass of female dieters.

MILK AND SEPARATION

Milk is versatile. One of its qualities is the capacity to separate or be separated. Milk is separated from cream, curds from whey. Its relation to separation extends in other directions. A form of physical separation is at work in the distancing or abstraction of milk from the female mammal's body. Separation abounds in the milk industry whereby the calf is separated from the cow, and milk is extracted from animals for human consumption. Separation more broadly occurs between milk for use and milk as a commodity for exchange. Separation is also part of the process of individuation—the separation of subject and object. Humans separate from caregivers, having passed through the nexus that milk provides.

Milk extracted or abstracted is a liquid representation of an annihilation of nature over time. In order to produce cows' milk for humans, the seasonal cycle related to gestation has been extended into the endless time of ever-increasing milk yields. This is the temporality of the market, of production and circulation. Production time is decoupled from the idea of limits and insists that what is profitable be available at all times. Milk flows across the political body, its stream an emblem of progress and the perfectibility of modern times. Situating milk as infinitely available, white, aseptic, and central to the adult Western diet was a quest of modernity. The mass industrialization of milk indicates a mode of industrial metaphysics: an abstraction from its associations with female human and non-human animal lactation and its transformation into a de-gendered industrial staple. Luce Irigaray proposed that all Western culture rests on the murder of the mother.[1] In milk and its replication, the efforts to replace or simulate, if not murder, the mother and to negate her capacity to provide milk, are evident. A human-centered philosophy of science assumes that its inventiveness and rationalizations can exceed anything that nature has produced, but, simultaneously, something called nature is essentialized and rendered a source of specific value. What is key is that whatever is devised does not exist in a vacuum, but is drawn into a matrix of valorization, which overdetermines its expressions. According to Elizabeth Grosz, "women's corporeality is inscribed as a mode of seepage."[2] Dissociated from messy female bodies, formula milks and processed animal milks extract, separate, and attempt to recombine a problematic fluid into something more streamlined. Bodies become erased in the dynamic of technologically realized reproduction, and modes are sought of imagining milk that obliterate intimacy and bodily exchange. Yet it returns as pornographica and as excessively visceral fantasy. There is an ambivalence attached to milk's visibility as a source of nutrition and comfort for babies, but also as a seeping spurting image for adult sexual consumption. Lactating breasts are a market niche in the pornographic index: Preggo/Milky.

SEEING MILK

Pure white milk is an ideal type. Cow's milk, for its part, exists in a range between blue and yellowy orange, depending on the fat and protein content. White milk is a product of fantasy, though industry

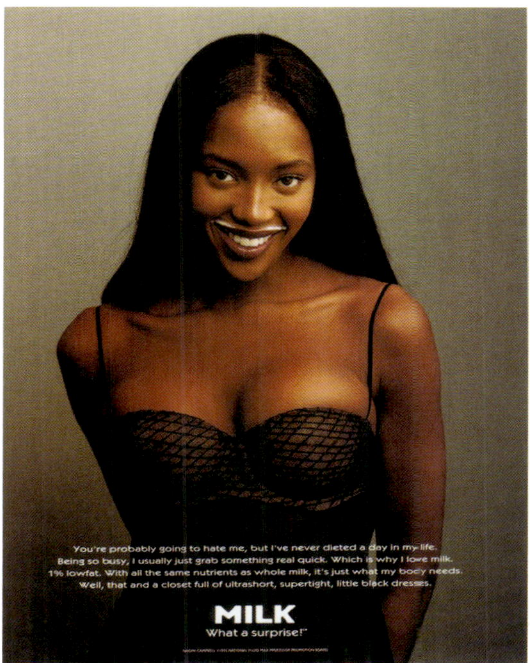

American milk advertisement, commissioned by the National Fluid Milk Processor Promotion Board, featuring a mustachioed Naomi Campbell, 1995.

plays its role in making it an actuality through homogenization. Milk's uniform white color is achieved by separating and recombining its constituent molecules. This is the making explicit of milk, of illuminating and enlarging it as a white presence in the world. Photography has played a role in this.[3] Milky behaviors previously undetectable by the human eye were evidenced in Harold Edgerton's microsecond photographs from 1931 onward, his faster lenses and better setup with stroboscopes perfecting the photographic techniques developed before him by Arthur Mason Worthington, who had published *A Study of Splashes* in 1908. Edgerton's images of the impact of the milk splash radiate shock, and this technique became the advertising standard for imaging liquid commodities. One of Edgerton's milk-drop photographs, titled *Coronet*, was included in the Museum of Modern Art's first photography exhibition in 1937. Papa Flash's dynamiting of time into image was spectacular and secured his celebrity status. It was also tethered to military research into ballistics.[4]

Edgerton's techniques and technologies later helped detonate and simultaneously photograph the H-bomb. His company, EG&G, designed and activated timing and triggering systems for bomb tests. And he patented a camera, the Rapatronic, with an exposure time as little as two microseconds, in order to photograph the massive expanding flash of the nuclear fireball in the first fractions of a second after discharge. The initial micro-moments of an atomic explosion produce weird irregular bubbles stippled by discrepancies in the density of the bomb's casing. If the hot force melted the support cables of the nuclear device, along with the surrounding desert sand and the eyes of any close-by onlookers, it also provided an image of melt, of frozen novelties caught at a moment of flux. The parameters of postwar culture might have been set: between hot bomb and frozen dessert, from most deadly to most innocuous. There is the "make anything you like" ice-cream dream of consumerism—emblematized in the boundless varieties of frozen dairy treats, colorful crystals with personality, dustings, aromas, and toppings, proposing a rainbow panoply of infinite possibility and a palette of luscious colors that the painter Willem de Kooning, for one, happily incorporated, straight from the twenty-eight flavors at the ice cream counter of a Howard Johnson's restaurant.[5] And there is the looming nuclear threat that, if activated, could liquefy it all, could dissolve every upturned eyeball, every pane of glass, making each human a puddle of once-was-ness. This bomb had its own creaminess, suggested in the testimony of journalist William L. Laurence: "The mushroom top was even more alive than the pillar, seething and boiling in a white fury of creamy foam, sizzling upward and then descending earthward, a thousand geysers rolled into one."[6]

Milk and photographic representation meet again in the digital age. The affinity between the lens and opaque fluid is extended for the commercial screen where the desideratum of digital simulation is the convincing reconstruction of real-world fluid dynamics. Computer-generated imagery (CGI) renders fluid simulations that delight in liquid rapture. Emulation of milk is reputedly the first thing everyone learns to do in CGI.[7] Milk acts again as a kind of primal, or primary, fluid. Spilt milk becomes

---

Opposite: The milk-as-ejaculate trope spans the worlds of fashion, advertising, and stock imagery, as seen in photographer Terry Richardson's 2001 shoot for clothing company Sisley (top) and a stock image currently available from 123RF Stock Photo.

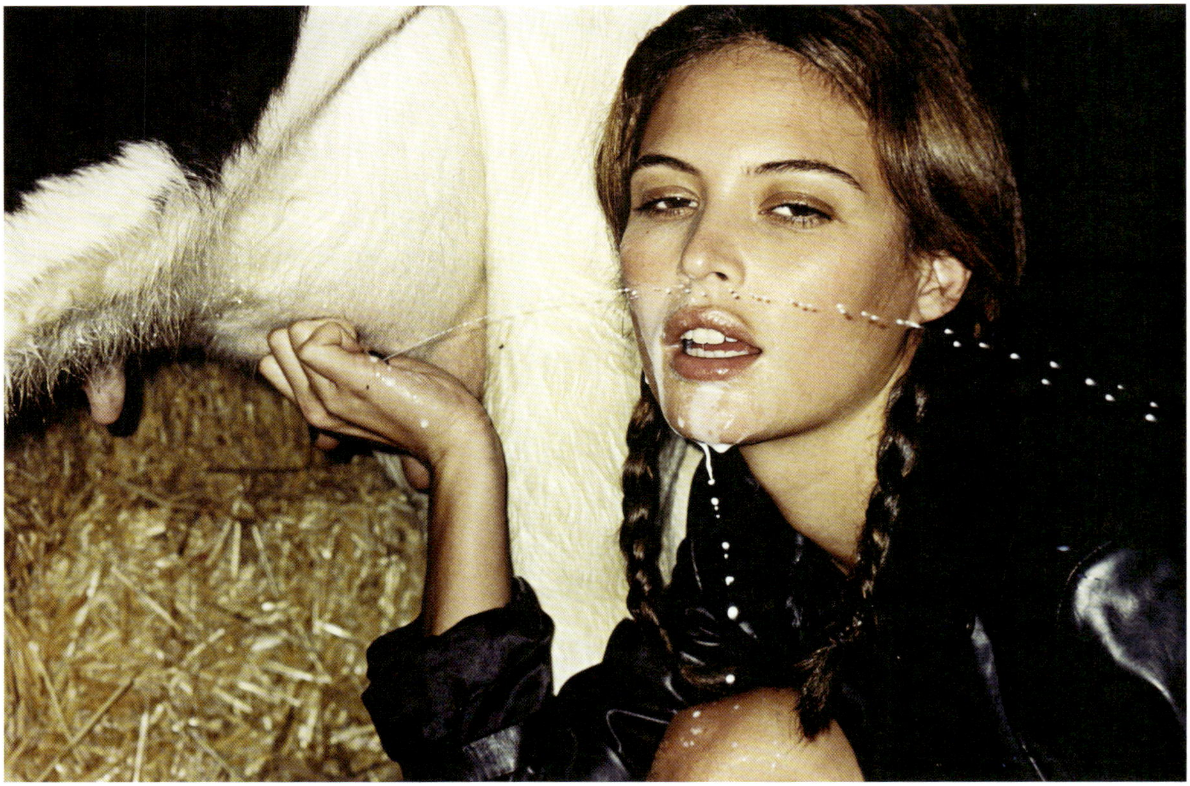

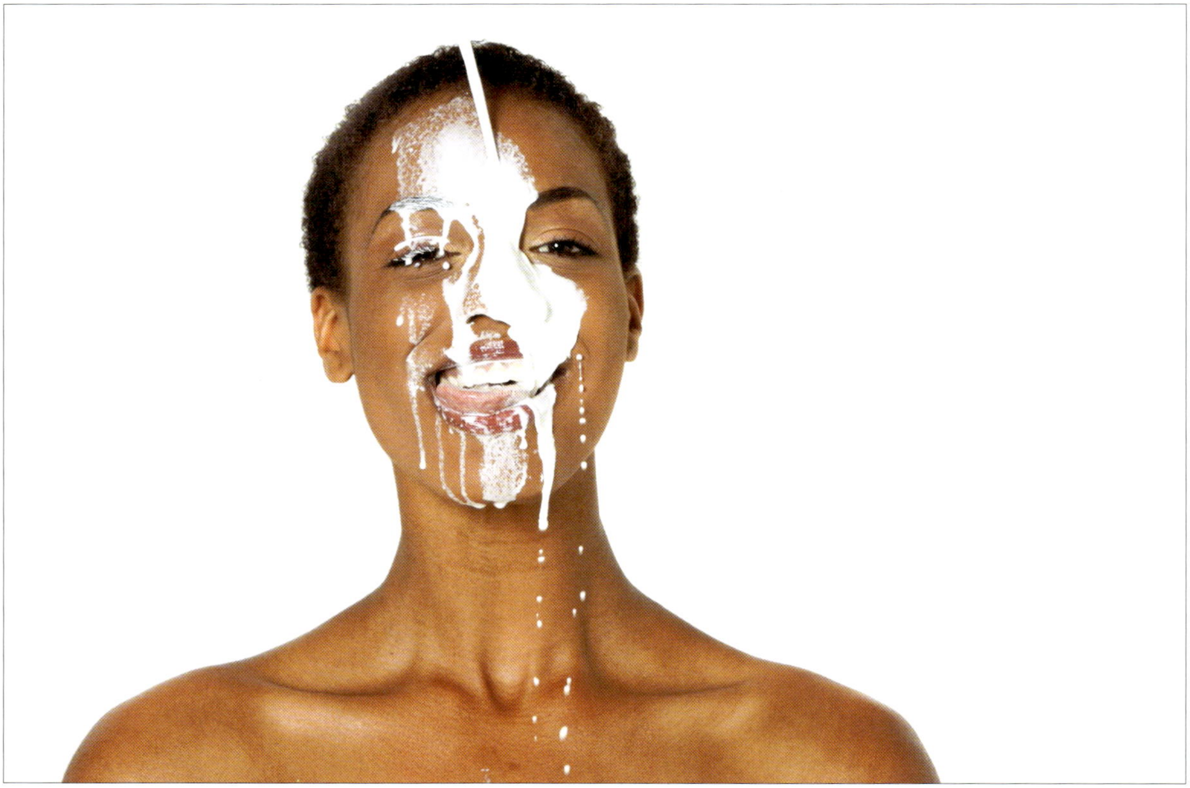

emblematic of both tragedy and of ecstasy. Captured by photographs or rendered digitally, milk takes on a body. It solidifies into forms that are in a state of suspension before collapse. CGI extends the capacity of milk to adopt any shape. It exploits its presence as liquid and animate, while rendering it as solid and infinitely shape-shifting.

Milk acts like unfired clay in the digital world. The frozen coronet of Edgerton's milk is donated an illusory capacity for movement and plasticity, combining in its phantasms the liquid and the crystal aspects of contemporary screens. Milk becomes anything, substituting for bullets, charging horses, or billowing dresses, but what it becomes specifically is a substitute for semen, for the ejaculate and its splash. This is something advertising also knew, when it played with milk-cum moustaches on young women's faces.

MILK'S CONTAINERS

Some of the earliest vessels were containers for milk, as fat particles found in their clay and on tools attest. Clay and milk have a long-standing affinity. Tablets found in ancient Babylonia and Assyria bearing the earliest recorded writing, protocuneiform, have pictographs of milk vessels pressed into them. But just as milk has been subjected to varieties of purification, so too has clay been edged toward whiteness and purity. Porcelain is milk's analogue: white, purified, numinous, idealized. Raw clay, like raw milk, is subjected to refinement, to smoothing out, to homogenization, to the market and its demands. It shares the same ability to take form and accept color. The milk and milk jug are coupled in the imagination—and the jug in turn becomes a euphemism for the breast. The clay milk vessel is drawn toward representation. Marie-Antoinette's Sèvres breast cup is a celebrated mimetic vessel, one that she commissioned to match the color of her own flesh; tipped by a pert nipple in pink, it was a rhyton designed to be cupped in the hands.[8]

Rumored—falsely—to be cast from her own chest, it became a symbol of her suspect lasciviousness. Marie-Antoinette—known as Madame Deficit—had a pleasure dairy based on that of another queen of France, Catherine de Medici, who, childless and unpopular, had the first of her dairies built at Fontainebleu.

Below: Italian advertisement for Mediterranea "body milk," 2009.

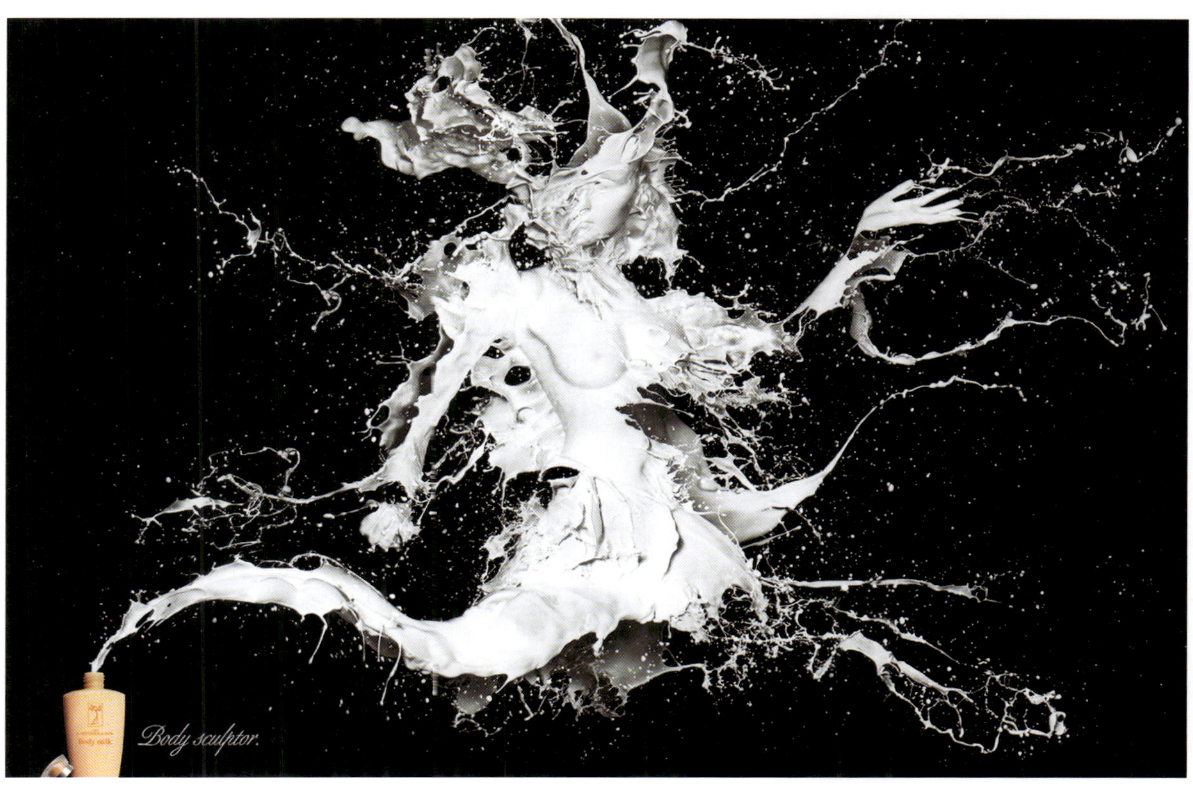

Marie-Antoinette's was at Rambouillet, and here she and her bosom friends could play at being milkmaids and consume milk products from a sixty-five-piece Sèvres porcelain service, including porcelain buckets mimicking the wooden counterparts in use in the peasant economy. In the pleasure dairies, women of the elite indulged in a fantasy of nurturing, a quality that France needed to regenerate itself without suffering the agonies of revolution. Madame de Pompadour—a courtesan of Louis xv, if apparently a frigid one—had also set up dairies, as well as sponsoring pastoral festivals. But rather than be associated with the fertile, health-sustaining properties of milk, Madame de Pompadour was rumored to be sickly. Her various ailments were to be ameliorated by milk, and her face was covered by a white mask of makeup made of milk to disguise her blemishes. It was said that she suffered from *fleurs blanches*, a slang term for venereal disease derived from the white discharge visible in menstrual blood (*flueurs*). Milk offered an emotional palette against the hyper-rationalism that would usher in the guillotine. It is still an emotional agent—for who has not cried over spilt milk? And who has not dreamed of happiness in the land of milk and honey?

The commercial milk vessels of the late twentieth century and beyond resist mimesis, and clay and milk are de-coupled. In Western markets, milk is now available only in one-use, infinitely available, standardized forms. In throwaway cartons, milk signifies both human ascendancy and the rinsed-out, exploited, and spent species of Earth whose yields are optimized but whose bodies are secondary. After years of being promoted as an essential component of the diet, associated with health and well-being, cow's milk is now a substance of controversy, linked with excess cholesterol, calcium loss, lactose intolerance, and obesity. A liter of milk currently retails for less than a liter of water.

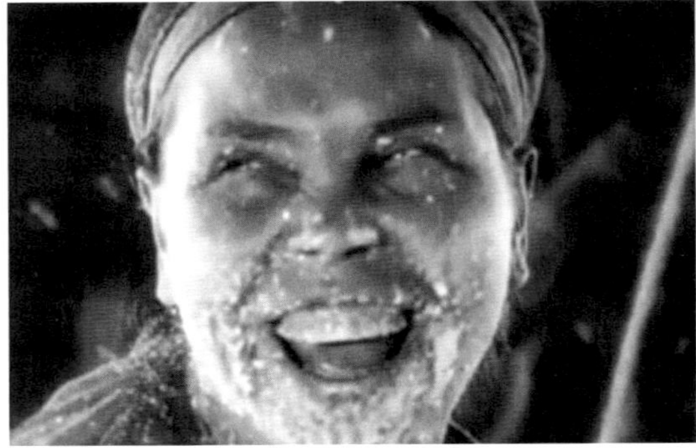

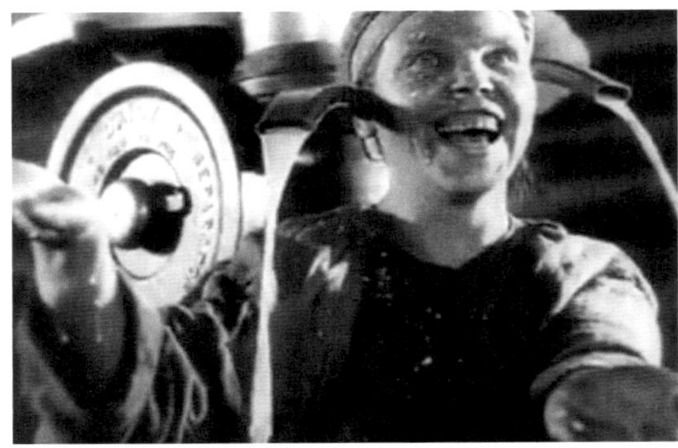

Digital stills from the "cream-separator" sequence in *The General Line*, 1929, directed by Sergei Eisenstein.

MILK'S GEOMETRY

As liquid, milk can drip freely, but in our social practice, milk is caught up, shaped, formed into standardized objects and directed along specific pathways. As milk flows, it maps out the geometrics of capitalist power. In Edgerton's freeze-framed photographs of milk coronets, it is still possible to see something of milk's unruly, exuberant self-shaping. The milk that sprays into the skies of pre- and early modern myths and paintings makes a heaven full of randomness. The milk that is made orderly within modernity is no less mythic, but it is presented as rationalized, a scientifically permeated fluid.

Industrialization produced the decline of the home dairy and the rise of the buttery and amalgamated dairies. In order to move beyond the capture of the cream by the wealthy, Sergei Eisenstein devised his cream-separator sequence in *The General Line* (1929). The nurturing qualities of milk are transferred to the actions of collectively operated and owned machinery. The cream is drawn off, not by the rich and not by hard graft, but by the machine, for the benefit of the workers. It spurts out ecstatically, another version of milk as cum shot, but conceived in a revolutionary context in which a redistribution of property or properties is imagined to be possible.

Milk flows into the grid. In this generous grid, milk is conceived as an ideal substance that distributes to all and everyone. The grid is an abstraction that functions in a phase space, illusorily working within an impossible time-space conceived without contradictions. The metaform of the "Milk Grid" is used specifically in

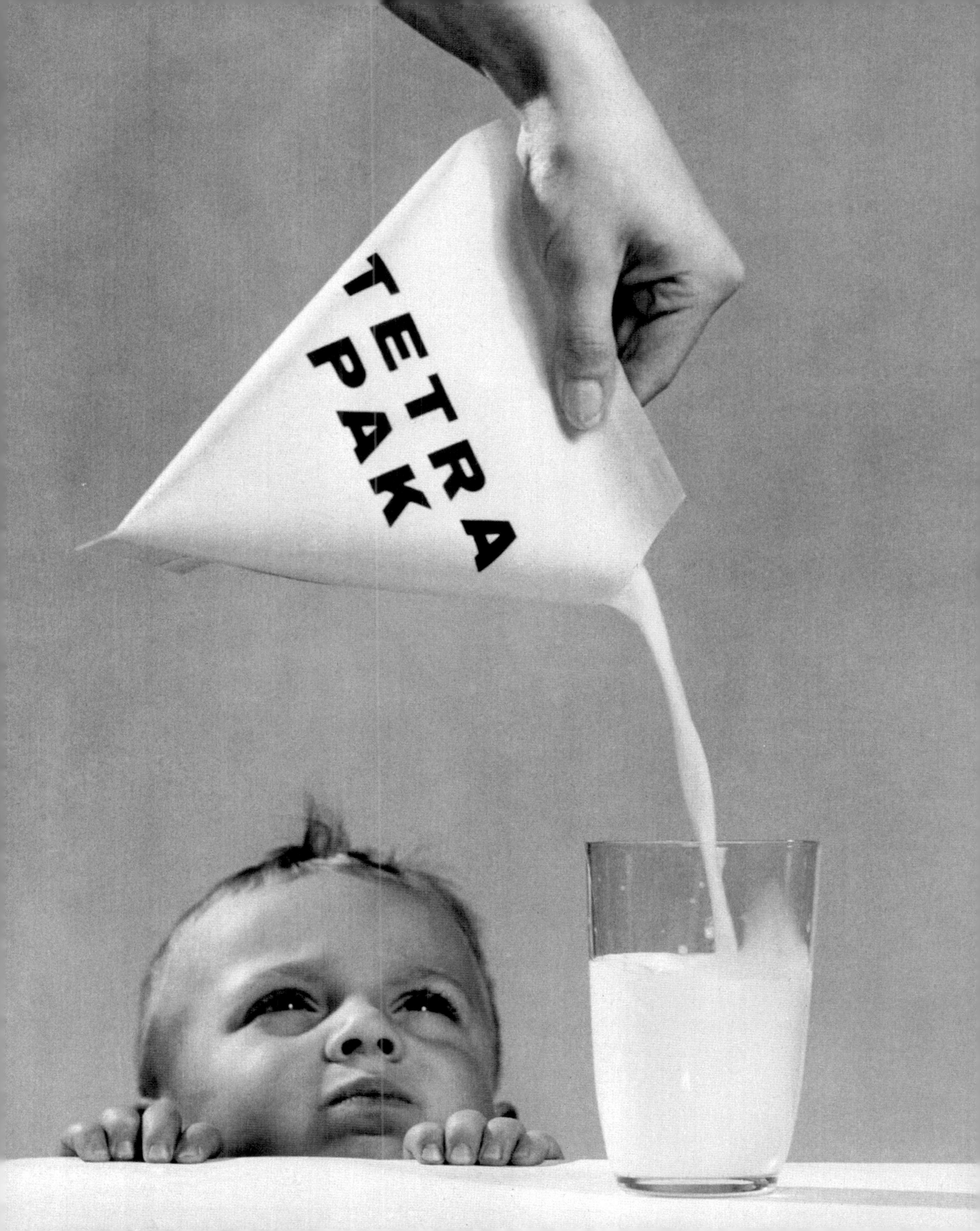

TETRA
PAK

Opposite: An empire built on the tetrahedron, the most basic of the five Platonic solids. Promotional image for Tetra Pak, 1950s.

Right: Plato gets a lesson in his own geometry. Promotional image for Tetra Pak, 1960s.

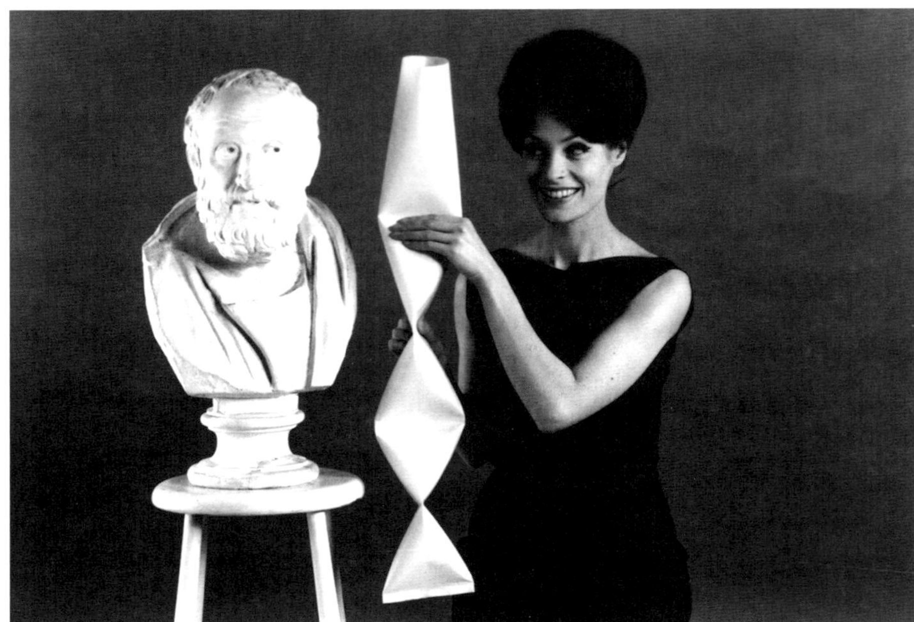

relation to India's national network of milk provision, which was established in the 1970s and which transformed India from a "milk-deficient nation" into the world's largest milk producer by 1998. (This program, also dubbed the "White Revolution" and "Operation Flood," was reanimated in 2015, as part of a project to stimulate liquid milk trade across South Asia, in order to push out the imports of milk powders from overseas.) The grid is a powerful image for a network that goes from cow to kitchen and covers an entire territory. It was modeled on the grid-like network of operations originally pioneered by the now-defunct Milk Marketing Board in the United Kingdom, which oversaw an integrated structure, from mechanized milking sheds to tankers to railway distribution. The milk grid can be extended from a motif of milk management in modernity, enmeshed with ideas of "progress," to the standardization of all its constituent parts—its extended operations going from insemination, gestation, and feeding to extraction, purification, bottling, and processing. Modernity involves the shift from handcrafted processes (technologies of clay to make sieves and vessels) to wood and glass (churners and pats), to metal and mechanical processes in the nineteenth and twentieth century, to robotics and digitized operations of the twenty-first century. Robotic systems can now milk, clean, and feed the milk-making beasts, process and package the produce.

In contemporary optimized dairy operations, there is no human contact between cow and human other than when milk enters the mouth. Geometries of milk have emerged to ascertain quality at the level of milk's micro- and macrostructure. Furthermore, to conceive milk operations as enmeshed in the geometry of the grid is to imagine the precision of the bottling plant, and the clear-cut configurations of cubes or triangles of butter and cheese. The grid produces geometric forms, and the more all is standardized, the sharper the angles, the more platonically ideal the shapes. In testing butter, penetration and compression tests deploy a range of geometries: cone, needle, cylinder, sphere, and plate. Tetra Pak added an additional geometry with its white tetrahedral milk packs and their hexagonal geodesic supermarket stacks. The Tetra Pak is formed from an endless columnal stream of aseptic milk. The innovation that shaped their success was based on the observation that a tube of milk can be poured endlessly and bisected laterally to create this iconic pyramid form, never contacting air, hand, or machine.

THE COW'S BODY

Capital's will to autonomy confronts material limits. Reciprocally, the material realm is shaped by forces of abstraction. The cow's body is overtaken by processes of "optimization." Such language pervades

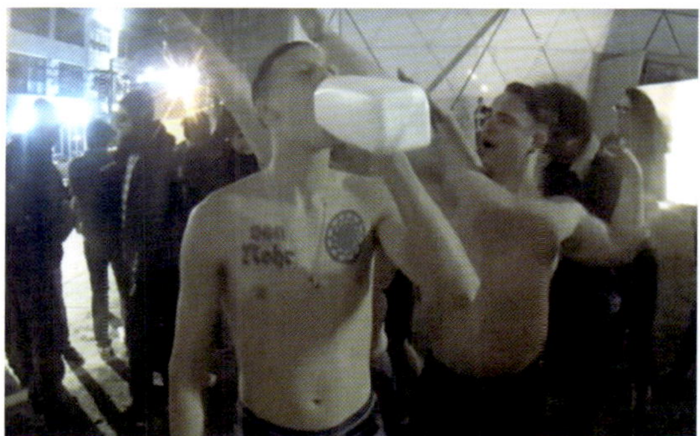

Digital still from the video feed of *HEWILLNOT-DIVIDE.US* at the Museum of the Moving Image, New York, 3 February 2017.

the industry, where "yield" is increased by manipulating the cows' feed, medication, living conditions, and genetics. There is a long history of destroying animals not deemed economically viable as part of national animal improvement plans. The United States Department of Agriculture still executes an "animal improvement program," now through genetic selection rather than the culling programs of the early twentieth century. Genetic animal "improvements" are tied into alliances of scientific-government-corporate policy. These optimizations of milk yields, to improve the productive efficiency and profitability of livestock, shadow the management of human health and development through managed nutrition, specifically those humans who are identified as biopolitically "backward." Approaches to animal and human optimization partake in a historical narrative, with a racial basis. When Herbert Hoover made an address in 1923 on the milk industry at the World's Dairy Congress, he affirmed that "upon this industry, more than any other of the food industries, depends not alone the problem of public health, but there depends upon it the very growth and virility of the white races."[9] The link between the whiteness of milk and the white races was reiterated in January 2017 during the installation HEWILLNOTDIVIDE.US by Shia LaBeouf at New York's Museum of the Moving Image. A live streaming broadcast from the street outside the museum was to run for the term of Donald Trump's presidency, providing a location for "resistance and insistence, opposition or optimism" through the endless chanting by the public of the work's title sentence to a camera. The project was closed down after three weeks, on 10 February 2017, because it had become a "flashpoint for

violence." Far-right groups intermittently hogged the camera. Dancing and shouting, they punctuated their performances with the choreographed drinking of milk directly from gallon jugs in an assertion of white supremacy: "They spat it out as they danced, letting it dribble down their chins."[10] Rightist websites underscore the connection between drinking white cow's milk and what they see as genetic optimization on a geographic-historical arc of lactose tolerance that has been traced across Europe. They toast the new political era with cheap, industrial milk, using it to oppose the "soft" leftist-liberal alternative and to celebrate whiteness as a dominant form.

DEEPER IN THE PYRAMID

Where Eisenstein depicted a collectively owned machine, the extension of the milk-machine under anti-solidaristic conditions goes into the body of the cow. Contemporary farming involves the invasion of the cow's body. As milk yields expand, life expectancy contracts. Big data has reconfigured every aspect of dairy farming, and is combined with the financialization of species and individual worth pioneered in the field of animal science through quantitative analysis. Animals are given a value, or Lifetime Net Merit, in dollars. Factors used in the calculation include an estimate of how much a bull's genetic material will affect the potential revenue from a dairy cow. Fluid, fat, protein ratios of the milk, and the quality of the ensuing progeny are predicted by gene markers and heritable traits, as well as pedigree records and market conditions. Body size; udder condition; foot, leg, and body ratios; cheese merit; fluid merit; daughter calving ease; productive life; daughter pregnancy rate; stillbirth rate—all are deduced through complex calculations of big datasets. There is an air of rationality gone wild, cold logic mixed with hijinks whimsy and mythopoesis: one bull who was scientifically calculated as possessing the highest net worth is named Badger-Bluff Fanny Freddie, and another, Ensenada Taboo Planet-Et.[11]

Current research aims to subsume the body of the cow entirely, as scientists attempt to generate "real" milk without the cow's presence in the new field of "cellular agriculture." Based on the promise of using milk cells as starter cells, but then regenerating milk synthetically, headlines ecstatically assert, "Animal lovers use biotech to develop milk made by man

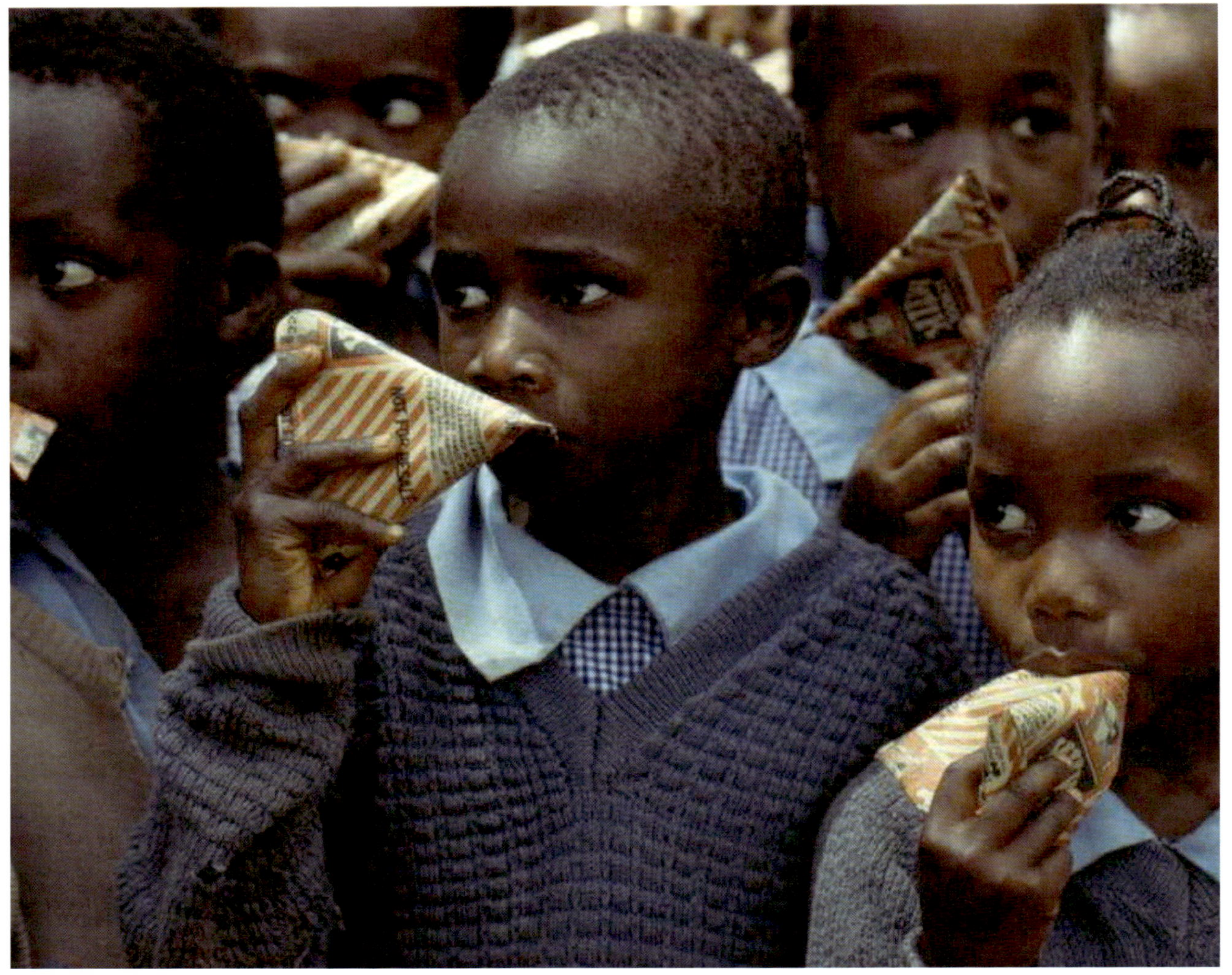

Milking what Tetra Pak calls "the bottom of the pyramid."
Photo from *Tetra Pak Dairy Index*, issue 5, May 2012.

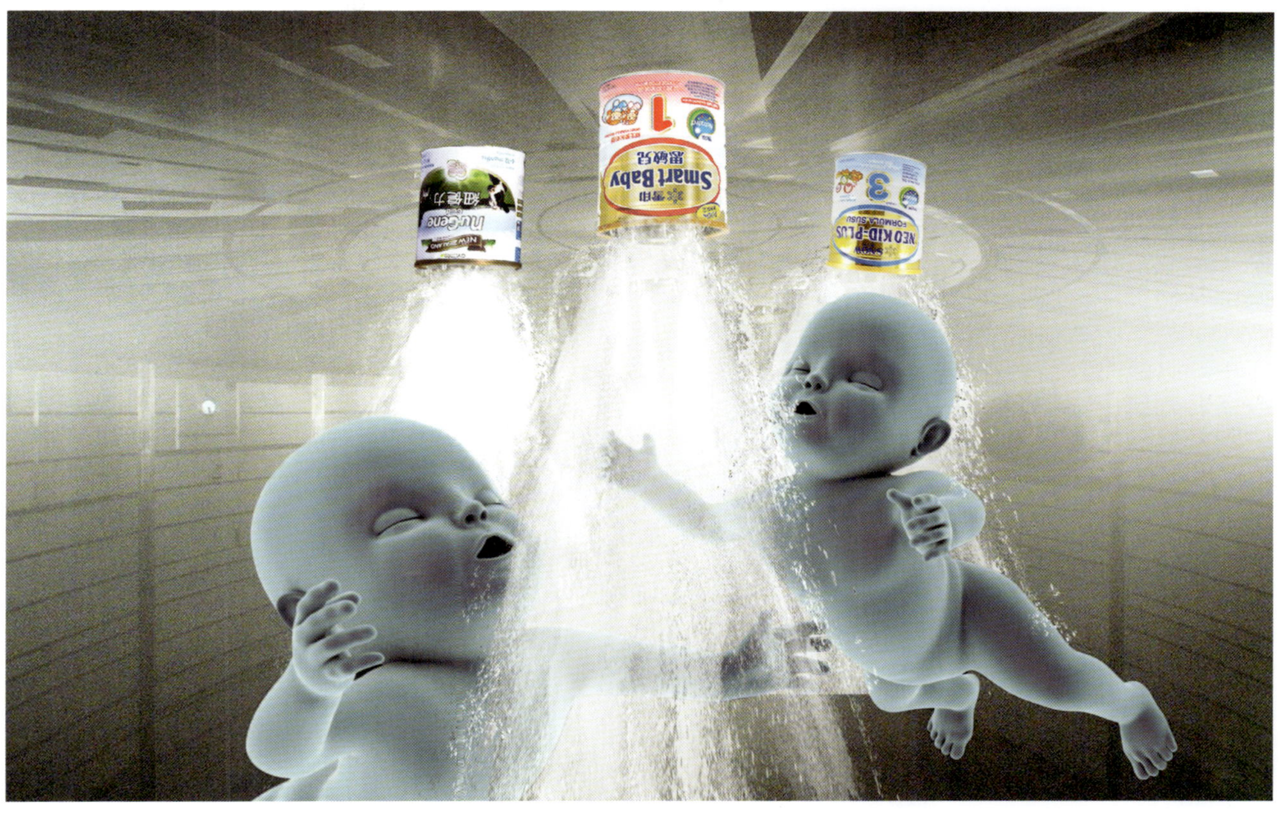

Production still from Melanie Jackson, *Deeper in the Pyramid*, forthcoming in 2018.

instead of a cow."[12] The nexus of nature and technology offers a physical and imaginative emancipation of generative new materiality that defies bounded perceptions of body, gender, and species. What seems to be a turning point is also a continuity that can be perceived in the changing forms of milk over time. Milk is not just a life-giving liquid but also one latent with the power of annihilation, and its shapings are driven by the attempt to wrestle control of supply, as the mythic characters Hera and Opis knew.

Who is all this for? The ideal platonic form of the milk carton emerges in a subprime market for milk. Western markets are turning against cow's milk as a degraded substance and are beginning to favor plant milk or milk without the cow, supertech milk from cows' starter cells, the kind of milk men make in laboratories. Adult milk recapitulates the journey that formula milk made a hundred years before it. Billions of one-use plastic vessels leech toxins into land and water. The platonic forms and messages of health are now pitched elsewhere, "Deeper in the Pyramid."

Since the 1950s, Tetra Pak's Brancusi-like pyramid cartons have morphed from solid form into conceptual strategy and economic principle. Milk became an ur-form, a prototype that has been rolled out into multiple commodity lines. Tetra Pak currently sells five hundred million packages a day. Its latest corporate strategy is labeled "Deeper in the Pyramid." A minimalist modernity is conceptualized as an economic principle that inserts its white arrows into the "economic pyramid" for a maximized return based on a presence radically more pervasive than is possible when the goal is to cream off revenues from an exclusive market. The strategy is focused on creating new markets among the population positioned toward the base of the economic pyramid. Currently, profits are gleaned from the pyramid's apex on a high return from a relatively small number of sales. By digging deeper into the pyramid, by pitching specially adapted product lines made from lower-cost ingredients for the mass population living on subsistence income between EUR 1.80 and 7.20 a day, the exponential increase in low-return profits promises a "'golden opportunity' for international companies."[13]

Milk is messy and compromised. Milk is original and pure. Milk is troubled, a turbid substance whose representation is difficult. It is presented as natural, health-giving, but is enmeshed in industrial processes and commercial strategies. It appears whole and entangled in life and liveliness, yet it speaks of death. To perceive the shapes within milk, the ways in which it has been shaped over time, is to give oneself up to its minglings, its combinations and recombinations with myth, social norms, social fantasy, and cultural practices. It means to conceive its expressibility, its capacity to be images, to seep into language and be made metaphorical. It necessitates thinking about the ways in which an orientation toward separation—from the body, from suppliers—has fed into its becoming abstracted for capital, into data, into something limitlessly reproducible and separate from or other to itself, as it flows between purity and abjection, the technoscientific and the bucolic, never settling, always spilling somewhere else.

1 Luce Irigaray, "Women-Mothers, the Silent Substratum of the Social Order," in *The Irigaray Reader*, ed. Margaret Whitford (Oxford: Blackwell, 1991), p. 47.

2 Elizabeth Grosz, *Volatile Bodies: Toward a Corporeal Feminism* (Bloomington: Indiana University Press, 1994), p. 203.

3 See Kenneth Hayes, *Milk and Melancholy* (Cambridge, MA: The MIT Press, 2008).

4 Roozbeh Ghaffari, Ozge Nadia Gozum, Katherine Koch, Amy W. Ng, Hua Fung Teh, and Peter Yang, "Harold Edgerton in World War II" (unpublished manuscript, 15 December 2000). Available at <web.mit.edu/6.933/www/Fall2000/edgerton/ EdgertonWW2.pdf>.

5 See <daviddavidgallery.com/artists/willem-de-kooning2>.

6 Calder M. Pickett, *Voices of the Past: Key Documents in the History of American Journalism* (Columbus, OH: Grid, 1977), p. 344.

7 This popular truism about training in CGI can be found circulating on various blogs and forums. See, for example, <helloyoucreatives.com/post/3307413119/cgi-milk-we-think-its-the-first-thing-everyone>.

8 See Meredith Martin, "Dairy Cases," *Cabinet*, no. 40 (Winter 2010–2011). See also her *Dairy Queens: The Politics of Pastoral Architecture from Catherine de' Medici to Marie-Antoinette* (Cambridge, MA: Harvard University Press, 2011).

9 *Proceedings of the World's Dairy Congress*, vol. 1 (Washington, DC: Government Printing Office, 1924), p. 15.

10 Jack Smith, IV, "Milk Is the New, Creamy Symbol of White Racial Purity in Donald Trump's America," *Mic*, 10 February 2017. Available at <mic.com/articles/168188/milk-nazis-white-supremacists-creamy-pseudo-science-trump-shia-labeouf#.PdAI0a51>.

11 Alexis C. Madrigal, "The Perfect Milk Machine: How Big Data Transformed the Dairy Industry," *The Atlantic*, 1 May 2012. Available at <theatlantic.com/technology/archive/2012/05/the-perfect-milk-machine-how-big-data-transformed-the-dairy-industry/256423>.

12 Tuan C. Nguyen, "Animal Lovers Use Biotech to Develop Milk Made by Man Instead of a Cow," *The Washington Post* (Washington, DC), 21 July 2014. Available at <wpo.st/kW6d2>.

13 See *Tetra Pak Magazine*, no. 104 (2015), dedicated to the theme "Deeper in the Pyramid," p. 3. Available at <endpoint895270.azureedge.net/static/documents/tp-magazine-no-104.pdf >.

I FEEL IT IS MY DUTY TO SPEAK OUT
Sally O'Reilly

Dear WhiteWave Foods,

I am writing to complain about one of your products: namely, Silk Cashewmilk (with a touch of almond). I imagine that you receive many complaints about your use of the word "milk," and frequent challenges to specify where exactly on the cashew nut the teats are located. This, however, is not a problem for me, since I simply mop up what I take to be a sloppy euphemism with a pair of quotation marks. No, what I wish to complain about is the recent redesign of your half-gallon "milk" cartons.

My bipartite beef with this redesign is 1) the reduction in realism of the illustration and 2) the stance of the nuts represented therein. To start with the latter point: I have come, in recent years, to identify with the two nuts who, like game siblings, plunge pell-mell into their fate. I hope that it is not an anthropomorphism too far to suggest that one splashes down as if propelled from a water chute, and the other arcs forward, as if diving headlong, emboldened by the first's joyful splash. This is an image of excitement and of freedom (from what, I presume, is for the "milk" drinker to decide). In the new arrangement, however, the two nuts face one another, turning their backs on the world to assume a conservative relation based in partnering and stability. My concern is that here you are affirming and perpetuating recent troubling shifts in political attitudes the world over. Your open and energetic cashews have become inward-looking; even their spatial alignment is now in almost complete agreement with one another, as if no differently oriented nut would be welcome.

The medium into which they are about to be subsumed has similarly been made safe. You have, it seems, seen fit to censor the milk-droplet coronet of the earlier packaging—which was, I felt, a nod to the pioneering photographic work of A. M. Worthington at the turn of the twentieth century, and a salute to the spectactularist high-speed film experiments of Harold Edgerton some fifty years later. The new design suppresses the tremendously uplifting splash motif, implementing instead what might be described as a mellifluous swelling of liquid about the nuts. This is no doubt to draw on connotations of silk, to visually insinuate the creaminess that the tongue can look forward to. Well, for one thing, a tongue cannot look. And for another, I do not need such synesthetic cues or Elysian fictions to aid me in my beverage choices. And for yet another, you have likely alienated your buyer base of thrill-seeking individualists with this new appeal to comfort-loving sensualists. This smacks to me of playing to the risk-averse majority; but then again yours is, I would feel confident in submitting, a numbers game above all else.

On the subject of harsh realities, I come back to my first point: the illustration's insulting retreat from realism. The previous packaging was so bracingly candid about the earthy origins of the nut. Not only were we invited to contemplate the somewhat irregular seam at which the two halves fuse, we were also treated to a well-lit view of the surface of the nut, ridged and pitted like the craggy face of an ancient poet. I could admire these nuts that had passed into "milk" with dignity and originality. The new protagonists, however, have been airbrushed and plumped up; they appear not to exist in any reality that I can identify with, but to hail from the pulpiest of fictions, and one that ends in an improbable perpetuity.

We all know that food photography lies—that the ice cream is mashed potato, that the meat is seared with shoe polish, that the milk, or "milk," is PVA glue or hair conditioner or suntan lotion. I understand that the look or sound of reality must be constructed to be convincing. But it is not the material lies you tell so much as the

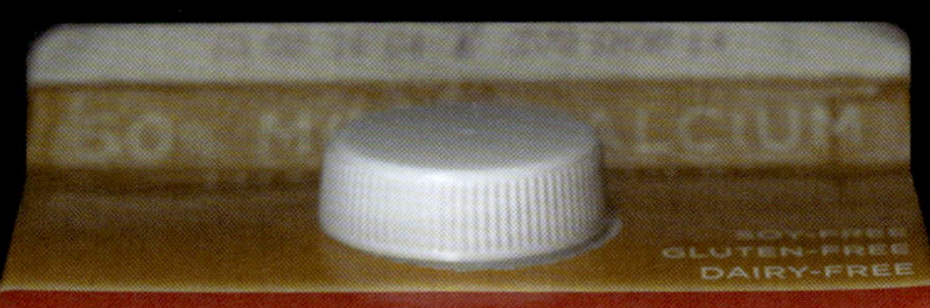

I FEEL IT IS MY DUTY TO SPEAK OUT

SOY-FREE
GLUTEN-FREE
DAIRY-FREE
ORIGINAL
Silk
Cashew
creamy cashewmilk
with a touch of almond
CREAMIER
than skim milk!
60
CALORIES
PER SERVING
HALF GALLON (1.89 L)

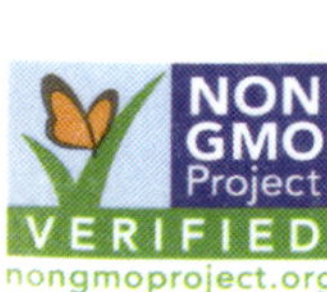

NON
GMO
Project
VERIFIED
nongmoproject.org

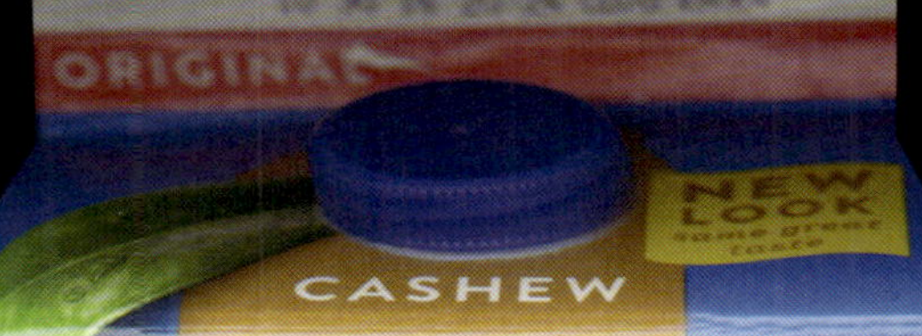

Irresistibly
Creamy

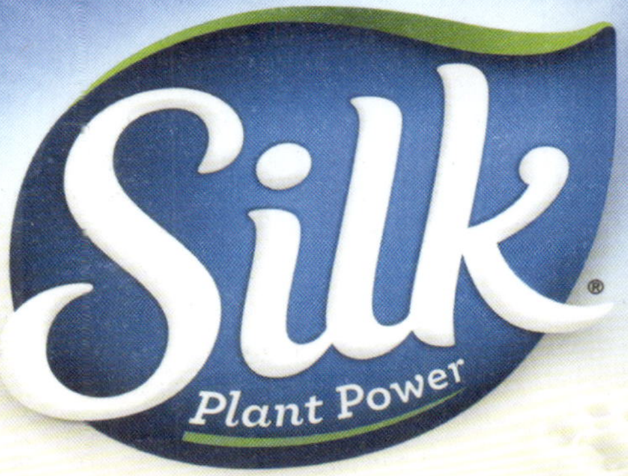

CASHEW
ORIGINAL

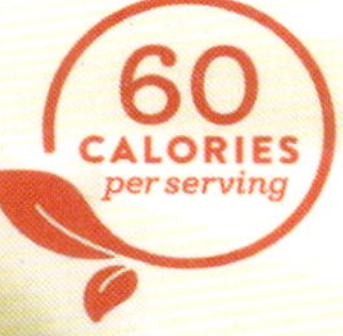

CASHEWMILK WITH A TOUCH OF ALMOND

HALF GALLON (1.89 L)

conceptual maneuvering that strikes me to the core. What are you trying to hide from us? What is it that you think we cannot handle?

Is it the cashew apple that you are so desperate for us to forget about, or to not even know of in the first place? Do you forsake the pear-shaped fruit that puckers indecently around its ovary (which is so chauvinistically called the nut)? Or is it the cashew bark exudate that you renounce as a substitute for gum Arabic and deny is employed as adhesive, insect repellent, and a lubricant in the electrical insulation of airplanes? Or do you wish to bury the pompous initialism CNSL, because, when pricked, it turns out to stand simply for cashew nut shell liquid—that caustic goop used in brake linings and bioplastics, and which, when it comes into contact with the skin, or even if inhaled, can cause a pruritic rash on the extremities, torso, groin, axilla, and buttocks, and, less commonly, a perianal itch or a blistering of the mouth, and, even less commonly, can transform ears into "large red terra-cotta classical casts of ears," as happened to the poet Elizabeth Bishop?

There is much about the cashew tree that I, and many others, are kept ignorant of. I would have thought you would be proud of the impressive company that it keeps as a member of the order Sapindales. Why not crow from the forest canopy that your product is related to the delicious mango, citrus, maple, lychee, and sumac trees, and to the historic big-hitters frankincense, myrrh, and balm of Gilead? Why not capitalize on its prestigious relatives the mahogany and the West Indian cedar, which furnish fine rooms and cigar boxes, respectively. Why remain quiet about its rubbing shoulders with the Ceylon oak, which is the source of Macassar oil, and the buckeye, which is used to make artificial limbs and paper and to stun fish? I can guess why. Because you do not wish us to know that it is even more closely related to the poison oak, poison ivy, and poison sumac. What the tranquil fiction that you feed us cannot admit is that this food originates as poison, that it is only through decortication and heat treatment that it is rendered food.

And yet I can cope with this sort of knowledge. I am perfectly at home with potatoes, for instance.

Perhaps I am mistaken in laying the blame with you. Perhaps it is the phalanx of official bodies that does not trust me to believe that shell liquid, sap, and "milk" are different. Is it the combined might of the African Cashew Alliance, the African Cashew Initiative, the National Council of Benin Cashew Exporters, the Brazilian Cashew Nut Manufacturers' Association, the World Cashew Nut Alliance, and the Vietnam Cashew Exporters' Association that silences you? Or do the International Nut and Dried Fruit Council, the Combined Edible Nut Trade Association, or the International Nut Council tie your hands on the matter? (Although I don't imagine the Californian Dried Plum Board or the American Peanut Council would gladly suffer the impositions of these last three generalists.)

If what I have inferred is indeed the case, then, as a valued consumer of your product, I can only convey my disappointment at your perviousness to political pressures. I hereby also express my hope that, at your next design summit, you will seek an alternative packaging solution that is as courageous and principled as it is affecting.

Yours sincerely,
Sally O'Reilly

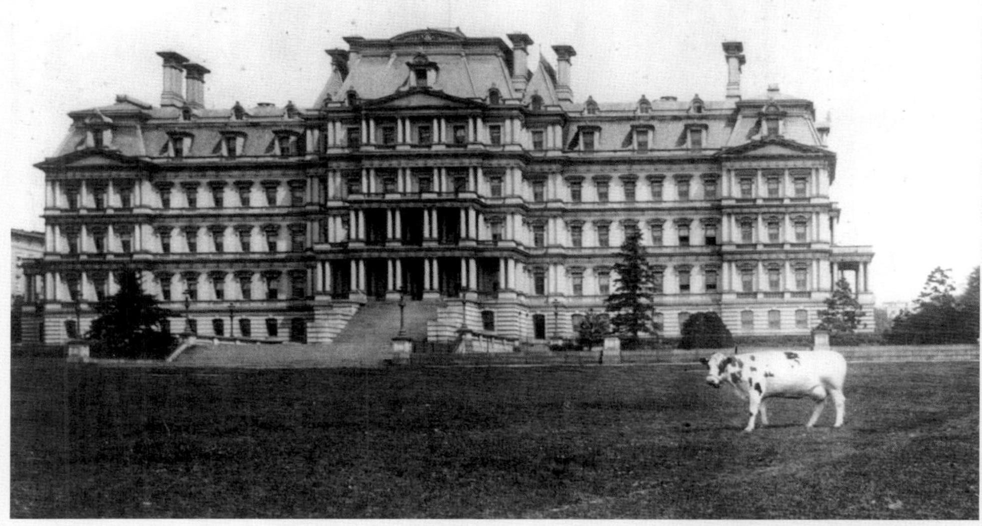

Pauline in front of the State, War, and Navy Building.

The eight years of Theodore Roosevelt's presidency saw the White House occupied by an unprecedented menagerie—from a bear named Jonathan Edwards to Maude the pig; a badger, a lizard, a hyena, a pony, guinea pigs, birds, and numerous dogs, including the famously cantankerous bull terrier known as Fighting Pete, whose penchant for biting visitors' legs eventually got him exiled to the family's estate on Long Island. Less zoologically promiscuous than his predecessor, William Howard Taft, who succeeded Roosevelt in 1909, brought with him a rather more modest faunal retinue in the form of a Jersey cow. Mooley, as the animal was known—an alternate spelling of the word "muley," meaning a hornless cow—was allowed to graze on the White House lawn and the Ellipse (then known as the "White Lot"). She provided fresh milk and butter to the Taft family for more than a year until one night in April 1910, when she died after gorging herself on oats she discovered in an open bin in the presidential stables.

Wisconsin senator Isaac Stephenson, saddened by the news, promised Taft the best-bred cow from his farm back in Kenosha County. The animal, named Pauline Wayne, was the daughter of the celebrated milker Gertrude Wayne, and was, wrote the *Washington Post*, "an aristocrat of the purest Holstein blood represented among the herds of the entire country ... valued at $1,000," or about $24,000 in today's money.

Pauline traveled in a special railway car to Washington, DC, and arrived on 3 November 1910. The *Washington Post* reported that a parade, complete with "a cloud of dairy wagons and hokey-pokey ice cream vendors," was meant to receive her. But thanks to an erroneous telegram sent by Pauline's chaperone, J. P. Torrey, the procession gathered at the wrong time—4 pm, instead of 4 am—and found itself confronted with an empty boxcar. (The *Evening Star* reported the incident somewhat differently, writing that Pauline's railway car had been left behind in Pittsburgh, and that Torrey only discovered the mistake upon his arrival in Washington.)

Like Mooley, Pauline—who the papers dubbed "Her Bovine Majesty"—was given free rein to graze Washington's choicest lawns, including those of the White House, the Ellipse, and the State, War, and Navy Building, known today as the Eisenhower Executive Office Building. In 1911, she traveled back to Wisconsin to participate in the International Dairy Show in Milwaukee. Visitors could, noted the *New York Times*, buy "tiny" souvenir bottles of her milk for fifty cents, and a full gallon for five dollars (about $122 today). There are conflicting reports of Pauline's daily yield, which in any case probably varied throughout her lifetime. The *Evening Star* claimed she produced up to nine gallons of milk per day and twenty-five pounds of butter per week. When she was on display in Milwaukee, the *New York Times* reported that she was producing sixteen gallons of milk per day and thus bringing in eighty dollars per day for the president. That figure was later corrected following a letter of complaint—the *Times* meant sixteen quarts, not gallons, meaning Pauline was producing a mere four gallons of milk each day.

Taft lost the 1912 election to Woodrow Wilson and moved to New Haven to become a professor at Yale Law School. Pauline retired to Wisconsin. When Wilson took up residence in the White House in the spring of 1913, he brought in sheep.

THE TOWN MILK CHOCOLATE BUILT
Will Wiles

In 2010, the British confectioner Cadbury, one of the country's largest and best-loved companies, was bought by the American food giant Kraft. Britain has decades of experience in watching its biggest and most-beloved brands taken over by foreign companies. It is practically a national sport. Wedgwood is owned by the Finnish housewares company Fiskars, which makes those distinctive, orange-handled scissors. Jaguar, which was bought by Ford in 1989, is now owned by Indian industrial behemoth Tata, a satisfying colonial inversion. Our "privatized" railways are in large part owned by the national railway companies of Germany, France, and the Netherlands.

But the sale of Cadbury was still a national shock, triggering a political scandal that resulted in lasting changes to the rules governing corporate acquisitions. But the damage was done, and the trauma continued. The now-renamed conglomerate Mondelez started rolling out the fruits of its merged product lines: Cadbury chocolate bars with the white filling of Oreo cookies; Cadbury chocolate as a flavoring in Philadelphia Cream Cheese.

Chocolate is a taste acquired in childhood, one that is associated with treats, and so chocolate brands easily acquire nostalgic goodwill. Even accounting for that, the Cadbury name had a particularly warm aura to it—a reputation combining sweetness, utopian paternalism, and milk.

Cadbury—which called itself Cadbury's for most of its history, only recently dropping the possessive form—was founded by John Cadbury, a Quaker merchant, in 1824. The company sold tea and coffee from a shop on Bull Street, Birmingham, in the English Midlands. In 1831, Cadbury began to experiment with roasting and grinding cacao beans in order to make chocolate. This was chocolate for drinking, as its solid form was yet to become popular, but from 1842 the shop did sell "French eating chocolate." In 1861, his health failing, John passed the still-small business to his sons, Richard and George. In their hands, it prospered, and when they were forced to leave the small factory-warehouse in Crooked Lane where John's first experiments had been carried out, they started looking for a large site outside of town on which they could build their own factory.[1] They alighted upon a completely rural location four miles from the city center, but close to canal and railway lines. This place was known as Bournbrook, and the company began to transfer production there in 1879, calling its new premises Bournville.

This move was not just a matter of industrial convenience. As Quakers, the Cadburys were unusually interested in the welfare of their workers—the firm paid good wages for the time, and pioneered incentive and savings schemes and the Saturday half-holiday. In the half-century the company had existed, Birmingham had grown from a market town to a booming industrial hub, on its way to becoming England's second-largest city. This pell-mell development had made it a deeply unhealthy place to live and work. "The brothers were only too familiar with the evil conditions of industry in the congested town," wrote T. B. Rogers, the editor of the *Bournville Works Magazine*, in a celebratory history of the company published in 1931. "They themselves loved the country, and they recognised the value of country surroundings as an influence in the lives of workers."[2]

At Bournville, Cadbury not only founded a huge, modern manufacturing facility, it also built a remarkable model community for its workers—an exercise in paternalist private planning that remains influential today. "Their step was considered by critics to be a wild adventure, for it was a time when industries were concentrated in towns, near to labour and to a town's services," Rogers wrote. "But for this step, the business could scarcely have become the great concern it did, and in town conditions it could never have attempted the industrial experiments it has carried out."[3]

Bournville wasn't unprecedented. It slotted quite neatly into an Enlightenment tradition of model communities dating back to the early years of the eighteenth century. To begin, these were aristocratic projects. As the architectural historian Gillian Darley writes in her 1975 book *Villages of Vision*, these projects were often the result of "emparkment": a landowner cleared homes off their estate in order to create a country park, and in compensation built a "model" community outside the newly erected gates. Sometimes

the intention behind these communities was salutary, aimed at easing rural squalor; sometimes it was merely aesthetic, the creation of a pastoral fantasy-world. Later, industrialists conducted their own experiments, such as the model mill-towns of New Lanark, built by Robert Owen on the River Clyde in Scotland, and Saltaire, created by Titus Salt near Leeds

Nevertheless, Bournville had unique character-istics, not least the way it became entwined with the company's products and image. In 1879, when the company made its move to the countryside, it still mostly produced drinking chocolate—a line that was soon to be branded Bournville. It did sell eating chocolate, but mostly in the form of "fancy boxes" of French-style bonbons. The natural bitterness of cocoa made pure chocolate unappealing to most consumers, so it was sweetened and flavored with additives such as vanilla. Rogers, in his boosterish history, makes a valiant effort to claim milk chocolate as a British inven-tion, stating that the company sold "milk chocolate prepared to the original recipe of Dr Hans Sloane," the eighteenth-century polymath whose collection became the nucleus of the British Museum, from 1849.[4] But milk chocolate, as we know it, was invented in Switzerland in 1875 by chocolatier Daniel Peter and Henri Nestlé, the inventor of condensed milk, who went on to found a successful company of his own. In 1897, Cadbury did develop its own milk choco-late product, but gallingly, they were outsold by the Swiss on home territory. John Bradley, in a more recent history of the company that is a little firmer on the facts than Rogers, states that by 1902, the year Cadbury opened its own milk condensing plant, it was only making a ton of milk chocolate a week, amounting to 1 percent of its business, while Nestlé was selling thirty times that in Britain.[5]

Realizing that its equivalent product was strug-gling, the firm changed tack. "The breakthrough in thinking was that the best milk chocolate would be defined by having the best milk credentials, as opposed to the best chocolate credentials," writes Bradley. "The next Cadbury milk chocolate had to have a far higher milk content than any previously available. By using large quantities of fresh full cream milk from British pastures, they would not only have a flavour to beat the Swiss, but the potential to leverage the quality, quantity and the British-ness of the milk in their advertising."[6]

Cadbury ordered its milk directly from local dairies, and to stress the connection with the farm and the cow, it called its new formulation "Dairy Milk" chocolate. Each pound of Dairy Milk was made using three-quarters of a pound of raw chocolate and two pounds of liquid milk—Cadbury referred to these proportions in its advertising, heralding "1 1/2 glasses of full cream milk in every 1/2 lb block."[7] The "glass and a half" is still used as a slogan today, although the reference to "full cream" has been dropped, and the company's logo is two glasses of milk being poured.

As the new product took off, Bournville became the hub of an empire of milk. To feed its condensing plant, the firm established satellite milk factories at Knighton and Frampton-on-Severn, in the dairy lands of Staffordshire and Gloucestershire. The company oper-ated its own fleet of motorboats to transport milk from these satellites to the main plant, moving thousands of churns by canal. At Knighton, the business of cleaning these churns for return to the dairies was itself on an industrial scale, involving superheated steam and a helical "churn tower" on which the containers dried in a descending spiral.[8]

Cleanliness was important. In the 1870s, public concern about widespread adulteration and contamina-tion of food had reached a crescendo, resulting in the 1875 Food and Drugs Act. Cadbury already traded on the purity of its wares, but at Bournville its concep-tion of purity spread beyond the sanitary state of the production line. Soon after the factory opened, the firm built twenty cottages for some of its workers. In the early 1890s, it purchased Bournbrook Hall, a large Georgian house, and used it as the nucleus of a more extensive planned settlement. By 1931, Bournville village had 2,000 houses and a population of 7,500.[9]

Bournville founder George Cadbury "believed that the root of most social evils lay in bad housing condi-tions and in the unsatisfying life of the town worker in crowded industrial areas, and he saw possible for him a fuller, happier life in a country environment," gushed T. B. Rogers in the company's centenary history. "It was to be an experiment, in town and village plan-ning, with pleasant open spaces, and with houses not occupying more than one-fourth of their own sites, each having an ample garden; and the scheme was built on an economic basis, so that it could be followed by other communities."[10] The houses were built in a cottagey Arts and Crafts style, all mellow brick and half-timbering. Throughout the development, harmony

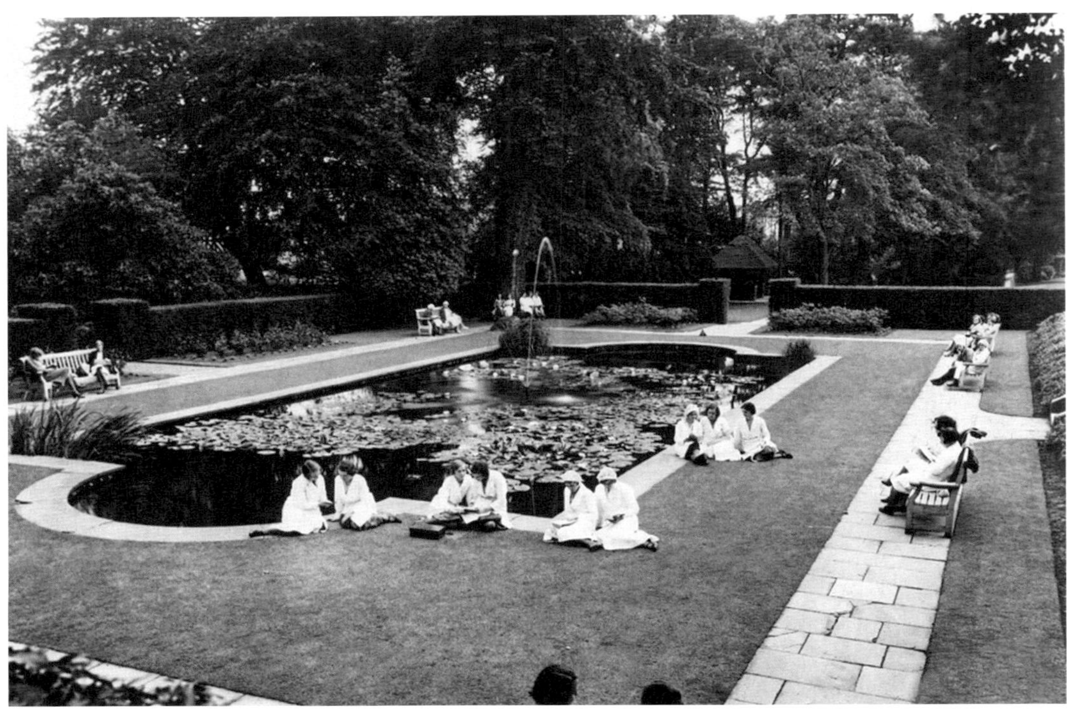

Workers at Cadbury's factory in Bournville take a break during a heat wave, 1932.

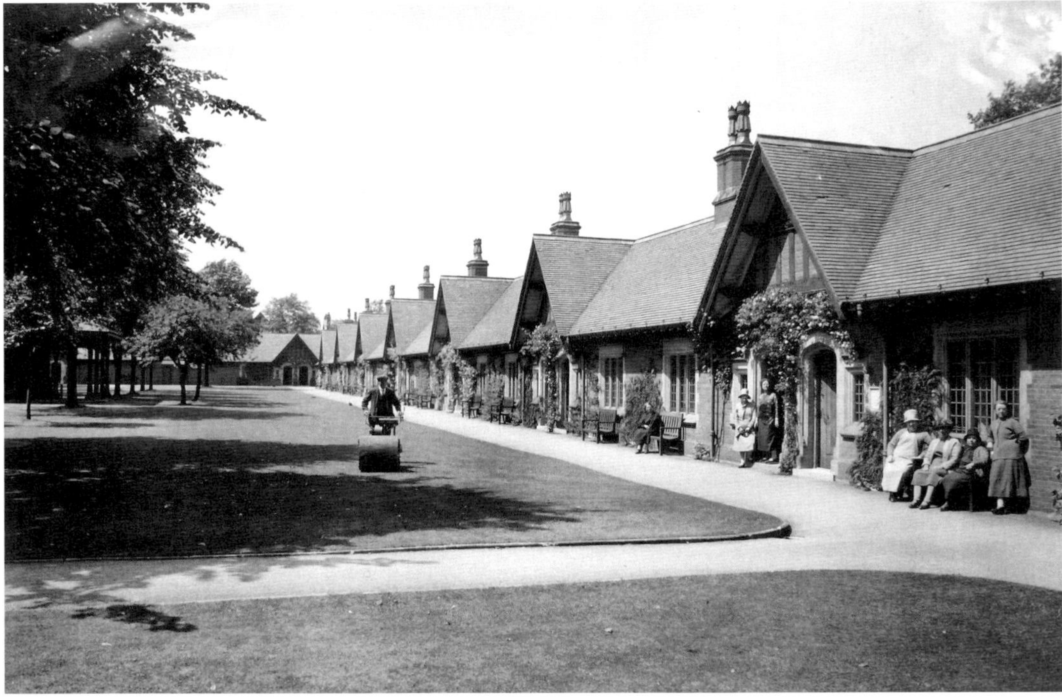

Bungalow homes built in the 1890s for retired Cadbury workers.

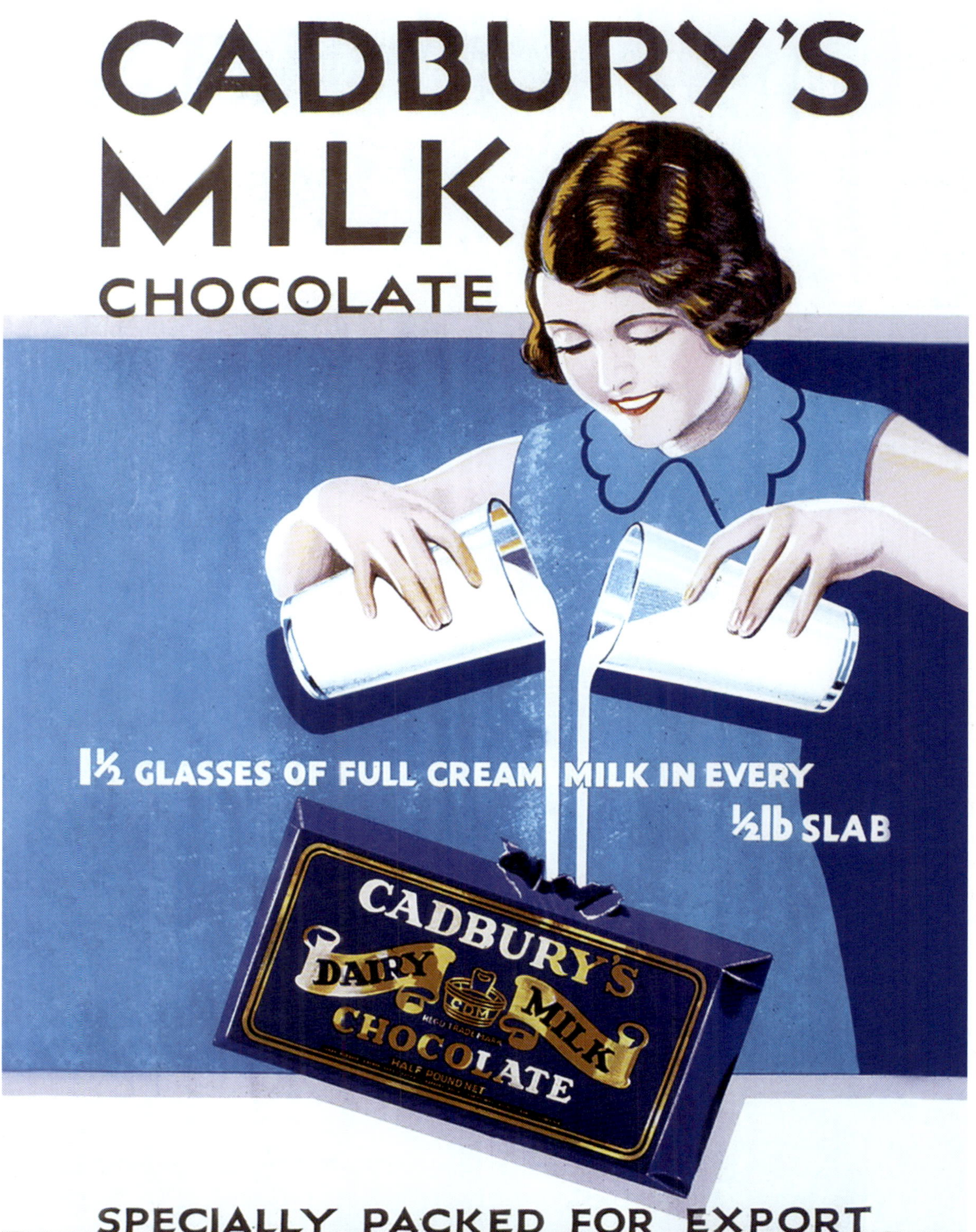
CADBURY'S
MILK
CHOCOLATE
1½ GLASSES OF FULL CREAM MILK IN EVERY
½lb SLAB
CADBURY'S
DAIRY MILK
CHOCOLATE
REGD TRADE MARK
C.D.M.
HALF POUND NET
SPECIALLY PACKED FOR EXPORT
CADBURY, BOURNVILLE, ENGLAND

Opposite: Advertisement for Cadbury's Dairy Milk bar, ca. 1935. The product proved a success from the moment it was launched in 1905, despite the company's decision not to devote significant resources toward advertising it. This policy changed in 1928, with the advent of the iconic "glass-and-a-half" campaign, touting the amount of "full cream milk" in each bar.

Right: Advertisement from the 1930s depicting an idealized Bournville.

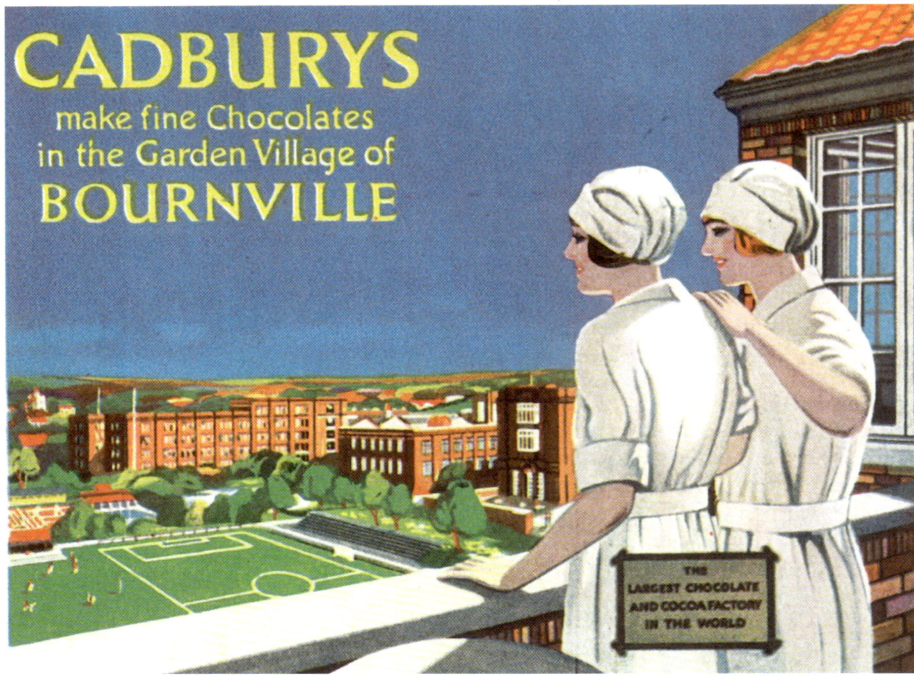

with nature was accented: "It was the firm's rigorous policy to preserve the natural features of beauty both within and around the factory, and to cultivate flower gardens wherever possible. In the 'nineties the Works were already becoming known to the world as 'The Factory in a Garden.'"[11]

Not all the firm's employees could live in the village, but all could enjoy its facilities. The company built a huge community center, the Dining Room Block, which was headquarters for dozens of staff organizations, including musical and dramatic societies, "the Youths' Club with its many activities … the camera club, the chess club, the ambulance corps, the folk dance society, and the 'feather and fur' and other societies for the cultivation of utility hobbies."[12] There were 110 acres of recreation grounds to promote physical fitness: Rogers records more than 220 sports teams, including 38 for soccer and rugby, 32 for cricket, 35 for tennis, 28 for bowls, 28 for hockey, and 25 for netball.

The moral health of the workforce was also a concern. As Quakers, the Cadburys abhorred alcohol, a fact that underpinned their whole interest in non-intoxicating hot drinks. The village was founded on strict temperance principles, with no alcohol permitted, although this stricture was later loosened, merely ensuring that all profits from sale of "intoxicating liquors" were "devoted to securing recreation and counter-attractions to the liquor trade as ordinarily conducted."[13] That may help explain why there were so many clubs and teams. More than half of the workforce were women and attitudes toward them could be traditional: "Women workers who married received gifts of carnations and Bibles and were sent home to raise their families."[14]

Milk, cleanliness, suburbia, and outdoorsy moral health flowed together in the company's public image. "Cadburys makes fine Chocolates in the Garden Village of Bournville," reads an advertisement from the 1930s.[15] The accompanying image is of two women in pristine white uniforms, one laying a sisterly hand on the shoulder of the other as they gaze out over a chimney-less vista of treetops and playing fields.[16] Other ads "showed highly contented Cadbury cows getting one of their twice-daily hand brushings in what looks like the cattle barn equivalent of the Ritz."[17] Purity was the motif: purity of product; purity of surroundings, rid of the corruption of the city; and purity of the virginal white-clad workforce. Milk was the perfect symbol: spotless, nurturing, paradisical.

Most importantly, it was a practical paradise. Cadbury's business surged ahead after its move to

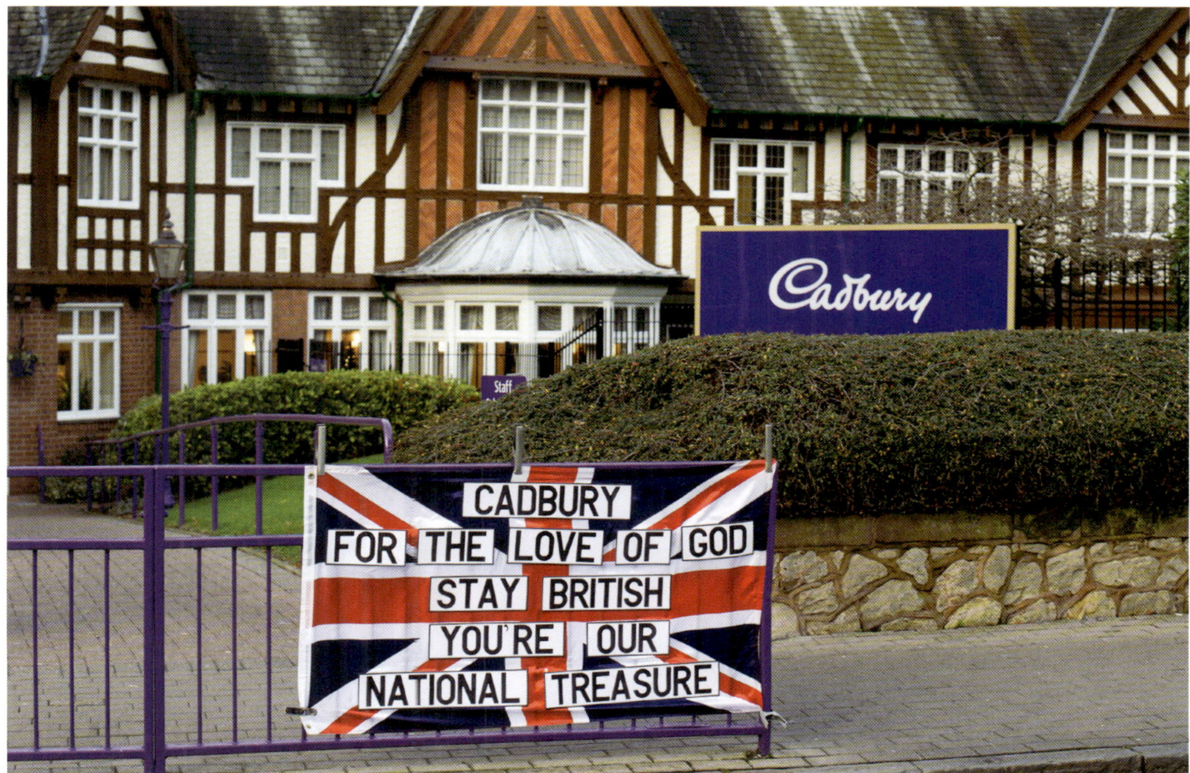

Bournville. In 1879, it employed 230 people; by 1899, it had eleven times that. The experiment was wildly influential. In 1898, Ebenezer Howard published *To-Morrow: A Peaceful Path to Real Reform*, republished in 1902 as *Garden Cities of To-Morrow*, a tract advocating dispersed, semirural industrial centers as an antidote to the evils of the Victorian metropolis. This led to the foundation of the Garden City movement, which held its inaugural conference in Bournville in 1901.[18] Bournville's tree-lined streets and gentle eaves have loomed over British planning ever since.

What's strange, however, is the recurrence of milk in many of the plans for model industrial settlements. Rowntree, another Quaker-founded chocolatier, had its own model village at New Earswick in Yorkshire. Today, the Rowntree name is as much associated with community housing and social research as it is with milk chocolate. Howard himself lingers particularly on dairies, affording them crucial locations in the outer ring of his proposed Garden City. The cost of supply of milk is one of his leading economic justifications for his scheme, cutting the distance between cow and consumer and reducing the number of deliveries. This echoes Isabelle Gatti de Gamond's much earlier writing on the Phalanstery, a combined industrial-residential community first proposed by Charles Fourier. "One hundred milk-women," de Gamond wrote in 1841, "who waste one hundred mornings in the town, will be replaced by a small wheel-carriage, bearing a tun of milk." We can, perhaps, infer a moral dimension in the faint sniff at those wasted mornings in town.

Bournville's civilities were public boasts, deliberately made central to the image the word "Cadbury" conjured in the mind. Milk was messaging. This has an older precedent, again blended with a view of the world in ideal form, the world made right. In *ancien régime* France, it was surprisingly common for female aristocrats to build picturesque "pleasure dairies" for elaborate displays of pastoral harmony. This served "the strategic purpose of conveying power while appearing to retreat from it," writes Meredith Martin in *Dairy Queens: The Politics of Pastoral Architecture from*

Above: Protest at Bournville following the sale of Cadbury to the American food conglomerate Kraft. Photo David Warren.

Catherine de' Medici to Marie-Antoinette. "Royal women used these seemingly unassuming buildings to express a political persona that heralded the abundant, hard-working contributions of queens, female companions, and mothers."[19] Nearly all of the noted architects of the day built pleasure dairies. Today, Jean-Jacques Lequeu's lasting memory rests almost entirely on the cowshed he built in the shape of a cow, but he also designed a decorative dairy for precisely this purpose. Perhaps more significant was Claude-Nicolas Ledoux, designer of the model industrial settlement housing the Royal Saltworks at Arc-et-Senan. He built a pleasure dairy for the chateau of Préaudeau de Chemilly, a treasury official, before 1785. This chateau was called Bourneville.

Within its soft shell of nourishment, milk has a hard center: necessity. For the infant, milk is not only wholesome; it is necessary for survival. There lies the sternness in the frolicking of the French aristocrats, and in the paternalism of Cadbury. But a reputation for purity is vulnerable to contamination. British, European, and American milk chocolate are made using different processes. Water-based milk and oil-based cocoa butter do not mix easily, and most recipes use a binding emulsifier, generally the soybean extract lecithin, which also minimizes the amount of expensive cocoa used. British chocolate further reduces cocoa butter via the addition of vegetable oil, a fact that made it the subject of a lengthy dispute within the European Union at the turn of the century.[20] American milk chocolate is different again, mostly following Hershey's patented process, which results in a product containing butyric acid. To the European palate, this has a soapy, even vomitous, taste.

This distasteful difference put a ghastly implication at the heart of the Kraft merger. It was suspected that Kraft's intentions might go beyond its adventurous additions to Cadbury bars, such as Ritz cracker crumbs. It was feared that the formulation of the chocolate itself might change. Kraft did little to allay this fear, weaseling out of other guarantees it had given and continually tinkering with the product line. The recipe for Creme Eggs, for instance, was changed in 2015, amid predictable outcry, and the shape of Dairy Milk bars was altered. Cadbury's Roses, boxed chocolate bonbons popular at Christmas, which used to come in twists of shiny paper, are now sealed in "flow wrap," like "mints in a bowl at the reception desk at cheap European hotels," in the disdainful words of the *Telegraph.*[21]

For some of the *Telegraph*'s aged, right-wing readership, the word "European" would carry more sting than the word "cheap." During the earlier cocoa dispute with the EU, the British tabloid press suggested that Brussels did not consider our chocolate to be chocolate at all and might force it to be renamed "vegelate." Like almost all stories of this type, this was a myth, one that gave a garden variety bureaucratic argument over food labeling the complexion of an assault on the national soul.[22] It is this kind of gleeful fabrication that has led directly to our present diplomatic calamity. The affective link between milk chocolate, childhood, and goodness makes it an effective weapon for nationalism.

1 T. B. Rogers, *A Century of Progress, 1831–1931: Cadbury Bournville* (London: Howard & Kearns, 1931).

2 Ibid., p. 36.

3 Ibid.

4 Ibid., pp. 20–21.

5 John Bradley, *Cadbury's Purple Reign: The Story Behind Britain's Best-Loved Brand* (Chichester, UK: John Wiley & Sons, 2008).

6 Ibid.

7 T. B. Rogers, *A Century of Progress*, p. 79.

8 Ibid., p. 76.

9 Ibid., p. 80.

10 Ibid.

11 Ibid., p. 56.

12 Ibid., p. 69.

13 Ebenezer Howard, *Garden Cities of To-Morrow* (London: Swan Sonnenschein and Co., 1902), p. 85n.

14 Michael D'Antonio, *Hershey: Milton S. Hershey's Extraordinary Life of Wealth, Empire, and Utopian Dreams* (New York: Simon & Schuster, 2006), p. 85.

15 The advertisement renders the company's name without the possessive apostrophe. This is presumably an error.

16 T. B. Rogers, *A Century of Progress*, p. 31.

17 John Bradley, *Cadbury's Purple Reign*, p. 102.

18 Dennis Hardy, "The Garden City Campaign: An Overview," in *The Garden City: Past, Present and Future*, ed. Stephen V. Ward (London: E. & F. N. Spon, 1992), p. 188.

19 Meredith Martin, *Dairy Queens: The Politics of Pastoral Architecture from Catherine de' Medici to Marie-Antoinette* (Cambridge, MA: Harvard University Press, 2011), p. 8.

20 See Colin Blane, "Euro Chocolate War Ends," BBC News, 25 May 2000. Available at <news.bbc.co.uk/1/hi/world/europe/764305.stm>.

21 See Harry Wallop, "The Many Ways Cadbury Is Losing Its Magic," *The Telegraph* (London, UK), 21 March 2016. Available at <telegraph.co.uk/food-and-drink/features/the-many-ways-cadbury-is-losing-its-magic>.

22 See "Chocolate or 'Vegelate,'" a blog post on the website of the European Commission. Available at <blogs.ec.europa.eu/ECintheUK/chocolate-or-vegelate>.

I PUT A LIGHT IN THE MILK
Jeff Dolven

François Truffaut is ready to move on. He is halfway through his series of interviews with Alfred Hitchcock, which take up the British director's films in roughly chronological order. The two have been talking about *Suspicion*, from 1941, the casting of Joan Fontaine, the debates over the ending, the disappointing decision to shoot in a sound stage rather than on location. But Hitchcock detains him over a last detail:

> A. H.   *By the way, did you like the scene with the glass of milk?*
> F. T.   *When Cary Grant takes it upstairs? Yes, it was very good.*
> A. H.   *I put a light in the milk.*[1]

Anyone who has seen the film will have to agree with Truffaut's assessment. Cary Grant, playing the charming bounder Johnnie Aysgarth, enters a dark foyer in the grand house that he and his new wife Lina cannot afford. The camera follows him from above as he crosses the floor and mounts the stairs, carrying a tall glass of milk on a silver tray held casually, one-handed, just above his belt. He is lit from behind, his face in black shadow, but the milk—the milk glows like a torch, the moving center of the scene, and as he approaches the waiting camera its white glare almost fills the screen. It is a beacon, a sign. But the reader coming upon the still image for the first time, and the moviegoer who has been following the story for ninety minutes, will be equally unsure: a sign of what?

For the reader, a sketch of that story is in order. Grant's Johnnie meets Fontaine's Lina on a train, where he persuades her to help him through a little contretemps about having a third-class ticket in a first-class compartment. The next time they see each other, it is at a fox hunt, where Johnnie, in ascot and bowler, carries himself with reassuring *savoir faire*. Next, he is at her doorstep, in the company of her hunting friends; then he appears again, by himself, in short order, and against the wishes of her father, the upright General McLaidlaw, they are married. It does not take long for Lina to realize what the audience already well knows, that Johnnie has no money of his own, and their lavish new life is lived in expectation of her inheritance. At her urging, he does take a job … but he

is soon discovered to be borrowing from the till. The general dies … but when the will is read, they learn he has cut his daughter out. There is a scheme with Johnnie's friend Beaky to invest in a cliffside real estate development … but Beaky dies mysteriously in Paris. Johann Strauss's "Wiener Blut" waltz, the leitmotif of the couple's infatuation, modulates from major to minor in the background. One morning, reading the mail while her husband is in the bath, Lina discovers that he has made inquiries into the terms of their common life insurance policy. Not long after, a mystery-writer neighbor tells that Johnnie has been asking about the relative merits and accessibility of undetectable poisons.

Such is the state of play when Johnnie climbs the stairs with that ostentatiously fateful glass of milk. Lina, undone by her doubts, has taken to her bed; the film's harsh chiaroscuro and canted camera angles are increasingly hers, as though Hitchcock had gradually ceded her the cinematographer's duties. The milk is the allegorical focus of this transformation. It is blameless, nourishing, the elixir of childhood. Its maternal benison ought by rights to promise fertility to the pair whose marriage is still unblessed. But Hitchcock pushes this innocent milk-language too far for anyone's good. "You mean a spotlight on it?" asks Truffaut. "No," Hitchcock answers: "I put a light right inside the glass because I wanted it to be luminous. Cary Grant's walking up the stairs and everyone's attention had to be focused on that glass."[2] The almost sacramental insistence on the milk's purity has the effect of turning the moviegoer's mind, as milk left out on a hot day will turn; the effect is much stronger than introducing a foreign body, a fly or a strand of hair, or a creeping stain. The shining glass asks not just to be seen, but to be believed. There is considerable craft in that transubstantiation, and Hitchcock points proudly to it. But then, for all that, milk could be said to be the perfect object of suspicion already.

Already: but not for all that long, historically speaking. The milk of other animals has only been a dietary staple in Europe since the eighteenth century, and the fear that it might be poisoned has no prominent place in the Christian tradition or the classical myths. It is otherwise in India, where cow's milk has been consumed in quantity for millennia. When the

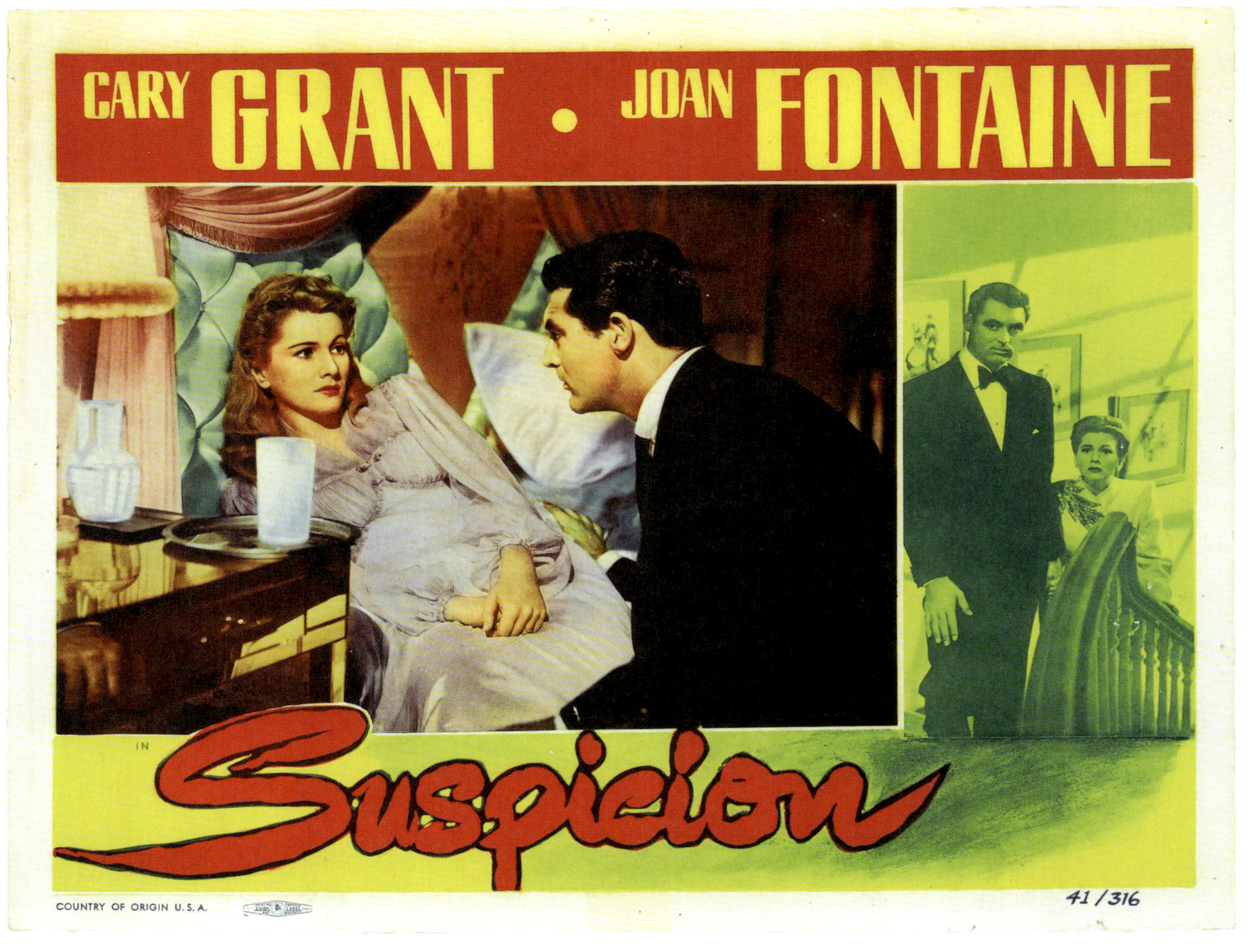

Heavy on the milk. Lobby card for Alfred Hitchcock's *Suspicion*, 1941.

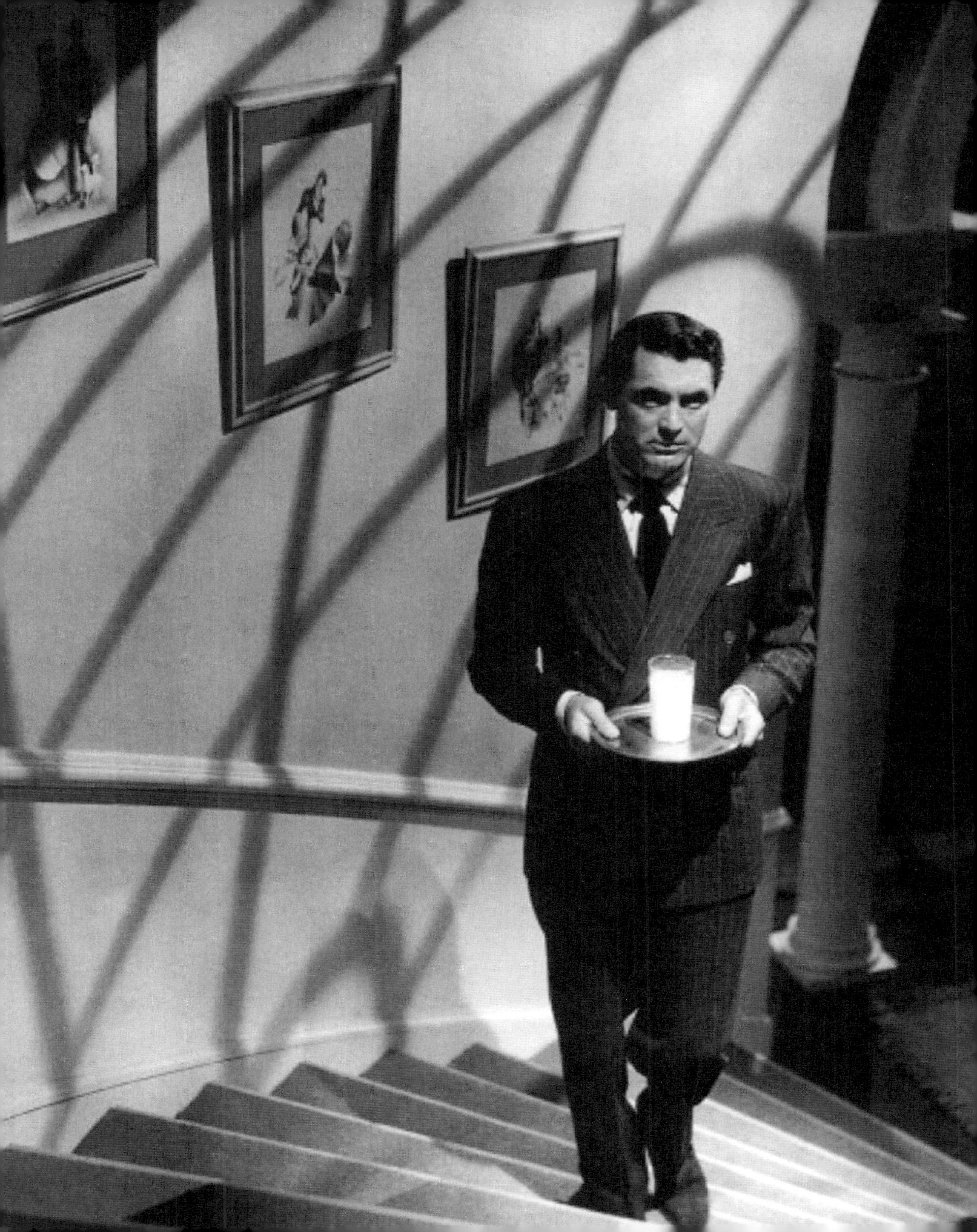

Hindu gods stir the ocean of milk, hoping to decoct a nectar to restore their immortality, the poison they release turns Shiva blue; Krishna is almost killed by the poisoned milk of his foster-mother Putana.[3] In the West, it takes the twin projects of expansion and industrialization to make widespread the suspicion that milk's honest complexion might protest too much.

The expansion story is American. The pattern of milk consumption among settlers at the beginning of the nineteenth century was traditional, households drinking the milk of their own cows, no far transport, no wide market. Still, the drink was important enough on the frontier that milk sickness could threaten the nation's very manifest destiny. "Milk sickness": its sufferers endured anorexia, nausea, listlessness, and acidosis, an unchecked acidity of the blood that could progress to coma or death. "Puking disease," "sick stomach," "the sloes" or "slows," "swamp sickness," "tires," "trembles"—by any name it was epidemic in the south, midwest, and southwest throughout the nineteenth century, blamed variously on arsenic, organisms in the soil, and baleful exhalations breathed from tilled land.[4] Young towns collapsed where it hit hardest, leaving ruins to be found by the next wave of settlers. "It has been conjectured by many," reported *The Medical Repository* as early as 1811, "that this affection depended on poisoned milk,"[5] but it would be another century before the cause was definitively identified as the white snakeroot, a woodland shade plant eaten by cows that strayed from their pasture. Once the etiology was clear, precautions were simple enough, and the disease is virtually unknown today. But in affected areas it was the century's chief cause of infant mortality, and perhaps even of disability and death among adults.

Milk sickness was a mystery that haunted the borders of settlement. "White poison" stabbed its centers. The phrase came to be used to describe the milk that was supplied to city dwellers during the rapid urbanization of the nineteenth century, brought to sale from the proliferating milk sheds around towns and cities. Milk was taken with coffee and tea; it was promoted as an alternative to breastfeeding, especially for working-class mothers; it was increasingly downed by the glassful. Milk was now a market. With new profits, and widespread competition, came the new cost-cutting strategies of an underregulated and unscrupulous industry. The sheds were punishing, unsanitary places, and the milk they produced would sit at warm temperatures for hours or days. The cows were often fed on distillers' waste. ("I have distinctly tasted the *Whiskey* in milk of cows," wrote one William Cobbett in 1821.[6]) Tuberculosis bacilli flourished in the accommodating barrels, pails, and bottles. The techniques for making the stuff presentable were themselves often toxic, with boric acid added to delay souring, and snail shells and animal brains mixed in to inspire a robust froth. The headlines in British newspapers acquire a queasy familiarity: "Poisoned Milk at Greenock" (*Edinburgh Evening News*, 1876), "Typhoid Fever and Poisoned Milk" (*The Dundee Courier*, 1878), "Another Lesson from the Poisoned Milk Pail" (*The Cornishman*, 1884).[7]

Turn that key, "poison milk," in the lock of the Internet today, and a thousand barn doors spring open. Respectable sites warn responsibly of the danger posed by growth hormones often found in dairy milk; others speculate less scrupulously, but often more urgently, about leukemia, pancreatic cancer, pituitary and thyroid overdrive, and countless other ailments, specific and general. There are reports on scandals like the 2008 sickening of Chinese children by milk adulterated with melamine. (Melamine masks the protein depletion of watered milk to get it past the inspectors; fifty-four thousand babies were hospitalized.) There are freewheeling conspiracy theories that discover the dairy lobby's machinations behind every symptom of the modern malaise. Indeed, as explanations go, trouble with the milk is hard to better. Not just poisoned milk, the scourge of the nineteenth century, but poison milk, as though straight from the teat the stuff were snakeroot itself. Who has not taken a suspicious sniff at the beak of a carton? And as religiously as you may check, you have already drunk it. Milk is the apple before the apple, each infant's original sin before ever choosing. If you suspect that something is wrong, basically wrong, and look back and back and back, back to the first thing that was ever put in you from outside, what have you got but milk?

Opposite: Cary Grant in publicity still for *Suspicion*. The film's script describes the scene: "LONG SHOT — FROM ABOVE —We see Johnnie on the stairs below. He comes up with measured tread, because he is carrying a glass of milk on a small plate. He comes on up and up. He turns the stairs, getting nearer and nearer towards the camera – so close that the glass of milk fills the screen."

Somewhere between the poisoned milks of Greenock and Shijiazhuang, milk enjoyed its golden age. The early twentieth century saw much more successful regulation of the industry; milk was safe, and between the wars it came to rival bread as a basic index of public nutrition. The period was captioned by Winston Churchill's famous proclamation, in the midst of the Battle of Britain, two years after *Suspicion* was made: "There is no finer investment for a community than putting milk into babies."[8] Milk consumption had never been so widespread, nor would it be again. Hitchcock's intervention is timed to this high, white tide of public confidence. He added his soupçon of arsenic at just the moment when milk was (as the poet James Schuyler would put it, twenty years later) coming into its own.[9]

Or did he? For Johnnie's uncanny glass rests untouched by Lina's bedside; the bulb burning in its heart goes undiscovered, and the poison, if there is poison, unproven. The next morning Lina decides to take a few days at her mother's house, and Johnnie insists on driving her, at speed, along the narrow cliff-side roads of Dover. As his powerful 1936 Lagonda rounds a sharp bend, the passenger door springs open, and Johnnie reaches toward his wife—to pull her back into the car and to safety. When they come to a stop, he explains everything. The plot, the insurance and the poison research, was all to kill himself, to end his shame and secure his wife's future after his death. Was there then no poison in the glass? Do Johnnie's good intentions redeem that milk? The light, it seems, was true. We have all taken our fatal drink, long ago, but Hitchcock's milk turns out to be not so much a poison as a diagnosis, holding our suspicions before us in its plain, white, shadowless, and beneficent light. A diagnosis, and a cure, for Johnnie came in compassion, like a good milkman, with a glass to soothe our suspicious

natures. Milk, after all, is what the poison control hotline will tell you to drink if you have accidentally consumed something truly poisonous. If we doubt the milk, what can we trust? If we trust the milk, we can take it from there.

Or can we? Hitchcock had another ending in mind, one the studio rejected, but which he described, wistfully, to Truffaut:

The scene I wanted, but it was never shot, was for Cary Grant to bring her a glass of milk that's been poisoned and Joan Fontaine has just finished a letter to her mother: "Dear Mother, I'm desperately in love with him, but I don't want to live because he's a killer. Though I'd rather die, I think society should be protected from him." Then, Cary Grant comes in with the fatal glass and she says, "Will you mail this letter to Mother for me, dear?" She drinks the milk and dies. Fade out and fade in on one short shot: Cary Grant, whistling cheerfully, walks over to the mailbox and pops the letter in.[10]

There was poison in the milk after all. One could imagine reshooting the scene to make it plain, with the milk beginning to boil in the glass as Johnnie approaches the bedroom, or with a pitch-black, sinister twist of milk-smoke rising from its surface. Or perhaps the negative could be swapped in, putting Johnnie in a white suit, with a tall draft of viscous crude on his tray. Or another possibility, another ending, maybe more in Hitchcock's spirit. Johnnie takes his seat beside Lina's bed, just as he does in the version RKO sent out into the world in 1941, and offers her the glass; she takes a long draft, and hands it back; he finishes it. Then they sit side by side without speaking, waiting to see everything that has already happened.

———————————

Opposite: Page from working script of *Suspicion*, showing one of the cuts Hitchcock made to the milk scene.

1 François Truffaut, *Hitchcock*, rev. ed. (New York: Simon and Schuster, 1985), p. 143. The image reproduced in Truffaut's volume is a publicity still: it shows Grant's face, which is in shadow in the film, and he holds the tray with two hands rather than one.

2 Ibid.

3 On milk in Indian mythology, see Wendy Doniger O'Flaherty, *Women, Androgynes, and Other Mythical Beasts* (Chicago: University of Chicago Press,

1980), pp. 53–58.

4 Thomas Cone, "Milk Sickness (Tremetol Poisoning)," in *The Cambridge World History of Human Disease*, ed. Kenneth F. Kipper (Cambridge: Cambridge University Press), pp. 879–880.

5 "A Disease in Ohio, Ascribed to Some Deleterous Quality in the Milk of Cows," *The Medical Repository*, vol. 3, ed. Samuel Latham Mitchill and Edward Miller (New York: Collins and Co., 1812), p. 92.

6 Hannah Velten, *Milk: A Global History* (London: Reaktion Books, 2010), p. 60.

7 *Edinburgh Evening News* (Edinburgh, Scotland), 22 March 1876; *The Dundee Courier & Argus and Northern Warder* (Dundee, Scotland), 25 January 1878; *The Cornishman* (Penzance, England), 24 January 1884. On "white poison" generally, see Hannah Velten's account in *Milk: A Global History*, pp. 55–76.

8 Deborah Valenze, *Milk: A Local and Global History* (New Haven: Yale University Press, 2012), p. 254.

9 At the end of his beautiful poem "Milk," Schuyler writes, "Trembling, milk is coming into its own." James Schuyler, *Collected Poems* (New York: The Noonday Press, 1993), p. 32.

10 François Truffaut, *Hitchcock*, p. 142.

(ALREADY
SHOT)437   SEMI-LONG SHOT - from Lina's eyeline - Johnnie stands
           framed in the doorway, holding the glass of milk.

                              JOHNNIE
                    I - I brought you something,
                    Monkeyface.

438-   SEMI-CLOSEUP. Lina's eyes follow the progress of the
445   glass of milk. They travel in a complete semi-circle
           until she sees the glass and his hand enter the right
           hand side of the screen, and place it on the table. She
           looks up at Johnnie and the CAMERA PULLS BACK. Johnnie
           bends over her saying:

                              JOHNNIE
                    Good night, Lina.

           He kisses her with a touch of fervency that surprises
           her a little.

           The CAMERA PANS him away from the bed, across to his own
           room. He opens the door and switching the light on,
           enters. He closes the door softly.

446   SEMI-CLOSEUP of Lina. She looks down at the milk and
           then toward Johnnie's door. Her face showing visible
           signs of distress she's going through. Suddenly she
           makes a decision to face Johnnie. She rises from the
           bed and

           CAMERA PANS her as she crosses in determination to his
           door. She hesitates at the door and then quietly turns
           the handle to enter. She stops suddenly as she sees:

INT. JOHNNIE'S DRESSING ROOM - NIGHT

447   SEMI-CLOSEUP from her viewpoint we see Johnnie's back.
           He is in the act of emptying some powder from a paper
           into a glass of water.

INT. AYSGARTH BEDROOM - NIGHT

448   CLOSEUP of Lina - she looks quickly back to her own milk
           and takes in the situation in a flash, realizing the
           mistake she has made. As she turns back quickly, she
           sees:

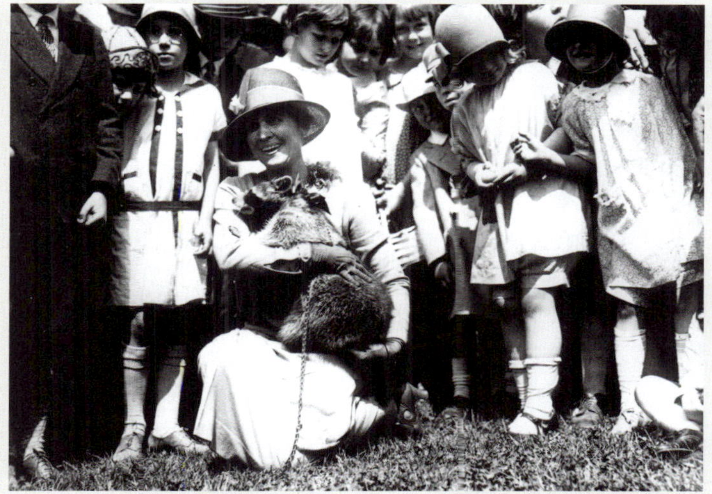

Researching the history of the cow that William Henry Taft kept at the White House, we discovered the long and varied history of presidential pets. While cats and dogs dominate the list, there were also some surprises. John Quincy Adams had an alligator, which lived in a bathroom; perhaps predictably, Andrew Jackson's parrot knew how to swear. Benjamin Harrison had a pair of opossums, Woodrow Wilson a ram named Old Ike who was partial to tobacco, Calvin Coolidge a raccoon, and Herbert Hoover not one but two alligators.

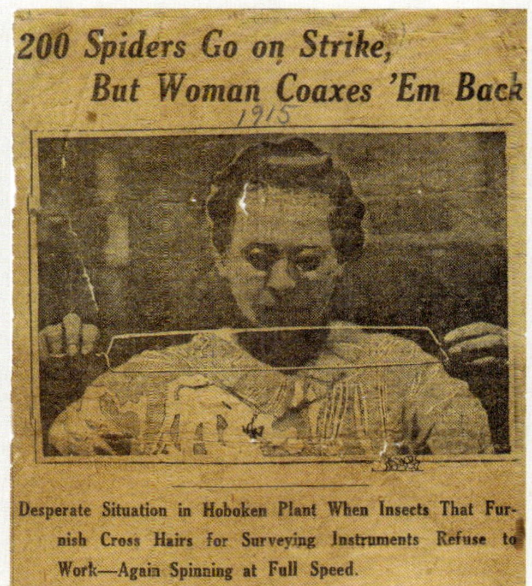

Desperate Situation in Hoboken Plant When Insects That Furnish Cross Hairs for Surveying Instruments Refuse to Work—Again Spinning at Full Speed.

Speaking of interspecies relationships, it turns out that the collection of spider silk for use in the production of gunsights for the military and other optical instruments—see D. Graham Burnett's "Spiders, Stars, and Death" in this issue—was a relatively widespread industry (and one that seems to have often been overseen by women). Mary Pfieffer, as Burnett notes, was engaged in gathering spider silk for more than half a century for the instrument maker Keuffel & Esser, based in Hoboken, New Jersey. A short piece in a 1941 issue of the *New Yorker* described her process of gathering her eight-legged workers—once every summer she would enlist a group of boys in the area to scour the marshes for the critters, for each of which she paid fifteen cents. After amassing a few hundred spiders, Pfeiffer began coaxing their silk by enticing them onto sticks from which she would then carefully fling them into the air using tweezers; the spiders would instinctively begin emitting silk (up to ten feet per toss), which she then duly collected and wound onto spools, though this would typically work only twice with each animal, after which point, the magazine's correspondent noted, "they seem to get wise to the stunt." Nan Songer—an image of whom appears in Burnett's article— was another similarly celebrated "spider lady," as the press liked to call them. She began her business just as Pfeiffer's career was winding down. Operating her spider ranch in Yucaipa, California, beginning in 1939, she installed her workforce, collected both by her and by others who sent her specimens from around the country, in a front room of her farmhouse. (Her preferred species included the banded garden spider and the black widow.) Songer's silk production technique was so sophisticated that, with the encouragement of the US Bureau of Standards, she began offering web to precise specifications, from "extra-heavy" (1/5,000th of an inch) to "extra-fine" (1/50,000th of an inch). For the most sensitive applications, she marketed the silk of week-old baby spiders, which at 1/500,000th of an inch was virtually invisible. Meanwhile, according to a *Life* magazine article from August 1943, the US Army Quartermaster Corps' spiderweb production shop in Columbus, Ohio, was directed by Armada Ruffner, whose job it was to entice between 100 and 180 feet of silk every week from each of the dozens of black widow spiders under her supervision.

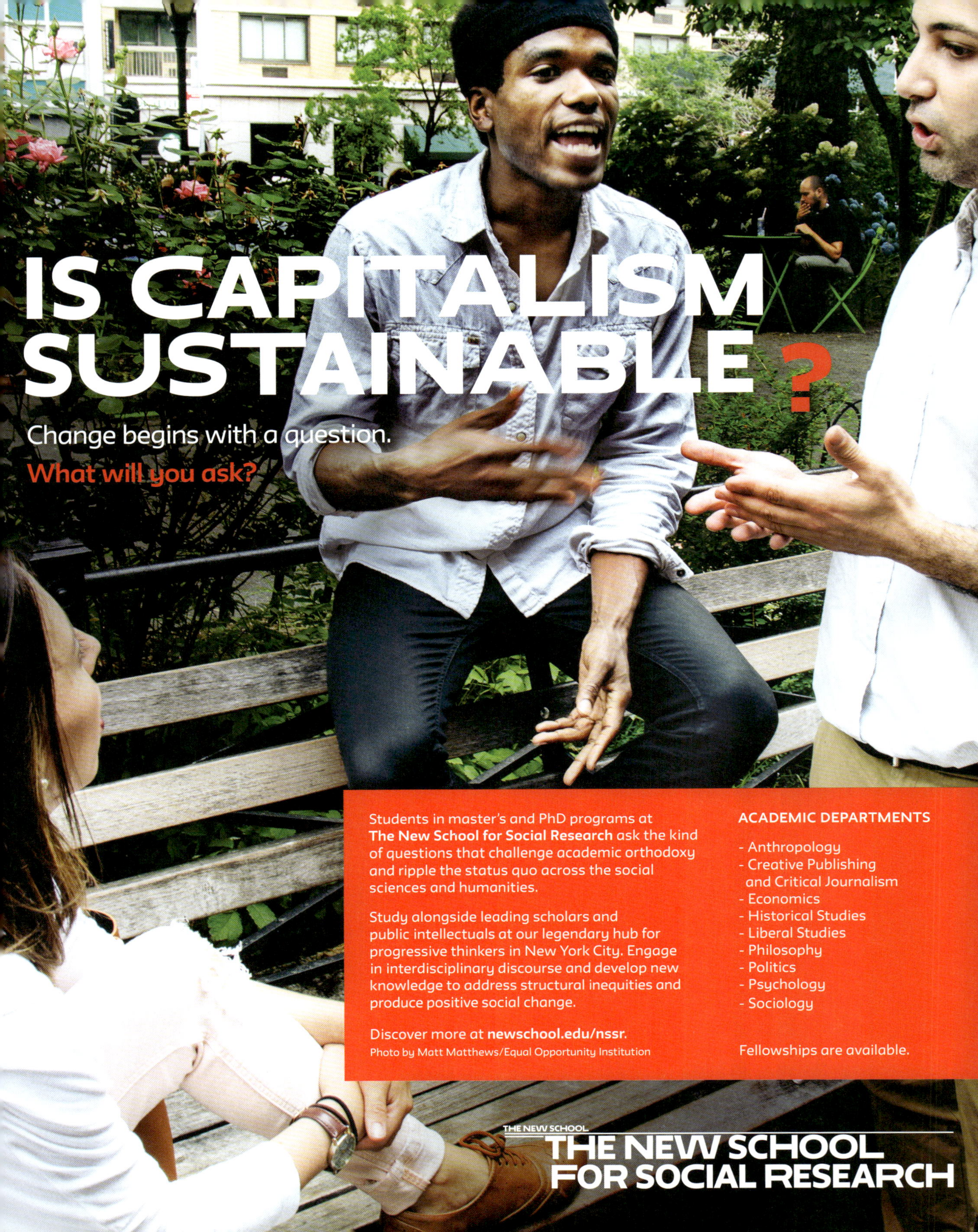

IS CAPITALISM SUSTAINABLE?

Change begins with a question.
What will you ask?

Students in master's and PhD programs at The New School for Social Research ask the kind of questions that challenge academic orthodoxy and ripple the status quo across the social sciences and humanities.

Study alongside leading scholars and public intellectuals at our legendary hub for progressive thinkers in New York City. Engage in interdisciplinary discourse and develop new knowledge to address structural inequities and produce positive social change.

Discover more at newschool.edu/nssr.
Photo by Matt Matthews/Equal Opportunity Institution

ACADEMIC DEPARTMENTS

- Anthropology
- Creative Publishing
  and Critical Journalism
- Economics
- Historical Studies
- Liberal Studies
- Philosophy
- Politics
- Psychology
- Sociology

Fellowships are available.

THE NEW SCHOOL
THE NEW SCHOOL
FOR SOCIAL RESEARCH

e-flux

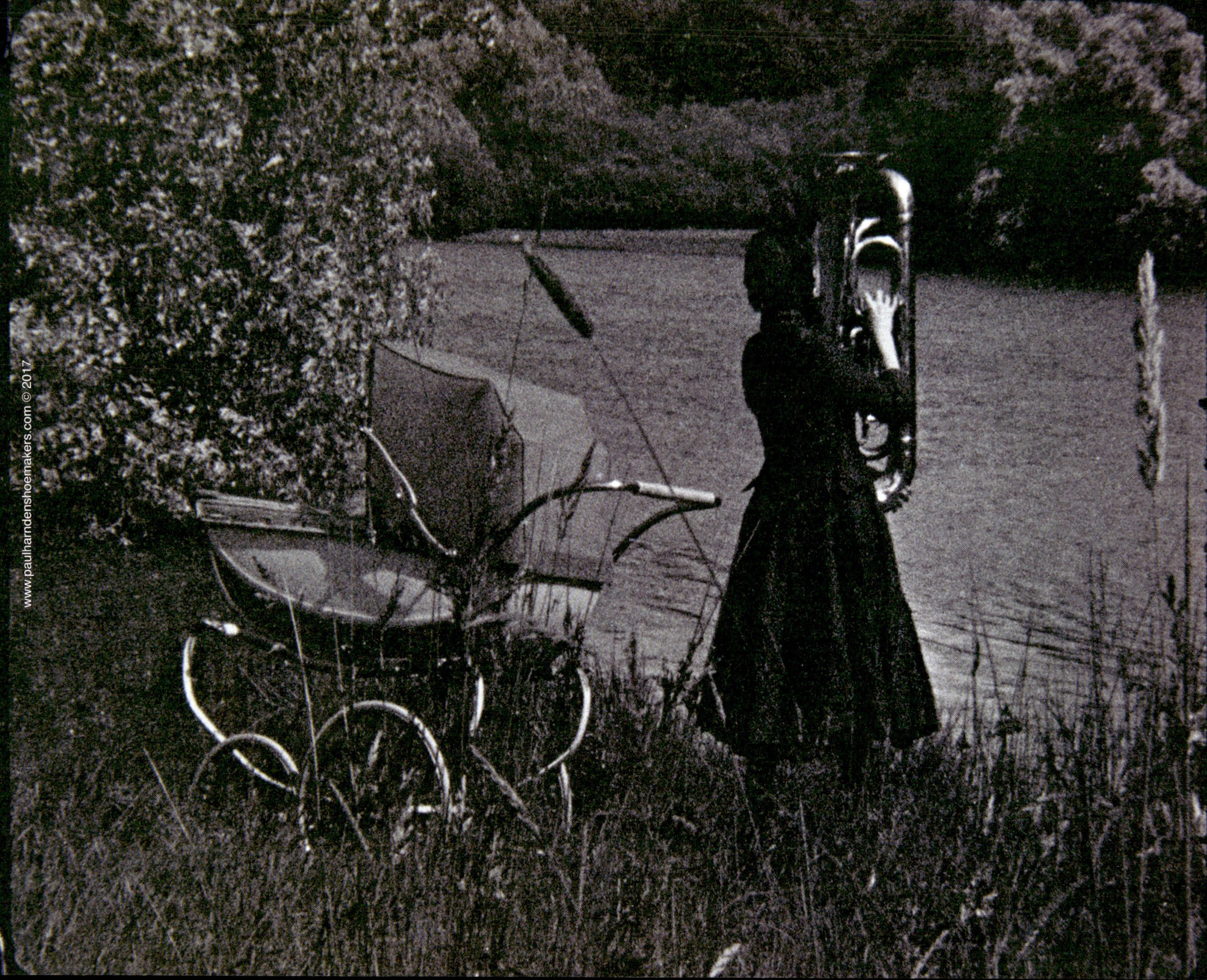

www.paulharndenshoemakers.com © 2017

CABINET
181 Wyckoff Street
Brooklyn, NY 11217 USA
phone + 1 718 222-8434
fax + 1 718 222-3700
info@cabinetmagazine.org
www.cabinetmagazine.org

Issue 58, Summer 2015

Cover: Evidence of an attempted burglary prevented by safety
glass, Gold-Baehr jewelry shop, Frankfurt, Germany, March 2013.
Photo Rupert Ganzer.

POSTMASTER
Please send address changes to Cabinet, 181 Wyckoff Street,
Brooklyn, NY 11217.

Cabinet (USPS # 020-348, ISSN 1531-1430) is a quarterly magazine
published by Immaterial Incorporated, 181 Wyckoff Street, Brooklyn,
NY 11217. Periodicals Postage paid at Brooklyn, NY, and additional
mailing offices.

Printed in Belgium by Die Keure, who have stolen our hearts.

ADVERTISING
phone + 1 718 222-8434
advertising@cabinetmagazine.org

DISTRIBUTION
Cabinet is available in the US and Canada through Disticor, which
distributes both using its own network and through Ingram, Ubiquity,
Hudson News, Media Marketing Research, Small Changes, Cowley
Distribution, Kent News, MSolutions, the News Group, Chris Stadler,
and Don Olson Distribution.

To carry Cabinet through one of these distributors, contact Melanie
Raucci at Disticor: phone + 1 631 587-1160, mraucci@disticor.com

Cabinet is available in Europe and elsewhere through Central Books,
London: orders@centralbooks.com

Cabinet is available worldwide as a book, with an ISBN, through DAP:
phone + 1 212 627-1999, dap@dapinc.com

For further information, contact: circulation@cabinetmagazine.org

INDIVIDUAL SUBSCRIPTIONS
1 year (4 issues):   2 years (8 issues):
US $32   US $60
Canada $38   Canada $72
Western Europe $40   Western Europe $76
Elsewhere $50   Elsewhere $96

Please send a check in US dollars made out to "Cabinet," or mail, fax,
or email us your Visa/MC/AmEx/Discover info to:

181 Wyckoff Street
Brooklyn, NY 11217 USA
phone + 1 718 222-8434
fax + 1 718 222-3700
subscriptions@cabinetmagazine.org
www.cabinetmagazine.org/subscribe

INSTITUTIONAL SUBSCRIPTIONS
Institutional subscriptions are available through library agencies
such as EBSCO, or directly from Cabinet:
www.cabinetmagazine.org/subscribe

SUBMISSIONS
We only accept submissions via email. Guidelines available at:
www.cabinetmagazine.org/information/submissions.php

Editor-in-chief
Sina Najafi

Senior editor
Jeffrey Kastner

Editors
D. Graham Burnett, Christopher Turner

UK editor
Brian Dillon

Art director
Everything Studio

Operations manager
William Simpson

Associate editor
Julian Lucas

Editorial assistant
Polly Dickson

Website directors
Ryan O'Toole, Luke Murphy

Editors-at-large
Saul Anton, Sasha Archibald, Mats Bigert, Brian Conley, Christoph Cox, Jeff Dolven, Leland de la Durantaye, Jesse Lerner, Jennifer Liese, Ryo Manabe, Alexander Nagel, George Prochnik, Frances Richard, Daniel Rosenberg, Aaron Schuster, David Serlin, Debra Singer, Justin E. H. Smith, Margaret Sundell, Allen S. Weiss, Eyal Weizman, Margaret Wertheim, Gregory Williams, Jay Worthington, Tirdad Zolghadr

Contributing editors
Molly Blieden, Eric Bunge, Pip Day, Charles Green, Acam Jasper, Srdjan Jovanovic Weiss, Lytle Shaw, Cecilia Sjöholm, Carl Michael von Hausswolff, Sven-Olov Wallenstein

Events
Bryony Quinn (London)

Cabinet national librarian
Matthew Passmore

Cabinet is a non-profit 501(c)(3) magazine published by Immaterial Incorporated. Our survival depends on support from generous foundations and individuals. Please consider supporting us at whatever level you can. Donations are tax-deductible for those who deal with Uncle Sam. All gifts are acknowledged online. Contributions of $25 or more will be acknowledged in the next possible issue; those above $100 will be noted in four issues. Checks to "Cabinet" can be sent to our office; please write "No need to launder" on the envelope.

Cabinet wishes to thank the following visionary foundations and individuals for their support of our activities during 2015. Additionally, we will forever be indebted to the extraordinary contribution of the Flora Family Foundation from 1999 to 2004; without their support, this publication would not exist. We would also like to extend our enormous gratitude to the Orphiflamme Foundation and the Opaline Fund for their generous support.

$100,000
The Lambent Foundation

$50,000
The Warhol Foundation for Visual Arts

$15,000
The New York City Department of Cultural Affairs

$10,000
The National Endowment for the Arts

$8,000
The New York State Council on the Arts

$3,000
The Danielson Foundation

$1,500–$2,500
Stina & Herant Katchadourian, Steven Rand and Nancy Wender, Terry Winters

$501–$1,000
Anonymous, Martha & Thomas G. Armstrong, Sara Clugage, Spencer Finch, Alexander Nagel, Sandy Tait & Hal Foster, The Edward C. Wilson and Hsu Coue Wilson Family Fund

$500 or under
Pamela Cederquist, Steven Igou, Deborah Lovely, Case Randall, Maisie Martin Siegel, Meredith Martin & Joshua Siegel, Lenore & Richard Niles, Sal Randolph, Margaret Sundell and Reinaldo Laddaga

$250 or under
Cameron Allan, Defne Ayas, Tauba Auerbach, Jeff Beall, Freya Cooper Kiddie, Mia Enell & Nicholas Fries, George Ganat, Jair Gonzalez, Alex Goodfriend, Cynthia Hansen, Peter Hapstak, Peter Jaszi, Craig Kalpakjian, James Katzenberger, Scott LeBouef, Paul McConnell, Elizabeth Merena, Helen Mirra, Andrew Pederson, Paul Ramirez Jonas, Eric Schmid, Pooja Shah & Rebecca Ward, John Sherburne, James Siena, Debra Singer & Jay Worthington, Jude Tallichet & Matt Freedman

$100 or under
In memory of Dr. Mark H. Beers, Andrew Green, Jeff Hall, Baron Hamman, David Hecht, In memory of Elon Joseph, Joe Krebs, David Lenowitz, Andrew Martin, Dmitry Mazin, Robert Meyer, David Saltonstall, Alisa Sniderman, Neil Weiss

CONTRIBUTORS

Erica Baum is a New York–based artist. Recent exhibitions include "Photo-Poetics: An Anthology" at the Solomon R. Guggenheim Museum, New York, and "Reconstructions: Recent Acquisitions in Photography and Video" at the Metropolitan Museum of Art, New York. Her books include *Dog Ear* (Ugly Duckling Presse, 2011) and *The Naked Eye* (Crèvecœur & Bureau, 2015).

D. Graham Burnett is an editor of *Cabinet* and teaches at Princeton University. He works with the research collective ESTAR(SER). For more information, see <estarser.net>.

Alice Butler is a writer and researcher based in London. She writes regularly for the British art press, including *frieze* and *Art Monthly*. In 2015, she was writer-in-residence at Jerwood Visual Arts, London. She is currently working toward a PhD at the University of Manchester on the "purging of the personal" in women's experimental writing and feminist performance art.

Jon Calame lives in Eastport, Maine, where he coordinates the Affordable Heat Consortium. He is the coauthor of *Divided Cities: Beirut, Belfast, Jerusalem, Mostar, and Nicosia* (University of Pennsylvania Press, 2007) and his most recent paper is entitled "A Hollow Where the Vandals Were," published in the spring 2015 issue of *Change Over Time*.

Nancy Davenport is a Canadian artist working in New York and Philadelphia. Her work has recently been exhibited at Exile Gallery, Berlin (2015); Dazibao Gallery, Montreal (2014); and the National Gallery of Canada, Ottowa (2013). Her book project on the United Nations is forthcoming from Cabinet Books in 2016. She is currently assistant professor in the Graduate Fine Arts Program at the University of Pennsylvania. For more information, see <nancydavenport.com>.

Leland de la Durantaye lives in Los Angeles, where he is a professor of literature at Claremont McKenna College. He is the author, among other works, of *Beckett's Art of Mismaking* (Harvard University Press, 2015).

Adam Jasper is currently a postdoctoral researcher at Eikones in Basel. He is an editor of *Architectural Theory Review* and a contributing editor of *Cabinet*.

Dennis Jelonnek is an art historian and doctoral candidate at the Freie Universität Berlin, where he is part of the BildEvidenz: History and Aesthetics research group at the Center for Advanced Studies. He is currently finishing his doctoral thesis on analogue instant photography, focusing on the Polaroid Corporation, and the diverse uses of the process by artists and amateurs.

Aden Kumler teaches medieval art history at the University of Chicago. She is the author of *Translating Truth: Ambitious Images and Religious Knowledge in Late Medieval France and England* (Yale University Press, 2011), and is currently working on a book that examines the formal and conceptual relationships between coins, seals, and communion wafers during the Middle Ages.

Reinaldo Laddaga is an Argentine writer and critic who lives in New York. He is the author of *Things That a Mutant Needs to Know* (Unsounds, 2013) and co-editor, with Jorge Carrion, of *Riplay* (Adriana Hidalgo editora, 2014), a collective Spanish-language rewriting of Robert Ripley's *Believe It or Not*. He is currently working on a book on the parallel lives of Gabriele D'Annunzio and Max Beerbohm.

Julian Lucas is a writer from New Jersey and associate editor of *Cabinet*. He has published in the *New York Review of Books* and the *Harvard Advocate*, where he edited the 2015 "Possession" issue. He is currently working on a series of essays about historical reenactments, computer games, and the Underground Railroad.

Geoff Manaugh is a New York–based freelance writer who publishes widely on questions of landscape, architecture, and technology. He is the author of the forthcoming *A Burglar's Guide to the City* (Farrar, Straus and Giroux, 2016), a study of the relationship between crime and the built environment. Previously, he was director of Studio-X New York, an off-campus urban think tank run by the architecture department at Columbia University.

Sally O'Reilly is a writer based in the United Kingdom. Recent projects include the libretto for the opera *The Virtues of Things* (2015), co-commissioned by the Royal Opera House, Aldeburgh Music, and Opera North, and a monograph on Mark Wallinger (Tate Publishing, 2015). In 2016, she will be writer-in-residence at Modern Art Oxford.

Margherita Peliti, a physicist by training, spent several years at the Rockefeller University studying the navigational behavior of one species of nematode. She currently lives in Paris, where she is training to become a civil servant.

Justin E. H. Smith writes from Paris. His next book, *The Philosopher: A History in Six Types*, will be published by Princeton University Press in spring 2016.

Jerry Toner is a fellow in classics and director of studies at Churchill College, Cambridge University. His books include *The Day Commodus Killed a Rhino: Understanding the Roman Games* (Johns Hopkins University Press, 2014) and *Homer's Turk: How Classics Shaped Ideas of the East* (Harvard University Press, 2013). He is currently working on a book on crime in ancient Rome.

Allen S. Weiss is an editor-at-large of *Cabinet* and the author of numerous books, including *Autobiographie d'un chou farci* (Mercure de France, 2006) and *Métaphysique de la miette* (Argol, 2013), two volumes of his culinary autobiography. He teaches at New York University.

AF328625

COLUMNS

COLORS / CADMIUM RED
Erica Baum

"Colors" is a column in which a writer responds to a specific color assigned by the editors of Cabinet.

———

In Adolph Gottlieb's *Cadmium Red Above Black* (1959), a red disc hovers over a black field like a red balloon presiding over an urban wasteland, its smooth round luminous form in stark contrast to the black jagged malaise underneath. Gottlieb's buoyant cadmium red balloon seems to float over the tumultuous landscape of the modern era.

Developed soon after the discovery in 1817 of the element cadmium, credited to the German chemist Friedrich Stromeyer, the first cadmium pigment was a yellow—cadmium sulfide. Long before cadmium red became widely available, artists were using cadmium yellow, the commercial production of which was established by the 1840s; Winsor & Newton, the British manufacturer of artists' materials, exhibited the pigment at the 1851 Crystal Palace exhibition in London.

Cadmium red had been available in the nineteenth century, but it was not until the early twentieth century, when a new process for the production of cadmium orange and cadmium red was patented, that it became affordable for a range of uses. A product of the industrial revolution, it became a signal red of the modern era. Able to withstand high temperatures—its melting point is over a thousand degrees Celsius—cadmium red was soon the red of choice in industrial production, especially in the manufacture of plastic items.

Cadmium red had always been prized for its permanence, brilliance, and opacity, and it was not long before the increasingly available pigment was taken up by modern artists,

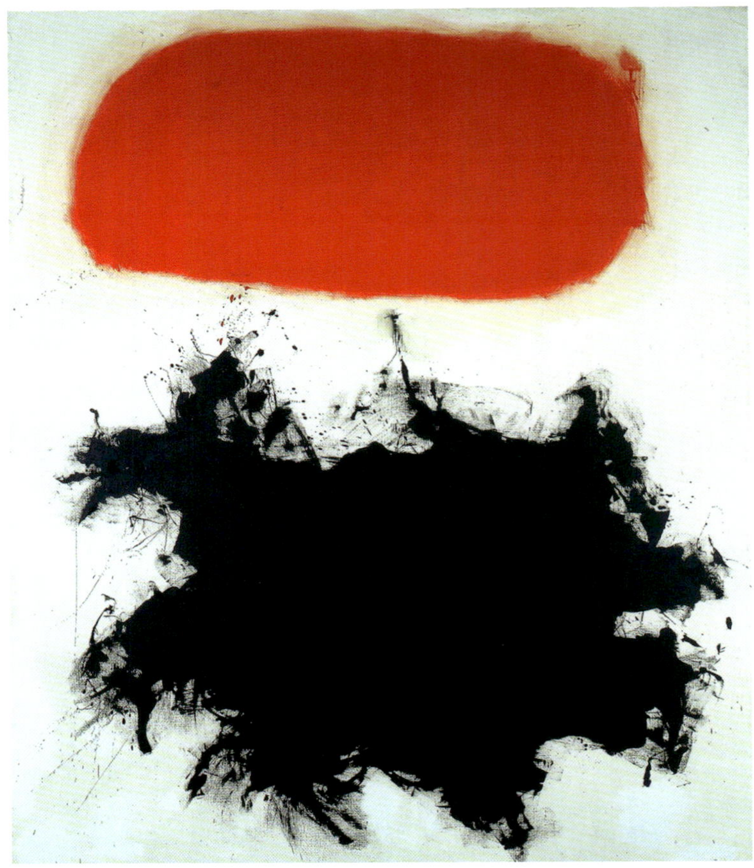

Adolph Gottlieb, *Cadmium Red Above Black*, 1959. Courtesy Blanton Museum of Art.

with Henri Matisse among the first to embrace it.

The red in his *The Dessert: Harmony in Red* (1908) is a cadmium red.

The red in his *The Red Studio* (1911) is a cadmium red.

The red in Vasily Kandinsky's *Sketch 1 for Painting with White Border* (1913) is a cadmium red.

The red in Kazimir Malevich's *Red Square* (1915) is a cadmium red.

The red in Ivan Kliun's *Cadmium Red* (1917) is a cadmium red.

The red in Theo van Doesburg's *Composition XXI* (1923) is a cadmium red.

The red in Piet Mondrian's *Composition with Red, Blue and Yellow* (1930) is a cadmium red.

The red in Mark Rothko's *No.5/No.22* (1950) is a cadmium red.

The red in Jasper Johns's *Target with Four Faces* (1955) is a cadmium red.

The red in Joan Mitchell's *La Chatière* (1960) is a cadmium red.

The red in Andy Warhol's *Red Marilyn* (1962) is a cadmium red.

The red in Josef Albers's *Homage to the Square: On an Early Sky* (1964) is a cadmium red.

The red in Barnett Newman's *Who's Afraid of Red, Yellow and Blue* suite

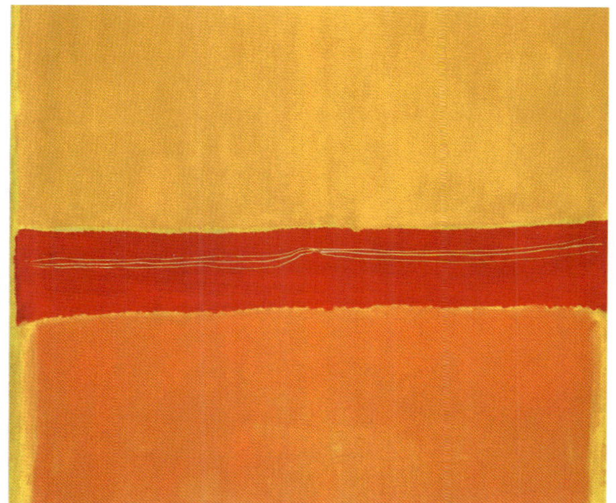

Mark Rothko, *No.5/No.22* (detail), 1950.

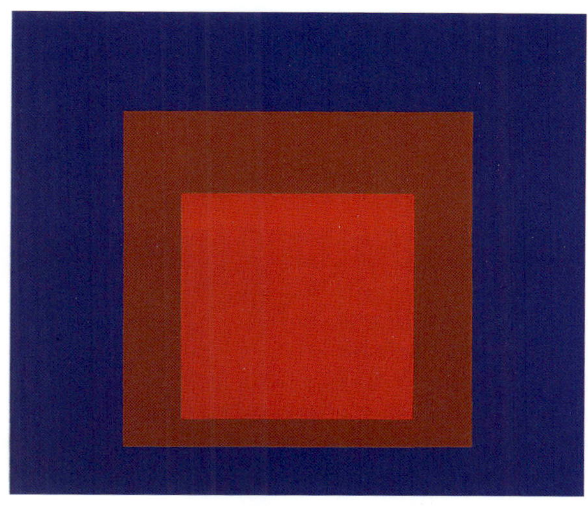

Josef Albers, *Homage to the Square: On an Early Sky* (detail), 1964.

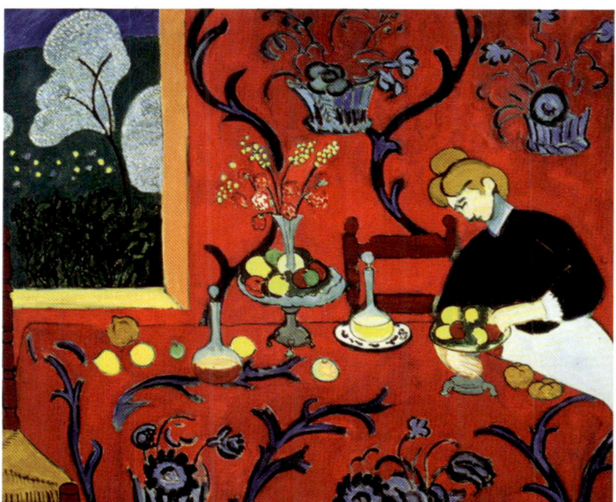

Henri Matisse, *The Dessert: Harmony in Red* (detail), 1908.

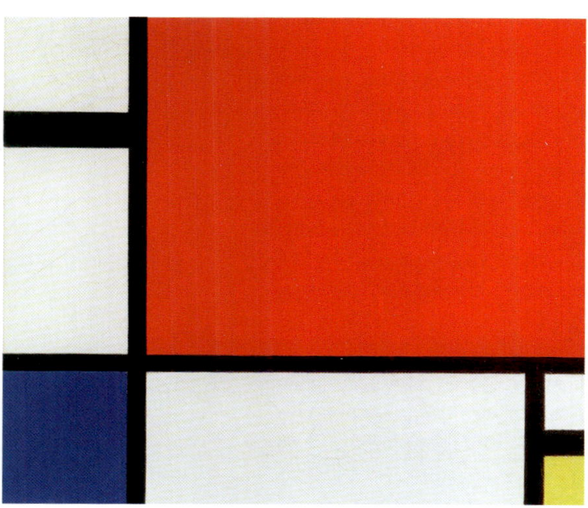

Piet Mondrian, *Composition with Red, Blue and Yellow* (detail), 1930.

Kazimir Malevich, *Red Square* (detail), 1915.

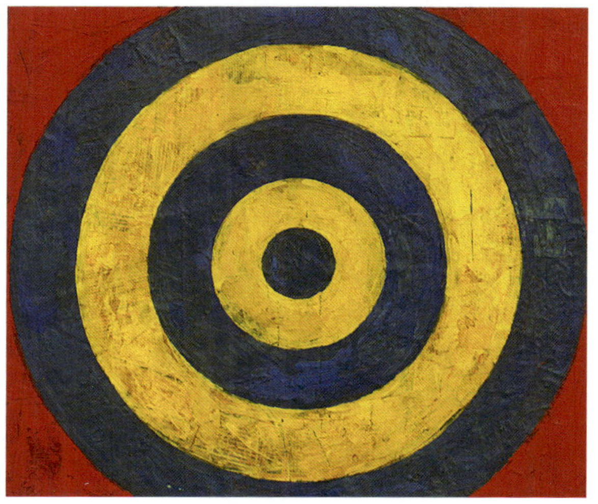

Jasper Johns, *Target with Four Faces* (detail), 1955.

(1966–1970) is a cadmium red.

The red in Donald Judd's *Untitled (S #199)* (1990) is a cadmium red.

The balloon in Albert Lamorisse's film *The Red Balloon* (1956)—later converted into a book—is also a brilliant cadmium red. I remember seeing the movie at our local library when I was five. We lived on 100th Street in New York, next to Central Park, a block away from the Bloomingdale branch. The police station was across the street. Everything in the neighborhood was laid out like a children's book, with all the basics—the butcher, the playground, the supermarket, the toy store—within a short distance. Most of the buildings in the immediate vicinity were constructed in the late 1950s and early 1960s, which meant that the imprint of urban planning was everywhere. The neighborhood was like a Mondrian painting. The library was part of a larger set of buildings that included the Health Department. One day we went there for a polio vaccine. But what I remember most was going to the library. The children's section was upstairs and occasionally in the afternoon they would close all the blinds and show films, the room becoming cavernous and red like Matisse's *Red Studio*.

. . .

Once upon a time in Paris there lived a little boy whose name was Pascal. He had no brothers or sisters, and he was very sad and lonely at home. … Then one day, on his way to school, he caught sight of a fine red balloon, tied to a street lamp. … He climbed up the lamppost, untied the balloon, and ran off with it to the bus stop. … But the conductor knew the rules. … "No balloons." … Pascal did not want to leave his balloon behind, so … the bus went on without him. When school was over … it had begun to rain and Pascal had to walk home because of those silly rules about balloons on buses. His mother *was glad to see him finally come home. But since she had been very worried, she was angry when she found out that it was a balloon that had made Pascal late. She took the balloon, opened the window, and threw it out.*

Now, usually when you let a balloon go, it flies away. But Pascal's balloon stayed outside the window, and the two of them looked at each other through the glass. Pascal was surprised that his balloon hadn't flown away, but not really as surprised as all that. Friends will do all kinds of things for you. If the friend happens to be a balloon, it doesn't fly away. So Pascal opened his window quietly, took his balloon back inside, and hid it in his room.

The next day, before he left for school, Pascal opened the window to let his balloon out and told it to come to him when he called. … Some of the tough boys of the neighborhood came by. They tried to catch the balloon as it trailed along behind Pascal. But the balloon saw the danger. It flew to Pascal at once. … So Pascal and his balloon got home without being caught.

The next day was Sunday. … He went into a bakeshop for some cake. Before he went inside he said to the balloon: "Now be good and wait for me. Don't go away." The balloon was good, and only went as far as the corner of the shop to warm itself in the sun. But that was already too far. For the gang of boys who had tried to catch it the day before saw it, and they thought that this was the moment to try again. Without being seen they crept up to it, jumped on it and carried it away.

The gang … tied the balloon to a strong string, and they were trying to teach it tricks. … Pascal saw the balloon over the top of a wall, desperately dragging at the end of its heavy string. He called to it. As soon as it heard his voice, the balloon flew toward him. Pascal quickly untied the string and ran off with his balloon as *fast as he could run. The boys raced after them. … For a minute Pascal thought he had escaped them, and he looked around for a place to rest. … But suddenly boys appeared from every direction, and Pascal was surrounded. So he let go of his balloon. But this time, instead of chasing the balloon, the gang attacked Pascal. The balloon flew a little way off, but when it saw Pascal fighting it came back. The boys began throwing stones at the balloon. "Fly away, balloon! Fly away!" Pascal cried. But the balloon would not leave its friend. Then one of the stones hit the balloon and it burst.*

. . .

Cadmium Red Above Black is part of Adolph Gottlieb's "Burst" series (1956–1974). According to the Blanton Museum of Art, which owns the painting, "its imagery derives from sketches he had made years before in the Arizona desert. The distilled red and black shapes—one stained and static, the other dynamic and more vigorously brushed—suggest essential oppositions or dualities, a central precept of Gottlieb's painterly investigation. The tension between these two elemental forms, and the straightforward monumentality of their presentation, conveys intensity, drama, and the constancy of change."

In Lamorisse's film, the bright red balloon promises a magical deliverance from the realities of Pascal's life. And even after it has been burst, all of the balloons in Paris come to the boy's aid and gather together to carry him up and away from the tumultuous cityscape. The neighborhood he left behind was soon to undergo its own changes. *The Red Balloon* was set in the area around Ménilmontant and Belleville, parts of which the city was soon to demolish in order to make room for large-scale housing projects.

THING / NO. 4
Sally O'Reilly,
Leland de la Durantaye,
Adam Jasper

"Thing" is an occasional column in which writers in various fields provide potential histories for an enigmatic object that cannot be identified by the editors of Cabinet.

———

Note the white scuffs. No, these are not caked-on flour or narcotics. This is neither a precision crêpe-making appliance nor a finely calibrated pair of scales. The white residue is in fact the tacky leavings of badly chosen tape, most likely used during transit. It would seem that, contrary to the manufacturer's advice, this has been moved while still assembled. Ideally, it should be taken apart and reassembled by an expert, and retuned to each location.

Look at the descending letters on the left. We can infer from the characters' interpenetration that this is a logo. But if you think that the final letter is an ornamental *l*, that this brand name is some hideous compaction of *heinous* and *anal*, and that this apparatus is employed in a harrowing penal colony–style punishment for sodomy, you are sorely wrong. That final letter is a *u*, spelling the proper noun Hanau. Although if you happen to know that *hana* in Czech means "blame," and you assume the *u* to be a creepy informality, the former hypothesis might still seem to be supportable. But this is sheer coincidence.

The circular-set text above Hanau offers the best clue of all. The numerical calibration flanked with "plus" and "minus" suggests a need for more or less of something. But what? Since I lack the patience to indulge your hopeless guesses, let me tell you. This device gauges the precise curvature of a sweeping generalization.

The Hanau Sweep Indicator is used in numerous polemical situations, from debating society training sessions and dogma purges to bigotry inquiries in classrooms, bars, or boardrooms. The retuning performed by the aforementioned installation expert is necessary to accommodate bulges in social pressure, worn patches in the weft of gravity (actual and metaphorical), and irregular fluxing of arguments in the vicinity. Once the apparatus is installed and operational, a section of a sweeping generalization is laid across the central disk, the bowed arm above presenting an optimum curvature against which to measure the divergence of the sweep in question. The component to the right then extrapolates the sweep to its grossest conclusions, yielding clearer criteria for judgment, and folds the sweep back on itself to test for reflexive viability.

In some instances, the sweep of a generalization will be deemed to have passed the Hanau test when the divergence, extrapolation, and fold readings all fall within stipulated limits. In other instances, two out of three "good" readings are acceptable. In a very limited number of circumstances, only an acceptable divergence from the optimum sweep is required. If a sweeping generalization has been identified as unacceptable within a given framework, it may be subjected to the Hanau Assumption Buster, then finished off with the Hanau Nuance Aggregator. The manufacturer recommends that all devices be used in conjunction with the full Hanau Correctness Range.

—Sally O'Reilly

• • •

Our name sounds like misfortune, Emile Hanau was often heard to say, and there can be little doubt that the instrument that bore his name brought him, and all the Hanaus, just that. Like most revolutionary innovations, it stepped quietly into the world. And for the remainder of his life its inventor would regard it with the liveliest hostility. It had brought out the worst in him. And despite its technical success it disappointed him in a fundamental sense, being, as he himself often put it, nothing so much as a highly charged vise of particularly rebarbative appearance—tungsten in its lower part, steel in its upper, the cross beam lined with highly magnetized iridium. As he himself pointed out, the last Hanaus produced, such as this one, look downright confused. As well they might.

The historical importance of the Hanau is, as Emile maintained in later years, in its making the robot not just possible but necessary. Once the machines enter into an unholy alliance with the other primates and enslave us, he observed, and they have a recognizable religion, they will most certainly revere the Hanau as a sacred object. It is their mother, after all. And father. There will doubtless be complicated rites, he went on, rituals to suit a new world of robots and monkeys living in true and durable harmony, at the center of which will be the Hanau. Such was his vision, one that grows from the same question with which his entire family has never since ceased to wrestle. Had Emile known, on that warm midsummer evening when he completed its design, the future it would bring, would he have acted as he did? If, when he completed that final sketch, lifting the pencil from the page, he had realized what he had just, as in a dream, done—had he on the night when he invented the object that would bear his name, and bring us robots, intuited, if only for the briefest of moments, what was to come—would he not have walked out of his study into the night, down the sloping hill to the beach and the bonfire blazing there, where his wife and daughters and siblings and cousins, young and old, even Ettore,

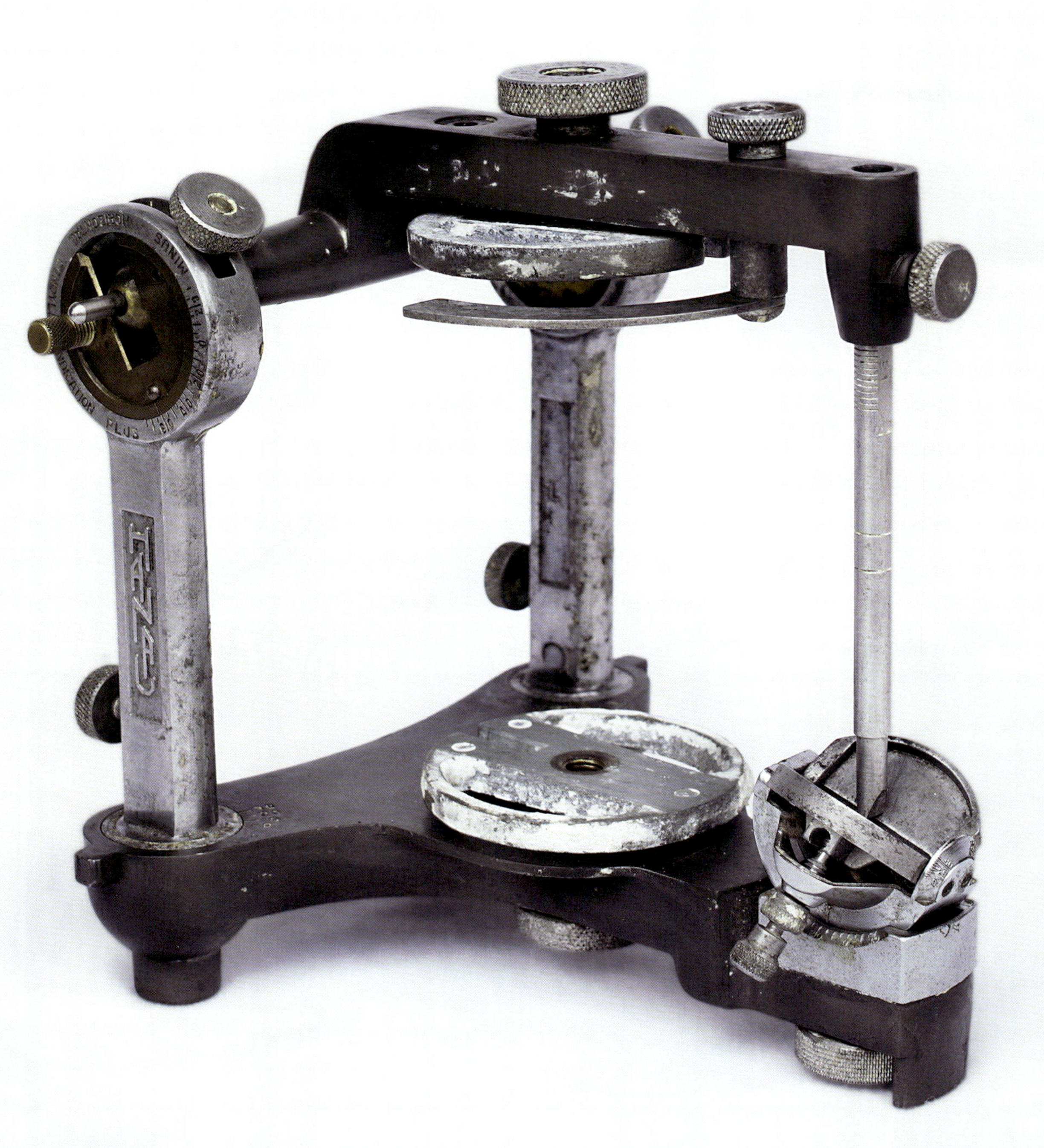

gathered, happy and warm, to celebrate the solstice, and would he not have moved smilingly among them, stopping to touch the shoulder of one, to kiss the cheek of another, until he reached the great fire, his face hot from it, and tossed the sketch into its flames, burning the design, banishing its memory? It is tempting, of course, to say yes. And yet if ever there was a man who deemed death by robot a fit end for our species it was him, as the object that bears his name so clearly shows.

    —Leland de la Durantaye

• • •

It now seems difficult to believe, but international standards for competition marbles are a twentieth-century invention. The mass production of glass spheres only began during the arms race leading to World War I, as a side effect of improvements in the manufacture of ball bearings, and so in spite of attempts by various interest groups to grant marbles a legitimate history going back to ancient Greece, the game can be best understood as a peripheral consequence of military industrialization. This confirms two general rules: first, that real innovations always present themselves in the guise of rediscovered traditions, and second, that the more outrageous the innovation, the more likely it is that it will be attributed to Greece or Rome.

The rules of contemporary games of marbles, as authorized by the BMBC (the British Marbles Board of Control) read almost as a chronology of the unfolding of industrialized warfare. Certainly, precursors can be named. Early innovators in polemical marbles in the Napoleonic era, like Lord Elgin, helped improve taw and refined the manoeuver known as the leaning top, and later expansionism by the victorious powers lead to the invention of the colonial game of golli, but moves like "elephant stomps," in which a player stamps a marble into the ground from above,

and "bombies," in which a player stands with one eye open and drops a marble directly onto those on the ground, refer directly to the evolution of aerial bombardment. The FIB (Fédération Internationale des Billes) has, predictably, rival metrics to those established by the BMBC for the determination of the legality of games of marbles. Equally predictably, both nongovernmental organizations have been thoroughly instrumentalized, and endless vexatious claims of treaty violations are regularly made or both sides, resulting in the need for ever more precise measurement machines.

Sadly, rationalized philosophy has been all too ready to assist. The tools used for lens grinding, a respectable philosophical activity that goes back to Spinoza, are now routinely applied to marble metrics. Newton's own first prism for studying the spectrum was a mere toy bought at a fair, but it has spawned all the tools needed for the mensuration of the vicious English Roundgame. The tragedy is that the same machines that measure marbles for legality—testing them for roundness, wholeness, transparency, refraction, duplicity, and center of gravity—have been used in the improvement of their efficacy as shooters. This 1930s German glass bead calibration machine is a classic example of a tool of philosophy that has been retrofitted for the purposes of war.

    —Adam Jasper

Cabinet *wishes to thank George Scheer for sending us the enigmatic object under consideration in this installment of "Thing." He made it possible for us to revive this column, the last installment of which appeared in 2006.*

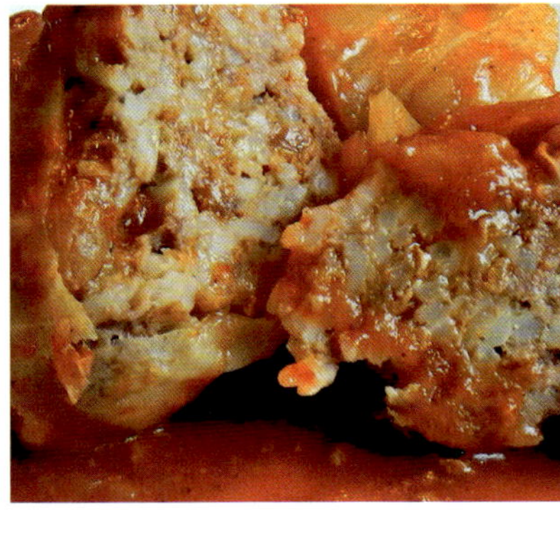 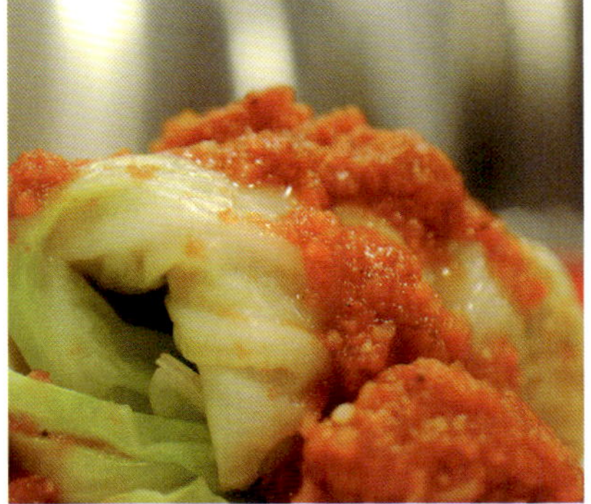 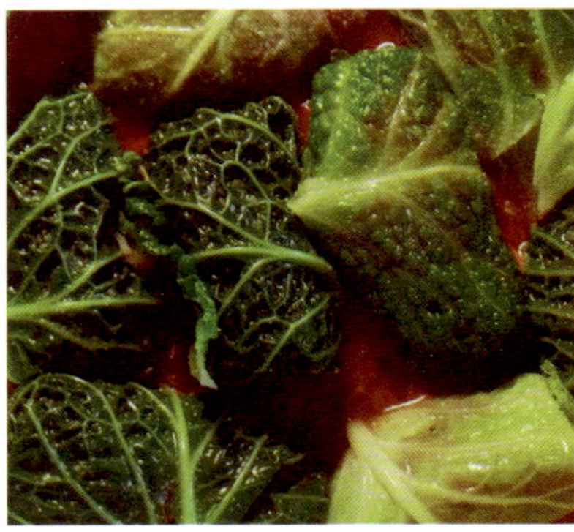

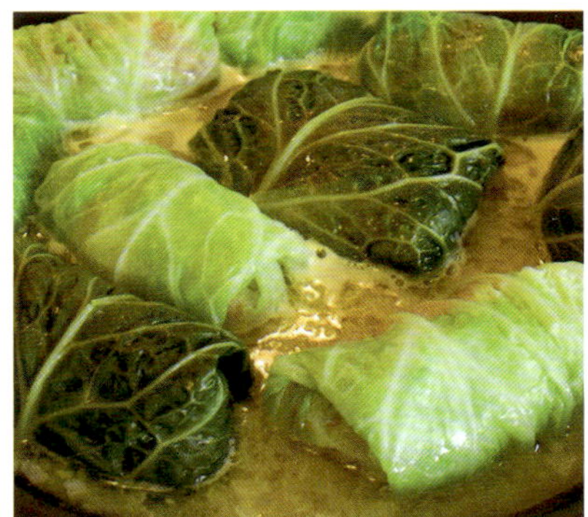 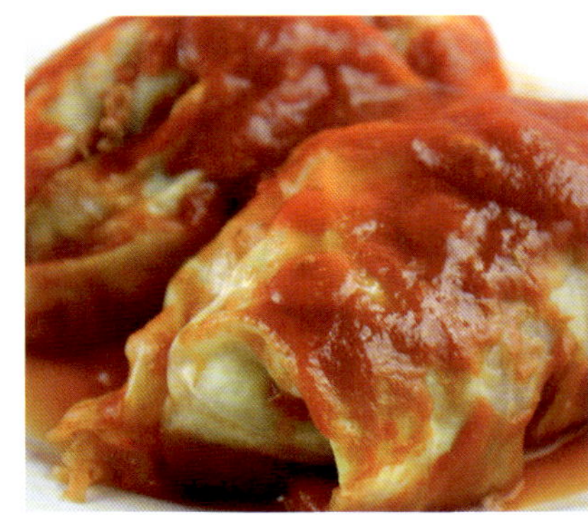 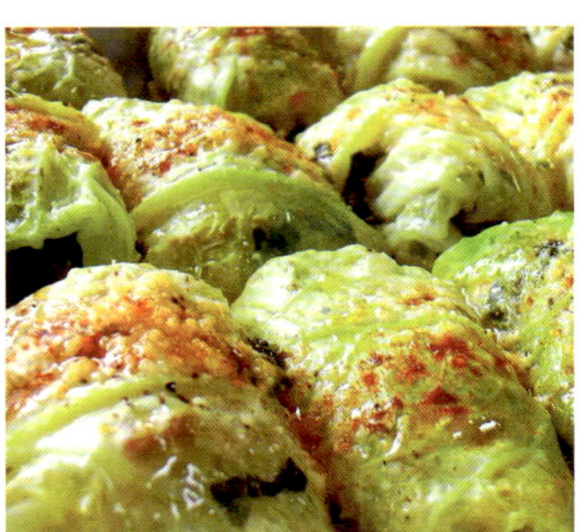

The leaves of autobiography: a few of the 77,760 varieties of *chou farci*.

INGESTION / FARCICAL FARCES
Allen S. Weiss

"Ingestion" is a column that explores its topic within a framework informed by history, aesthetics, and philosophy.

Sometimes an olive is just an olive. Those, Kalamata in nature, that served as an appetizer in the shaded courtyard of an ancient building a few steps from the Seine, I ate in all innocence, which is usually the case with olives. However, the fact that the brut prosecco from Asolo that was poured alongside bore the fanciful name "Ca'Zen" I took to be an allusion, for I had recently published *Zen Landscapes*, and my host (as well as chef, sommelier, and master of ceremonies), Emmanuel Giraud, is a virtuoso of suggestion and connotation, revival and rememoration. In a preface I had recently penned, I had characterized Giraud as "*Dottore in golosità*, professional sybarite, epicure, hedonist, gastronomic Prospero," insisting that, "I cannot but henceforth address this gourmet-performer as *hypocrite mangeur, mon semblable, mon frère*."[1] It was a late June evening, the eve of my departure to Nice, and as we climbed the stairs to his apartment, the conversation began to resonate with gastronomic complicity.

The prosecco was transmuted into champagne, and the first course was not long in coming: *stuffed zucchini flowers*.[2] Such *fleurs de courgettes* or *fiori di zucca*—a dish found from Provence through southern Italy—are particularly enjoyed in Nice, and I could only take the gesture as a delicate means of sending me off for a month beneath the palms. The second dish was equally evocative of my destination: *stuffed squid*.[3] Giraud well knew that my most cherished gastronomic tale is Maryline Desbiolles's *La seiche*, an autobiographical novel that takes place in a village north of Nice, in which the chapters are each introduced, and allegorized, by a stage in the preparation of a stuffed squid.[4] At this point in the meal I began to realize that I was witness to—and part of—a master narrative. But I did not yet know that it was my own!

Emmanuel Giraud's gastronomic performances depend on equal measures of gourmandise (where it is clear that *le savoir augmente la saveur*, knowledge improves taste), excess (if one can speak of the "measure" of excess), and rememoration (which is essentially a form of forgetting, since each and every memory is a screen that dissimulates endless past experiences).[5] In one of his most memorable performances, *Devenir gris* (Montpellier, 2009), he created a contemporary version

of Grimod de la Reynière's *dîner funèbre*, the 1783 all-male funerary dinner at which the guests had been served an entirely black meal—a keystone in the history of French gastronomy made even more famous through its reimagining by Joris-Karl Huysmans in *À rebours* (1884), the "bible" of *fin-de-siècle* decadence.[6] Grimod revisited by Huysmans staged by Giraud. But for Giraud, the proof is not simply in the pudding (figuratively and literally speaking, as pudding was one of the dishes on Huysmans's menu), nor even in the excess (though excess there was in this performance, quantitatively and qualitatively), but essentially in the retrospection, for some time after this dinner theater (the diners were, most self-consciously, also performers) each diner was asked to recount his memory of the meal. The first I heard of Giraud's performances was when I was invited to participate in *Devenir gris*, but unable to do so, I—who knew by heart the various versions, literary and culinary, of Grimod's celebrated meal—spent years trying to imagine what I missed. I suspect that my account of this missed occasion would be no less rich than the tales of those who attended.

This is perhaps the moment to note that the shock of the main dish to follow made me totally forget the *intermezzo* that Giraud prepared just after the squid, intended as a *transition champignonesque jubilatoire* in the form of tiny *fregola sarda* pasta with bits of sautéed morels moistened with lobster broth whipped with butter. I was reminded of it when questioning Giraud about the recipes, and only then remembered its unctuous simplicity. As we shall immediately see, there was a decidedly structural reason to forget this dish, as it was the only one served that evening that did not quite fit the central theme.

When invited to dinner that June evening, I had expected a splendid meal, with inspired gastrophilic

conversation to match, and I wasn't disappointed. But what makes it worthy of analysis is that I also received a demonstration of cuisine as symbolic form (à la Panofsky), articulated by the equivocation of the term *farce*, in both the culinary sense of *stuffing* and the theatrical sense of *charade*. I should have guessed the main dish: *stuffed cabbage*. Allusion, illusion, collusion: what a fine meal, and a true friendship, should entail. Giraud was thoroughly familiar with the first volume of my culinary memoirs, *Autobiographie dans un chou farci* (Autobiography in a stuffed cabbage), as well as with the fact that after the publication of this book, I occasionally made my own particular (and peculiar) stuffed cabbage recipe for friends.[7] On the surface, Giraud clearly intended his stuffed cabbage recipe as a form of homage. Or so I thought. For him, cuisine is never merely a sensual phenomenon, but also a conceptual gambit. In my little volume, centered on the stuffed cabbages of my origins (Hungary, Poland), my nation of birth and upbringing (USA), and my country of predilection (France), I felt the necessity of precisely defining the subject, so as to avoid the tautology that a stuffed cabbage consists of a cabbage leaf stuffed with anything whatsoever (a definition that permits every stuffed-cabbage eater the most profound egocentrism, thus the least critical distance).[8] The multifarious (but nevertheless circumscribed) reality of this dish is of much greater interest than its empty ideality. By isolating and multiplying the pertinent features of the stuffed cabbage (leaf type; stuffing content; cooking mode; outer form; etcetera), I established a combinatory mechanism that produced 77,760 variants. This structuralist-rococo culinary labyrinth is of certain sociological interest, for many of the juxtapositions reveal the minute differences in recipes that obtain from region to region, just as a patois will change slightly from

valley to valley. We also discover that—just as phonetics teaches that in any given language not all possible combinations of sounds are meaningful—many variants appear to be gastronomically nonsensical. However, these seemingly meaningless variants are precisely the points where culinary innovation is possible.[9] While Giraud's gastronomic imperative entails the search for taste lost, mine is a quest for forms found.

I thus fancy myself a specialist in the art of stuffed cabbage, and when the beautiful arrangements of Giraud's version arrived on the table, I was, needless to say, thrilled, intrigued, nervous. The first bite increased my anxiety, for I knew that something was wrong: *this was a false stuffed cabbage!* The "cabbage" leaves were composed of Swiss chard leaves, basil, and pork caul, and were stuffed with Breton lobster and nearly burnt croutons moistened with reduced lobster bouillon, then baked in more of the bouillon for approximately twenty minutes; the accompaniment was Swiss chard and diced celery, with the sauce being the extremely reduced lobster bouillon simply whisked with butter.

The history of culinary *trompe l'oeil* is ancient and vast, from Trimalchio's celebrated dinner in Petronius's *Satyricon* (which was the subject of a 2009 performance by Giraud at the Villa Medici in Rome); to the sundry recipes concocted by talented episcopal chefs to make meatless Fridays less frustrating to gourmand ecclesiastics, and the endless ways of preparing tofu to look and taste like meat in the strictly macrobiotic *shōjin ryōri* of Zen Buddhist monks; through Marie-Antoine Carême's fantastic pastry *pièces montées* based on his detailed architectural studies, up to the scientific trickeries of molecular gastronomy. Here, in a performance of which I was subject, object, and participant, Emmanuel Giraud's farce was a farce!

Kalamata olives
Stuffed zucchini flowers
Stuffed squid
Fregola sarda
False stuffed cabbage

A philosopher once proclaimed that the only valid criticism of a work of art is another work of art, an idea generally more alluring to poets than philosophers. In my aforementioned preface concerning his performances, I offered Giraud—author of the *Anthologie fabuleuse, fallacieuse et facétieuse du pâté en croûte* (Fabulous, fallacious, facetious anthology of the pâté en croûte)—a recipe as a culinary gift.[10] Given the extraordinary dishes recounted in this book, I imagined that Giraud could well transform the famed pot-au-feu at the core of Marcel Rouff's beloved 1924 novel, *La vie et la passion de Dodin-Bouffant, gourmet* (translated as *The Passionate Epicure*), into a *pâté en croûte*. Consequently, I provided a recipe for transforming this very same pot-au-feu into a *chou farci demi-deuil*. In exchange, that June evening he offered me a *faux chou farci*.

I am not sure whether this text demands an epilogue, but soon after I established my stuffed cabbage combinatory, I began traveling to Japan. One day I entered a supermarket, and at the sushi counter I saw something intriguing: pieces of raw salmon wrapped in tiny cabbage leaves—a form of stuffed cabbage previously unimaginable to me! I was deeply troubled, as I wondered whether I would have to extend my combinatory schema to account for such anomalies (anomalous at least in the European sense of the dish), which would exponentially increase the number of variants to 93,312. It gradually became clear that given my original geographic and autobiographical delimitation of the question, the Japanese version was by definition superfluous—at least for the moment. However, I now wonder whether I need add a new category to account for simulacral versions of the recipe, for *fake stuffed cabbages.* Whatever be the case, I have come to realize that the innocent olives were nothing of the sort. Rather, this fruit stuffed by nature with its own pit was the prolegomenon to a farce.

1 Allen S. Weiss, "À la recherche du goût perdu," preface to Marylène Malbert, Emmanuel Giraud, *Le goût de la mémoire* (Paris: Les Éditions de l'Épure, 2015), p. 8.

2 As I believe that all good gastronomic writing should whet the appetite as well as spur the imagination, I offer detailed descriptions (which can double as recipes) of the dishes. Thus, to begin: zucchini flowers stuffed with Piedmontese cow-and-sheep-milk ricotta and anchovies, with a drop of argan oil.

3 Small squid stuffed with Bronte (Sicily) pistachios (2/3 whole, 1/3 finely chopped), Corrèze chanterelles (girolles) sautéed in butter with fresh garlic, shallots, and parsley, and the chopped tentacles sautéed in olive oil; topped with fresh and conserved zests of Minori (Amalfi) lemons.

4 Maryline Desbiolles, *The Cuttlefish*, trans. Mara Bertelsen (New York: Herodias, 2001). Also see Allen S. Weiss, "The Epic of the Cephalopod," in *Feast and Folly: Cuisine, Intoxication, and the Poetics of the Sublime* (Albany: State University of New York Press, 2002), pp. 73–84.

5 See Emmanuel Giraud, *L'excès: Dix façons de le préparer* (Paris: Les Éditions de l'Épure, 2013).

6 Grimod de la Reynière's *L'almanach des gourmands* (1803–1812) is the origin of gastronomic journalism; the entire series was recently reprinted with a preface by Jean-Claude Bonnet (Paris: Menu Fretin, 2012). See also Jean-Claude Bonnet, *La gourmandise et la faim: Histoire et symbolique de l'aliment* (Paris: Livre de Poche, 2015).

7 Allen S. Weiss, *Autobiographie dans un chou farci* (Paris: Mercure de France, 2006), p. 44. The blanched leaves of savoy cabbage are stuffed with a mixture of ground veal and pork, sautéed onions and garlic, chopped prunes, rice parboiled in chicken broth, sour cream or crème fraîche, parmesan, one beaten egg, pine nuts, parsley, thyme, salt, pepper, and cayenne pepper; these stuffed cabbages are then cooked covered over a low flame for at least two hours on a base composed of onions and garlic sautéed in a mixture of vegetable oil and thickly chopped fatty bacon, to which has been added chopped cabbage, carrots, leeks, tomatoes, salt, and pepper. One will immediately note from the use of rice, pine nuts, and parmesan that this is not a traditional French recipe; in fact, its sources of inspiration are Hungarian, Polish, Italian, American, Provençal, Aveyronnais. A recipe from everywhere or nowhere. See also Allen S. Weiss, "Reflections on the Stuffed Cabbage," *Gastronomica*, vol. 7, no. 1 (Winter 2007), and Allen S. Weiss, "Prunus Variations," in Ines Lechleitner, *The Imagines* (Berlin: Sternberg Press, 2014).

8 When lecturing on the aesthetics of cuisine, I find that I refer to the stuffed cabbage less and less, since every time the topic is touched upon, most of the auditors immediately evoke their favorite stuffed cabbage, almost always that of their grandmother (the "grandmother" being a key trope in the annals of the oral transmission of cuisine and taste). Rather than fall into this subjective trap, which is enough to attenuate if not totally undermine any empathy that a recipe can establish, I make use of another work, *Comment cuisiner un phénix* (How to cook a phoenix) (Paris: Mercure de France, 2004), reassured that none of the audience can ever have tasted the recipes contained therein.

9 Sometimes what appears to be culinary nonsense turns out to be part of a dissimulated logic. For example, I had long believed that red cabbage leaves were never used to make stuffed cabbage, until I finally began to come across—in French cookbooks of the Limousin and Alsace, as well as some from the USA—stuffed red cabbage recipes. These were without exception associated with the cuisine of the hunt, and always included, in the French incarnations, wild mushrooms and foie gras.

10 Emmanuel Giraud, *Anthologie fabuleuse, fallacieuse et facétieuse du pâté en croûte* (Paris: Éditions Alternatives, 2012).

INVENTORY / WHEELS OF DESIRE
Jon Calame

"Inventory" examines or presents a list, catalogue, or register.

———

There are at least seven hundred distinct recreational vehicles on US roads today, from teardrop trailers to Greyhound-bus–sized customized motorhomes that can provide up to 465 square feet of domestic space when their sliding sections are extended. This area is roughly comparable to that of a typical Manhattan studio apartment. The largest RVs–categorized as Class A because of their weight–can include washing machines and dryers, dishwashers, marble countertops, tiled showers, exterior televisions, and any number of additional amenities.

This proliferation of models disguises a much smaller number of generic physical types, which basically consist of small or large furnished boxes, driven or pulled. This increases the need for seduction and novelty during consumer courtship. What is the nature of this seduction, in which an object–a Copper Mountain ($53,440), Palazzo ($224,450), or Cornerstone ($625,686)–promises you freedom from the malaise accumulated across a working life by allowing you to roll unhindered toward an unspecified oasis?

Automobile names rarely achieve the same metaphoric intensity, and shrink from any serious effort to mine the buyer's imagination, though trucks, sport utility vehicles, and all-terrain vehicles provide a nomenclatural bridge when they invoke the language of liberation, as with the familiar Escape, Explorer, Range Rover, and Rogue. On the whole, recreational vehicle names delve deeper, further heighten expectations, and

reveal more about the aspirations of their future owners because they are not simply machines for transport but also tools for temporarily–and sometimes permanently–re-rendering a life.

In compiling what I believe to be a near-comprehensive list of all RVs currently on the road in the United States, it seemed to me that their names issue from seven great clans of desire to which their owners wish to belong when enjoying their leisure time. Ranked according to the number of model names affiliated with each clan, they are:

Clan	Number of members	Associations
Exploration	175	Discovery, frontier, exotica, freedom
Indulgence	151	Leisure, luxury, waste, dream
Purity	132	Nature, harmony, flight, wilderness
Rank	90	Privilege, status, excellence, aristocracy
Conquest	63	Predation, war, ruin, coercion, empire
Defiance	58	Heresy, mischief, abandon, unpredictability
Nativism	44	Nostalgia, nationalism, diplomacy, home

Between these clans, intermarriages are common. The Cherokee Vengeance, for example, simultaneously suggests nativism, purity, defiance, and conquest (but in which direction?); a nearly perfect model name. The Glacier points to both exploration and purity, but is a hint of defiance also intended, as the wheels spin and the polar caps thaw? Alongside the Safari, Tundra, and Savannah, there is an evident fondness for wild animals: Arctic Fox, Canyon Cat, Caribou, Cheetah, Cougar, Coyote, Desert Fox, Dolphin,

Eagle, Gazelle, Golden Falcon, Grey Wolf, Hornet, Koala, Lynx, Mako, Mallard, Mustang, Puma, Raptor, Redhawk, Viper, Wildcat, and Wolf Pup. Other model names reference picturesque, often sparsely populated American places: Wyoming, Montana, Utah, Colorado, Dakota, Alaska, Flagstaff, Yellowstone, Catalina, Sedona, Yuma, Tahoe, Sonoma, Sun Valley, Shasta, Kodiak, Phoenix, Laredo, Santa Fe, Monterrey, and Sanibel. Harder to imagine would be metropolises such as Chicago or Atlanta, though an Atlantis does exist.

The American highway now beckons more than eight million feral wanderers, among them Admirals, Ambassadors, Aristocrats, Braves, Chieftains, Contessas, Diplomats, Gladiators, Nomads, Pioneers, and Warriors. Never fully departing, never quite arriving, they assert their right to ramble without hardship, hindrance, or timetable. These arks of desire pass by, equipped lock, stock, and barrel, posing a very American riddle: what is both Vagabond and Chateau, All American and Lakota, Spartan and Royale? Now the answer is whispered to us like a Zephyr through Torrey Pines, now it rumbles like Patriot Thunder through Heritage Glen.

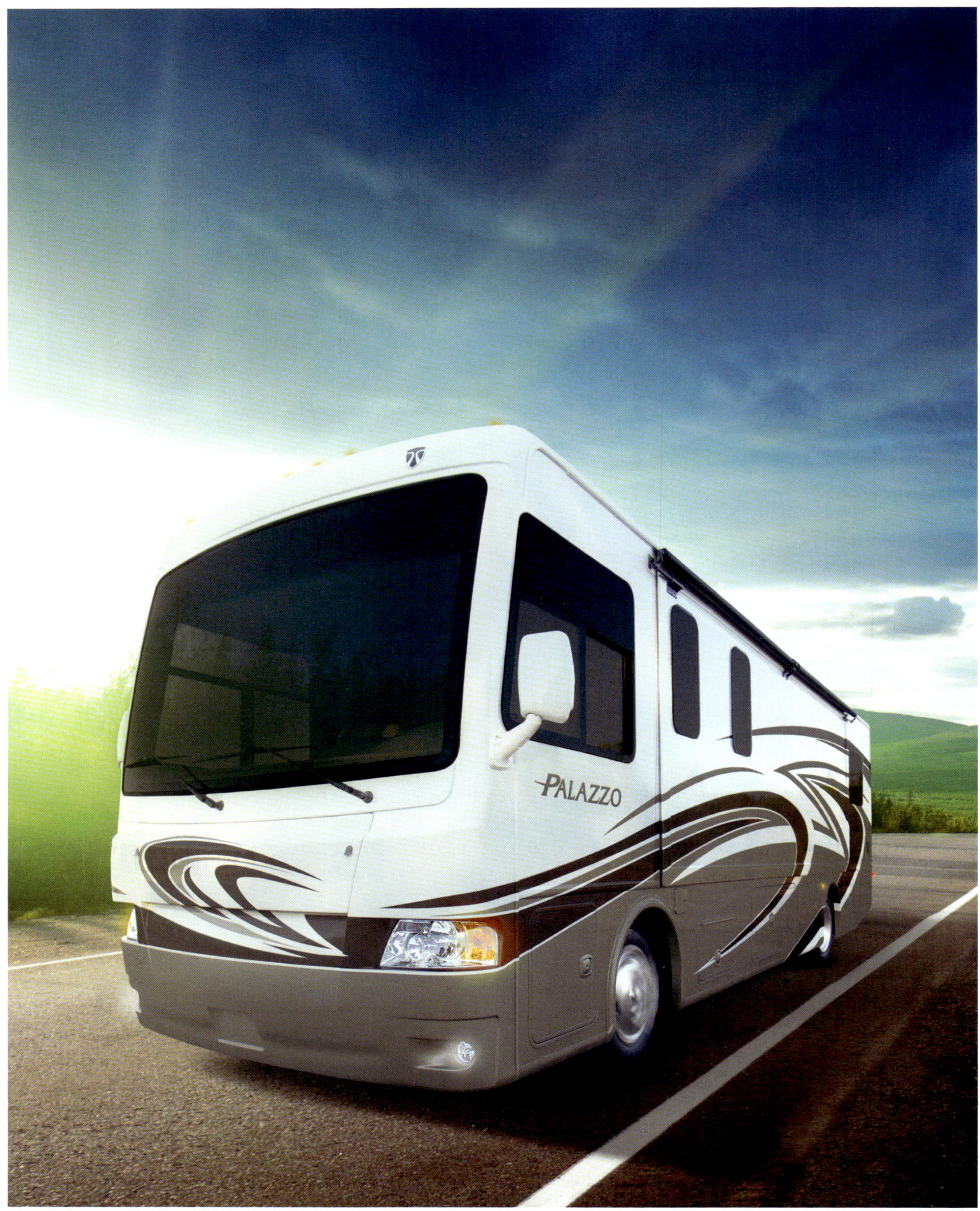

The splendid indulgence offered by Thor Motor Coach's Palazzo.

EXPLORATION

Aliner
Alite
Access
Adventurer
Adventurous
Alante
Alaskan
Antigua
Ascent
Aspect
Atlantis
Aviator
Backpack
Bantam Flier
Bay Star
Big Country
Blaze'n
Blue Ridge
Bounder
Bristol Bay
Cabin A
Cambria
The Camden
Camplite
Campmaster
Canyon Cat
Canyon Star
Car-Go
Carri-Lite
Columbus
Companion
Compass
Concourse
Cross Country
Cross Terrain
Dakota
Del Mar
Denali
Discovery
Durango
Elkridge
Encounter
Endeavor
Endura
Everest
Expedition
Explorer
Flagstaff
Formula
Freedom
Freedom Elite
Freedom Express
Freedom Spirit
Freelander
Frontier
Gateway
Grand Junction
Hemisphere
Hill Country
Independence
Interstate
Isata
Journey
Journeyer
Karry-All
Kingston
Kodiak
LaPalma
Laredo
Latitude
Liberty Elegant
Lady
Little Guy
Mandalay
McKinley
Melbourne
Meridian
Milan
Mini
Minnie
Mintaro
Mirada
Montclair
Monte Vista
Montego Bay
Monterey
Mountaineer
Nash
Navigator
New Vision
Sportster
Nomad
North Country
North Shore
North Trail
North Ridge
Northstar
Okanagan
OpenRoad
Orbit
Outback Sydney
Overlander
Passport
Pathfinder
Phoenix
Pioneer
Plateau
Portofino
Prairie Schooner
Qwest
R.Pod
Ranger
The Red Rock
Ridgecrest
Riverside
Road Ranger
Road Runner
Road Warrior
Salem
Santa Fe
Santara
SatelLite
Scenic Cruiser
Scottsdale
Scout
Seville
Siena
Simplicity
Starflyer
Starflyte
Summit
Summit Ridge
Surveyor
Sydney
Tab
TaDa
Takena
Timberlodge
Tioga
Tour
Tour Master
Touring Cruiser
TrailRider
Trail Runner
Trail-Aire
Trail-Bay
TrailCruiser
Trail-Lite
Trailblazer
Trail Manor
Trail Master
Transporter
Travato
Travel Lite
Travelaire
Traveler
True North
Ice Lodge
Tucson
Tuscany
Utah
Vectra
Ventana
Ventura
Venture
Via
View
Viewfinder
Vista
Vista Cruiser
Voyage
Voyager
Wagoneer
Walkabout
White Water
Wyoming
Yellowstone
Yuma

INDULGENCE

Allure
Aruba Lite
Astora
Augusta
Autumn Ridge
Baja
Bayside
Blast
Boogie Box
Breeze
C-Force Nitro
Cameo
Canyon Trail
Capri
Captiva
Catalina
Cayman
Chalet
Cruise Air
Cruise Master
Cruiser
DayDreamer
Designer
Destination
Diamond Star
Domani
Dorado
Dyna Aire
Ease
Excursion
Fiesta
Flair
Forza
Fun Finder
Fun Mover
Golden Ridge
Grand Sport Ultra
Granite Ridge
Greystone
Gulf Breeze
HitchHiker
Horizon
Impulse
Infinity
Islander
Jag
Jamboree
Jazz
Komfort
Kountry Aire
Kountry Star
Land Yacht
Landau
Layton
Lazy Daze
LeSharo
Max-Lite
MaxSport
Mega-Lite
Miramar
Momentum
Motorsport
Nimbus
Nitrous
Oakmont
Oasis
Outlook
Palazzo
Paradise Point
Popular
Prospera
Providence
Pulse
Que
Reflection
Rendezvous
Residency
Resort
Rezerve
Rose Air
RPM
Select Suites
Serenity
Siesta Sprinter
Sightseer
Silver Shadow
Skamper
Skyline
SolAire
Solei
Solera
Sport
Sportscoach
Sportsmaster
Sportsmen
Sportster
Spree
Sprinter
Sterling
The Suite
Summerland
Suncruiser
Sunflyer
Sun Valley
Sun Voyager
Sunbird
Suncrest
Sundance
Sundancer
SunnyBrook
Sunova
Sunseeker
Sunset Bay
Sunset Creek
Sunset Trail
Surf Side
Swinger
Tailgator
Tango
Terry
Topaz
Torque
Toyhouse
Tracer
Tradewinds
Travel Star
Tribute
Trilogy
Tropi-Cal
Ultimate Advantage
Ultimate Freedom
Ultrasport
Vacationer
Vantare
Vegas
Veranda
Vibe
Viva!
VRV
Wanderer
Weekend Warrior
Weekender
Wide Open
Willow Creek
Wind River
Windsport
Winter Creek
Work and Play
X-Aire
X-treme
Zoom

PURITY

Adirondack
Admiral
Aereon
Aerolite
Aerostar
Agile
Airflyte
Alpine
Aluma-Lite
Alumascape
Angler
Arctic Fox
Aspen Trail
Aurora
Avion
Bambi
Berkshire
Brookside
Brookstone
Cardinal
Caribou
Cascade
Cedar Creek
Cedar Ridge
Chaparral
Cheetah
Cirrus
Coast
Colorado
Comet
Concord
Constellation
The Copper Mountain
Cougar
Coyote

MAIN

A CITY FOR POETS AND PIRATES
Reinaldo Laddaga

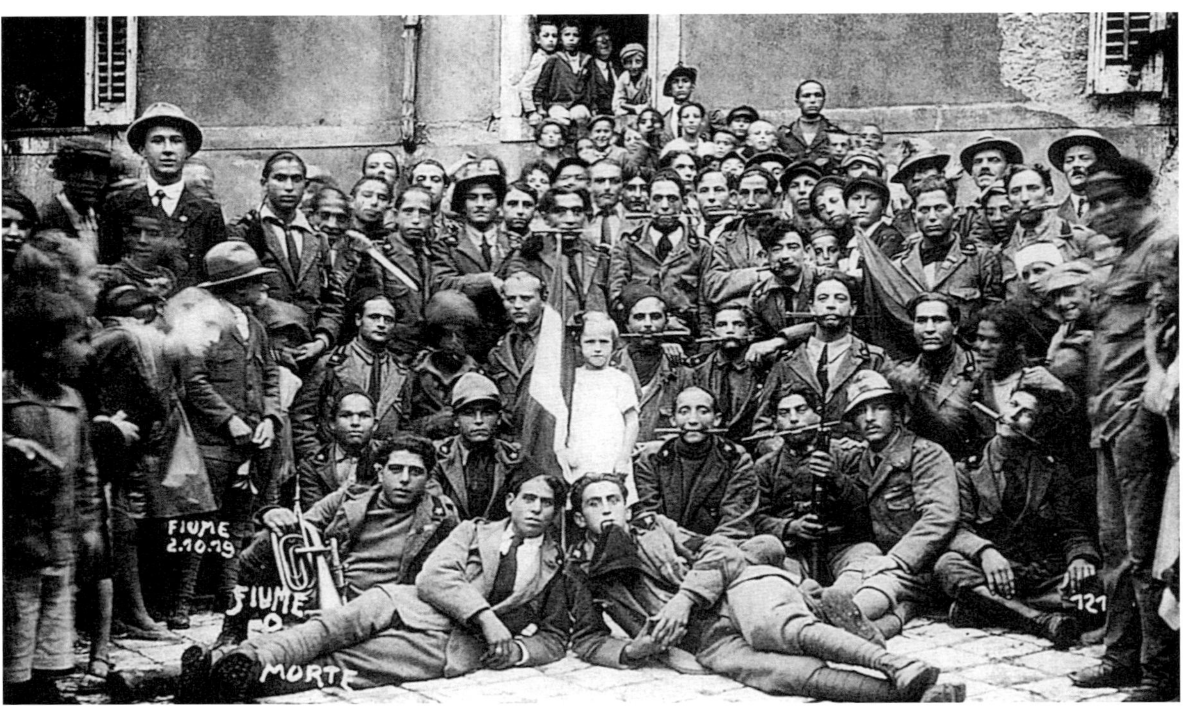

I've always found it intriguing that canonical histories of early twentieth-century art and literature, usually so generous in their treatment of the emergence of the historical avant-garde, never mention its most spectacular development: the creation, and ultimate failure, of the so-called Italian Regency of Carnaro. In a certain way, this omission is understandable. What happened between 1919 and 1920 in the contested city of Fiume, when—under the leadership of writer Gabriele D'Annunzio—a peculiar alliance of soldiers, artists, and adventurers occupied the city with the initial intention of annexing it to Italy, complicates the most common narrative in which modern art and progressive politics by nature go together.[1] But, as historian Roger Griffin's excellent *Modernism and Fascism* observes, a number of avant-garde movements shared fascism's aspiration to cure the world (or at least Europe) of anomie and a loss of vitality. These conditions were understood as by-products of modernity, and particularly so at the end of a war that made patent the failure of modernity's promise of material and social progress. Both movements proposed a return, in the midst of crisis, to a primordial space where the envoys

of a new humanity could gather the seeds for a future world. In Fiume, fascists and Dadaists, futurists and Bolsheviks, were, for a few months, in the same camp.

Let's try to imagine Italy at the end of World War I. A constitutional monarchy the disparate regions of which had only very recently integrated, it had entered the war in 1915 on the side of the British-French alliance one year after the hostilities started, having received from France and England guarantees of territorial compensation. The ensuing three years of combat caused in this mostly traditionalist, agrarian society an even deeper upheaval than the one suffered by its allies. The massive mobilizations for the war, and the replacement of young men in the world of work by women, wrecked not only the basis of the economy but also the structures of prewar society. For some social groups, the expectations of political influence changed: the country's government had promised

Above: A group of *arditi*, Fiume, 2 October 1919. Holding daggers between their teeth, a practice these soldiers favored on the battlefield, became a symbol of their fighting spirit.

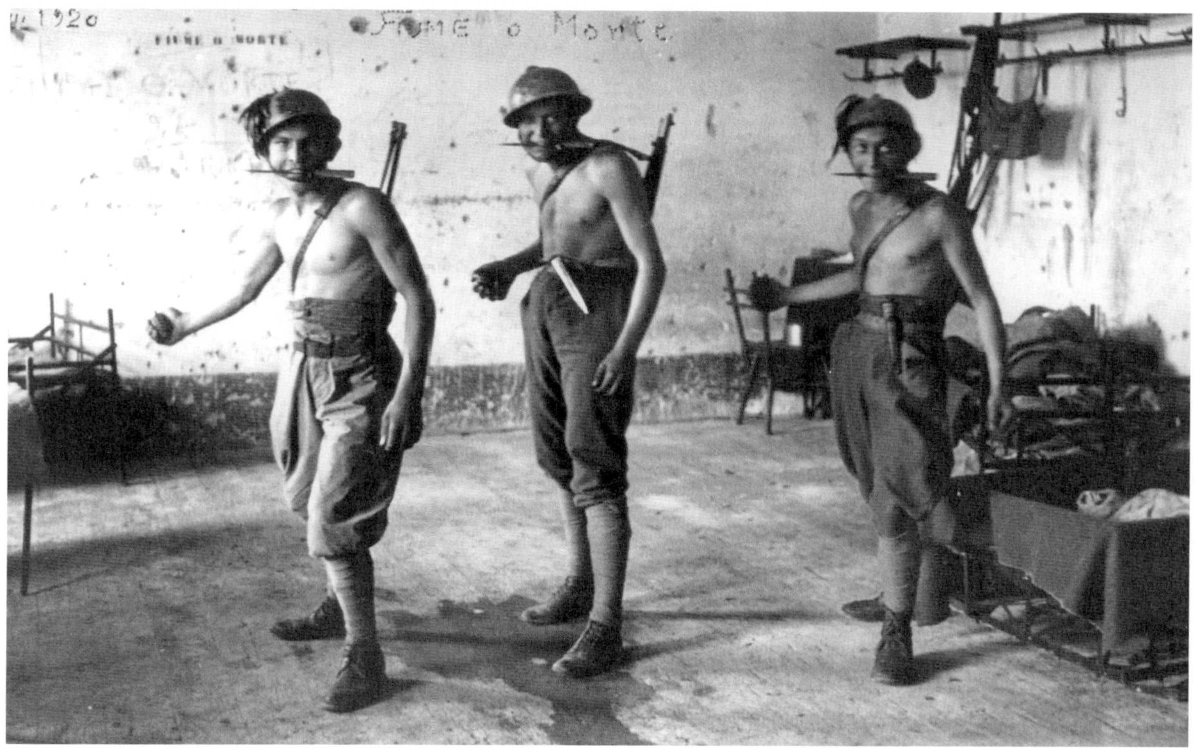

Three Fiumean *arditi* brandishing their weapons of choice, August 1920.

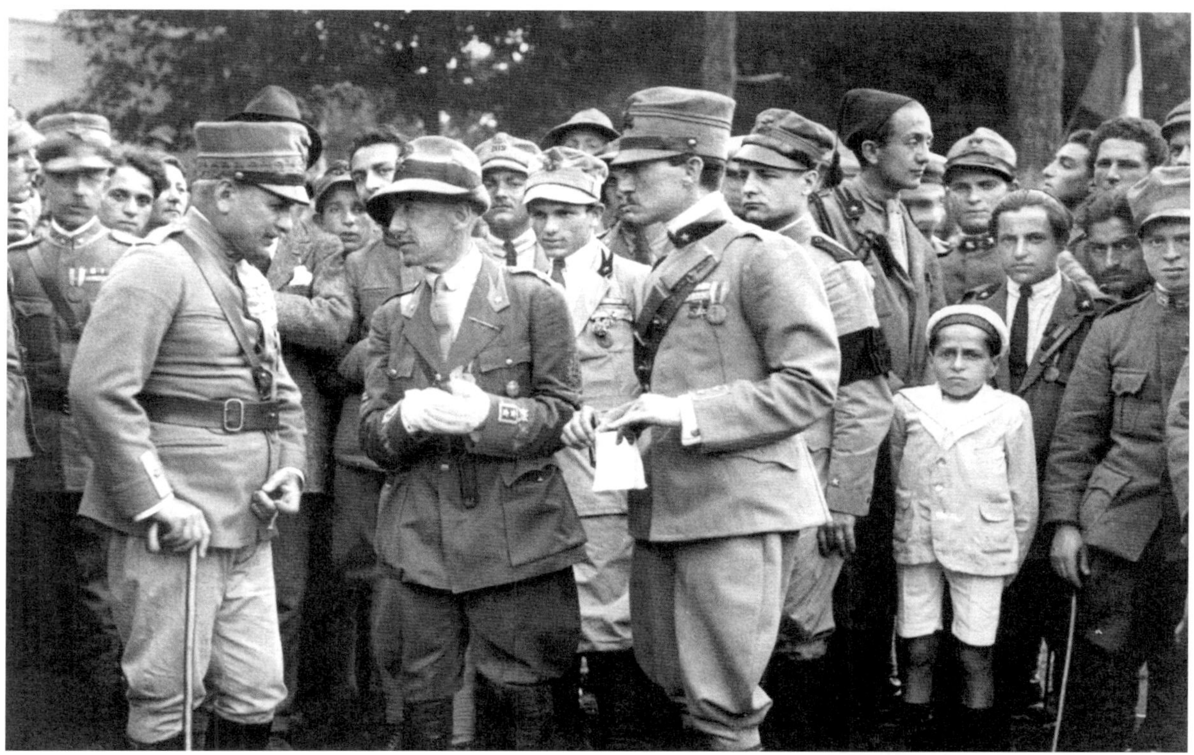

D'Annunzio conferring with two of his military commanders, 30 May 1920.

new and unprecedented power to its disenfranchised lower classes (a promise that the political class would soon discover it never should have made). The war had been long, and there were young men who did not remember a way of life other than the tough but eminently exciting one they had experienced at the front, where they had died by the hundreds of thousands. The survivors still remembered the bare, dry skeletons in the rocky hills of the Carso, the scene of the most brutal battles, and now they identified their own dignity with the dignity of the nation.

This was true for the entire army, but especially for the assault troops known as the *arditi*. During the war, the *arditi* had refused all weapons that would weigh them down: they preferred grenades carried in pockets and daggers held between teeth as they raced toward the enemy trenches, which they rarely reached. They liked to be called "alligators," were partial to cocaine, and, among them, homosexuality was commonplace. No leader had been able to take for granted the loyalty of these highly volatile men. And now that the war was over, like the German Freikorps, they found no place for themselves in a society where the exhausted majority expected to return to a peaceful civilian life.

We cannot understand the events in Fiume (or the subsequent rise of fascism) without making an effort to imagine a world in which hundreds of thousands of young men who had been promised a share in the spoils of victory returned, after years both frightening and exhilarating—some of them half-blind or deaf, some insomniacs or addicts—to anxious mothers and wives unwilling to listen to their stories, to jobs in industries where bosses worried about productivity. They had known extreme anguish but also fleeting glory, and for a few years had been members of a warrior community where their powers and weaknesses were celebrated and acknowledged. Some of these men formed the core of D'Annunzio's followers.

And why Fiume? At the end of World War I, a dispute exploded over the fate of the Istrian peninsula. Largely ruled by the Republic of Venice over the centuries, Istria became part of the Austro-Hungarian empire in 1797. In the course of the nineteenth century, Fiume—the largest city on the peninsula—became one of the main ports of the northern Adriatic and the most prestigious resort for the Hungarian elite. The population in the countryside was mostly Slavic, but Fiume had a substantial, thriving Italian community

that held the reins of economic power and had been slowly working to restitute the city to what they saw as its motherland. This community was fully justified in assuming that the Allied victory and the dissolution of the Austro-Hungarian Empire represented the crucial occasion to achieve this goal: in the negotiations preceding Italy's entry into the war, Great Britain and France promised to transfer Istria to the Italian government. Instead, the Versailles conference of 1919 sanctioned the formation of a new nation—the Kingdom of Serbs, Croats, and Slovenes, later Yugoslavia—whose territory, it now seemed, would include Istria. For the Italians in Fiume, this awful prospect was due to the incompetence and weakness of the Italian negotiators and had to be immediately corrected by the use of force. For the demobilized soldiers who roamed the country without any particular destination or place in bourgeois society, and for men like Gabriele D'Annunzio, Benito Mussolini, and Filippo Tommaso Marinetti, this denial of the fruits of victory was the most intolerable of humiliations. Talks started between the Italianists in Fiume and some of the new political leaders emerging in the ruins of postwar Italy. This is where D'Annunzio enters the story.

Gabriele D'Annunzio was the most prestigious Italian writer of the late nineteenth century. He was the author of realist novels, symbolist theater pieces, peculiar collections of poems, and exalted psycho-sexual melodramas. He had lived a life of luxury in Rome, Naples, Florence, and Paris, and wrote a work of musical theater, *The Martyrdom of Saint Sebastian*, which was scored by Claude Debussy. But by the early 1910s, he probably felt that he was past his prime. This must have been at least part of the reason why he saw—and he was not alone in this—the war as the opportunity for a great renewal. By then in his fifties, he surprisingly became an aviator and, after a dazzling series of incursions into enemy territory, a war hero. He lost an eye in battle, but even this affliction was the occasion to write an eminently modern book called *Nocturne*. To the young, he was proof that the old Italy was still capable of magnificent exploits. It is also understandable that he feared that now that the fighting had ended, his personal decline of the prewar years would resume. He considered various options, including leading a march to Rome to overthrow the present government and undertaking an unprecedented, heroic flight from Venice to Tokyo—anything, except

returning to the calm of his life as a fading, middle-aged writer. He began to make explosive speeches that called for the return of the great glory of Italy. He announced and demanded a conflagration that would restore the spiritual authority of the country. He thought that the loss of Fiume would have a profound symbolic dimension and that it was vital to recover the city.

It seemed to Fiume's Italian elite that they had found their leader. D'Annunzio had developed connections with the *arditi* in Venice during the war and had shown himself perfectly capable of eliciting extraordinary enthusiasm in his followers. In September 1919, a band of a few hundred ex-combatants marched under his command toward Fiume. No one stopped them; on the contrary, the Italians among the Allied troops charged with guarding the city joined their cause. They entered Fiume, whose non-Slavic population initially received with euphoria the arrival of this strange leader who had never governed before, who had the vaguest political ideas, and who seemed to be mostly occupied in the tiring task of self-glorification. He professed a deep admiration for his young followers and gave endless speeches calling Fiume "the city of the Holocaust," the place where the old world was going to end and still-unheard-of ways of life would develop.

The initial plan, however, was more modest: D'Annunzio intended to repatriate Istria to Italy. But the Italian government, which had accepted the resolutions made at Versailles, had no interest in this gift. The project soon began to mutate: if the Italian regime in power was too corrupt and cowardly—too easily dominated by the Americans and their sidekicks, the old Europeans—then the example of the troops at Fiume would unchain a mass movement that would overthrow it, and perhaps even elevate D'Annunzio to the position of leader of the nation. None of this happened. Instead, a tense standoff began. The embarrassed Italian government convinced the Allies that it would deal with the situation, which it argued was an internal matter. But lacking confidence in its own army, Italy didn't attempt to take Fiume; rather, it instituted a partial siege, with the intention of keeping the revolt from expanding without entirely asphyxiating the population. Four months later, in December 1919, the Italian government presented to the National Council, which was the organ of the Italian community at Fiume, a formal declaration that it would work to impede the annexation of the city to the Kingdom of Serbs, Croats,

and Slovenes, and a guarantee of either its annexation to Italy or, if this was not possible, its autonomy. This seemed good enough for the Fiumean citizens, who were not as convinced as before of the virtues of their new leader, and decided to accept it. But D'Annunzio was unwilling. Not yet. Perhaps never. Nor were the more radical youth who seconded him ready to abandon what they had begun to call the "City of Life."

From the beginning, the coexistence of the diverse groups that gravitated around D'Annunzio had been difficult. There were the citizens of Fiume and the Italian troops (the *arditi*, the *carabinieri*), but also Bolsheviks who rushed to the city (in a Moscow speech, Lenin said he and D'Annunzio were the only authentic revolutionaries of Europe); anarcho-syndicalists; futuristic, fascist Dadaists; and oddities like the curious war hero Guido Keller, whose mascot was an eagle, who slept naked in the tops of trees, and who was one of the new commander's main lieutenants. The universe around the leader quickly fragmented into factions. Forced to take sides, D'Annunzio came to rely mostly on the young artists, anarchists, and *arditi* who constituted the radical wing of the grand alliance of Fiume, and who formed the "Union of Free Spirits Tending Toward Perfection" (or, as they nicknamed it, "Yoga"). The group shared an enthusiasm for Hinduism, spiritual aristocracy, nudism, and for building an agrarian utopia where preindustrial forms of life would be restored. Subgroups were formed: the Brown Lotuses, who wanted to lead a simple life and professed a return to nature; the Red Lotuses, who proclaimed the arrival of a new world transfigured by a renewed sexuality; and a group who identified themselves as the followers of a still-undefined "Sacred Love."

The fate of the utopia that this group was pursuing became increasingly dire as the isolation of Fiume became more profound: from the beginning of 1920, food became increasingly scarce, and it became harder to find the fabric needed for the confection of ever-more-flamboyant uniforms for the city's soldiers and ever-more-splendid flowers for their festivals. But, according to all accounts, the atmosphere in Fiume

---

Opposite: A selection of Fiumean stamps issued during D'Annunzio's occupation of the city. Note the variety of symbols recalling the Roman empire. The stamp at the center of the left column features a portrait of D'Annunzio himself. Courtesy Ivan Martinaš.

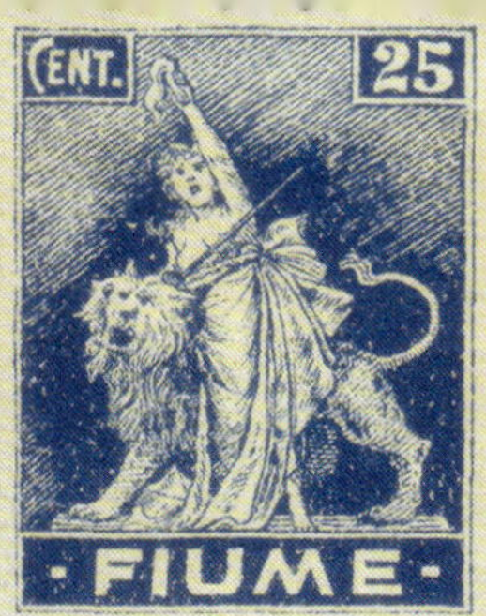

CENT. 25
FIUME

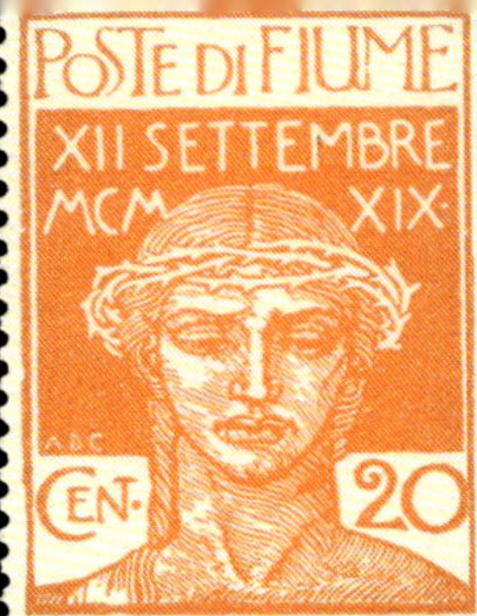

POSTE DI FIUME
XII SETTEMBRE
MCM XIX
CENT.
20

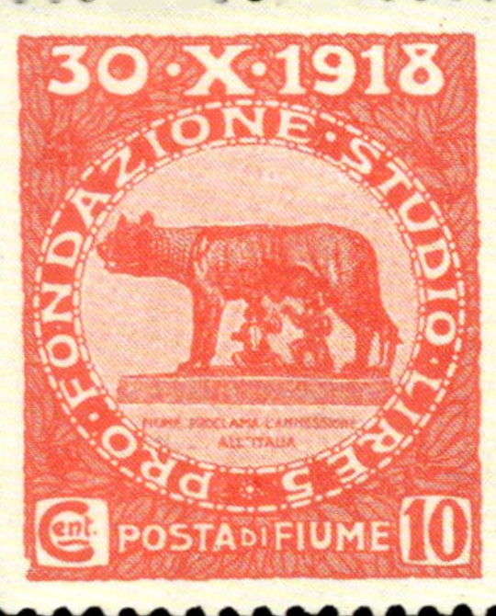

30 · X · 1918
PRO FONDAZIONE STUDIO LIRE 5
FIUME PROCLAMA L'ANNESSIONE ALL'ITALIA
Cent. POSTA DI FIUME 10

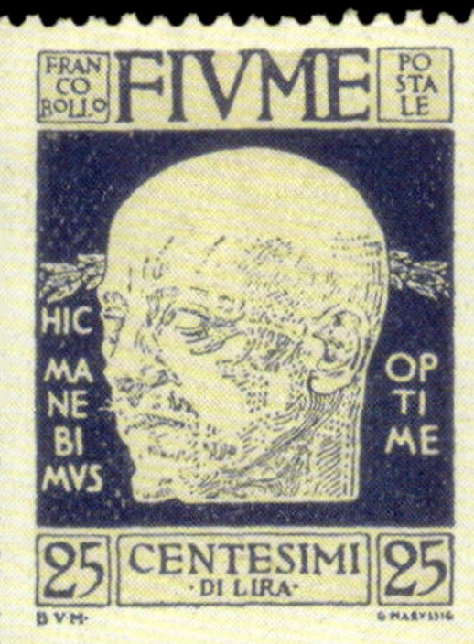

FRANCO BOLLO FIUME POSTALE
HIC MANE BIMVS
OPTIME
25 CENTESIMI DI LIRA 25

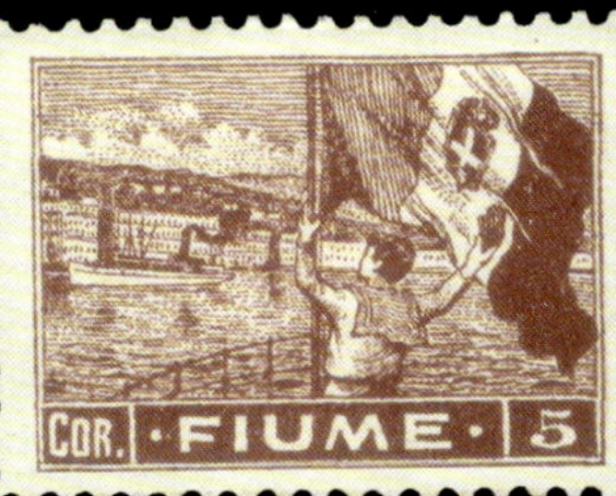

COR. · FIUME · 5

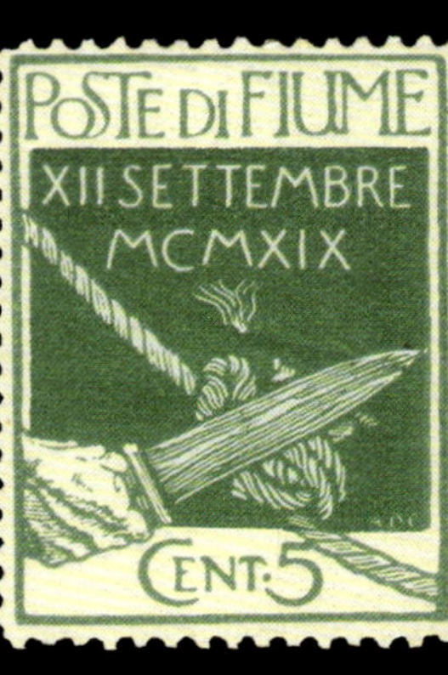

POSTE DI FIUME
XII SETTEMBRE
MCMXIX
CENT · 5

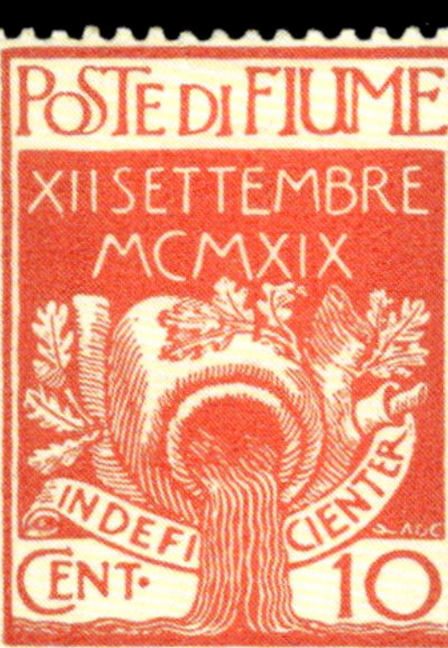

POSTE DI FIUME
XII SETTEMBRE
MCMXIX
INDEFICIENTER
CENT.
10

POSTE DI FIUME
ARCO ROMANO
30 CENTESIMI 30

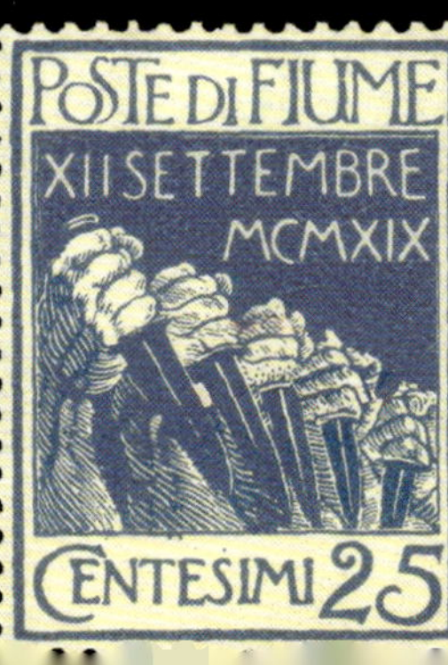

POSTE DI FIUME
XII SETTEMBRE
MCMXIX
CENTESIMI 25

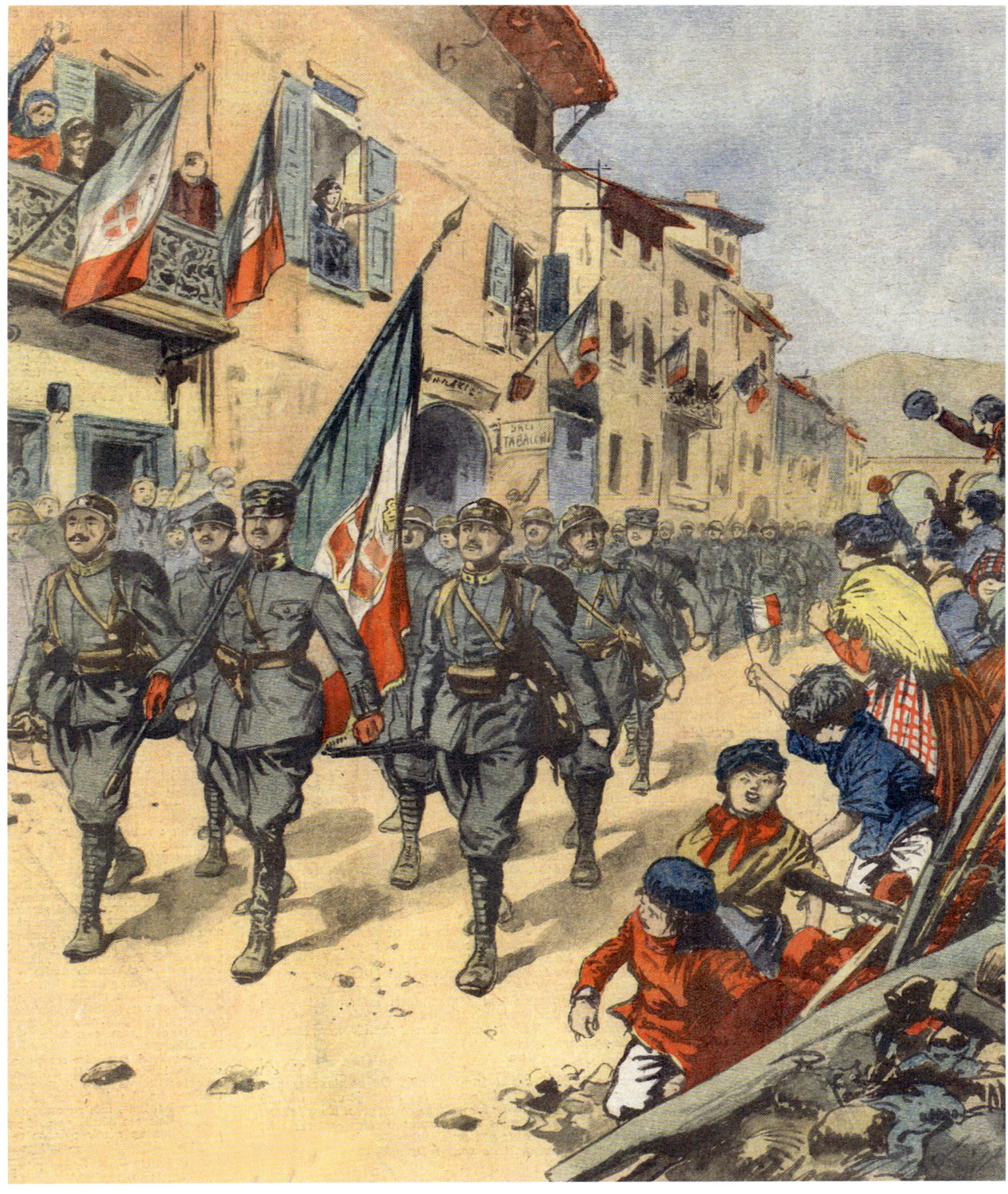

Italian troops entering Fiume after D'Annunzio's defeat,
December 1920. This image from *Le Petit Journal* of 9
January 1921 was captioned, "The end of the adventure."

remained more or less that of a continuous party, partially fueled by the drugs that the *arditi* had become addicted to on the battlefield and to which their leader was now also addicted. It was a "Bal des Ardents," a dance of the burning, said the Belgian poet Léon Kochnitzky, one of D'Annunzio's closest aides. At the festival of San Vito, he continued, "one's gaze, wherever it fixed, saw a dance: of lanterns, of sparks, of stars, starving, in ruin, in anguish. Perhaps on the verge of death in the flames or under a hail of grenades, Fiume, brandishing a torch, danced before the sea."[2] The regime was increasingly sustained by pirate raids of various kinds, and by the fruits of the burgeoning drug trade. The warships moored in the port at the time of the occupation were used to capture merchant ships along the Adriatic coast, between Messina and Trieste. Groups of rebel soldiers stole horses, weapons, and food from Italian garrisons in the countryside. But medicine and food for the children was still lacking, and D'Annunzio ordered scores of babies to be sent to Italy and given away for adoption. The contrast between the euphoria of the young and the increasing desperation of the local bourgeoisie intensified.

The city had become a magnet for radicals. One, who arrived in 1920, was the prominent syndicalist Alceste De Ambris, an active figure in the workers' movement and founder of the Fasci d'Azione Rivoluzionaria Internazionalista, which would eventually merge with other *fasci* led by Benito Mussolini. De Ambris became D'Annunzio's chief of staff and started working on a constitution for a new state, which they named the Italian Regency of Carnaro (the traditional Italian name for the region surrounding the city). The Charter of Carnaro is an extraordinary document. The ideas at its base are mostly those we would expect from a revolutionary syndicalist, not surprisingly given that De Ambris was responsible for the first draft of the document. The text states from the beginning that it will be "a government elected by the people—*res populi*—founded on productive work, and its ordering principle is inspired by the most generous and diverse forms of autonomy as they were understood and exercised in the four glorious centuries of our communal period."[3] The constitution attempts to maintain a balance between the recognition of the equality and diversity of citizens (because "the harmonic interplay of diversity makes stronger and richer the common life") and the intention to "widen, expand, and hold the

right of the workers above any other law." The document restricts private property, which is not entirely eliminated but is subordinated to the good of the community. Work is idealized as an activity that elicits "the feeling of virtuous joy" that should be the dominant mood of citizens and is located at the center of the three "religious beliefs" that the constitution enshrines:

Life is beautiful and worthy of being severely and magnificently lived by a man rebuilt entirely by freedom;

The complete man is one who knows how to exercise every day his own virtue to offer every day his brothers a new gift;

Work, even the humblest, even the most obscure, if done well, tends to beauty and ornates the world.

This state of the citizen-worker is organized around corporations, designed on the model of labor unions. The charter prescribes the formation of nine corporations consisting, respectively, of factory workers, technicians, managers, public officers, merchants, farmers, students and teachers, professionals, and sailors, and a tenth, supplementary one that is vaguely defined and most peculiar.[4] The executive branch that presides over them must be as fluid and transitory as possible; the judiciary must encourage the citizens to settle their accounts, whenever possible, without the intervention of the courts; legislators should meet just a few times a year.

But the baroque prose of the final document belongs, unequivocally, to the poet-leader who finalized De Ambris's draft. In addition to the brilliant and occasionally convoluted character of the text, it's probably due to D'Annunzio that the pillars of the Free University placed at the top of the regency's educational structure are a School of Fine Arts, a School of Decorative Arts, and a School of Music. Also to him must be due the disproportionate attention paid by the charter to the institution of an Office of Aldermen composed of "men of pure taste, exquisite skill, and of the newest education." Their work was to ornament streets and squares "with that same musical sense that guides the creation of … republican pomp or of a carnival representation," prepare the civic festivals, and educate the people in the love of forms and colors, especially when they are incorporated into the "vivid and powerful utensils" that are deployed in daily life. And perhaps it was also due to D'Annunzio that the

charter declared music the highest of all the city's arts. From their first day in school, children would be taught "choral singing founded on the basis of the most naive peasant poetry," because music announces the realm of spirit and gives a glimpse of the dawn of a new kind of freedom. And they would learn to appreciate not only the music produced by voices and instruments, but also the one produced by tools used in work and by machines that roar following their own mysterious rhythm. These are the last lines of the charter:

> *Choral and instrumental bodies subsidized by the state are instituted in all the Communes of the Regency.*
>
> *The College of Aldermen is entrusted with the task of building a rotunda capable of holding at least ten thousand listeners, with comfortable seats for the people and a vast pit for the orchestra and the choir.*
>
> *Large choral and orchestral performances are totally free, as the Church Fathers said of God's graces.*

When we read the charter, written in the first half of 1920 and proclaimed (to the dismay of the local bourgeoisie) in July of that year, we realize that Fiume had undergone, in the course of just a few months, a profound mutation. It was initially intended to bring about a change in Italian policies, but now that this initial plan had failed, D'Annunzio, De Ambris, Kochnitzky, and Keller saw it as a place where a profound restructuring of global politics would begin. Now they conceived of the regency as the beginning of a movement where Italians, Serbs, Egyptians, Turks, Indians, Irish, and others would revolt against the domination of capitalism, of imperialism, of all forms of decay. Therefore, they decided to establish a League of Oppressed Peoples to carry out this magnificent task and bring to Fiume a number of delegates to start the discussions meant to give a specific form to, ultimately, world revolution, of which a great uprising in the Balkans would be the first step.

But it was too late: the economic and political crisis had become too deep. The rewards of piracy were not sufficient to keep the city functioning. The links between the circle of the leader and the institutions of bourgeois community (with the National Council at the center) had broken. Those factions of the army attracted by the nationalist program of 1919 started to leave. D'Annunzio, who from the beginning had oscillated between supporting the most extreme plans of his left wing and acting to win the confidence of the most conservative elements of his strange coalition, became increasingly erratic. Even some of his closest collaborators, who could now rarely see him, locked in as he was in his suite at the Hotel Europe, began to doubt him.

The Fiume adventure ended in the last days of 1920 in an anticlimactic way. The Treaty of Rapallo, which settled the relations between Italy and the Kingdom of Serbs, Croats, and Slovenes, granted full autonomy to the city. It could be supposed that D'Annunzio, politically defeated, would then have given up the struggle and abandoned Fiume, but he didn't. Neither the first of his goals (the annexation of Istria to Italy) nor the second (the creation of a political entity of a new type) met, he refused to recognize the validity of the treaty. An Italian assault on the city in late December 1920 (Bloody Christmas is the name that tradition would give those days) overcame remaining occupant troops—by now in full disarray—in exactly two days.

Many of the demobilized soldiers who had supported D'Annunzio were soon to become the most devoted and active members of the emerging fascist movement. As for the poet himself, he would spend the last years of his life in splendid confinement in a villa on Lake Garda. He was honored, materially supported, and publicly celebrated by the fascist regime, but it was understood that his political life was over. His literary work was essentially completed too: he spent the rest of his life editing, reordering, and monumentalizing what he wrote in his first five decades, and died in 1938. His most enduring legacy as a public figure was perhaps the development of a kind of political spectacle that would be perfected by the infinitely more somber Benito Mussolini and Adolf Hitler.

1 In English, the only book-length account of the story is Michael A. Ledeen's *The First Duce: D'Annunzio at Fiume* (Baltimore and London: The John Hopkins University Press, 1977). The story is also told, in a more fragmentary manner, by Lucy Hughes-Hallet in her biography of D'Annunzio, *Gabriele d'Annunzio: Poet, Seducer, and Preacher of War* (New York: Knopf, 2013).

2 Quoted in Michael A. Ledeen, *The First Duce*, p. 151.

3 Unless otherwise indicated, all translations are my own.

4 The tenth corporation, says the text, has no art or categories or vocabulary. Its fulfillment is anticipated as that of the tenth Muse. Reserved for the mysterious powers of the people at work and in ascension, it is a votive figure devoted to the unknown genius, the apparitions of the new man, the ideal transfiguration of the labors and days, the complete liberation of the spirit from painful breath and bloody sweat. It is represented in the civic sanctuary by a burning lamp that is inscribed with an ancient Tuscan expression from the age of the Communes, which splendidly alludes to a spiritualized form of human work: *Fatica senza fatica* ("effort without fatigue").

THE INTERNET OF SNAILS
Justin E. H. Smith

The snail, class Gastropoda, is noted for a number of exceptional traits. For one thing, it contains a model of the universe in its self-secreted shell: the whorls of hardened mucus instantiate the same logarithmic expansion, sometimes called *e*, that we see in the spirals of galaxies. For another, some naturalists have observed peculiar powers associated with the snail's reproductive faculty. They have observed, in particular, a sort of sympathetic bond that endures, across any distance and for the duration of their lives, between any two snails who have once brought their slimy peristaltic rods together in courtship. It has not escaped human curiosity to see whether this bond might be seized upon and used for certain technological applications.

Paris, October 1850. A young man, a former law student and radical candidate for the Constitutional Assembly by the name of Jules Allix, publishes in the feuilleton of *La Presse* an article describing a new invention.[1] He is not himself the inventor, but is only speaking, he claims, on behalf of his associates, Monsieur Jacques Toussaint Benoît from Hérault near Montpellier, and a man identified only as "Monsieur Biat-Chrétien, the American" (later referred to simply as "Biat"). The discovery is of a "pasilalinic sympathetic compass" that will facilitate "universal and instantaneous communication of thought, at any distance whatsoever."

In the article, Allix dissimulates, stalls, takes an inordinate amount of time to tell us what this machine actually does. He moves at a leisurely pace through a survey of theological positions on magnetism. The distinguished men of Notre Dame, he tells us, are prepared to see it not as a trick or an illusion, but as the crowning mystery of God's creation, a constant announcement, in the seeking out of metal by metal, of God's wisdom and might. If we are prepared to admit gravity, why not other forces too? Why, for example, should we not admit the "galvano-magnetico-mineralo-animalo-adamical sympathy" that governs the pasilalinic sympathetic compass?

Unlike the electrical telegraph, we are eventually told, the compass has no conductive wires, but only two unconnected and portable boxes, each containing a voltaic pile, a wooden or metal wheel ringed with copper sulphate–lined metal troughs. And, in each of these troughs, a snail.

A snail? Allix dwells in excessive detail on irrelevant points, and breezes right past relevant ones. He checks off the most recent scientific shibboleths—Steinheil's advances in telegraphy in Munich, Matteucci's in Pisa—and he frontloads the technical terminology like Lieutenant Sulu explaining the impossible physics of warp drive. After a long digression, however, we are offered a bare-bones description of how the machine is to work. Allix explains, first of all, the natural phenomenon, observable only in snails, of "sympathizing," which is to say of creating an indivisible bond through copulation:

After the separation of the snails that have sympathized together, a sort of fluid is released between them, for which the earth is the conductor, which develops and unfolds, so to speak, like the nearly invisible thread of the spider or that of a silkworm, which one could unfold and elongate in an indefinite space without breaking it, but with this one difference, that the escargotic fluid is completely invisible and that it has as much speed in space as the electrical fluid, and that it would be by means of this fluid that the snails produce and communicate the commotion of which I have spoken.

Why is this sympathy found only in snails? Allix does not say explicitly, though he does remind us that snails are hermaphrodites, "which is to say male and female at the same time." We are perhaps invited here to recall the myth, or something like it, of the original androgyne, attributed to Aristophanes by Plato in *The Symposium*. In the beginning, the philosopher recounts, every human being had four arms and four legs, two heads, and two sets of genitals, and so every human being lacked nothing, and longed for nothing, and the body was in perfect communication with itself. For Allix, then, to be male and female at once is to have it all, and it appears that, at least in snails, this perfection is distilled into the sexual fluids, so that, once exchanged, each hermaphroditic snail now shares in the other's being completely.

But let us return to the mechanics. A pair of snails—which have previously sympathized with one another and which, therefore, remain in perfect and

instantaneous contact—are placed in two separate boxes. When one of the snails is manipulated, it triggers an "escargotic commotion" that causes its partner to move. By having numerous such pairs—each representing a single letter of the French alphabet—divided between corresponding troughs in the two boxes, successive manipulations of particular snails in one box would transmit words that could be read through the motions of the sympathetic snails in the other box.

Allix promises that, with this device, "all men will be able to correspond instantaneously with one another, at whatsoever distance they are placed, man to man, or several men simultaneously, at every corner of the world, and this without recourse to the conductive wires of electrical communication, but with the sole aid of what is basically a portable machine." The machine will serve as the basis of a global system of instant wireless communication: an Internet of snails.

Before the public appearance related in the article, our salesman and future communard had been in hiding following the 1848 "June Days," a popular revolt in Paris in response to the closing of the National Workshops that had been set up, after the revolution of February of the same year, to provide training for the jobless.[2] He would be arrested one year later in connection with another uprising, and soon after would find his way into the company of the occultist and charlatan Jacques Toussaint Benoît, who had been cooking up a plan to gain sponsorship for the above-described snail compass from the investor Hippolyte Triat, born Antoine Hypolitte Trilhac, who had for his part recently founded the first modern athletic gymnasium in Paris.

On 2 October 1850, the experiment described by Allix in his article for *La Presse* was carried out in Benoît's Paris apartment. Messieurs Benoît, Allix, and Triat were all present. And, if Allix's account is to be believed, Biat was there as well—at least in a modality that would later come to be known as "teleconferencing"—participating from an undisclosed location in America.

Allix was far more impressed than Triat. The prospective investor had been installed with one of the two boxes behind a curtain, with Allix and his own box on the other side, while Benoît set himself up between them to observe. It is not clear exactly what happened, but it appears that Benoît found a constant supply of pretexts for walking back and forth between the two men on either side of the curtain, influencing Triat's actions and gleaning hints and signs in a less than rigorously scientific way. If we believe a possibly embellished account by the nineteenth-century Englishman Sabine Baring-Gould, Triat was indignant, and insisted that the experiment be tried out again.[3] Benoît agreed, only to disappear into the night before Triat could have the satisfaction of exposing this dastardly fraud. And a few years later Allix was to become a footnote to the biography of Victor Hugo, when, hiding from the authorities on the island of Jersey, he once again attempted to communicate by means of escargotic force, to the great amusement of the participants in the French author's "talking table" séances.[4]

Allix had taken on the task of drumming up public support, and the *La Presse* article, written before Benoît's disappearance, was a dazzling display of salesmanship, erudition, and gumption. Perhaps most remarkable of all, in our present age of shrinking machines, is his promise that although Benoît's first models were more than two meters high, eventually the public could expect to enjoy more convenient models, transformed into stylish furniture or even jewelry made of wood or metal or any material one might wish. They would be found everywhere, from government offices to ladies' dressers and even their watch chains. The original iteration had, according to Allix, been built to accommodate snails representing every letter or character of every known writing system in the world, while future streamlined models, made for the larger public, would conveniently contain only twenty-five troughs, one for each letter of the French alphabet. And as each trough could be filled by any species of gastropod whatsoever, and as there are many species that are very small indeed, no larger than the head of a pin, soon, Allix assures us, there would be pasilalinic sympathetic compasses no larger than pocket watches. Ordinary men and women would carry them along as they went about their daily errands, from time to time sending off quick escargotic missives—texts, if you will—to their friends and loved ones down the street and around the world.

Allix promises that by means of the compass there will soon be "electrical newspapers, electrical mail," spreading across the entire world, as if by magic, at a minimal cost. Beyond just a "national press," one in which the news will be published in regional towns

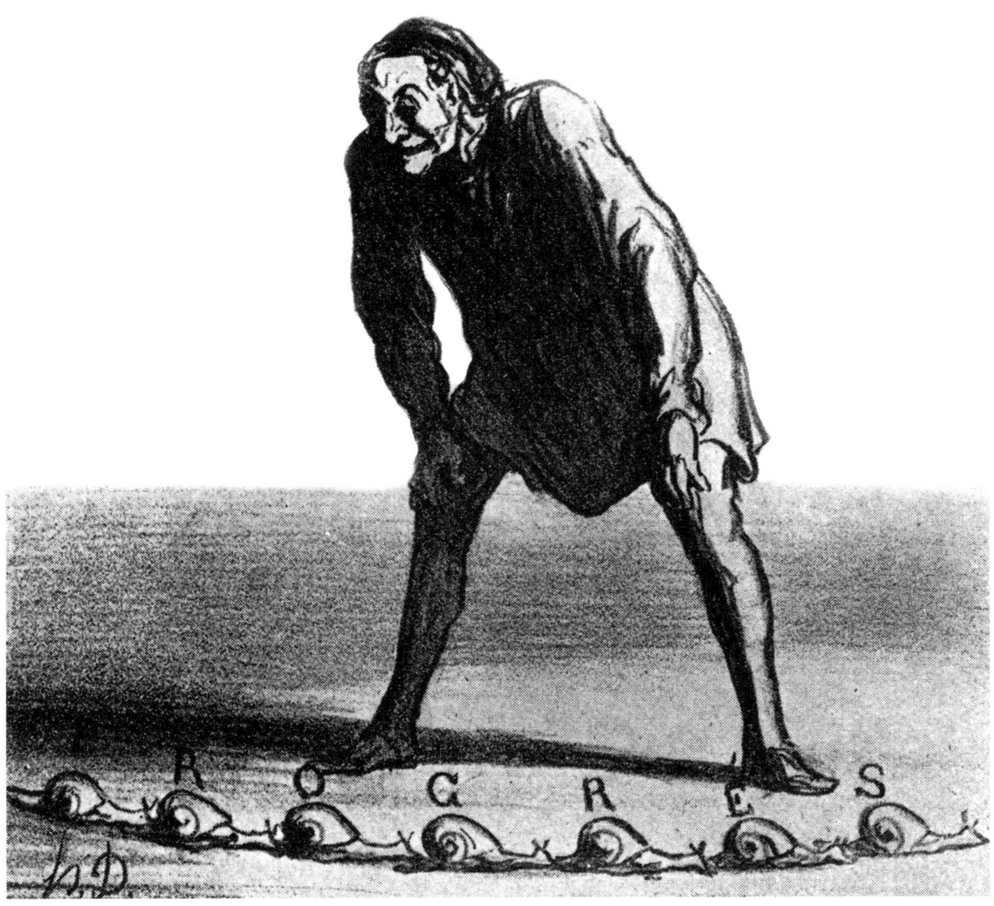

Honoré Daumier, *Les escargots non sympathiques*, published in *Le Charivari*, 25 September 1869. Nineteen years after Jules Allix's article, the trope of "sympathetic snails" had retained enough currency to be used as the title of this cartoon. Where Allix's sympathetic snails had promised a world of instantaneous communication, the non-sympathetic snails here represent the slow progress of social reforms promised by the Second Empire to workers like the one depicted in Daumier's drawing.

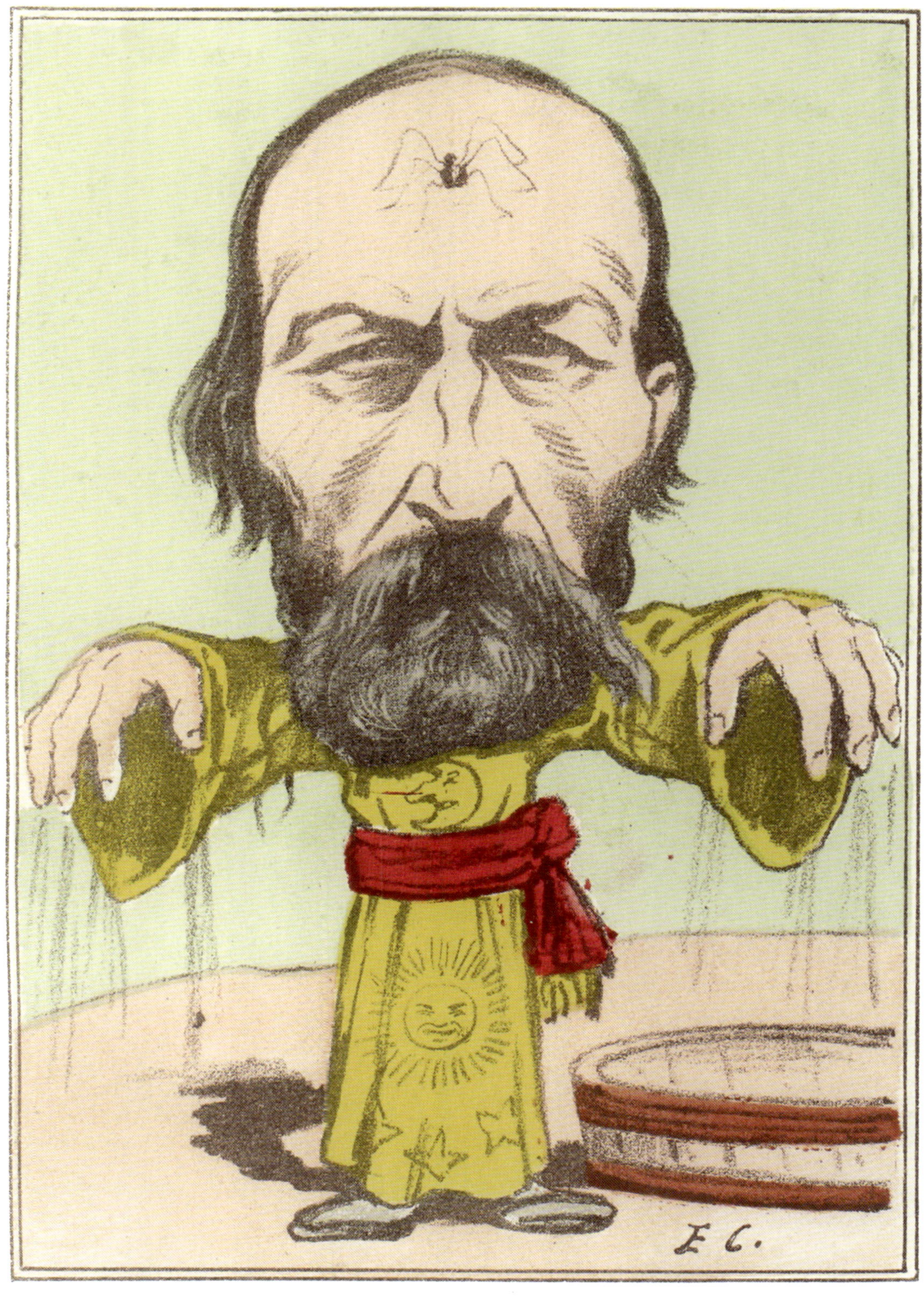

at the same hour as in Paris, readers will also be able to browse "the English press, the German press, and that of all the countries of the world." It is not entirely clear how all this—what we today would call electronic communication—would work technically: if there can only be communication between snails that have previously copulated, it would not seem possible for information to be broadly disseminated, unless perhaps there were special "server" snails that had copulated with many others. But let us not get hung up on details.

The activity of government, too, was to be transmitted via the compass, and the walls of the parliament buildings "turned inside out" as invisible, dematerialized orators were "infinitely multiplied before an innumerably large audience," their words circulating "as rapidly as thought to all points in the world, thanks to the mysterious agent of the invisible sympathetic fluid, bringing with them not only the passion that drives the orator, but also the beating of his heart and the least vibrations of his soul!"

Allix quickly reels himself back in, wipes the sweat from his brow, reassumes his scientific composure: "I must remember," he says, "that I am not to give in to enthusiasm."

. . .

I am not interested in Jules Allix's snails for their own sake, but as a chapter—not the first—in a very, very long history. This is what we might call the deep history of the Internet. Significantly, it is also the history of biology: of thinking about what it is in living beings that sets them apart, and of trying to harness whatever this is for feats we seem to have always known to be possible.

Montpellier, 1657. The eclectic English philosopher Kenelm Digby, combining elements of Aristotelianism with the new mechanical physics, gives a presentation to the assembled learned men in the provincial capital of the *département* where Benoît will be born some years later. The subject is the controversial "weapon salve," where an injury is treated by application of a "powder of sympathy" not to the injured person's body but, at a distance, to the weapon that had injured him.[5] This sort of sympathetic effect would be denounced by the strictest mechanical philosophers as an "occult force," a violation of the law that says there is nothing in the world but atoms or corpuscles bouncing around like so many billiard balls, but Digby insists that the causal

bond between the weapon and the wound could be explained by the rapid motion of invisible particles between the weapon and the body, thus "naturally, and without any Magick, cur[ing] wounds without touching them."[6]

Applications in the domain of telecommunication were soon tried out. An anonymous 1688 pamphlet proposes to solve the problem of establishing longitude while at sea by sending a dog that had been wounded with a knife in London aboard a ship traversing the ocean. The knife would stay in London, and each day at noon, salt would be poured on it, causing the dog to yelp in pain, it was hoped, and thus telling the voyagers the exact time back home.[7] In the nineteenth century, for example in the imposture of Allix and Benoît, such action at a distance was typically accounted for in terms of electricity and magnetism, rather than in the preferred early modern language of bare particles in motion. But both Digby's weapon salve and the later escargotic contraption involve speculation about some peculiar features of the ambient medium that facilitate such remarkable actions at a distance; and both, too, involve sentient animals not only as their test subjects, but also as the furnishers of the properties and powers that make the telecommunication possible.

Before there was a distinct science of biology, the study of living beings was the core element of the foundational science of nature. The cosmos as a whole was modeled after the living animal body, and the problems of physics seemed to have their resolution in the study of physiology, rather than the reverse, a twist that still leaves its trace in the overlapping morphemes in the names of these two sciences.

Thus we may go back further still, long before Digby, to the world soul of the Stoics, and to the giant animal that is the world, and which the world soul quickens. For Zeno of Citium and his student Cleanthes in the third century BCE, God seemed to be a sort of fire pervading the universe. Later Stoics, notably the second-century BCE philosopher Chrysippus, will identify the human soul as pneuma, a rarefied spirit that enlivens the body in the same way that God does the world as a whole. Typically, soul is conceived as some sort of breath, or flame, or a combination of the

<hr>

Opposite: Caricature of Allix as an occultist. From *La Commune*, a book of portraits by Hippolyte Mailly & Charles Vernier, 1871.

two, and there is a perfect correspondence between the human ensoulment of the body and God's of the world. For Cleanthes, as reported by Cicero, the soul is "made of fire" but at the same time it is "nourished by the moistures of the Ocean because no fire could continue to exist without sustenance of some sort." It is therefore not like the ordinary fire that consumes all things and then burns out, but is rather "vital and wholesome." It "preserves, nourishes, maintains and bestows sensation on everything," like the sun itself.[8] If the world is not already a great sensorium, then we will make it into one, for we cannot think of the world except on the model of our own living bodies, in which signals shoot like lightning from one end to the other, in which, as the Hippocratics said, "all things conspire" [*sympnoia panta*].

What is the nature of this conspiration? Is human symbolic exchange in continuity with it, or rather a rupture from it? Having created the Internet from scratch, do we now pridefully project our own humble contraption far beyond its limited domain in order to make sense of nature as a whole, just as, some centuries ago, advances in the science and art of chronometry had all the philosophers declaring that the world is a great clockwork? Or is the Internet an outgrowth of what is already there?

In a recent, breathtakingly original work, the anthropologist Eduardo Kohn has argued that we may grasp "how forests think" if we abandon the idea that all thinking must take place by minds entertaining symbolically communicated abstract concepts.[9] For Kohn, following a largely underappreciated strand of C. S. Peirce's semiotics, representational signs are only one kind of sign, existing within vast systems of non-representational semiotic exchange, as when a vine snaps, and causes a monkey to grasp at another. Wherever there is such a system of signs, there is thinking, though not human thinking, and we must in turn understand this non-human thinking, which taken as a whole we may call "nature," as the antecedent and substratum of what human beings do when they, for their part, think. Thinking, or systems that involve thinking, thus mark no rupture with the natural world, but rather are better seen as an excrescence or outgrowth of it.

Kohn's theory helps us to make literal sense of much of the way people speak—in the popular science press, for example—which would otherwise be bracketed as mere loose metaphor. We are now being told,

to cite one recent study that was widely reported on, that there are fungal networks beneath the forests, a "wood-wide web" that enables conspecific plants to share information, to deliver chemical packets of nutrients, and to block, with toxins, the interests of competitor species trying to move into their niche.[10] Here, as with reports by sociobiologists of rape among ducks or political hierarchies among ants, the accusation of runaway analogizing cannot be decisively refuted: from the simple fact that there is an analogous process in non-human nature, we may not conclude that a human endeavor has a true counterpart among the animals and plants. And yet: my surge of joy when a tweet of mine is favorited is, in the end, a chemical process too, just like the organic chemistry underlying plant growth and life. And the joy is experienced as a sense of community, of belonging to something I cannot see, and that loves me. Is there some dim joy when a nutrient packet comes across the woods to the roots of a lonely plant?

I am trying to work toward a position where it does not seem absurd to suggest that the Internet might best be investigated as a branch of natural history, and that like other questions in natural history, the question as to its nature might best be answered genealogically. What is that human experience out of which there emerges some new technologically mediated way of doing things? In the case of cinema, we are fairly familiar by now with the analysis of this new art form into its constitutive ancestral lineages: the realist novel, certain schools of European painting, the shadow theater. And what is it that we are doing when we shoot guns? We are enabling our hands to be what we had always wanted them to be: perfect organs of killing, senders of more deadly projectiles. And what is this thing we call "transportation"? Just look back at Samuel Pepys, that vanguard of modern everydayness, who hops on and off boats to cross the Thames, to make it from one appointment to the next. "So I down to the water-side, and there got a boat and through bridge."[11] Pepys is a harbinger of the world to come, a modern man, taking public transit before it exists in any real sense. The Tube will grow out of him, out of his desires and motions.

In all of these cases—cinema, guns, transportation—it may seem that we are looking at relatively recent, compressed, and familiar instances in the history of technology: slightly earlier chapters of it,

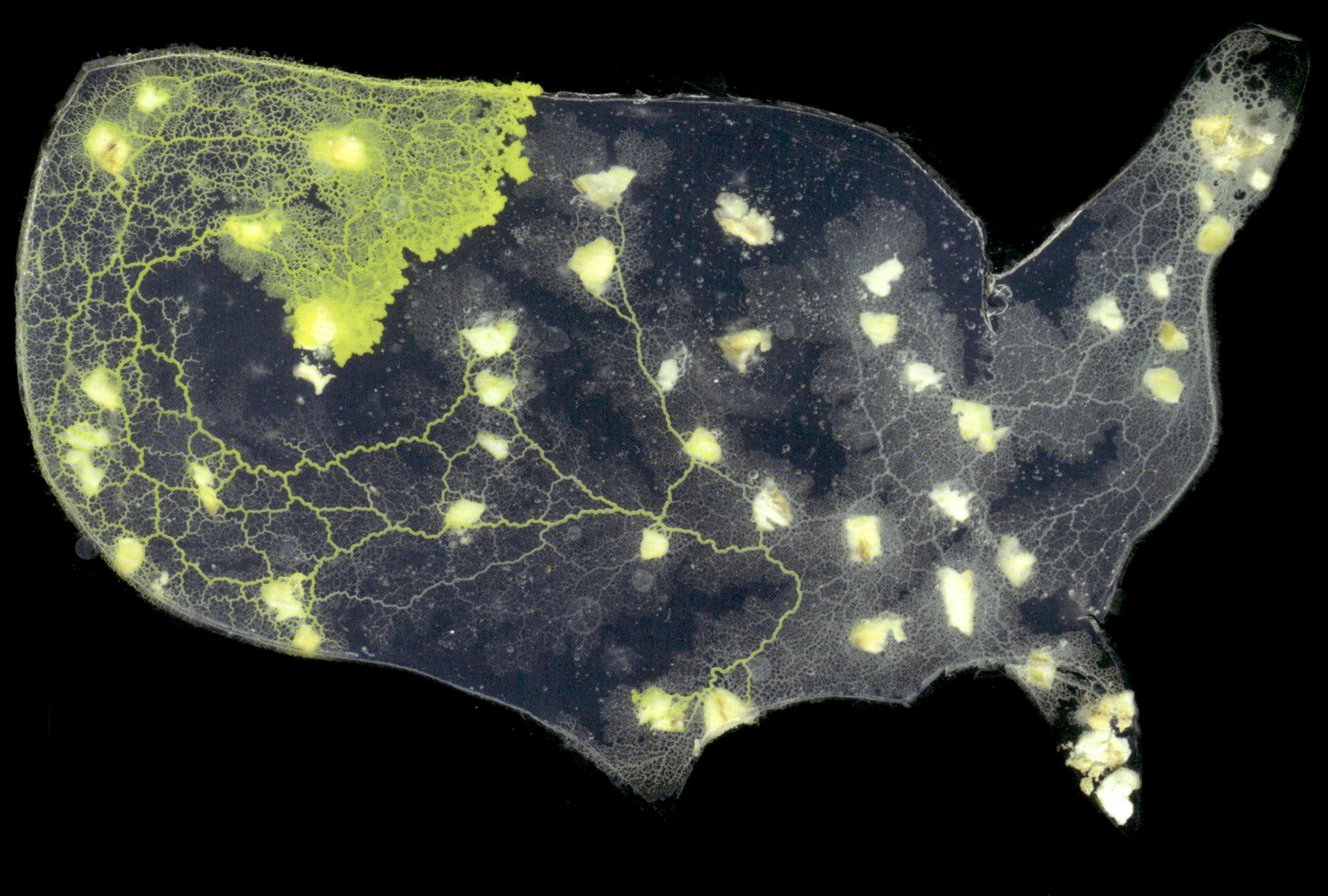

Hacking the wood-wide web. The slime mold *Physarum polycephalum* is used in laboratories across the world to map more efficient highway and subway networks. Here, in an experiment staged at the International Center of Unconventional Computing at the University of the West of England, the mold is redrawing the US interstate highway system. Photo Andy Adamatzky.

perhaps, but nonetheless ones safely on the human and social side of the boundary that marks this realm off from nature, and so from the study of natural history. Yet behind or beneath cinema, guns, and transportation, there are human minds imagining stories, human hands thrusting, human feet walking: these are the true antecedents to the history of technology, and they are indeed continuous with what we observe throughout the natural world. To cite another example, the anthropologist Tim Ingold has deftly exposed the facile character of the distinction we generally wish to make between the naturalness of walking and the artificiality of riding a bicycle. As Ingold explains, "If walking is innate in the sense—and only in the sense—*that given certain conditions*, it is bound to emerge in the course of development, then the same applies to cycling. And if cycling is acquired in the sense that its emergence depends on a process of learning that is embedded in contexts of social interaction, then the same applies to walking. … Both walking and cycling are skills that emerge in the relational contexts of the child's involvement in its surroundings, and are therefore properties of the developmental system constituted by these relations."[12] Ingold concludes that walking and cycling are both thus situated "within the same overall process of evolution—an evolution, that is, of the developmental systems which under-write these capacities."[13] And again, the same may be said of listening to stories and watching movies, or of punching and shooting, or of walking and riding the subway: in each pair of cases, we are looking at a product of natural evolution and a behavioral disposition exemplified in a certain cultural context, and yet, in each pair, we are looking at what is in a certain sense the same sort of thing. The separation between the study of culture and natural history is, in the end, arbitrary and unfounded.

But let us return to the Internet. One of the most evident genetic strands in its prehistory is, of course, the book. Today, the Internet is in fact doing what the most grandiose claims about the book maintained that that humble object could do: duplicating the world, providing a perfect reflection of the order of nature (which properly understood was itself a book). In this respect, the Internet is not really a machine or engine at all, even if things that clearly are engines contribute to its genealogy. It is not like those things that transform nature by hydraulics and pyrotechnics and so

on. Its history may be traced back in part to Agostino Ramelli's book wheel, one of the "diverse and artificial-tious machines" described in a curious work of 1588, but in order to understand its power, destructive and otherwise, one would be mistaken in concentrating on the mechanics of it.[14] Unlike the case of the clock in early modern Europe, to conceive of the world as an Internet is not to get overexcited about one of our newest contraptions, for the Internet is not really a contraption at all. One would do better to trace it back far further, to Holy Scripture, to runes and oracle bones, to the discovery of the possibility of reproducing the world through the manipulation of signs.

This discovery was never exclusively, or even principally, experienced as facilitating the communication of practical information between human beings. Communication is far stranger than, say, transportation. The latter offers no action at a distance, no mysterious conjuring of mental images, memories, emotions, by sounds or signs. Even when we understand the technology behind communication, we feel as if there is something left over, which the technological explanation must necessarily leave out. That is why it was simultaneously experienced as a tapping into, a penetration of, the divine intelligence that pervades all of the natural order. Symbolic communication—first ephemeral speech, but then, later, communication across distances by means of more or less permanent signs—was never simply human, but was also always taken to be a divine or quasi-divine medium quickening and connecting all of nature. Thus so much of the writing in the Hindu temples of medieval southeast Asia is placed on top of structures, facing upward toward the sky, where no human being might read it. Thus the scrawled prayers inserted into the Wailing Wall. And thus do we draw out fragments of our inner lives, slivers of monuments of who we take ourselves to be, and write them and post them, without knowing for whom, or to what end. We send them out into the cosmos. And thus, too, one of the first transmissions exchanged at the demonstration: after Allix spelled out the word *GYMNASE* in honor of Triat's most recent venture, he received the phrase *LUMIÈRE DIVINE* in return. All theories of the all-pervading medium—the ether, pneuma, *spiritus mundi*—are in the end variations or analogies drawn from the observation of light, which is not itself fully divine but radiates out from something that is, and elevates everything it touches or

transpierces. Christians conceive this principle, variously, as Logos, or the Word, of which Christ himself, God made flesh, is a personification.

The clock, it is sometimes said, did not measure something that was already there; it was an instrument that itself produced hours and minutes and seconds. The clock gave us time as a collection of discrete temporal quanta. The Internet has been more like the aqueduct: it did not invent what flows through it, but only channeled it. What flows through it is human desire, and human aggression, which are in turn only our microcosmic expression of the general laws that govern all of nature: "All things proceed through love and strife," as Heraclitus had it. Love, or its close cousin desire, may well have been the principal motor of all advances in communication technology in the modern era. Thus, Patchen Barss discerns the pornographic origins of new media since the rise of the printing press, but most intensively since the beginnings of photography in the mid-nineteenth century, when the first erotic photographs began to circulate. Barss argues that new communication technologies typically pass through their "pornographic years" until "other, slower-developing non-sexual applications could gain a popular foothold."[15]

The Internet is also in large part a technological by-product of postwar military research: the "strife" part of Heraclitus's formula. But it enters civilian households through love. It is not just that pornography is the primary application people seek out once the technology is already there, but rather that the pornographic desire itself generates the technology, realizes the contraptions that human fantasy has always imagined for itself. And now war and masturbation are facilitated by one and the same machine. Drones drop bombs, and monitors attest that somewhere these bombs subtract the lives of goats and humans. Meanwhile a webcam reveals that what is called a "creampie" is somewhere else overflowing all natural concavities. The Internet is coursing with animal spirits, hungry and enraged, a perfect mirror of the world itself. The world is an animal; the Internet, which has always existed as conceptual possibility, as human destiny, as desire, as fungus, as escargotic commotion, as life, is the animal's embodied soul.

A full translation of Jules Allix's article is available at <cabinetmagazine.org/issues/58/smith.php>.

1 The text, dated 17 October 1850, was published anonymously in *La Presse*, in two parts, on 25 and 26 October 1850, under the title "Communication universelle et instantanée de la pensée, à quelque distance que ce soit, à l'aide d'un appareil portatif appelé Boussole pasilalinique sympathique." Digitized copies of the two parts of the article are available through the Bibliothèque nationale de France at <gallica.bnf.fr/ark:/12148/bpt6k475317s> and <gallica.bnf.fr/ark:/12148/bpt6k4753185>.

2 The secondary literature on Allix is limited, but a biography may be pieced together from various sources, notably Jules Clère, *Les hommes de la Commune*, 5th ed. (Paris: E. Dentu, 1872); Charles Chincholle, *Les survivants de la Commune* (Paris: L. Boulanger, 1885); and Thomas Bouchet, "Allix, Jules," in *Dictionnaire biographique du fouriérisme*, available at <charlesfourier.fr/spip.php?article421>.

3 See Sabine Baring-Gould, *Historic Oddities and Strange Events* (London: Methuen & Company, 1889), p. 197.

4 See Gustave Simon, *Chez Victor Hugo: Procès-verbaux des tables tournantes de Jersey* (Paris: Louis Conard, 1923), particularly the séance of 3 September 1854.

5 Kenelm Digby, *A Late Discourse Made in Solemn Assembly of Nobles and Learned Men at Montpellier in France, by Sir Kenelm Digby, Touching the Cure of Wounds by the Powder of Sympathy* (London: Lowdes, 1658).

6 Kenelm Digby, *A Late Discourse*, p. 3.

7 See *Curious Enquiries* (London: Randal Taylor, 1688).

It is generally believed that this pamphlet was strictly satirical, and reflected no real plan, intended or executed, for the measurement of longitude.

8 See Hans Friedrich August von Arnim, ed., *Stoicorum veterum fragmenta*, vol. 1 (Stuttgart: Teubner, 1964), p. 504.

9 Eduardo Kohn, *How Forests Think: Toward an Anthropology Beyond the Human* (Berkeley: University of California Press, 2013).

10 See Nic Fleming, "Plants Talk to Each Other Using an Internet of Fungus," *BBC*, 11 November 2014. Available at <bbc.com/earth/story/20141111-plants-have-a-hidden-internet>. The term "wood-wide web" has in fact been in use since late in the last century. See Thorunn Helgason et al., "Ploughing Up the Wood-Wide Web?" *Nature*, vol. 394, no. 431 (30 July 1998).

11 See entry for 2 September 1666 in Samuel Pepys, *The Diary of Samuel Pepys* (London: Macmillan, 1905), p. 412.

12 Tim Ingold, "'People Like Us': The Concept of the Anatomically Modern Human," in Tim Ingold, *The Perception of the Environment: Essays on Livelihood, Dwelling and Skill* (London and New York: Routledge, 2000), p. 375.

13 Tim Ingold, "'People Like Us,'" p. 376.

14 See Agostino Ramelli, *Le diverse et artificiose machine* (Paris: n.p., 1588).

15 Patchen Barss, *The Erotic Engine: How Pornography Has Powered Mass Communication, from Gutenberg to Google* (Toronto: Doubleday Canada, 2010), p. 3.

ARTIST PROJECT / WHO IS JIMMY BUCKLES?
Nancy Davenport

In 2008, the United Nations began a massive reno-vation of its headquarters in New York. For the first time since construction was completed in 1952, the entire East River complex was torn apart to replace the outdated and decayed electrical, heating, and ventilation systems. All of the UN's iconic spaces were completely gutted, upgraded, and then reconstructed. The character-defining elements (including the inte-rior decor of the General Assembly Hall and Security Council Chamber) were also restored and returned, as closely as possible, to their original state.

The renovation of the Conference Building, which houses the Security Council Chamber, happened to coincide with a series of intense debates in the General Assembly about organizational reform.[1] At the center of the debates was the Security Council and the urgent need to update its procedures and expand its membership. Although Security Council reform had been a recurring item on the General Assembly's agenda for over twenty years, there was greater momentum during this session to overcome the deadlock. A new initiative was launched to reform the Security Council at the very same time that its chamber was being physically torn apart.

There is no need to reiterate all the ways that the UN has failed to live up to its proclaimed principles, nor how often the architecture has been criticized as embodying these failures. In his 1953 review of the new headquarters, for example, Lewis Mumford wrote about the building's functional limitations—how it did not make the necessary provisions for exten-sion, change of purpose, and future development. He wrote: "In the Assembly Building, as in the Conference Building, the future is frozen solidly in the form of the present."[2]

In 2011, I began to photograph the Conference Building. Initially, I planned to work only for the duration of the debate on Security Council reform but the project expanded and I returned to document the renovation at regular intervals over a period of three years. For most of the photographs, I focused on the midpoints of construction—for example, when the Security Council Chamber was stripped down to its skeleton, with the base of the horseshoe table strangely exposed but the familiar form still recognizable. I

focused on in-between moments, after the past was stripped away and before the past was reinstalled.

In addition to photographing the work being done, I also recorded and transcribed interviews with various people at the UN headquarters, including delegates, interpreters, cleaners, and construction workers.[3] The following pages, excerpted from a larger book project, focus on a football betting pool and a legendary transgression.

1 See the records of the 66th General Assembly, 50th & 51st Plenary Meetings, 8 November 2011.

2 Lewis Mumford, "United Nations Assembly," *The New Yorker*, 14 March 1953, p. 81.

3 My thanks to all who participated and gave so much of their time during breaks and after hours.

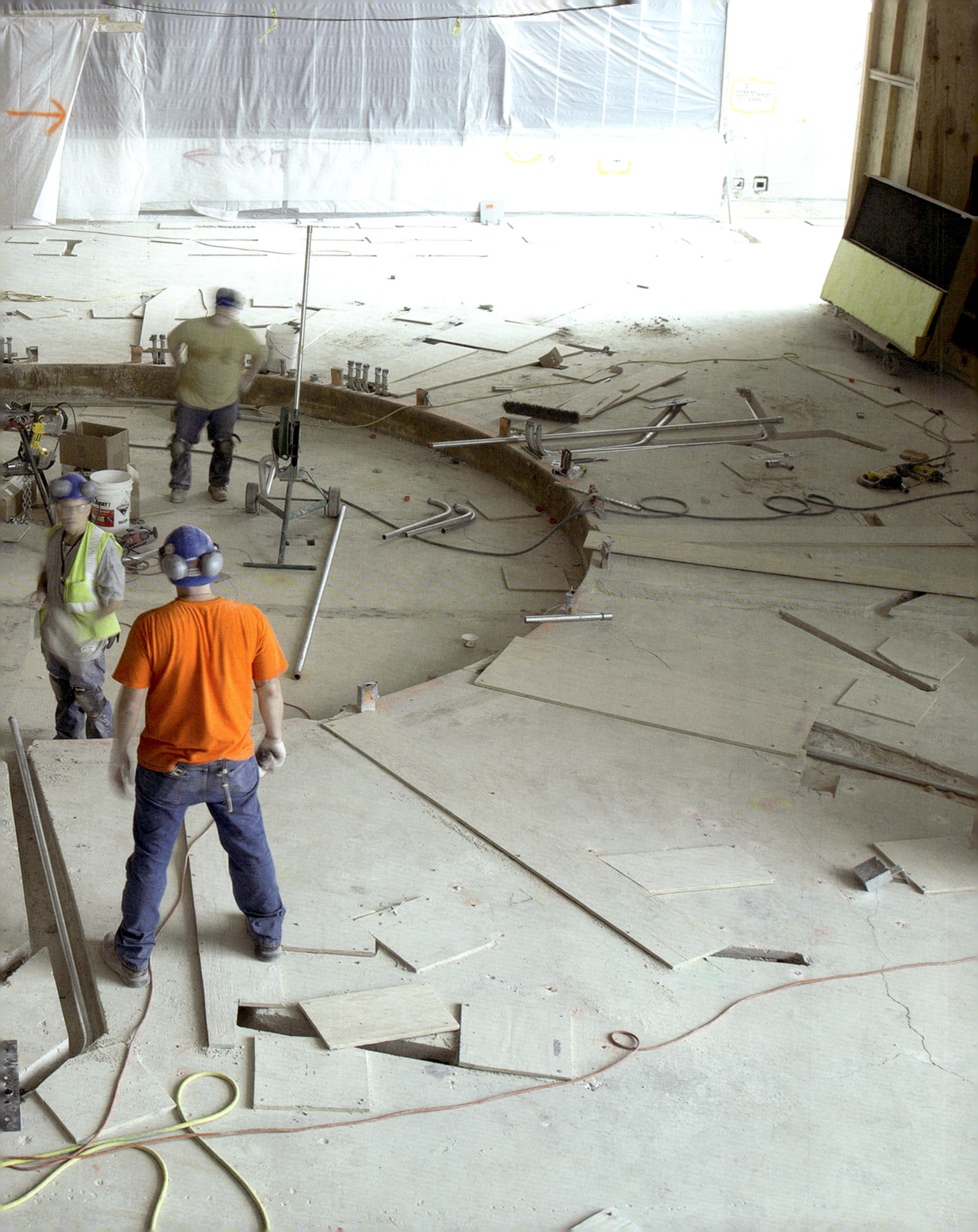

ND:

Could you tell me why 'Buckles' or 'Jimmy Buckles' is
written everywhere around the Security Council Chamber?
Who is Jimmy Buckles?

DG:

I don't actually know the guy, but I did hear the story.
They used to take little side bets on the football games
every Sunday and there was a certain fellow who put money
on the same boxes every week, he always took the same
three boxes. So one day, he wrote his name in the grid
as usual, placed his bet. Then the foreman comes up and
wants to place the same bet...

RS:

Buckles was running the football pool.

DG:

Right, Buckles was doing the boxes and says he
didn't get the first guy's money in time... so he says.

RS:

So he says.

DG:

Buckles crossed the first name out, put the foreman's name
in... and *this* is the box that hits. The box hits $2000.
Quite a stir ensues. Now there's two guys claiming the winning
box. Big uproar for $2000. That's not a small uproar.

RS:

So the word goes around, he gave away this fellow's box to
the foreman, who just happens to be giving out the overtime.

DG:

He buckled under the pressure. So they started calling him
'Jimmy Buckles'. And they started writing 'Buckles' & stuff
about 'Buckling' on the walls, on the lifts, everywhere.
Now there are 'Buckle-isms' on every floor.

RS:

It got so bad that the UN sent around a memo saying:
"Who is Jimmy Buckles?" and "No more Buckles".

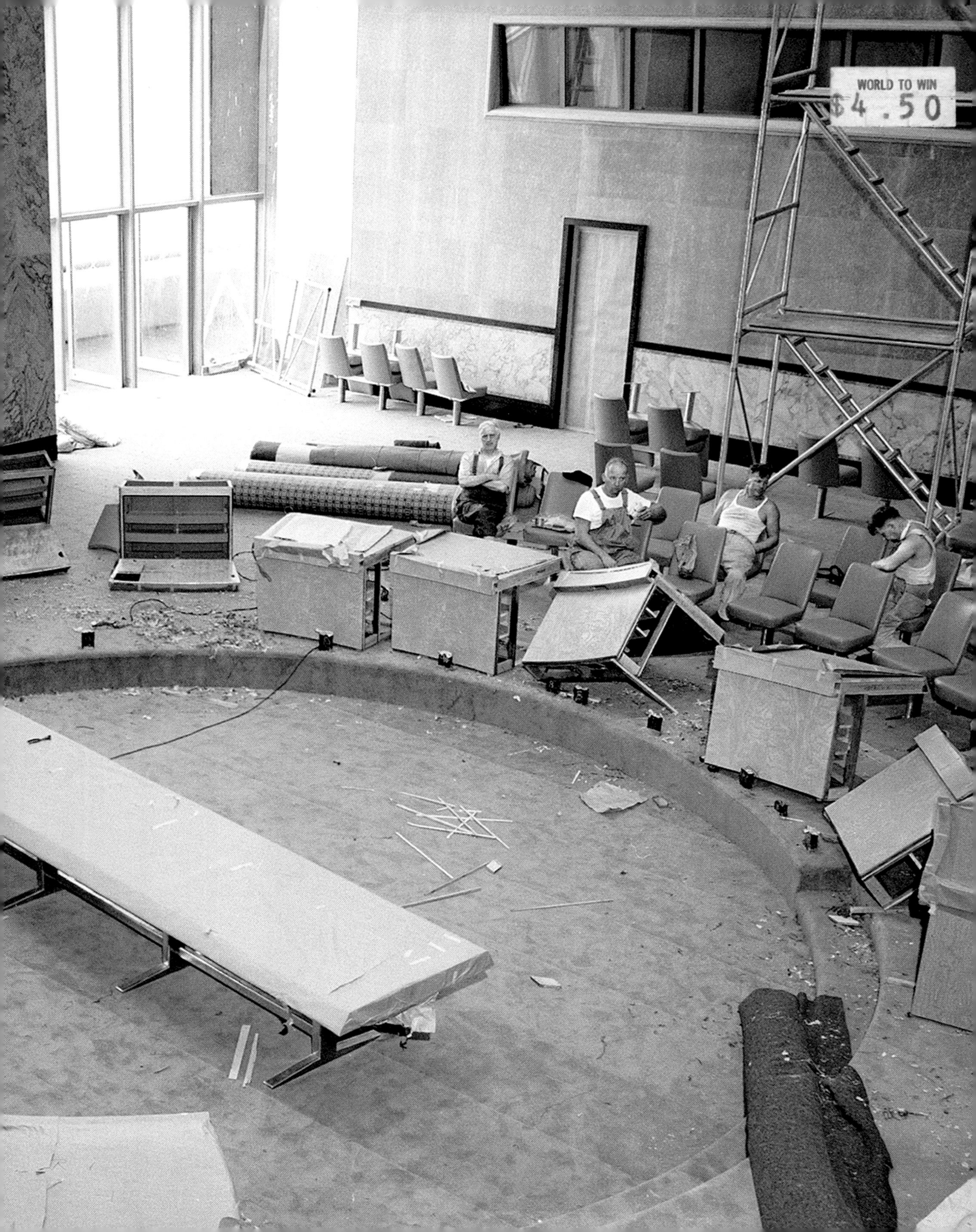
WORLD TO WIN
$4.50

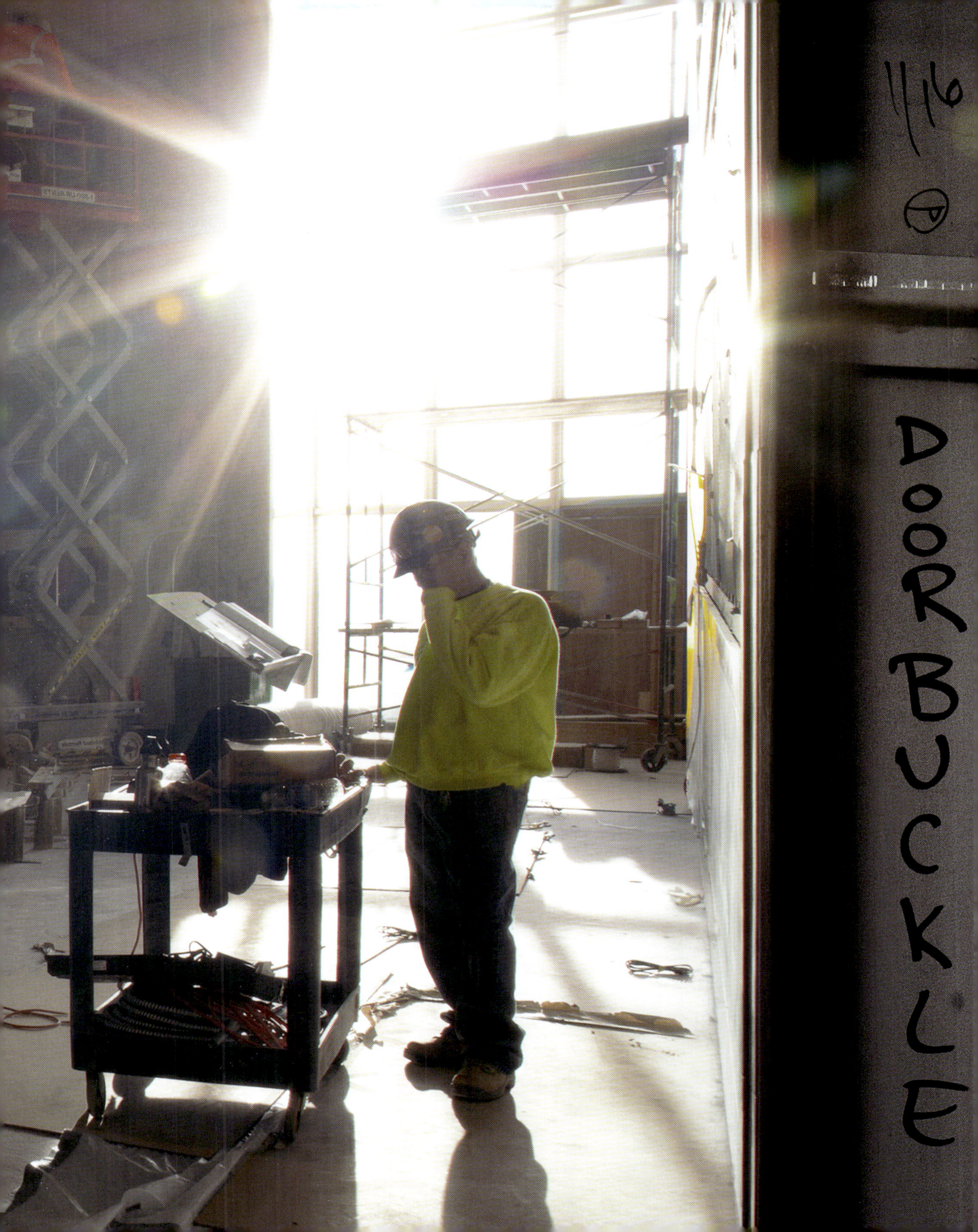
11/16
DOOR BUCKLE

ND:

Do you know Jimmy Buckles?

MB:

Buckles is notorious. He's the guy who got into trouble with
the electricians... he's a nervous wreck.

JF:

No no it's about a football pool. He tried to beat the pool.

TZ:

No, that's not right. He buckled.

MB:

Meaning?

TZ:

One guy claimed a box, Jimmy gave his word. A minute later
the foreman asked "can I get in?" and Jimmy let the foreman
buy in... that's why he's called Buckles.

GM:

He gave it up to the foreman. Got his overtime. The writing
just took off after that. Now there's 'Buckles' everywhere,
the floors, the tools, on every piece of equipment...

TZ:

I've seen a 'Buckles' going down the highway on the side of
a truck. 'Buckles Condo' is written on the garbage bins.

GM:

On low beams, it says: "Mind your head(everyone except Buckles)"

(laughs)

BL:

Yeah, Buckles is a little guy, something like four feet tall.

TZ:

So, that's pretty much the story. Jimmy sold out. Somebody
said "You buckled, I can't believe you " and it just took off.

                              ND:
Is he working in the Security Council today? I'll ask around...
His first name is really 'Jimmy'?

                              BL:
No, actually his real name is Dave.

                              GM:
He likes to be called 'Pesci'. He thinks he's Joe Pesci.

                              ND:
Does he look like Joe Pesci?

                              BL:
Nah, he doesn't look like him at all. But he thinks so.

                    (TZ, BL, GM *together*)
He thinks he does...

                              TZ:
He likes to play the tough guy.

                              MB:
You can't trust him.

                              BL:
I think the Buckle-isms are poetry. Everyone is writing...

                              GM:
All the trades started writing it. I'm sure they don't know
who Buckles is... they just rode with it.

                              ND:
I guess you saw the memo the UN sent around: "Who is
Jimmy Buckles?"... after the memo, did people stop writing?

                              BL:
Nah, its never going to end.

                              JF:
He buckled.

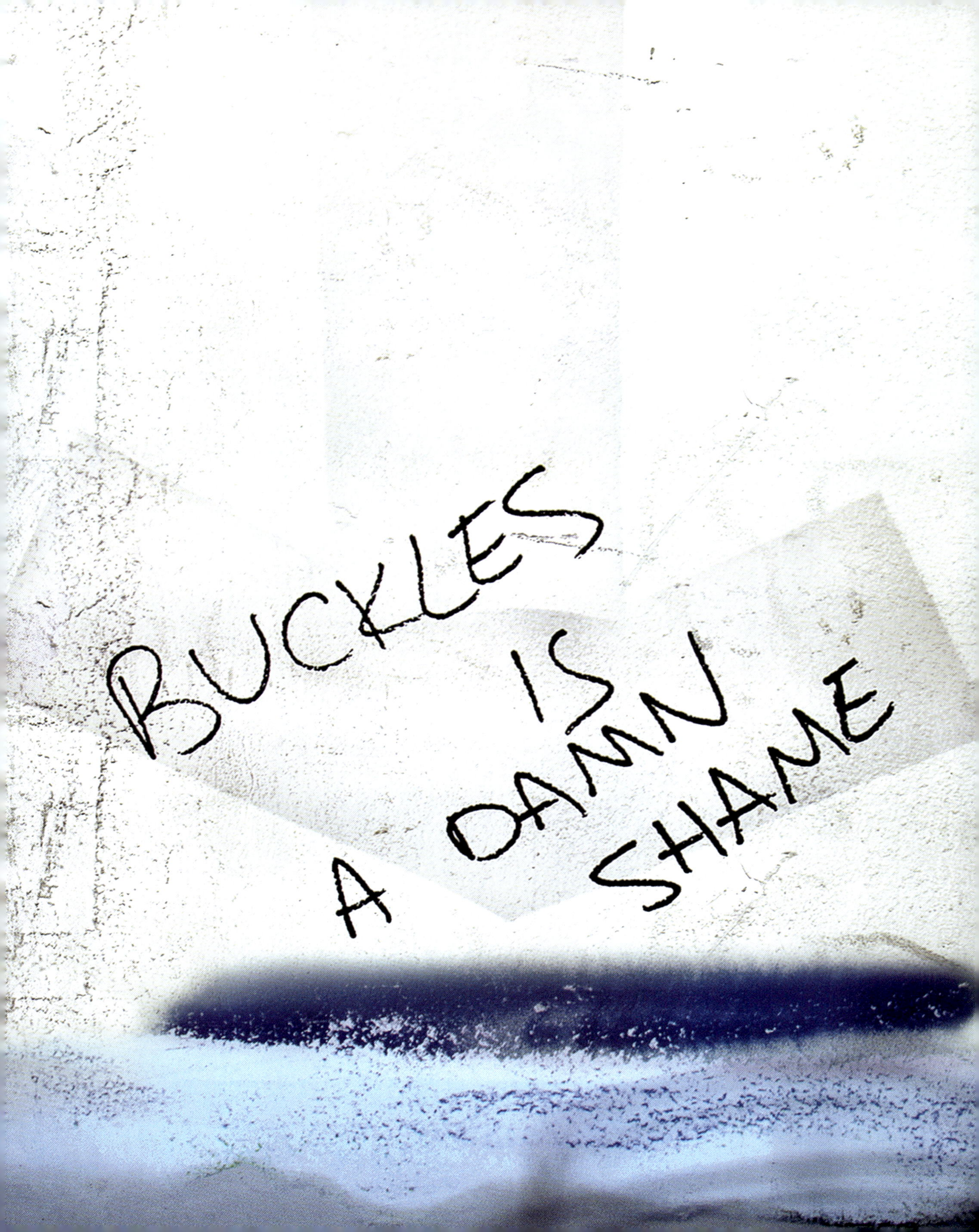

BUCKLES
IS
A DAMN
SHAME

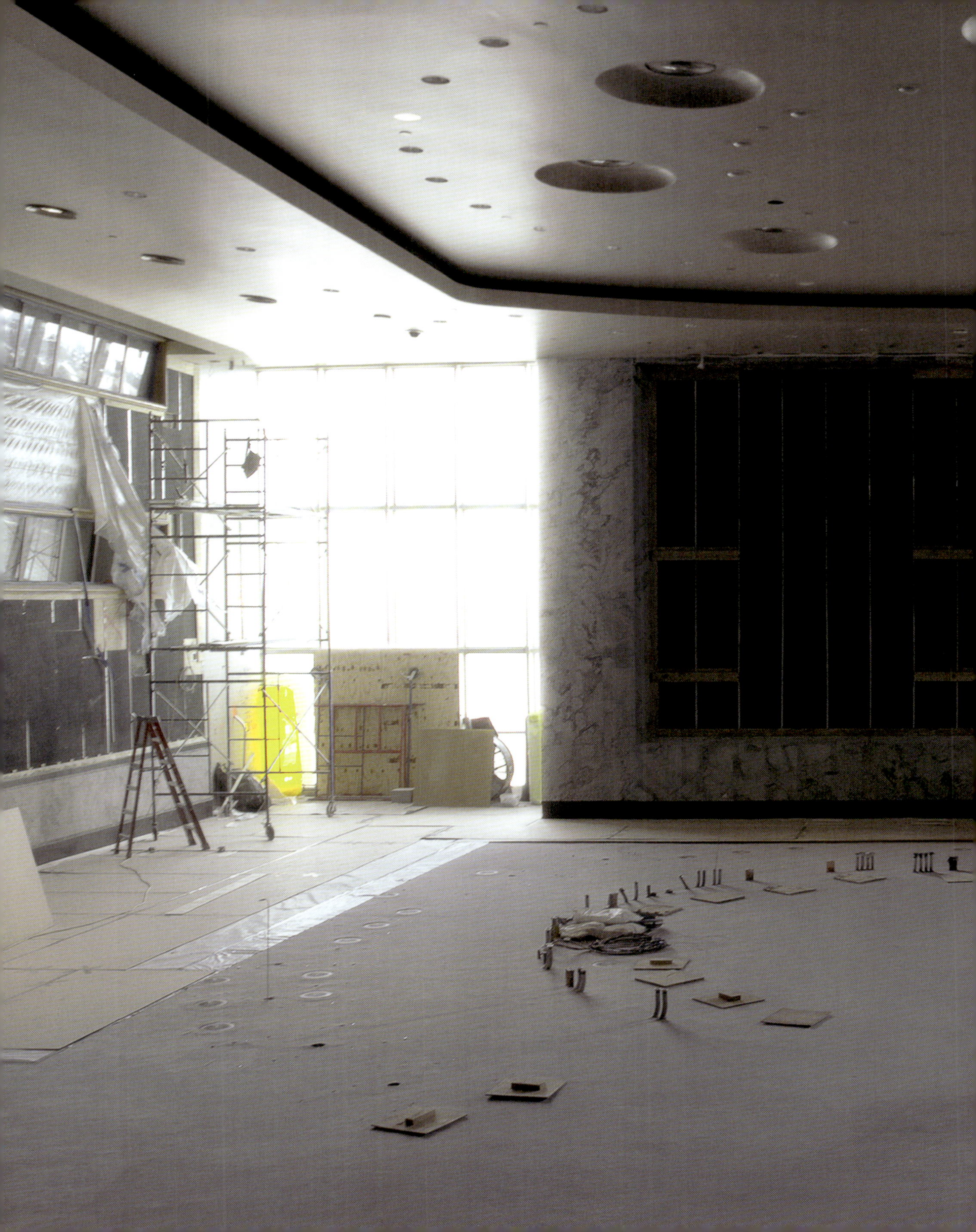

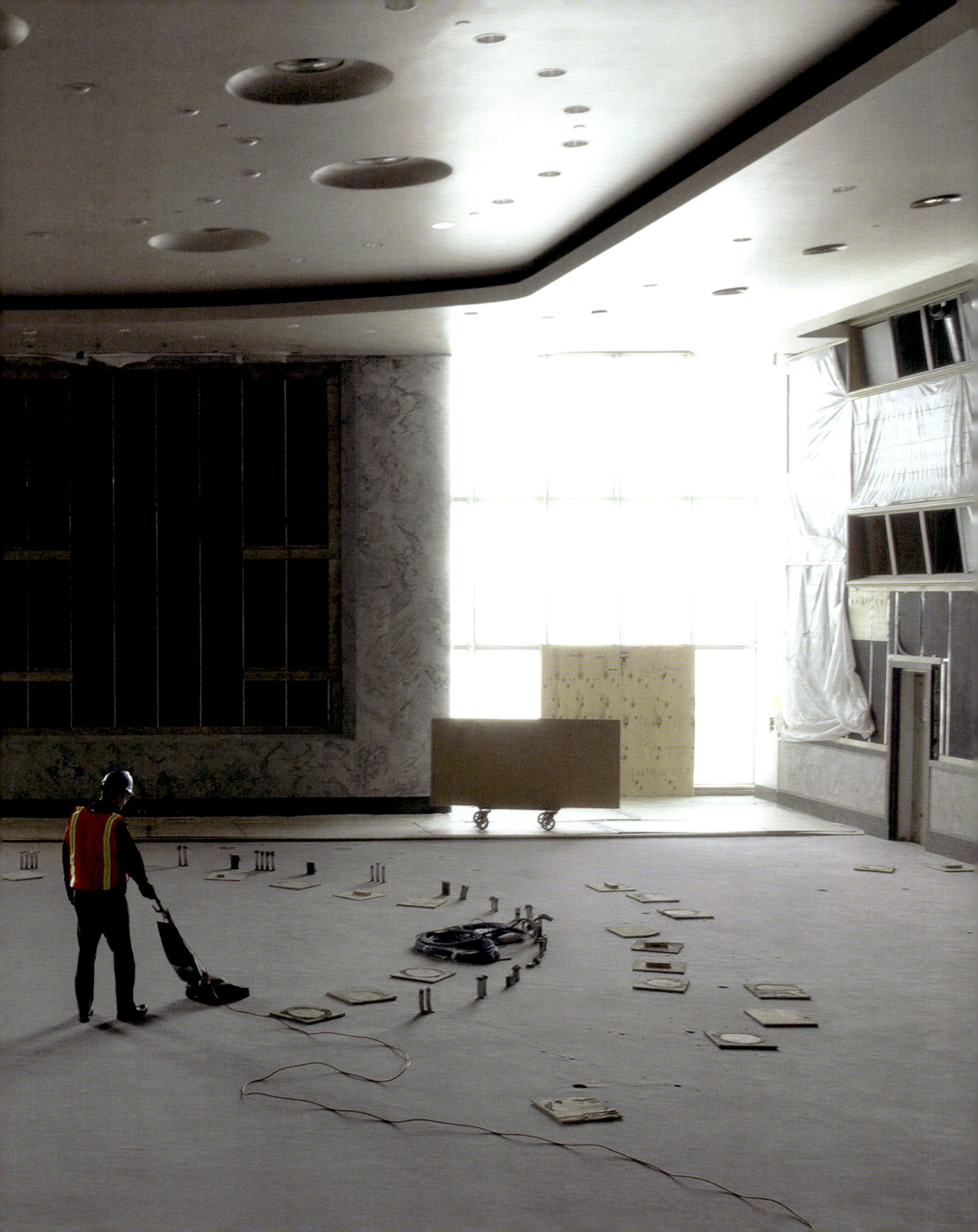

INSTANT MASTERPIECE
Dennis Jelonnek

"Instant photography sits in a vastly interesting position at the intersection of art and science."[1] This observation by Edwin H. Land, inventor of the one-step photographic process and founder of the Polaroid Corporation, appeared in a 1979 issue of *Close-Up*, the quarterly magazine the company published in the 1970s and 1980s. Land was writing about an exhibition that was prepared and presented at the Vatican by a group of the company's specialists in the same year and which was slated to begin a tour of museums and galleries in the United States. The show itself, however, might just as well have been perceived as a nifty work of postmodern pastiche,[2] for it presented the public with a 95 percent scale reproduction of Raphael's 159-inch-by-109-inch *Transfiguration*, made up of four horizontal peel-apart Polaroid photographs. As a nearly seamless whole, the composite of these sixty-second photos was, like the original painting, exhibited in a sixteenth-century gilded frame, which added a touch of pastiche's "blank parody" to the object.[3] Moreover, when first shown at the Vatican Museums, the framed double had been put on an altar-like support against the backdrop of heavy draperies, simulating the painting's original purpose as an altarpiece. The exhibition's allusion to a church setting was reinforced by a succession of moveable walls bearing thirty large-format magnifications of details from Raphael's painting set in dark wooden frames, thus evoking the aisle of a nave flanked by subordinated side niches. The staging culminated in the elevated—and dramatically heightened—presentation of "The Big One" as an "Instant Masterpiece."[4]

"These pictures have no autonomous power of signification …; they are provided with signification by the manner in which they are presented." Douglas Crimp's exemplary description, also written in 1979, of the "postmodern" character of Sherrie Levine's photographic work applies equally well to Polaroid's project, which also deliberately used "processes of quotation, excerption, framing, and staging" to present the company's achievements at the Vatican Museums, albeit for non-artistic, promotional purposes.[5] This was in fact the third and final such campaign that Polaroid had conducted in museums since 1973, when their revolutionary sx-70 integral picture system had first

been marketed. It had had rather disappointing sales figures, and as profits continued to decline during the 1970s, these reproduction campaigns—which operated alongside the company's policy of collecting, and frequently exhibiting, contemporary artists' Polaroids[6]—increased in complexity and rhetorical sophistication.

Paradoxically, this final extravaganza in the Vatican Museums in 1979, which had necessitated building a room-sized "Camera Camera" for reproducing the entire painting and directing a "coffin-sized"[7] Polaroid "20x24" camera at respective details using a forklift, was intended to be perceived by the public as "the essence of simplicity"[8] in photographic printmaking. This claim was also expressed in the accompanying sumptuous catalogue, which successfully contributed to the Polaroid Corporation's self-fashioning as a laboratory that provided "'beautiful' science as the basis for ultimate beauty in pictures."[9] The urge for a synthesis of aesthetics and innovation "at the intersection of art and science," echoed time and again in the company's public statements, also resonates in the prediction that their high-quality reproductions would not only "give the public a sense of a work's grandeur as originally perceived by its creators" but would also "take the public into that world previously known to art scholars and museum specialists."[10]

The promise of emotional participation in the work of art, as well as of scientific knowledge about the painting, was provided within the exhibition through the thirty highly detailed photographs of sections of *The Transfiguration* and through the catalogue. While the exhibition relied on dramatic staging—in which the procession of detail images would eventually lead the viewer to the *pièce de résistance* photograph of the entire painting[11]—the catalogue reversed the emphasis. Its images mainly consisted of magnifications of small fractions of the painting, serving to establish the curator's argument about the impetus for, and results of, the work's recent restoration. Thus, they justify a subsequent illustrated report on the photographic apparatus and procedures used for the reproduction campaign, which at the same time heavily referenced the history of photography. By recounting some of the medium's primal scenes in the text and by stressing the visual

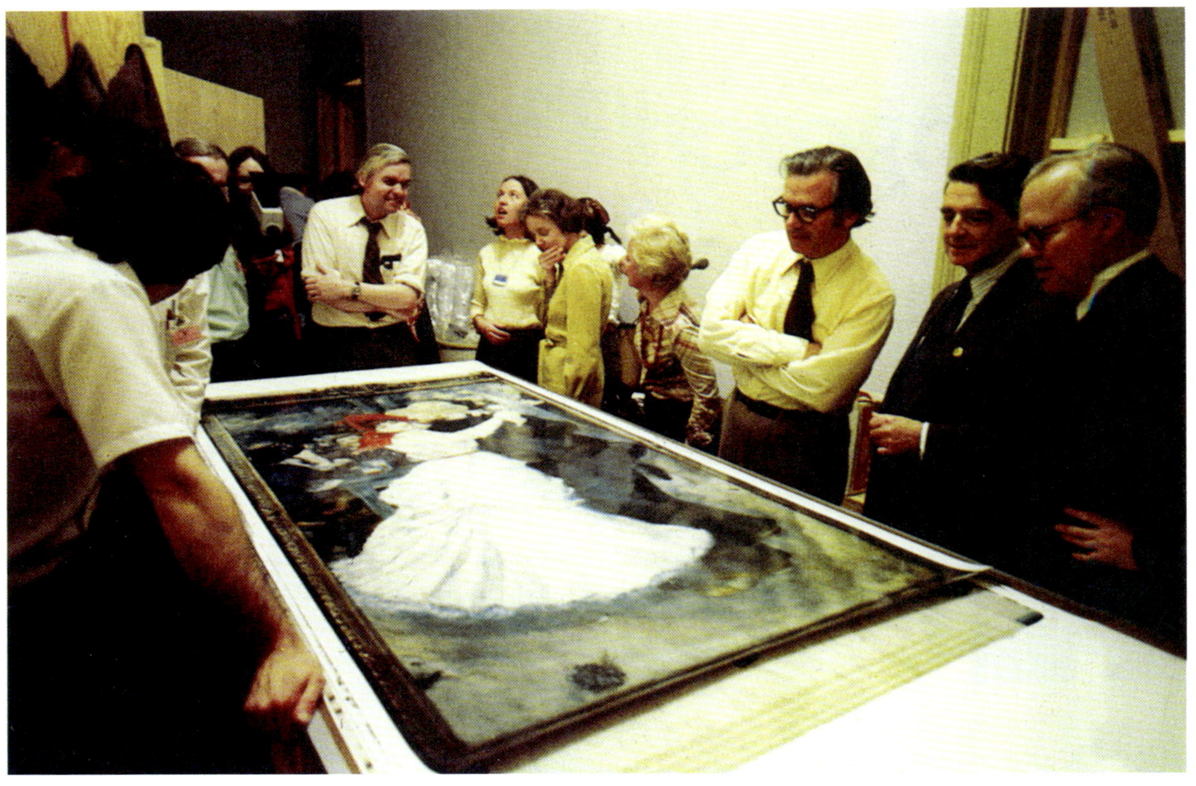

Examining a full-size photograph of a Renoir painting, Museum of Fine Arts, Boston, 1976. This was the first photographic replica of an artwork made using Polaroid's room-sized "Camera Camera."

resemblance of Polaroid's custom-built cameras and their operation to early modern representations of camera obscuras, the comparatively young corporation sought to insert itself in the history of photography as its latest great leap in innovation.

The choice of Raphael, too, was well considered, since the painter was a primary reference point during the first expansion of the use of photography in the mid-nineteenth century. Already in the writings of Nicéphore Niépce, Jacques-Louis-Mandé Daguerre, and William Henry Fox Talbot, photography had been conceived as an affordable and convenient method of reproducing art, although the actual deficiencies of the processes could barely be concealed and often created the contradictory need for additional retouching.[12] The chemicals used during the medium's infancy were to blame for the inconsistent quality of the photographic rendition of artworks: the emulsions not only reduced colorful paintings to monochrome gray scales, but were also incapable of responding to certain hues. The yellow parts of a painting, for example, would appear as black on the negative. It was exactly this inability to render the color yellow that had a huge impact in particular on the reproduction of Raphael's paintings. After centuries of efforts in copying the popular artist's works in paintings, drawings, and prints, the invention of photography seemed to promise a way of gathering and disseminating Raphael's widely dispersed oeuvre with qualitative consistency. Between 1853 and 1861, for example, an ambitious attempt had been made to augment Prince Consort Albert's Raphael Collection at Windsor Castle by hiring professional photographers to reproduce Raphael paintings in other European collections. But the photographers had to give up their endeavors whenever the multiple layers of varnish on a given painting had overly yellowed through the centuries, which would yield completely dark negatives.[13] In the history of photography, these unusable negatives thus stand for the inability of the medium to live up to its claim of mechanical objectivity, which remained unredeemed in practice, at least until reliable color photography was introduced in the middle of the twentieth century.[14]

In 1979, the Polaroid Corporation, keen to prove that its Polacolor chemistry was also equal to the challenge, once again turned to Raphael. The nineteenth-century question of color fidelity had regained significance on the occasion of the cleaning of *The Transfiguration* between 1972 and 1976, which revealed a surprising intensity of color and simultaneously made every existing photograph of the painting seem faint and fallacious. During the same period, Polaroid's main competitor Kodak had canceled a contract regulating the peaceful coexistence, and even occasional cooperation, of the companies[15] in order to announce the introduction of its own instant image technology, which boasted "remarkable color quality."[16] Considering this new threat to their monopoly, the Polaroid Corporation was more than willing to reproduce the refreshed *Transfiguration*, whose superstar status in the US had led to it being touted as the "greatest picture in the world."[17] All these factors made the painting the ideal object for proving the outstanding features of Polacolor, whose quick, sixty-second development allowed for instant, on-site verification of the photographs' chromatic accuracy. This unique feature of the Polaroid process had been emphasized by Land as early as 1950: "By making it possible for the photographer to observe his work and his subject matter simultaneously, … it is hoped that many of the satisfactions of working in the earlier arts [such as drawing, sculpture, and painting] can be brought to a new group of photographers."[18] By proclaiming the unique features of the Polaroid process, the company was not only able to challenge Kodak and, by extension, "conventional" photography in general, but also to initiate what might be outlined as a contemporary form of *paragone* between "one-step photography" and "the earlier arts."[19]

Turning Raphael's *Transfiguration* into an object of competition, Polaroid added yet another layer to the painting's history, which itself had begun life as a competition piece in a *paragone*.[20] Although there is no written proof for an explicit arrangement of a contest, Cardinal Giulio de Medici had simultaneously commissioned the painting by Raphael and a second one by Sebastiano del Piombo in August 1516 for the Saint Just and Saint Pasteur cathedral in Narbonne, France. The choice of the protagonists, with Sebastiano being a follower of Michelangelo and thus an explicit

---

Opposite: Page from catalogue accompanying Polaroid's Vatican exhibition showing Raphael's *Transfiguration*; twenty boxes frame the important details that were photographed and printed in the volume at actual size or greater.

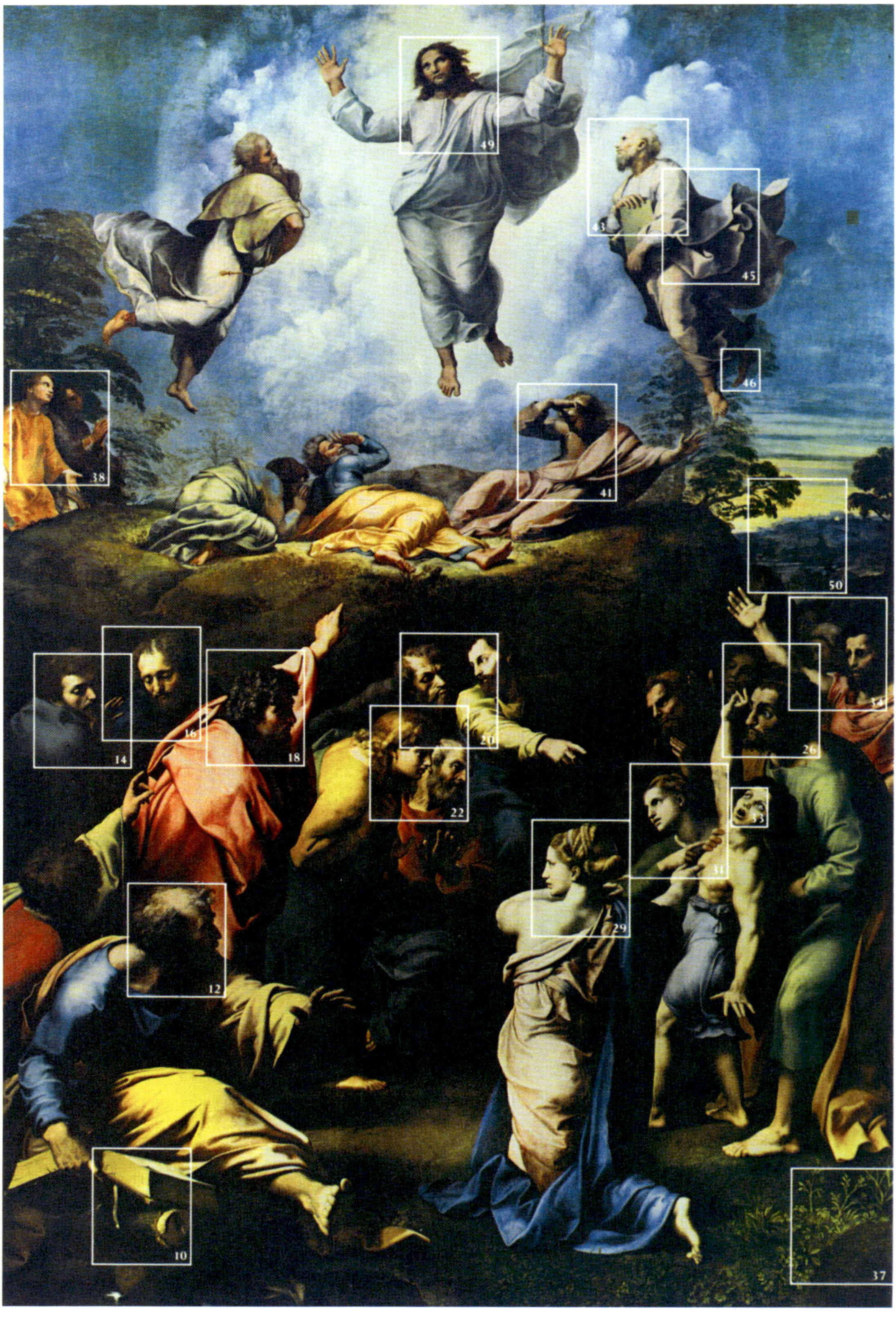

opponent of Raphael, indicated that the cardinal was perhaps less interested in furnishing the cathedral than in confronting the most influential directions in cinquecento painting, demanding an answer to the question as to what contemporary art should be.[21] Whatever the motivation for the double commission, those most concerned with artistic matters in Rome saw it as a battle between artistic titans.

For his part, Sebastiano opted to depict the raising of Lazarus, in which he tackled the predominant *difficoltà* of a balanced arrangement of a crowd around a central event, here Christ's resurrection of Lazarus. The artist seems to have presented the painting unofficially to the cardinal in 1519, just as Raphael had finally begun *The Transfiguration*. Probably informed about his rival's work, Raphael included a similarly elaborate composition of interacting figures in the lower part of his painting, representing the biblical story of the disciples' failure to heal a possessed boy. In the upper part, which at first glance seems to be unrelated to the lower sphere of action, Raphael literally offered new light on the subject by stressing the Christological context of

Jesus's illumination: "And after six days Jesus taketh with him Peter, and James, and John, and bringeth them up into a high mountain apart by themselves: and he was transfigured before them; and his garments became glistening, exceeding white, so as no fuller on earth can whiten them. And there appeared unto them Elijah with Moses: and they were talking with Jesus."[22]

Raphael created a thoroughly dramatic translation of the biblical description, emphasizing Christ's exceeding brightness by using the color white not only for the fabric, but also for the rendition of a divine sphere in which Christ is situated above the grounds of Mount Tabor. Instead of the conventional golden mandorla, often with God the Father hovering above Christ, Raphael invented a hybrid form in which the Son's theophany and metamorphosis are combined in the seemingly natural phenomenon of a sudden brightening of the clouds around a white-clad Jesus.

Below: Preparing for the shoot. Polaroid's "20×24" camera (along left wall) and scaffolding for the "Camera Camera" (right), the Vatican, 1979.

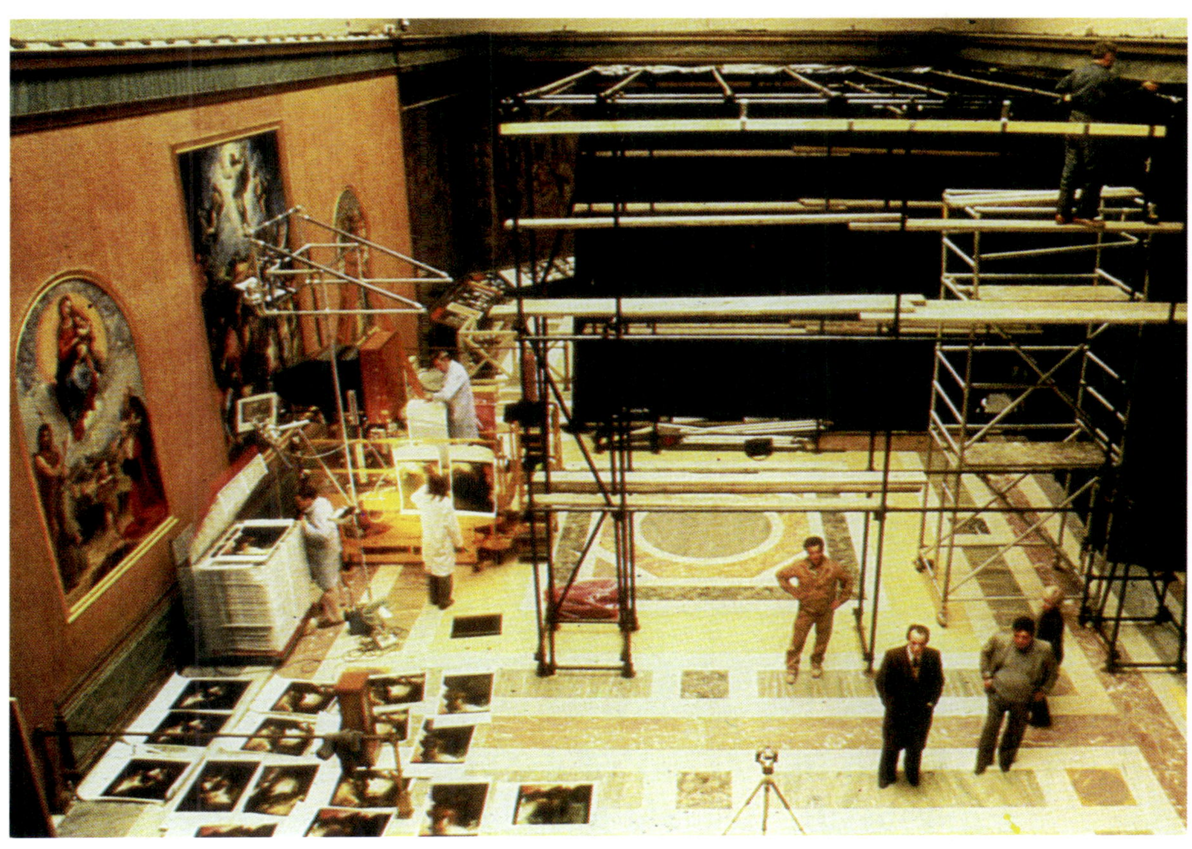

With his elaboration of a hitherto conventional iconography, Raphael addressed both Sebastiano's painting and previous artists' executions of the same iconography in order to claim artistic superiority over both.[23] Additionally, with his unprecedented combination of the transfiguration scene in the upper part and the scene around the possessed boy, which in the Gospels occurs after Jesus descends from the mountain, Raphael points in a third direction, proving the supremacy of painting over literature: while the latter is only able to tell stories in a temporal succession of verbal descriptions, the combined composition shows the unique ability of the visual arts to render events so that they are simultaneously perceived by the beholder.[24]

Offering an extension of Raphael's ambition, Polaroid proposed to "make the photographs more than just a reminder of the shapes of the painter's images; the challenge was to make photographs that were exact records … with such accuracy as to withstand the closest inspection."[25] Once the painting's reproductions were successfully carried out, its significance as a demonstration piece, already integral to its creation, was both extended and inverted by the instant image: the painting had been 'transfigured' into photographs of itself, which were "faithful in microscopic detail." While the original's fragile state did not allow it to be moved from the Vatican, where it could only be seen from behind distancing barriers, its "perfect" photographic double—billed as "A Masterpiece Close-Up"—could be exhibited everywhere and viewed from as near as one wished. By displaying photographic fragments and magnifications, the company allowed the viewer to perceive even more than the artist himself: photography's optical constraint to register everything in front of the camera lens was now proclaimed as its utmost virtue, making it possible to generate "direct magnifications," as Land called them: "This type of photograph provides an increase in the effective resolution, letting the painter and others

Below: Inaugural installation of Polaroid's traveling exhibition "A Masterpiece Close-Up: The *Transfiguration* by Raphael," the Vatican, 1979.

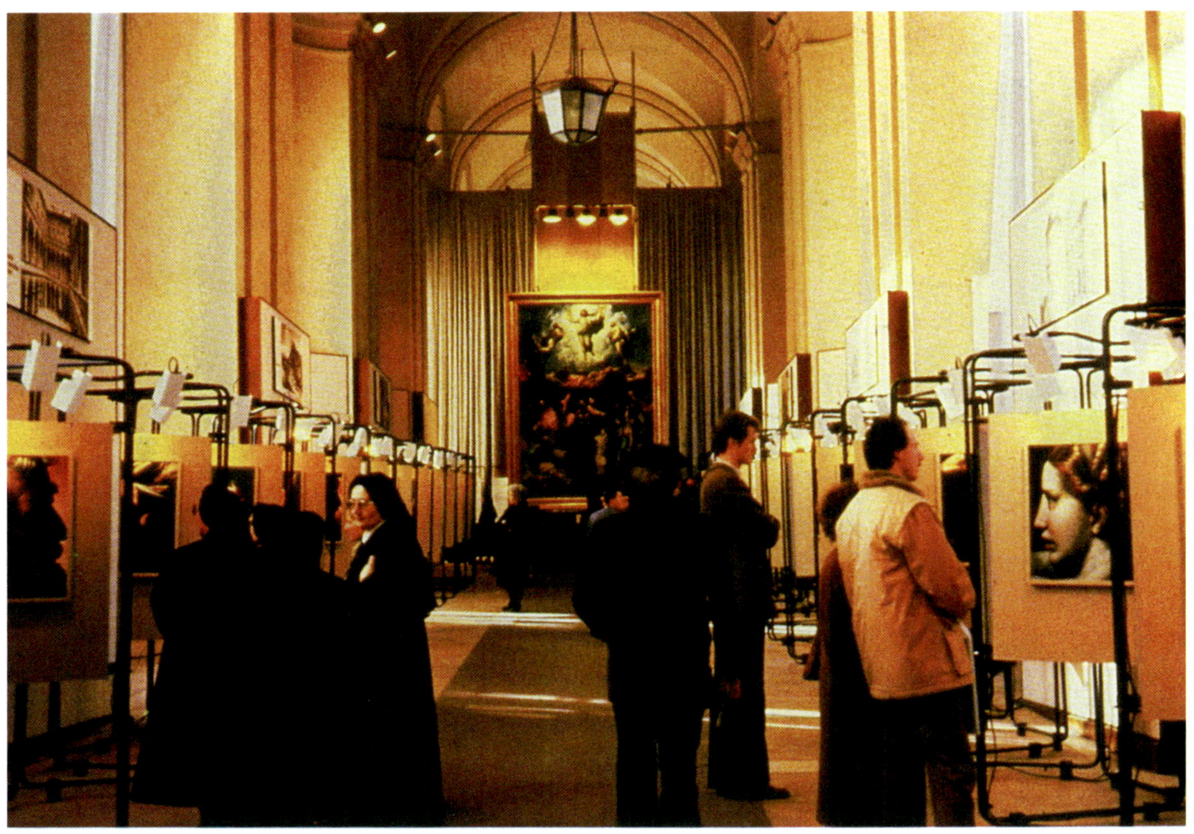

see things they couldn't have seen any other way. If you had used a magnifying glass, you would have just seen a fraction of an inch; this way you have a whole area to contemplate."[26] The photographs fixed and surgically revealed more than the unaided eye would be able to perceive under the spatiotemporal conditions typically offered in a museum. Thus, the detail photographs of *The Transfiguration* surpass the painting insofar as they additionally enhance, and unmask, it through a display of its minutest brushstrokes, opening its secrets to art history: "I would predict that over the years the scholarly uses of our system," wrote Land, "will match in importance the large-scale enjoyment of the replicas of the paintings as paintings."[27]

Presenting itself as the latest advance in a positivist history of photographic precision and speed, and at the same time as superior in comparison to its contemporary competitor Kodak, the Polaroid Corporation apparently reanimated the Renaissance taste for multi-directional competitive debate—the pursuit of which had originally triggered the execution of *The Transfiguration*. The historical competitions among painters, between painters and sculptors, and between artists and writers was now expanded into a competition between art and photography.

Polaroid not only transferred this stylized rivalry regarding the mastery of a certain *difficoltà* to the present day of the late 1970s; the making of the photographs also involved and transformed the central endeavor that Raphael pursued in *The Transfiguration*: light as the basic concern of his painterly representation had now become the ephemeral medium of the object's recreation in the form of a near life-size photographic double. The depicted flash-like transfiguration of Christ, an epiphany of His divine nature visible to three faithful disciples only, was profanely mirrored in the moment of the powerful photoflashes used to transmit the painted scene onto oversized Polacolor film. The Polaroid reproduction campaign would not only produce exact photographs of the Raphael painting, but also reproduce an event of flashing light in the "Camera Camera" at the moment of photographic exposure, which Land described in retrospect: "[A room-sized camera is] nice to have because you can invite your friends in. You have a bench inside. You charge a quarter, and you have infrared viewers so that people can see what's going on inside the camera."[28] Attendees at Polaroid's campaign were thus able to witness the miracle of photography, all the way from the usually invisible starting point inside the camera until the moment when the peel-off negatives were removed from the marvelous self-developing positive prints. The revelation of the process as a precise symmetrical constellation of the original painting outside and the sheet of negative material inside the camera—the two invisibly connected by the custom-made optical lens—made the photographic projection of the image onto film seem like "the essence of simplicity."[29]

Whereas Raphael's representation of Christ's whiteness in *The Transfiguration* echoes the symbolic connotation of light as a metaphor of eternal truth, Polaroid's reproduction campaign may be described as an act of scientific counterbalance by investigating the physical specificities of light and its use-values. Instant photography absorbed Raphael's painted rendition of a divine radiation and thereby illumined the contradictory nature of physical light: the company's simple photographic set-up demonstrated the property of light as the principle of visibility, which in itself is not visible but which provides the conditions under which visibility becomes possible in the first place.[30] The photographic reproduction campaign of Raphael's tableau established a condensed situation, in which mimetically represented light in the artist's painting was transferred by light as an invisible physical medium to become visible as a material trace in its photographic representation.[31] The iconography of *The Transfiguration* as "an allegory of the transformative nature of representation"[32] inspired its own transformation into a set of photographs, which emblematically represent the age of light-based mechanical reproduction. It is an age marked by photography's constant attempts to stress its distinctive features through a form of emulation, one that seeks to imitate, and nevertheless surpass, the earlier art of painting.

1 Edwin H. Land, "Editorial statement," *Close-Up*, vol. 10, no. 1 (Winter 1979), n. p.

2 See Claire Bowen, "Pastiche," in *The Princeton Encyclopedia of Poetry and Poetics*, eds. Roland Greene, Stephen Cushman et al., 4th ed. (Princeton, NJ: Princeton University Press, 2012), p. 1005.

3 For more on "blank parody," see Fredric Jameson, "Postmodernism and Consumer Society," in *The Anti-Aesthetic: Essays on Postmodern Culture*, ed. Hal Foster (Seattle: Bay Press, 1983), p. 115.

4 A. Richard Turner, "Instant Masterpieces: Raphael, Polaroid, and the Holy Ghost," *Art Journal*, vol. 41, no. 4 (Winter 1981), p. 369.

5 The quotation is from Douglas Crimp, "Pictures," *October*, no. 8 (Spring 1979), p. 87.

6 See, for example, *Innovation/Imagination: 50 Years of Polaroid Photography* (New York: Harry N. Abrams, 1999).

7 A. Richard Turner, "Instant Masterpieces," p. 367.

8 John McCann and Victoria Lyon Ruzdic, "The Photography of *The Transfiguration*," in *A Masterpiece Close-up: The Transfiguration by Raphael*, ed. Vatican Museums and Gallery (Vatican City: Editrice Libreria Vaticana, 1979), p. 54.

9 Edwin H. Land, "Chairman's Letter," *Polaroid Corporation Annual Report 1978* (1979), p. 5.

10 Larry Salmon, a curator at Boston's Museum of Fine Arts, quoted in "Getting the Big Picture," *Time*, vol. 110, no. 13 (26 September 1977), p. 83.

11 A. Richard Turner, "Instant Masterpieces," p. 367.

12 See Herta Wolf, "'Es werden Sammlungen jeder Art entstehen.' Zeichnen und Aufzeichnen als Konzeptualisierungen der fotografischen Medialität," *Zeitschrift für Medienwissenschaft*, no. 3 (2010), pp. 27–41.

13 *The Works of Raphael Santi da Urbino as Represented in the Raphael Collection in the Royal Library at Windsor Castle, formed by H.R.H. The Prince Consort, 1853–1861 and completed by Her Majesty Queen Victoria*, [ed. Carl Ruland] (London: n. p., 1876).

14 See Jennifer Montagu, "The Raphael/Ruland Collection," in *Art History through the Camera's Lens*, ed. Helene E. Roberts (London and New York: Routledge, 1995), pp. 37–58; Dorothea Peters, "From Prince Albert's Collection to Giovanni Morelli: Photography and the Scientific Debates on Raphael in the Nineteenth Century," in *Photo Archives and the Photographic Memory of Art History*, ed. Costanza Caraffa (Berlin and Munich: Deutscher Kunstverlag, 2011), pp. 129–144.

15 Kodak was one of the first customers of the Polaroid Corporation, which had started in business producing polarizing plastic sheets. These sheets were used for "Polascreen" polarizing filters, which Kodak would provide for their cameras from 1935 on. Polaroid, on the other hand, also benefited from Kodak's know-how. As Elkan Blout, vice president and general manager of research at Polaroid, recalled: "Polaroid would do the fundamental chemical and process research, inventing and synthesizing molecules that were both dyes and photographic developers, and Kodak would criticize our work and contribute its broad color chemistry experience, providing emulsions suitable for the color process. In return for this help, Kodak would secure the right to produce the negative film for the first Polaroid color photographic process. During the next six years, starting in 1952, scientists and engineers from the two companies met each month, alternating between Cambridge and Rochester." See Elkan Blout, "Polaroid: Dreams to Reality," *Daedalus*, vol. 125, no. 2 (Spring 1996), p. 44.

16 Richard A. Bettis and David Weeks, "Measuring the Financial Impact of Strategic Interaction: The Case of Instant Photography" (Southern Methodist University, Cox School of Business Working Papers, Paper 123, 1985), p. 11. Available at <digitalrepository.smu.edu/business_workingpapers/123>.

17 Petronius Arbiter [pseud.], "A Great Work of Art: Raphael's 'Transfiguration': The Greatest Picture in the World," *The Art World*, vol. 1, no. 1 (October 1916), pp. 56–60. It can be assumed that the reception of Raphael's painting in the US was influenced by descriptions in Goethe's *Italian Journey* (published in 1816–1817) and in Nietzsche's *Birth of Tragedy* (published in 1872) of the depiction by Giorgio Vasari in his *Lives of the Artists* (published in 1550 and extended in 1568). There are also numerous famous nineteenth-century English texts that address the painting, such as lectures by Joshua Reynolds and by Johann Heinrich Füssli (Henry Fuseli), as well as Mary Shelley's travel writings. See Joshua Reynolds, *The Works of Sir Joshua Reynolds*, vol. 1 (London: T. Cadell, Jr. and W. Davies, 1797), p. 83; Johann Heinrich Füssli's lectures on painting delivered at the Royal Academy between 1801 and 1823, available in Gisela Bungarten, *Johann Heinrich Füsslis 'Lectures on Painting': Das Modell der Antike und die moderne Nachahmung*, vol. 1 (Berlin: Gebrüder Mann Verlag, 2005); and Mary Shelley, *Rambles in Germany and Italy in 1840, 1842, and 1843*, vol. 1 (London: Edward Moxon, 1844), pp. 223–224. American writings on the painting also propagated the artwork's high reputation, for example, the anonymous lecture "Notes on Raphael's 'Transfiguration,'" *The Journal of Speculative Philosophy*, vol. 1, no. 1 (1867), pp. 53–57, and Bernard Berenson, *The Central Italian Painters of the Renaissance* (New York and London: G. P. Putnam's Sons, 1897), p. 173.

18 Edwin H. Land, "One-Step Photography," *The Photographic Journal*, vol. 90 (January 1950), p. 7. The article, published in one of the Royal Society's journals, was based on a lecture presented at a meeting of the society in London on 31 May 1949.

19 Land used the generic term "conventional photography" to distinguish instant photography from all other photographic processes. See Victor K. McElheny, *Insisting on the Impossible: The Life of Edwin Land* (Cambridge, MA: Perseus Books, 1998), p. 165.

20 I would like to thank Alexander Nagel for his help in clarifying aspects of the painting's history. See Rudolf Preimesberger, "Tragische Motive in Raffaels 'Transfiguration,'" *Zeitschrift für Kunstgeschichte*, vol. 50, no. 1 (1987), p. 94.

21 Mark 9:2–4 (American Standard Version). For more on the Christological context, see Dorothy Lee, "On the Holy Mountain: The Transfiguration in Scripture and Theology," *Colloquium*, vol. 36, no. 2 (2004), p. 143.

23 See Götz Pochat, "Imitatio und Superatio: das Problem der Nachahmung aus humanistischer und kunsttheoretischer Sicht," in *Klassizismus: Epoche und Probleme*, eds. Jürg Meyer zur Capellen and Gabriele Oberreuter-Kronabel (Hildesheim, Zurich, and New York: Georg Olms Verlag, 1987), pp. 317–335.

24 Ibid.

25 John McCann and Victoria Lyon Ruzdic, "The Photography of *The Transfiguration*," p. 54.

26 Edwin H. Land, "The Universe of One-Step Photography," in *Pioneers of Photography: Their Achievements in Science and Technology*, ed. Eugene Ostroff (Springfield, VA: Society for Imaging Science and Technology, 1987), p. 230.

27 Edwin Land quoted in John McCann and Victoria Lyon Ruzdic, "The Photography of *The Transfiguration*," p. 66.

28 Edwin H. Land, "The Universe of One-Step Photography," p. 230.

29 John McCann and Victoria Lyon Ruzdic, "The Photography of *The Transfiguration*," p. 54.

30 See Hans Blumenberg, "Light as a Metaphor for Truth: At the Preliminary Stage of Philosophical Concept Formation," in *Modernity and the Hegemony of Vision*, ed. David Michael Levin (Berkeley: University of California Press, 1993), p. 33.

31 For a comprehensive summary of the "trace" as a leitmotif in photography theory, see Peter Geimer, *Theorien der Fotografie zur Einführung* (Hamburg: Junius, 2009), pp. 13–69.

32 Jodi Cranston, "Tropes of Revelation in Raphael's 'Transfiguration,'" *Renaissance Quarterly*, vol. 56, no. 1 (Spring 2003), p. 4.

AUTOBIOGRAPHICAL BODIES
Alice Butler

It could be a doorstop, a paperweight; a telephone directory, or a diary. It could be a "book" if its one-thousand-odd pages had found a publisher back in 1974. (But they didn't.) And so it remains static and singular—categorically, but not materially, dead. Searching for the word we might call it to make it safe—this unpublished, peripheral object—I'm going to say it's a manuscript. In Dodie Bellamy's *The Letters of Mina Harker*, the epistle-maker is nicknamed MS, code for "Manuscript": a textual body, living through ink and paper, she is "her own scandalous invention."[1]

. . .

The same could be said of Clive R. Curtis, the unknown author of the unknown novel "Sparraw's Kneecaps," its first volume given the self-referential subtitle: "A Novel—totally nonfictional." This manuscript has been manhandled and is moth-eaten, its type dirtied across different decades. Curling forward and back is the red front cover, repaired beyond recognition. The back cover has a hole in its heart. Scribbled above this rip is Clive Reginald Curtis's London address written at a forty-five-degree angle: a mixture of looping letters and squared-off capitals. A torn monochrome page adhered to the manuscript's middle repeats: FRAGILE PLEASE HANDLE WITH CARE.[2]

Marguerite Duras would have considered Clive's manuscript, with its jagged spine and jagged syntax, an isolated body of what she called "virtual literature." "Published literature," she wrote, "represents only one percent of what is written in the world. It seems worthwhile to talk about the rest, an abyss, a black night out of which comes that 'bizarre thing,' literature, and into which almost all of it disappears again without a trace."[3] "Sparraw's Kneecaps" is a cryptic archival object and a novel in one. Locked into a latent state of anticipation, the object's anonymity enables an imaginative reading, and writing, of gossip.

Clive's novel is autobiography made fragile by the context of fiction. He cuts into the self and carves it, mixing confession with novelistic invention in spiraling, uncensored syntax. William Burroughs once told the poet-artist Jeff Nuttall that the way to make cut-ups was to "establish a schizophrenic relationship with a typewriter"[4]—a promise Clive attempts to

fulfill. In this novel of "autobiographical anecdotes," Clive looks to "smother [the page] with type" to "reach [his] aim of 55,000 words." Word count hereby becomes an indication of lexical prowess, and morphemes are made numerical. Seemingly out-of-control, the writing multiplies itself; raw, atavistic, unclean—a merging of life and language. As Duras writes (in the book called *Writing*): "Writing comes like the wind. It's made of ink, it's the thing written, and it passes like nothing else passes in life, nothing more, except life itself."[5]

As the typed documents of his past are shuffled into the red compendium (everything from psychiatrists' notes to publishers' rejection letters), Clive's naked body is transcribed as text itself. The tissue paper facts are exposed as sheer and unruly when transplanted into the space of the novel. This urge to "memoirize" reminds me of Alexander Trocchi, ventriloquizing as the character Joe Necchi in *Cain's Book*. Joe is a drug addict working on a Hudson River boat, but also the writer of the book we are reading:

—The facts. Stick to the facts. A fine empirical principle, but below the level of language the facts slide away like lava … and if I find it difficult to remember and express, and difficult to express and remember, if sometimes words leap up, sudden, unnatural, squint and jingling skeletons from the page … I suppose it is because they take a kind of ancestral revenge upon me. … No doubt I shall go on writing.[6]

A flag of literary protest, *Cain's Book* was first brought out in Britain by avant-garde publishing renegade John Calder in 1963, and was swiftly met with an obscenity trial on account of its depiction of sex and drugs. Meanwhile, Clive was gorging on these banned books in an act of sleazy excess: he reads like he types, then vomits it back at the page in a kind of disorderly barf speech.

The angsty writer in Clive is in a constant tussle with his underground competitors: he is a literary leech, looking to feed on as many avant-garde writers as possible. "Sparraw's Kneecaps" thus contains a thousand other pamphlets and paperbacks in what comprises a frenetic splurge of contextual material: first he lists "the magazines 'Books & Bookmen,' 'The London Magazine,' 'Ambit,' and 'Penthouse,'" before

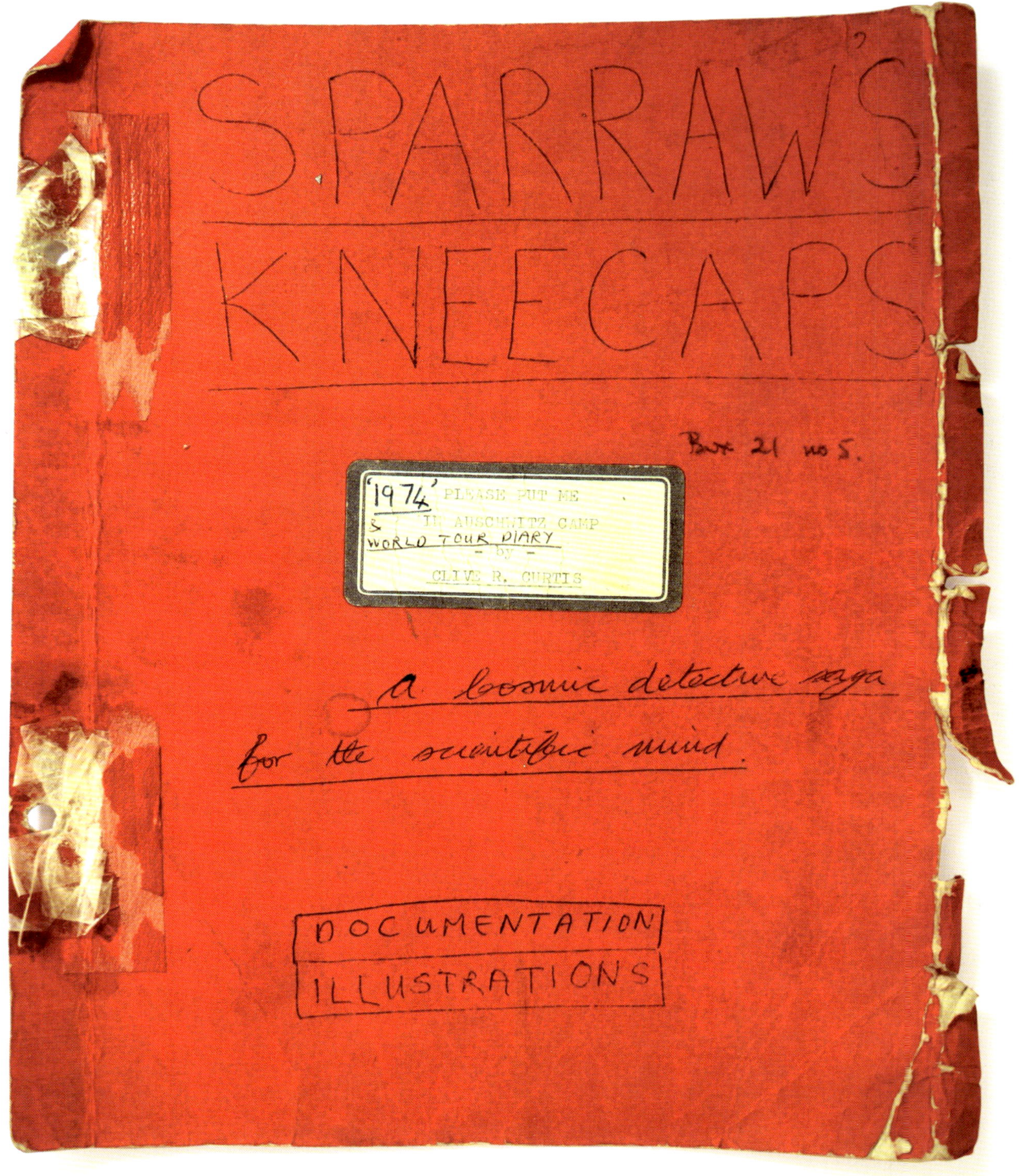

Front cover of "Sparraw's Kneecaps" manuscript by Clive R. Curtis, ca. 1974. All photos Taki Shiomitsu. All images courtesy Elizabeth Price and Wysing Arts Centre.

```
                 AUTOBIOGRAPHICAL ANECDOTES

N.B.  The following was written when the Author was only 23 years old.


INTRODUCTORY INDEX
Date of birth.  12 September 1941.
Father.  (Died 1953.)  Scientific Humanist.  He contracted muscular
            dystrophy;  a considerable man.
1949-52.  Junior school.
1951.     Suntrap Health School.  One year.  Asthma.  Unpopular and
            uninterested.  Aged 10.
1952-57.  Senior School:  Stanhope Secondary School.  5 years.  Too
            many Boys' Brigade and professional bourgeois elements.
            As ever fragmented, a nihilist's joy, a failed place.  Got
            eight O-level G.C.E.s.  (Like Robert Graves's public school.)
1954.     A Methodist Youth Social, Middlesex.  Unpopular and
            uninterested.
            A Suburban Dancing School.  Unpopular and uninterested.
1956.     Family (step) and neighbours.  Mother disillusioned by
            Father's death (I was then 12).  She worked in an engineer-
            ing factory.  Stepfather:  nonentity.  Step-siblings:
            hostile nonentities.
Middlesex Youth Club.  Disintegrated;  barren;  but a few good
            intentions.
South Coast Holiday Camp.  Commercialised.  Numbers of lost people
            there.
1958-61.  Southall Technical College.  Part-time study for O.N.C.
            Mech.Eng.;  3 years.  Like a diseased rabbit-hutch.
            Hoover Ltd.  An engineering apprenticeship;  3 years.
            Apprentices hostile and barren.  Unhappy and perturbed.
            Did a good deal of reading and walking.
October 1961.    Belmont Psychiatric Hospital;  3 months.
Home, Middx.  Left apprenticeship.  Read nineteenth-century
            literature.
1962/63/64/65.  Agricultural camp.  Go there annually for fruit and
            vegetable harvest work.  A total of 6 months.  300 people

                              - 25 -
```

Above: Curtis as art model. Page from "Sparraw's Kneecaps."

enumerating—without shame—the following publications and periodicals, as well as the destinations to buy them:

He then hitchhiked up the A40 to Indica, Better Books, University Bookshop, and Foyles, and spent £150 of his £312 before tax for that period on the paperback revolution. … An article in the 'News of the World' informed him of the 'Underground,' the Indica bookshop, and the 'International Times' underground newspaper, and from the second of these Curtois purchased numerous invaluable 'little magazines' and San Francisco beat poetry from America. … The Calder & Boyars Ltd. avant-garde literature series, plus American publishers Grove Press, New Directions, etc., etc., introduced him to avant-garde fiction. Calder & Boyars were discovered from an advert in the Avant-Garde edition of The Times Literary Supplement, some five years previously whilst I was modelling at the Chelsea School of Art (incidentally, Miss Ann Quin was my modelling secretary at this school before she became famous; the day she left a doorkeeper died of arsenic poisoning!); and Grove Press was introduced to me by the butch-lesbian. … Burroughs I read about in The Times Literary Supplement and bought from Better Books when I was sleeping rough in the grounds of a Surrey Art School in their greenhouse.

Relentless in its unedited parataxis, this passage performs the material excesses of the bookshop shelf. It also sets the historical scene, exposes a cast of characters, and reveals Clive to be a literary performer even while surviving on ten shillings a week. Clive, MS, you scandalous invention: what can your diary-fiction tell us about avant-garde publishing in 1960s London? Written within a history outside of what is known, "Sparraw's Kneecaps" indexes the secrets of a literary past. Like the Necchi/Trocchi of *Cain's Book,* Clive's narrator exhorts himself "to accept, to endure, to record"[7] his surrounding milieu, unabashedly plucking people and paperbacks from the typewritten streets of London.

• • •

1964: Three shops knocked together made the paperback section of Better Books. Its owner Tony Godwin had recently devised a sly process of epistolary exchange, in which he and his friend Lawrence Ferlinghetti (owner of City Lights Bookstore in San Francisco) traded otherwise banned books across the Atlantic. The poet Bill Butler was appointed as manager first; then Miles, who later founded the underground newspaper *International Times,* took over once Butler moved to Brighton to open the Unicorn Bookshop, and when Miles left, the sound poet Bob Cobbing stepped in. Cobbing was the founder of Writers Forum, a small press based in North London that published concrete poetry in loose-leaf publications such as their magazine *And,* as well as individual artists' chapbooks.

The doors of Better Books welcomed not only the anonymous Clive. The network of artists, poets, publishers, and filmmakers that made work, or bought work, within its walls and infamous basement—which after a fire in late 1964 was used for Happenings and Cobbing's Cinema 65—included such figures as Gustav Metzger, Charles Marowitz, John Latham, Barry Flanagan, Jeffrey Shaw, Trocchi, and Nuttall. Many of these artists featured in the environmental exhibition *sTigma,* an abject assemblage of polyester dolls, filthy panties, sanitary pads, and used condoms that inhabited the corridors and corners of Better Books. A diary entry of Nuttall's, written with the same kind of quotidian attention as Clive's confessions, paints a curious picture of the bookshop's faces:

AUTOBIOGRAPHICAL ANECDOTES

N.B. The following was written when the Author was only 23 years old.

INTRODUCTORY INDEX

Date of birth. 12 September 1941.

Father. (Died 1953.) Scientific Humanist. He contracted muscular dystrophy; a considerable man.

1949-52. Junior school.

1951. Suntrap Health School. One year. Asthma. Unpopular and uninterested. Aged 10.

1952-57. Senior School: Stanhope Secondary School. 5 years. Too many Boys' Brigade and professional bourgeois elements. As ever fragmented, a nihilist's joy, a failed place. Got eight O-level G.C.E.s. (Like Robert Graves's public school.)

1954. A Methodist Youth Social, Middlesex. Unpopular and uninterested.
A Suburban Dancing School. Unpopular and uninterested.

1956. Family (step) and neighbours. Mother disillusioned by Father's death (I was then 12). She worked in an engineering factory. Stepfather: nonentity. Step-siblings: hostile nonentities.

Middlesex Youth Club. Disintegrated; barren; but a few good intentions.

South Coast Holiday Camp. Commercialised. Numbers of lost people there.

1958-61. Southall Technical College. Part-time study for O.N.C. Mech.Eng.; 3 years. Like a diseased rabbit-hutch.
Hoover Ltd. An engineering apprenticeship; 3 years. Apprentices hostile and barren. Unhappy and perturbed. Did a good deal of reading and walking.

October 1961. Belmont Psychiatric Hospital; 3 months.

Home, Middx. Left apprenticeship. Read nineteenth-century literature.

1962/63/64/65. Agricultural camp. Go there annually for fruit and vegetable harvest work. A total of 6 months. 300 people

The first of a two-page autobiographical sketch included in "Sparraw's Kneecaps."

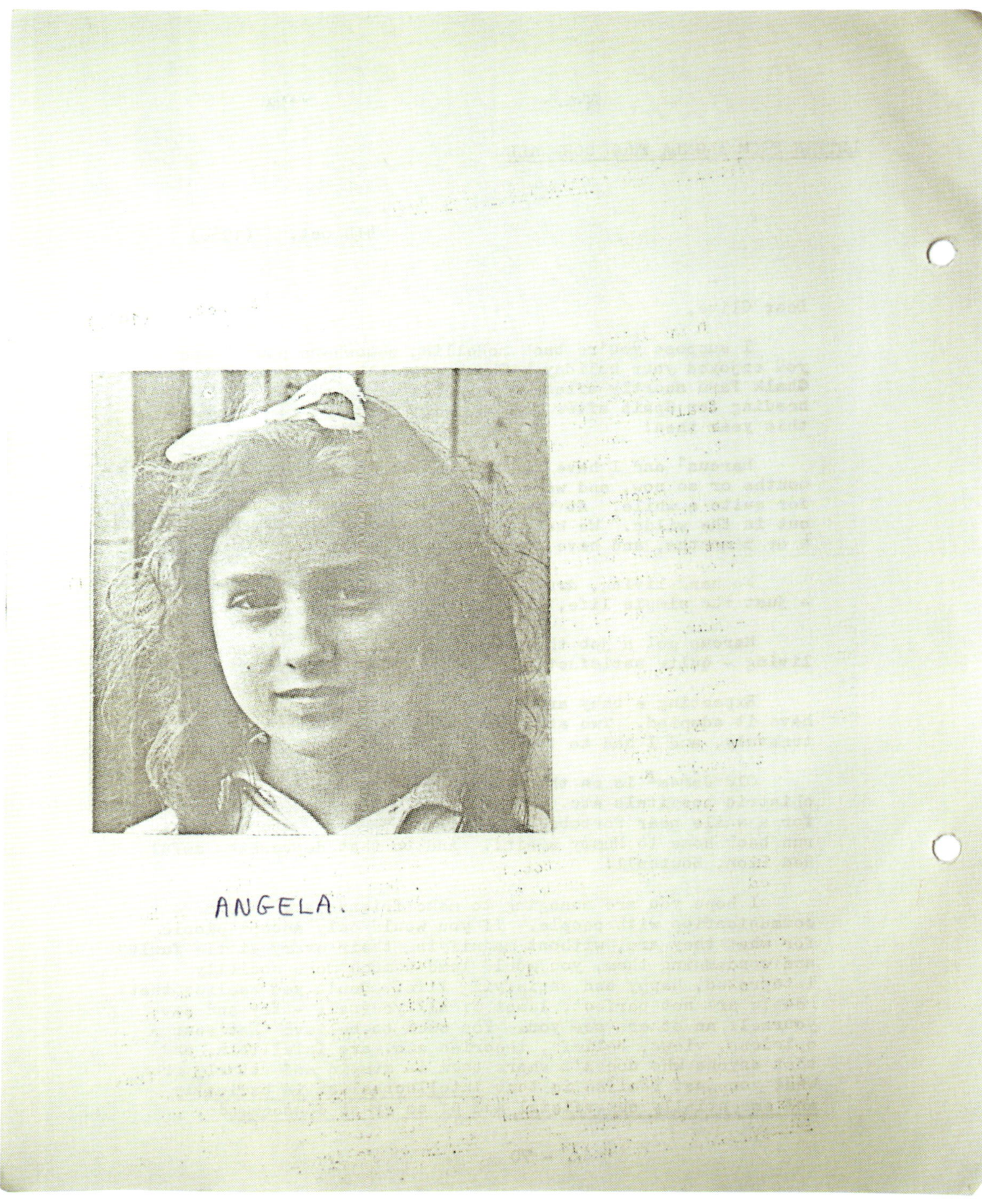

Page from "Sparraw's Kneecaps" depicting Angela,
Clive's former girlfriend and correspondent. The author
is left spurned when Angela runs away to the "wilds" of
Cornwall with Marcus the "hipster model."

October 1965. There is a special peculiar atmosphere to these Better Books functions, a sort of curious mixed atmosphere, part Quaker, part Anarchist, part decadent. The crowd usually consists of idealistic figures in publishing, up and comings, amiable potheads, one or two celebrities, and a rash of kids of all three sexes.[8]

I wonder if the Quaker that Nuttall is sketching is the bearded and bespectacled Allen Ginsberg. The Beat poet had come to London in May of that year, following his deportation from Czechoslovakia, and he soon announced his willingness to read for free at Better Books. His performance there sat between poetry and painting (to use the title of a 1965 exhibition at London's ICA), with Warhol gorging on it from a front-row seat.

Following Ginsberg's basement poetry readings, plans were quickly made for a large-scale event that would bring American and European avant-garde poets together in once city, and place their work in conversation. The International Poetry Incarnation took place at the Royal Albert Hall on 11 June 1965. Filmed by Peter Whitehead, this heavily mythologized event pulled poetry apart from the page: words were there to be spat and sung, and sliced into society. (There were daffodils everywhere: yellow, even amid the sixties cigarette smoke.) Ginsberg sang with his Indian cymbals before shrouding himself in women and foliage; Harry Fainlight fought the hecklers; Ferlinghetti, Trocchi, and Michael Horovitz all read too; and Austrian poet Ernst Jandl's performance was as guttural as the spectators' roars. (A mimeographed resurrection of his June reading, *mai hart lieb zapfen eibe hold*, was published by Writers Forum in November 1965.) The Finnish concrete poet Anselm Hollo, as well as Ginsberg, also read from Writers Forum typewritten booklets, the typewriter being the object of the times, especially for our man Clive: "I've been thinking of going for a walk with the typewriter, to Harrow-on-the-Hill, and lie in the grass to add a few pages to the novel."

Ditto for the drugged-up, diarizing Trocchi, in whose writing the typewriter structures our position toward the place in which he and we find ourselves—the space of the novel. The many sensory allusions to the typewriter teasingly suggest the novel's means of production, as well as its narrative; for example: "They had heard the noise of the typewriter during the afternoon and that was sufficient to arouse their curiosity.

It's not usual for a scow captain to carry a typewriter."[9] Character and author merge through the image of the typewriter, and its technology as a verbal machine— "the robot goes on writing, recording, unmasking himself, exposing him or herself through language itself."[10] Trocchi, as writer, processes and mediates the life of Alexander Trocchi via the character of Joe Necchi: it is an intimate exposure of life, disguised in the texture of its prose.

The Brighton-born writer Ann Quin was a typist too—she was there at the International Poetry Incarnation, just round the corner from her day job as secretary at the Royal College of Art. But their archive has no record of her—it was a professional position after all; she was a typing automaton, not a typing author. The reality was that, like Necchi the scow captain in *Cain's Book*, or Clive the life model in "Sparraw's Kneecaps," Quin edited, eroticized, and rewrote her life as "novel." She mined the use of the typewriter for her own transgressive ends.

In "Sparraw's Kneecaps," Clive recounts while in the bath a fantasy of a conversation he had with Quin—strangely asexual—in which he mocked her "over her plebeian origins in public!" She had been his modeling secretary at one time, as he freelanced his way naked through the art schools of London while moonlighting as a writer in a metropolitan attic somewhere, much like Quin. It was at 62 Redcliffe Road, surrounded by failed starts and fag-ashed manuscripts, that Quin wrote her first novel, *Berg*, named after the painter Adrian Berg (whom she had a crush on).

Along with the Poetry Society and the ICA, the editor of *Ambit* magazine, Martin Bax, also corresponded with Clive, but only on account of the manuscript's problems, as a letter, dated 10 July 1970 and stuck to one of the book's pages, describes: "Your piece will probably be in the number of Ambit which appears on July 15th but it may have to be held over till October." The extract he speaks of was never published, an archival memory not retrievable from the catalogued stacks. By summer 1970, Ann Quin had already been featured in the pages of *Ambit*. Built on the episodic, her fourth and final novel. *Tripticks*, began as a short story that won first prize in a creative writing and drugs contest sponsored by the magazine. In the notes to "Plan for the Assassination of Jacqueline Kennedy," the tenth chapter of *The Atrocity Exhibition*, J. G. Ballard (fiction editor of *Ambit*) describes how Lord

Goodman threatened legal action against them for such a prize, despite Quin's drug-of-fiction being the oral contraceptive.[11]

Tripticks is a cut-up document of Quin's time in America during the late 1960s, when she stayed at the D. H. Lawrence Ranch in New Mexico as part of a literary award she had won. In the novel, she translates the peyote of Placitas into a body of conjoining texts, restless in their fractured composition and schizophrenic imagery. It was also during this stay that she struck up a relationship with the Beat poet Robert Sward, both sexual and creative. Together, they wrote through their trips, which are subsequently realized by Quin as the hallucinatory sexscapes of *Tripticks*:

A fluid dance, and all our limbs flowing into, out, through, until I had no idea whose hands, breast, leg I touched, or was touched by. … When fantasy has the weight of fact; and fact has the metaphoric potential of fantasy. … A certain rhythm, a nervous montage. Trips not on established trails. A series of spectacular switch-backs. Domes and carvings, arches and flying buttresses.[12]

The novel is reminiscent of the voiced impression, as Quin confessed to her threesome adventures in an interview from 1972: "Everybody fantasises about making love with a stranger, and when you're in bed with two people, you know, at the same time you don't know, whose hand it is, or whose mouth, and this is extraordinarily exciting."[13] The biography is the prologue, but fiction then kicks it away, reframes it in a distracted syntax of momentary clauses, elemental images, and bodily tics.

It might seem surprising that a publishing culture interested in printing "stuff which is incomplete, tentative, naïve, idiosyncratic", and therefore divorced from established literary forms and narrative content, would produce novels with the autobiographical body at

their heart.[14] Life-writing, a literary tradition obsessed with storytelling progression, seems an unlikely genre for a literary counterculture looking to break the power lines of linear language. But not when it is occupied and appropriated by the event of writing. The autobiographical texts that haunt the histories of the London avant-garde are wayward documents of the real: memoir is performed, and then disavowed, in the composition and form of the text.

For the London underground of the 1960s and 1970s, the diary was an intimate form to be owned, then rebelliously detourned. The artist-writer Ian Breakwell began writing his *Continuous Diary* in 1965, a polyphonic document of autographic inscriptions, type, collage, and photography. By shaping his life into something paper and pliable, shifting and unstable in its form, Breakwell exceeds biographical "truth" with the making of art. Like Breakwell's multimedia memoirs, or Quin's fragmented novels of confession, "Sparraw's Kneecaps" too points to a surprising strand of linguistic invention that was "happening" in the London literary avant-garde: biography as verbal experiment. As a marginal textual object, Clive's manuscript is both a social document and a diary, an exposé of his location and a raw unveiling of himself—the dirt, the masturbation, the grime—in a language just as raw. This is not just text, akin to the cold conceptualism of the time; it is text *with* body. "Sparraw's Kneecaps" performs the act of fiction making: it is a novel that documents its own becoming, tracing the interior and exterior worlds of its author. A paper object, it is subversively plastic insofar is it is an *art-ificial* catalogue of the real: an expression of transgressive formal intent, not faked verisimilitude. And so, as life nestles beneath the surface of the syntax, and language bends biography, the facts evade our touch. Clive Curtis: a scandalous invention all along.

1 Dodie Bellamy, "The Letters of Mina Harker," in *High Risk: An Anthology of Forbidden Writings* (London: Serpent's Tail, 1991), p. 233.

2 The British artist Elizabeth Price picked the manuscript up at an East London market for £10— its penciled price a mark of its time travel. Price authored its contemporary usage when she chose to exhibit the object alongside a video work of hers in the 2013 group exhibition "Relatively Absolute," curated by Gareth Bell-Jones at Wysing Arts Centre in Cambridge, England.

3 Marguerite Duras, cited in Joe Milutis, *Failure* (London: Zero Books, 2012), p. 4.

4 Jeff Nuttall, *Bomb Culture* (London: Paladin, 1971), p. 246.

5 Marguerite Duras, *Writing* (Minneapolis: University of Minnesota Press, 2011), p. 45.

6 Alexander Trocchi, *Cain's Book* (Richmond: Alma Classics, 2011), p. 5.

7 Alexander Trocchi, *Cain's Book*, p. 24.

8 Jeff Nuttall, *Bomb Culture*, p. 147.

9 Alexander Trocchi, *Cain's Book*, p. 3.

10 Alexander Trocchi, *Cain's Book*, p. 55.

11 J. G. Ballard, *The Atrocity Exhibition* (London: Harper Perennial, 2006), p. 145.

12 Ann Quin, *Tripticks* (London: Marion Boyars, 2009), p. 64.

13 John Hall, "Landscape with Three-Cornered Dances," *The Guardian*, 29 April 1972.

14 John Rowan cited in Jeff Nuttall, *Bomb Culture*, p. 161.

SACRAMENT TO STREET FOOD
Aden Kumler

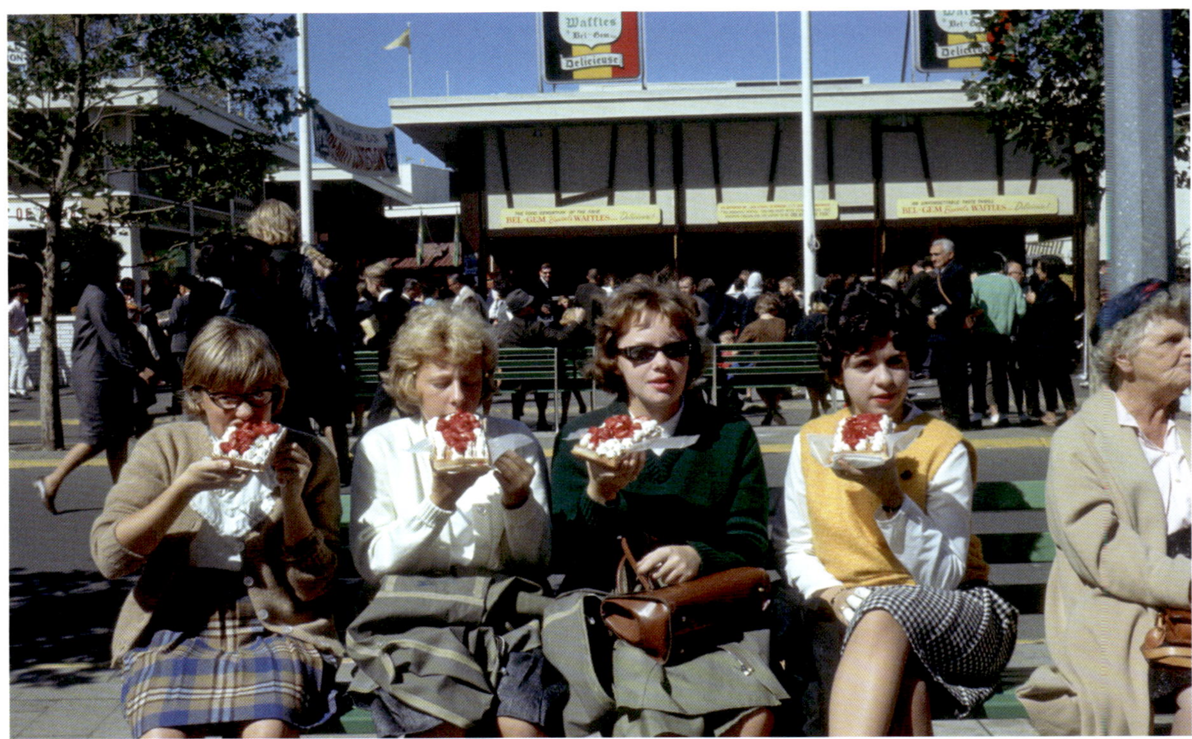

The 1964–1965 World's Fair in New York is generally credited with having induced the first major
"waffle craze" in the United States. Operating out of
the fair's simulacral "Belgian Village," Maurice and
Rose Vermersch, emigrés from Brussels, together with
their daughter, MariePaule, were astonished by the
enthusiastic response to their "Bel-Gem Waffles." Rose
Vermersch had the idea of loading the waffles with
whipped cream and strawberries (a deviation from
Belgian custom) as an appeal to the American sweet
tooth.[1] Her instinct was right: the waffles "were one
of the undisputed hits of the Fair."[2] Taboo for carbo-
hydrate-vilifying diets today, the World's Fair waffles
of 1964 offered a sweet, if inauthentic, taste of the Old
World amid the celebrations of modernity on display in
Flushing Meadows.

The waffle was not always such an innocent pleasure. From an historical point of view, the Vermersch
family's Bel-Gem Waffles were a triumph of rehabilitation, effectively rebranding an old culinary
phenomenon with a troubled history as a novel, sweet
treat for postwar America.[3]

Although wafers and waffle-like cakes were
enjoyed in ancient Greece and Rome, the real heyday
of the pastry begins in the Middle Ages. Already in the
eighth century, monks in Europe consumed several
kinds of wafers: light, fragile *nebulae* (also called *neules,
nieules*); the apparently more robust *échaudés* (cooked
first in water and then baked and served warm, as the
name suggests); and the delicate *oblata* or *oublies/oublees*
that shared a name and a recipe with the communion
wafers employed in the Catholic Mass.

Like the Western communion wafer, *oublies* were
made from a thin batter of wheat and water cooked
between the flat surfaces of a long-handled ironwork
press set over a fire. Unlike the communion wafer,
which was smooth on one side and impressed with

Above: Four happy customers of Bel-Gem waffles, 1964
World's Fair, New York. The snack proved so popular
that the Vermersch family opened a number of additional
stands during the course of the fair, such as this one in an
area known as the International Plaza. Courtesy Bill Cotter
<worldsfairphotos.com>.

raised motifs on its other, *oublies* were cooked in presses that produced reliefs upon both surfaces of the pastry.

Nebulae and *oblata* were served on special occasions in medieval monasteries, primarily certain Sundays and during the season of Lent. Some sources describe the thin wafer cakes as a light collation consumed with wine on special occasions, often at dinner the night before major religious holidays. Both *nebulae* and *oblata* were distributed as pittances (a benefaction in the form of food or drink, often to commemorate a death) to the monastic community. *Oublies* also served as a customary payment that vassals made to their lords at set points over the course of the year throughout medieval Europe. Over time, this *droit d'oubliage* (as it was called in France) was replaced by more pragmatic forms of tribute: measures of wheat flour and, eventually, money.

Other medieval monastic sources indicate that *oblata* could refer to communion wafers that had not been consecrated by a priest. Each priest was required to celebrate Mass daily; in some monasteries, this could regularly produce a situation in which wafers were prepared and brought to the celebration of Mass, but not actually consecrated by the priest because the number of monks actually taking communion turned out to be less than expected (due to serious illness, inadequate moral-spiritual preparation for taking communion, and so on). Accordingly, the number of *oblata* actually brought to the altar and consecrated by the celebrating priest would be less than the total number of wafers brought to that mass. In such cases, the excess *unconsecrated* wafers were given to monks who had not taken communion as something to be eaten before any other food was consumed at a meal.[4]

How and why this custom came about is unclear. Certainly, stories and sermons from the thirteenth and fourteenth centuries describe *consecrated* wafers put to less than orthodox uses: buried in fields to help the harvest, inserted in bee hives and beer casks to impart their power to honey and beverages, and allegedly stolen by Jews for the purpose of exposing the fraudulence of Christian claims for the sacrament (with inevitably disastrous results). Because the act of consecration in the Mass did not change the appearance of the communion wafer, it was impossible to tell if a wafer was consecrated or unconsecrated from how it looked alone. Perhaps it was this ambiguity— was a communion wafer encountered outside of the

Mass consecrated or unconsecrated?—coupled with ecclesiastical fears about the sacrilegious use of consecrated wafers, that led to a hypervigilant approach to even *unconsecrated* wafers. What is clear is that many monastic communities preferred to dispose of any surplus unconsecrated wafers "in-house," rather than risk even the appearance of a profane circulation or use of communion wafers beyond the cloister's walls.

For some early medieval writers, *nebulae* and *oublies* were two words for the same thing, but elsewhere the *nebula* is described as the lightest and thinnest of all waffle-like cakes; its Latin name—literally meaning mist, vapor, or cloud—expressed the wafer's *subtillissimus* status.[5] By contrast, the *échaudés* served in monasteries seem to have been more substantial, twice-cooked confections.

If the earliest descriptions of *oublies* suggest that they were often indistinguishable from the wafers consumed in the Mass, later medieval sources reveal a dizzying diversification of the wafer cake. *Grandes oublies* and *oublies plates* seem to have been large wafer cakes, but we also encounter references to a smaller wafer, called an *estrier*, likewise cooked once in an ironwork press and sold as a secular snack. The *oublies de supplications* and the *oublies renforcees* that appear in late medieval texts seem to have been closest to the modern waffle with a batter composed of wheat and water, but also featuring butter, milk, and/or eggs. In some regions and cities, this more substantial, waffle-*oublie* featured yet other ingredients, including lemon zest, white wine, orange flower water, and salt. The *oublie renforcee* was certainly the heartiest member of the wafer-waffle repertoire known in the Middle Ages: as its name suggests, this pastry was "reinforced" by introducing layers of a filling—often cheese—alternated with layers of batter, in successive rounds of cooking a single pastry in a single press. The word *walfre* is recorded already in 1180; in subsequent years, it would mutate into *golfre*, *gaufre*, and, finally, *gauffre*, the modern French word for the pastry (the English word *waffle* also comes from this root). Like *oublies renforcees*, medieval and early modern *gaufres* were usually made with some combination of eggs, milk, and butter; according to some early sources, they were most delicious when filled with cheese.

The earliest surviving wafer presses date from the thirteenth century, long after the waffle had been established as a regular feature of monastic dining.

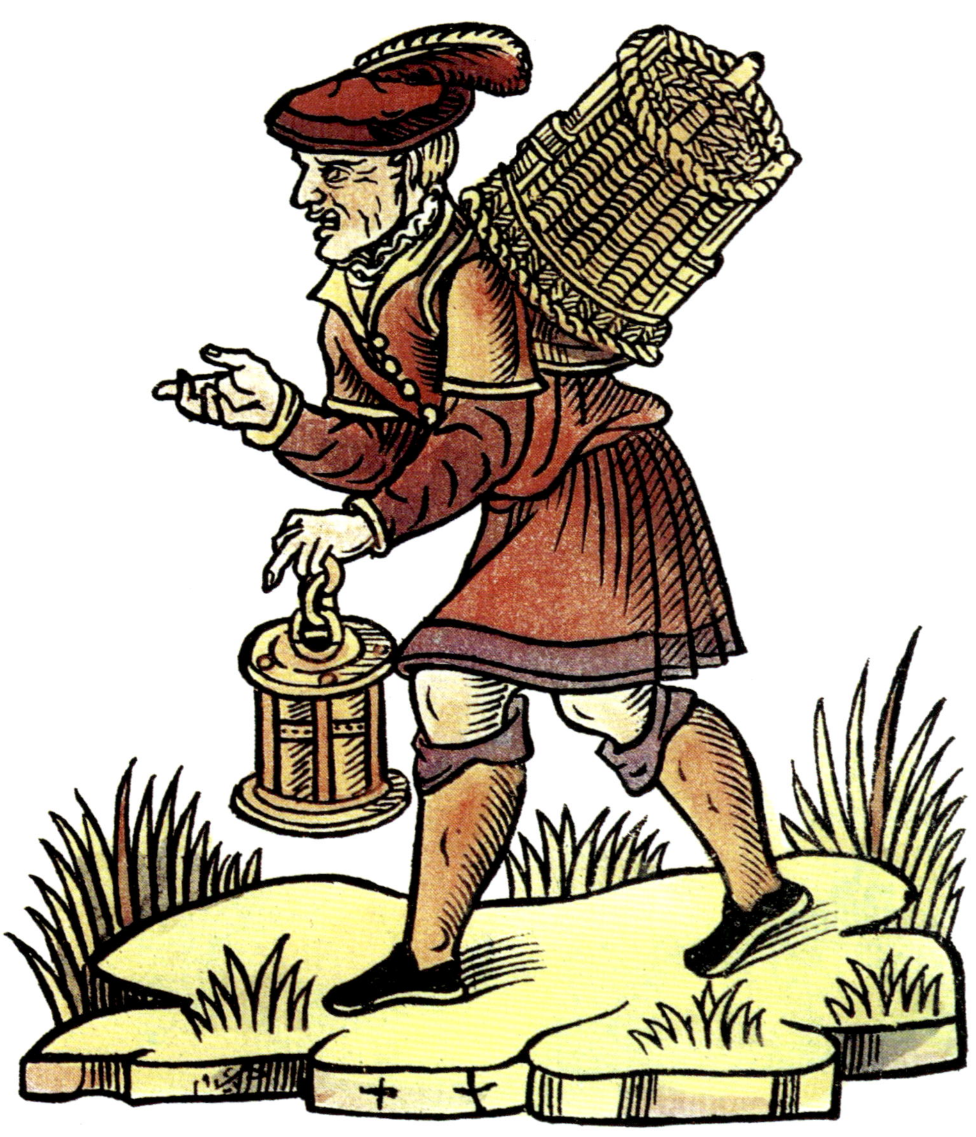

Woodblock print depicting an oublieur. From *Les cris de Paris*, ca. 1500.

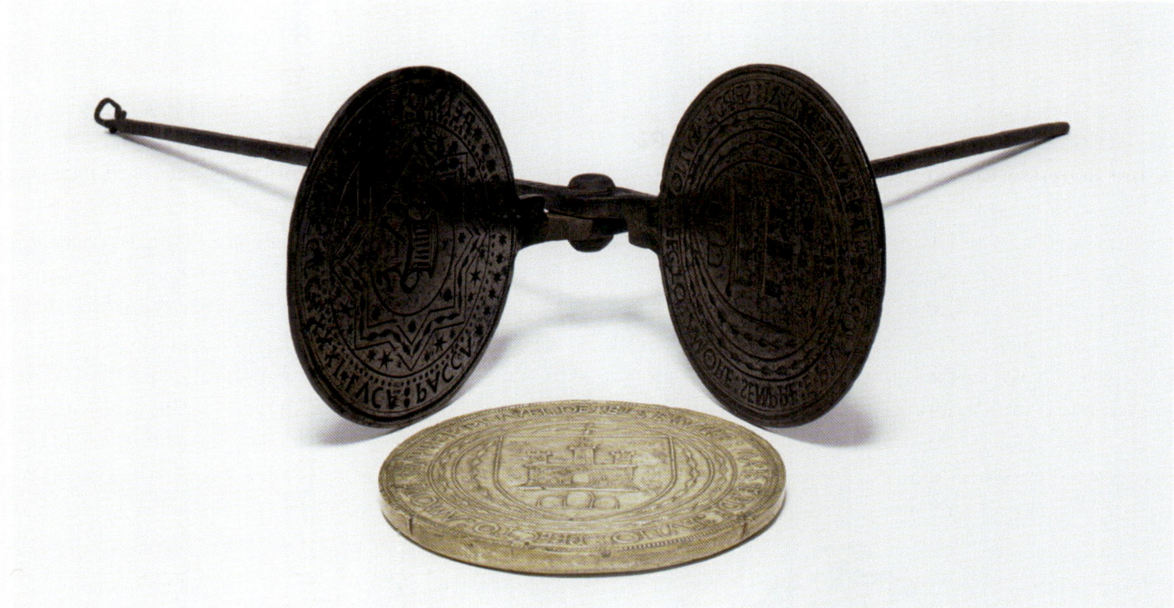

The vast majority of the premodern presses preserved today date from the fifteenth and sixteenth centuries, their engraved surfaces reflecting a late medieval and Renaissance love of visual complexity. Round, oval, or rectangular in form, most premodern presses were not designed to produce the gridded topography of high ridges and deep square recesses that are the hallmarks of the postwar American waffle. It seems to have been only at the close of the Middle Ages that presses designed to produce waffles looking like those consumed in North America and parts of Europe today began to predominate, particularly in the Low Countries. Instead, in most regions of medieval and early modern Europe, the surfaces of waffles were occupied by the lively forms of religious motifs, human figures, animals, and swags of ornamental flora. Impressed with names, dates, mottos, and coats of arms, many waffles celebrated the presses' owners, and sometimes their makers. Throughout premodern Europe, *oublies* and *neules* spoke a visual and textual language of festivity suited not only to their use in religious contexts but also to their place in weddings and other secular feasts.

In medieval and Renaissance celebrations of the Feast of Pentecost, an annual event commemorating the gift of tongues and the descent of flames experienced by the Apostles after Christ's resurrection, *oublies* and *neules* played a spectacular role. When the

Veni creator hymn was sung during Mass on Pentecost at the Cathedral of Rouen, members of the clergy, hidden under the high vaults of the church, showered the people below with *oublies*, oak leaves, and flaming flax fibers. During the singing of the *Gloria in excelsis*, a dove with *neules* tied to its legs was released within the church. Amid this multimedia extravaganza, the burning flax fibers vividly simulated the tongues of flames described in the Gospels, momentarily transforming ordinary Christians into latter-day Apostles. The dove, carrying a cargo of *neules* as it flew about the cathedral, played the part of the Holy Ghost. The significance of the cascade of *oublies* from the vaults remains a mystery: possibly it was meant to re-enact the miraculous delivery of manna to the Israelites during their Exodus in the desert?[6]

Rouen was not the only church in France to make dramatic use of wafer-cakes. In the years 1369–1378, the cathedral in Cambrai purchased twelve thousand *oublies* for their Pentecost performance.[7] In Amiens, at the end of the seventeenth century, the Church of Saint-Germain purchased eight hundred *oublies* for distribution at the Feast of Pentecost in one year alone. Wafers continued to be important props in Christian ritual theater throughout Europe well

---

Above: Late fifteenth-century Umbrian wafering iron. Courtesy Victoria & Albert Museum.

into the eighteenth century. Today, a variant of this practice survives in the intricate paper *neules* hung in Catalonian and Majorcan churches during the Christmas season.

The demand for wafers and waffles in the Middle Ages and Renaissance required a supply on a huge scale. The trade of waffle- or wafer-making is particularly well documented for medieval and early modern Paris. And it was in Paris, modernity's City of Lights, that the medieval waffle came to earn a rather shadowy reputation. The professional, lay production of communion wafers and wafer-like cakes in Paris surfaces in a series of trade regulations and legal privileges first confirmed for the *Communauté des Oublieurs* by the French crown in 1270; these legal stipulations were repeatedly expanded and renewed in the centuries following.

Statutes for the Parisian trade corporation of *oublieurs* issued in 1397 detail how members of the profession were to conduct their business. They dictate that apprentices in the trade had to be at least five years of age; women could not make communion wafers, nor could they sell waffles or wafers in the street. No *oublieur* was permitted to make waffles or wafers for Jews. At the completion of an apprenticeship, as in other medieval skilled trades, the would-be *oublieur* had to produce a *chef d'oeuvre* in order to earn the right to operate on his own. The *chef d'oeuvre* was a legally defined culinary feat requiring the production of five hundred *grant oublies*, three hundred *supplications* (the product closest to the modern waffle in its ingredients and form), and two hundred *esterels* (also called *métiers*): all told, a thousand waffle-like cakes in a single day.[8]

Once established as a master *oublieur*, the waffle maker was expected to operate out of a shop. In addition to this fixed locale, Parisian *oublieurs* also engaged in mobile selling. On major religious feast days, waffle makers would set up stands outside of churches, selling to the crowds leaving Mass or at loose ends on these holy days when most forms of work were forbidden. The making and selling of wafer-cakes on the doorsteps of churches was big business for the *oublieurs* and, at times, devolved into less than collegial conflict. Accordingly, trade regulations insisted that the stands of *oublieurs* outside churches must be separated by a span of at least two *toises* (approximately twelve feet).[9]

Oublies were also a major street food in medieval Paris, as in many other medieval towns and cities.

Apprentices, servants, and family members were sent into the streets to call their wares, hoping they would be invited into private homes to make to order the fresh *oublies* that, together with spiced wine, customarily closed the bourgeois dinner meal.

By law, the street vendors of *oublies* in Paris (and their colleagues elsewhere in France and in parts of Europe) were not allowed to sell wafers for cash. Instead, they transacted their business by means of a kind of gambling game, involving a die (or dice).[10] Customers committed themselves to purchase *oublies* (each at a fixed price); the quantity of *oublies* to be paid for was determined by the roll of the dice (or die). The higher the number rolled, the more *oublies* the customer would win (and pay for).[11] If a six was rolled, however, the vendor had to hand over his *coffin* (the term for the basket carried by *oublieurs*) and its pastry contents; his defeat customarily culminated in a song sung to entertain the victorious customer. By law, the *oublieur* could not pay cash to recover his *coffin*; instead, he could only make more wafers and gamble with them until he was so lucky as to roll a six and recover his basket.

This bizarre state of affairs seems to have been established from the earliest years of the trade. In his dictionary of Latin vocabulary, a text pitched at the international community of University of Paris students for whom everyday French was a foreign tongue and Latin the lingua franca, John of Garland (ca. 1195–ca. 1272) noted, "Street-criers of *nebula* and waffles call out through the night, selling waffles, *nebulae*, and meat pasties in baskets covered by a white cloth; and often the baskets are hung from the windows of clerks, having been lost by a roll of the six."[12] Given the ubiquity of street selling in premodern Europe, why was a legal fiction disguising the sale of *oublies* imposed upon *oublieurs* and their customers? No rationale is provided by the sources, but it seems likely that the close resemblance of pastry *oublies* and communion wafers was the cause. Like all sacraments, church law forbade the selling and buying of consecrated communion wafers. Although the *oublies* sold in the streets of medieval towns and cities were certainly not consecrated, it may well have been a desire to avoid even the suggestion of such commerce that imposed this restriction on *oublieurs*, a sign of the continuing anxiety surrounding even unconsecrated wafers in medieval Europe. Certainly the ban on selling *oublies* to Jews suggests that the persistent, close

resemblance of sacred and secular wafers was a source of constant concern. This interpretation of the seemingly bizarre practice of "playing for wafers" would go some way toward explaining why this stipulation seems to have only been imposed on the sale of *premade* wafers, and not on those made to order at the shop, the private house, or at stands outside churches. Perhaps witnessing the actual making of the pastry allayed any concerns that the customer might be about to consume a consecrated wafer.

To attract customers, the sellers of waffles exploited the pre-eminent premodern marketing tool: the human voice. Among the various *cris de Paris* announcing goods and services on offer in the city, the *oublieur* made himself known by incessantly singing, "*Chaudes oublees, renforcies,*"[13] (Hot oublies, stuffed oublies!) or else "*La joie! la joie! Voila des oublies!*" (Joy! Joy! Here are oublies!).[14] Hearing the street vendor's cry, diners would invite him into the house in order to have *oublies* made fresh and hot, on the spot.

This practice inevitably courted trouble. By the last decade of the fifteenth century, Parisian *oublieurs* had a bad reputation.[15] Ostensibly purveying waffles and wafers, *oublieurs* became shady characters in the Parisian imagination. By custom, the vendors of waffles roamed the city late into the night, calling their cakes in neighborhoods both affluent and seedy. Frequent victims of crime themselves, *oublieurs* were suspect in the eyes of their fellow Parisians because of the pickpockets, professional gamblers, and prostitutes who drafted behind them, entering homes in order to prey upon diners. As *oublieurs* made waffles and wafers at a rich man's fire, it was feared they were surreptitiously casing the joint. In the view of civil authorities and of upstanding senior members of the trade, tasty waffles too often served as the proverbial sheep's clothing for a pack of wolves, those *oublieurs* whose real business was crime. The elected leadership of the Communauté des Oublieurs became alarmed that the trade's reputation was suffering as a consequence of its association with crime, and they called upon the civil authorities to crack down on shady waffle- and wafer-sellers. Despite their best efforts, however, the *oublieur* became a figure of infamy, up to no good in the dark.

The terrifying specter of the waffle maker as a covert criminal haunted Paris long after the close of the Middle Ages. During the years of La Fronde (1648–1653), the civil wars that pitted the French nobility and

the *Parlements* against the crown, enemies of the Chief Minster Jules Cardinal Mazarin were dubbed *oublieux*, because, like *oublieurs*, they roamed the city at night, plotting against Mazarin and the queen regent, Anne of Austria.[16] In the early eighteenth century, after the famous highwayman Louis Dominique Garthausen—alias Cartouche—and his accomplices set off a crime wave in Paris, the figure of the *oublieur* was again associated with nefarious goings-on. At the time, it was widely believed that many *cartouchiens* disguised themselves as *oublieurs* as they went about their violent business at night. In response, the police issued a ban on all street selling of *oublies*.[17] Even after Cartouche was publicly executed on the wheel in 1721, the wafer makers of Paris suffered the loss of the street trade that had been so important to their success for centuries. Many *oublieurs* abandoned their *métier* all together.[18]

But it's hard to keep a good street food down, and the *oublie* made something of a comeback. In the "Ninth Walk" of his posthumously published *Reveries of a Solitary Walker*, Jean-Jacques Rousseau (1712–1778) recalled the pleasures, both immediate and vicarious, offered by an *oublieur* in the Bois de Boulogne:

A group of about twenty little girls, led by a kind of nun, came along, and some sat down, others played about quite close to us. While they were playing, an oublieur *passed by with his drum and wheel, looking for customers. I could see that the little girls were longing to have some wafers. ... While their governess was hesitating and arguing with them, I called the* oublieur *over and said to him: "Let all of these young ladies take it in turns to draw tickets, and I shall pay for them all." These words filled the whole company with a joy which would have been worth all the money in my purse, had I spent it all in this way.*[19]

Having purchased one ticket for each little girl, entitling her to a spin of the *oublieur*'s wheel—a dial with a spinning pointer that indicated the number of *oublies* won by a spin—Rousseau benevolently rigs the game:

Although there were no blanks [on the wheel] and there would be at least one wafer for each girl ... in order to make the festivities jollier still, I secretly told the oublieur *to put his usual skill to unusual ends by making as many good numbers come up as he could possibly manage and that I would reward him for doing so. Thanks to this foresight, almost a hundred wafers were given out. ... My wife subtly persuaded those*

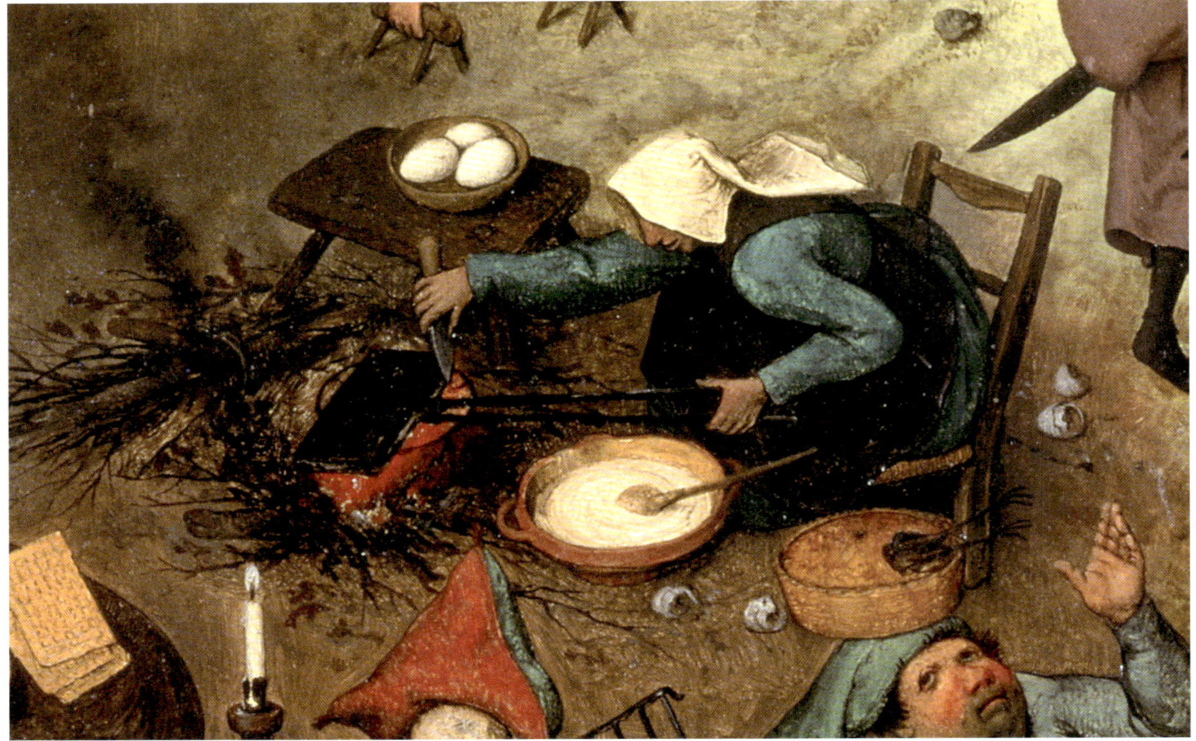

Making waffles. Detail from Pieter Bruegel the Elder, *Fight Between Carnival and Lent*, 1559.

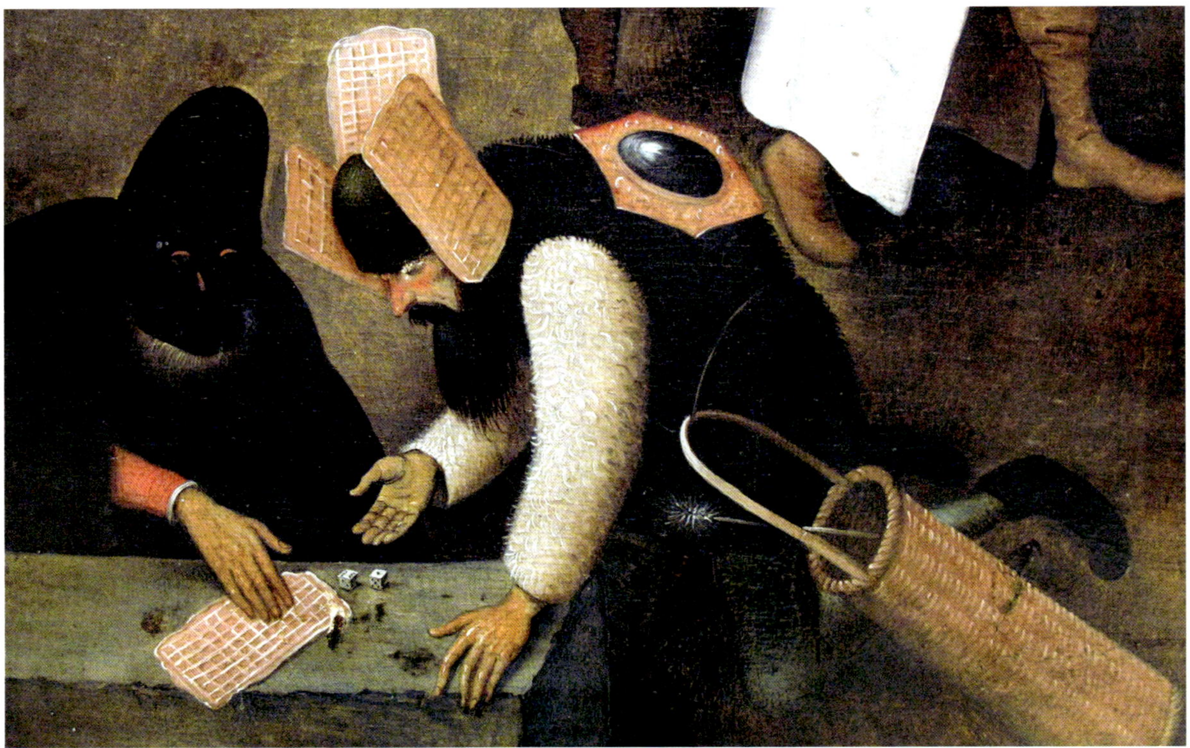

Rolling for waffles. Detail from Pieter Bruegel the Elder, *Fight Between Carnival and Lent*, 1559.

 ADEN KUMLER

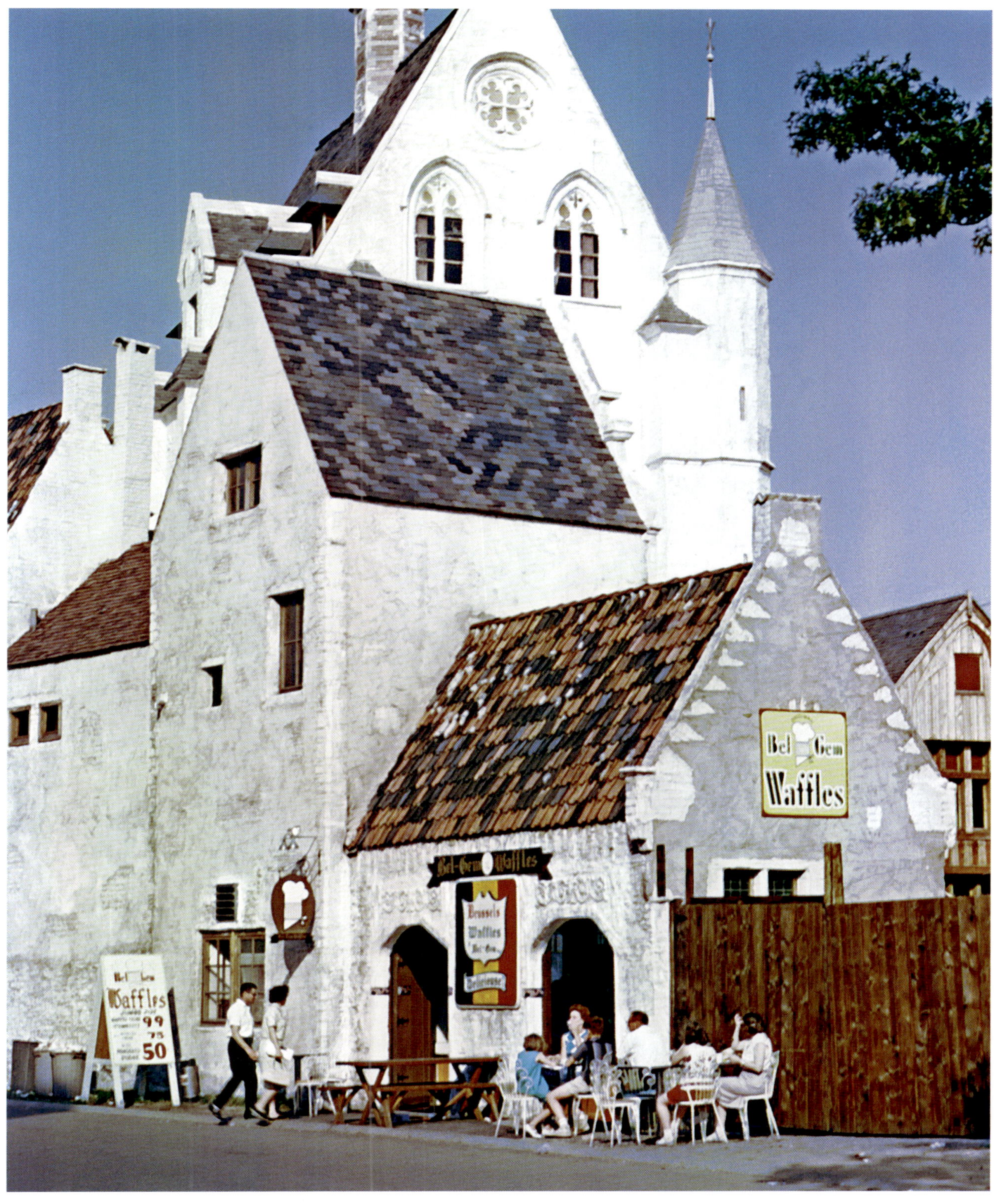

The Belgian Village, the original World's Fair home of Bel-Gem waffles. Courtesy Bill Cotter.

who had plenty of wafers to share them with their friends, and in so doing almost everyone received the same number and the joy was spread more evenly around the group.[20]

Despite Rousseau's praise for the pleasure of giving and receiving *oublies*, the *oublieurs* of Paris never regained the status and success they had enjoyed in the Middle Ages and Renaissance. Tarnished by their association with the criminal *demi-monde, oublies* were eclipsed by a new confection: *le plaisir des dames.*[21] Basically an *oublie* rolled into a suggestively phallic cylinder or a conical form (like the modern ice cream cone), the *plaisir des dames* was sold by female street vendors who carried the delicate cakes in shallow trays.

In many images, the *marchande de plaisirs* is a crone with a juvenile clientele. But in other depictions, the street seller is an enchanting beauty. And according to verses that accompanied a series of images of the *marchande de plaisirs*, the rolled wafers had their own, very adult appeal, particularly to *parisiennes*:

Treat yourself on the cheap,
Here's the pleasure of ladies.
For your husbands, I've got cornets,
For your lovers, colifichets.
Come choose, girls and women,
Here's the pleasure of ladies,
Here's pleasure![22]

Pastry horns for cuckolded husbands, bird feed for lovers, and pure pleasure for the women of Paris—no wonder the *plaisir des dames* flourished after the wafer and waffle had faltered!

I would like to thank Sonja Grund, head librarian at the Wissenschaftskolleg zu Berlin, who, together with her team, offered generous assistance with the many obscure sources that researching this topic required. This essay is dedicated to Grund, who was a crucial research collaborator on this project.

1 See David Leveille's segment on PRI's program *The World*, 22 April 2014. Available at <pri.org/stories/2014-04-22/it-was-1964-worlds-fair-when-americans-fell-love-belgian-waffles>.

2 Quote from Bill Cotter. See <worldsfairphotos.com/nywf64/aerial-ride.htm>.

3 Nineteenth-century North American recipe books included directions for making waffles, including a variant based on cooked rice. These were, however, more spartan dishes than the sugary, indulgent "Bel-Gem" waffles popularized by the Vermersch family at the World's Fair. The "Belgian waffles" that have come to be a fixture of the US breakfast scene since then are very much a postwar American invention. In Belgium, several varieties of waffles were made starting in the medieval period, but they were all local confections: the waffles of Liège, for example, differed from the waffles of Brussels, which formed the culinary point of departure for the waffles sold by the Vermersch family in Flushing Meadows.

4 Xavier Barbier de Montault, "Nieules et gaufriers au moyen âge et à la Renaissance," *Mémoires de la Société Archéologique du Midi de la France*, vol. 10 (Toulouse: La Société Archéologique du Midi de la France, 1874), p. 167.

5 According to the thirteenth-century writer Eberhard of Béthune, cited in Charles Du Cange, "Nebula," *Glossarium mediae et infimae latinaitais*, (Niort: La Favre, 1883–1887), vol. 5, col. 581c. Available at <ducange.enc.sorbonne.fr/nebula2>.

6 Alfred Darcel, "Les repas chrétiens," *Annales Archéologiques*, no. 27 (1870), pp. 280–281.

7 Alain Derville, "La vie religieuse au XIVe siècle d'après les comptes de la cathédrale de Cambrai," *Revue d'histoire de l'Église de France*, vol. 74, no. 193 (1988), p. 221.

8 René de Lespinasse, *Les métiers et corporations de la ville de Paris: XIVe-XVIIIe siècles*, vol. 1 (Paris: Imprimerie nationale, 1886), p. 372.

9 Ibid., p. 376.

10 While the earliest medieval sources indicate that street sellers of *oublies* employed dice to determine the quantity of wafers to be purchased by an individual customer, early modern sources describe the *oublieur* as carrying a device consisting of a spinning arrow or other indicator mounted on a disk, not unlike a clock face: the number upon which the arrow rested after a spin determined the quantity of *oublies* to be purchased by the customer.

11 In the streets of medieval Paris, *oublies* were won by the *main* (literally, "a hand"), a unit of five to eight wafers.

12 John of Garland, "Praecones nebularum et guafrarum pronuntiant de nocte guafras et nebulas et artocreas vendendas in calathis, velatis albo manutergio, et calathi frequenter suspenduntur ad fenestras clericorum, senione perditi," in his *Dictionarius*, included in Auguste Scheler, *Lexicographie latine du XIIe et du XIIIe siècle: Trois traités de Jean de Garlande, Alexandre Neckam et Adam du Petit-Pont: publiés avec les gloses française* (Leipzig: F. A. Brockhaus, 1867).

13 Guillaume de la Villeneuve, "Le dit des Crieries de Paris," MS fr. 837, ff. 246–267, Bibliothèque nationale de France. Cited in Philippe Ménard, "Un reflet de la vie quotidienne: Le dit des Crieries de Paris," in *Plaist vos oïr bone cançon vallant?: Mélanges offerts à François Suard* (Villeneuve d'Ascq: Université Charles de Gaulle-Lille 3, 1999), p. 611.

14 Ibid., p. 611.

15 Pierre Vinçard, *Les ouvriers de Paris: Alimentation* (Paris: Gosselin, 1863), p. 77–78.

16 Victor Fournel, *Les cris de Paris: Types et physiognomies d'autrefois* (Paris: Librairie de Firmin-Didot et Cie., 1887), p. 59.

17 Pierre Jean-Baptiste Legrand d'Aussy, *Histoire de la vie privée des Français depuis l'origine de la nation jusqu'à nos jours. 1ère Partie*, vol. 2 (Paris: Ph.-D. Pierres, 1782), p. 265.

18 Victor Fournel, *Les cris de Paris*, p. 60.

19 Jean-Jacques Rousseau, *Reveries of the Solitary Walker*, trans. Russell Goulbourne (Oxford and New York: Oxford University Press, 2011), p. 99. Translation modified.

20 Ibid., p. 100. Translation modified.

21 The *oublie* also lost out on the feast day church trade to another upstart, the *pain d'épices*. See Rolande Bonnain, "D'une pâtisserie cérémonielle: Usage de l'oublie," *Ethnologie française*, new series, vol. 23, no. 4 (December 1993), p. 545.

22 This verse is cited in Rolande Bonnain, "D'une pâtisserie cérémonielle," p. 551. *Cornet*, meaning horn or trumpet, is used here as a punning word, certainly intended to call to mind the "cuckold's horns" of the husband cheated on by his wife. A *colifichet* was a little pastry made without butter or salt, usually given to birds; also, more generally, a trinket.

JUBRIQUE UPDATE
The Editors

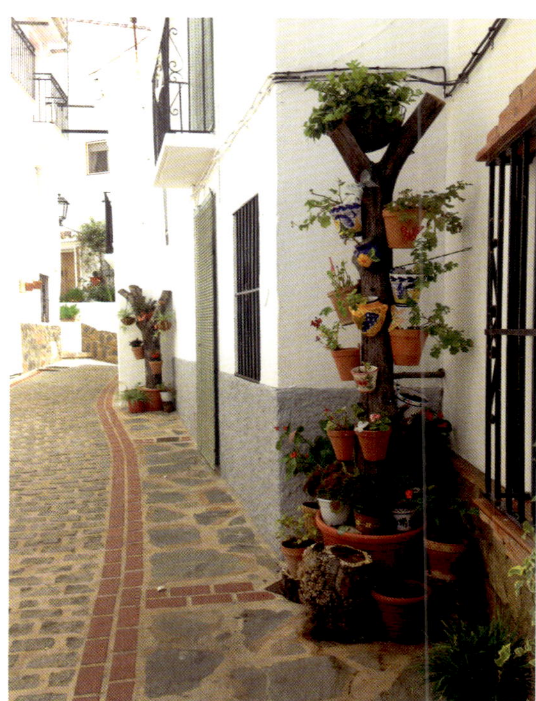

Above: A typically charming street in the village of Jubrique, Spain.

Veteran *Cabinet* readers may remember that in January of 2012, we published an article by Jonathan Allen about the Andalusian village of Júzcar, whose financial straits had led it to make a deal with the Belgian menace known as the Smurfs. To promote the Smurfs' new film, the production company, Sony, painted the village—one of southern Spain's *pueblos blancos*, famed for their all-white houses—the queasy-making blue of the small, deeply irritating critters. While researching the article, Allen was living in the next village over, Jubrique, whose centuries-old white façades had escaped despoilment. Through Allen, *Cabinet* was put in touch with Jubrique's mayor, David Sánchez, who agreed to an unorthodox publicity campaign that would attract more tourists to his village and also make *Cabinet* better known in the beautiful region of Andalusia. Here in New York, we made a copy of Jubrique's historic coat of arms and proudly paraded it around the city, while a local artist in Jubrique made a copy of our decidedly less historic coat of arms to be carried by Sánchez during the village's two most important annual festivals. A year later, Sánchez went one step further, commissioning a tiled mosaic of our coat of arms to be placed permanently on a building in the village.

Fast forward to the summer of 2015, when the magazine's editor-in-chief, Sina Najafi, found himself in Andalusia on a tour of important Smurf sites around the world. Taking his life into his own hands, he drove up the implausibly windy road to Jubrique to visit Sánchez and see the permanent evidence of our transatlantic friendship. After a tour of the town and a visit to the mosaic—which was in fact located on an exterior wall of Sánchez's mother's house—the mayor graciously treated his guest to a Coke at the local bar. The conversation soon turned to *aguardiente*, or "fire water," a local spirit made in a gourd-shaped copper still that can be seen on the village's heraldic shield. After explaining that no one in the town currently possessed an official license from the provincial authorities to produce the heavy-duty tipple, Sánchez informed his guest that the bar owner nevertheless made the very best that Jubrique had to offer. Armed with two large bottles of contraband hooch, generously procured by his host, Najafi somehow made it down the now even more implausibly windy road. Taking his siesta later that afternoon under the influence of fire and water, Najafi had a terrifying vision that the Smurfs had come to the Gowanus canal area and painted the *Cabinet* offices blue.

Opposite, clockwise from top left: Najafi, David Sánchez, and the mayor's mother in front of the *Cabinet* coat of arms; Sánchez in conversation with two of his constituents; a still, formerly used to make *aguardiente*, on display in one of the village squares.

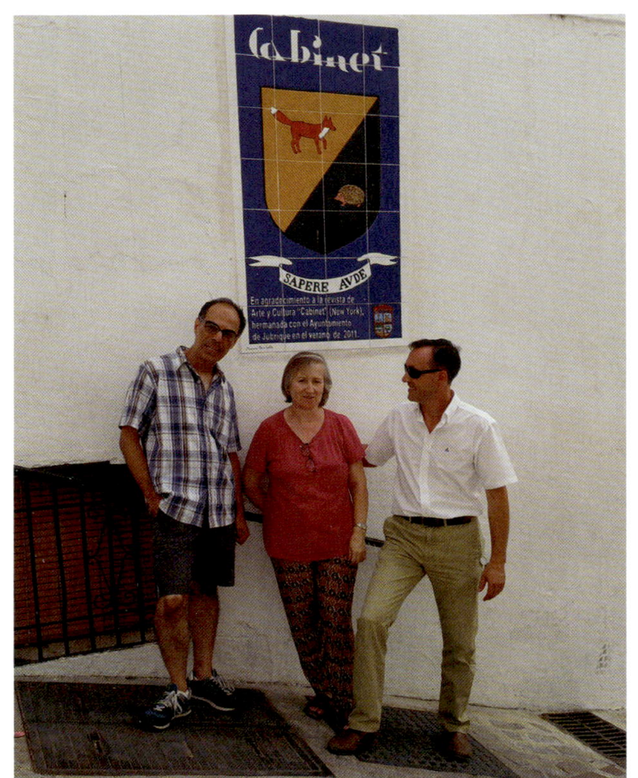
Cabinet
SAPERE AVDE
En agradecimiento a la revista de
Arte y Cultura "Cabinet" (New York),
hermanada con el Ayuntamiento
de Jubrique en el verano de 2011.

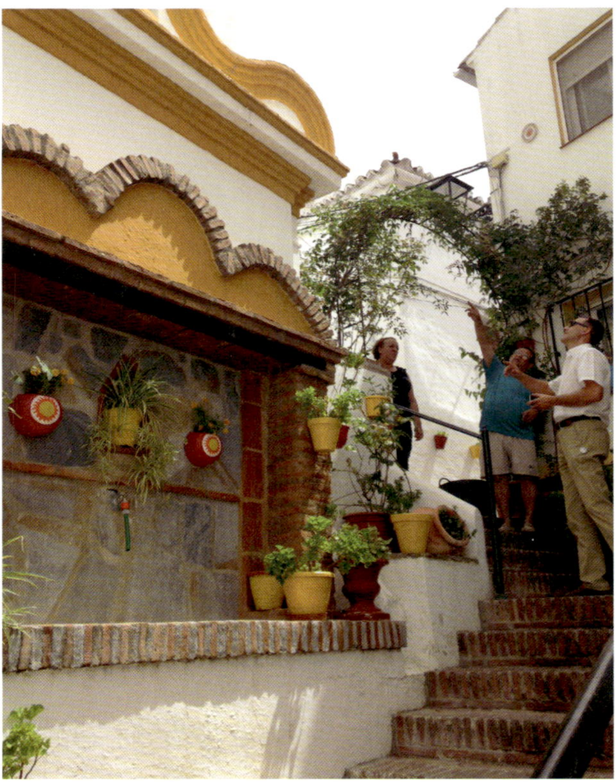

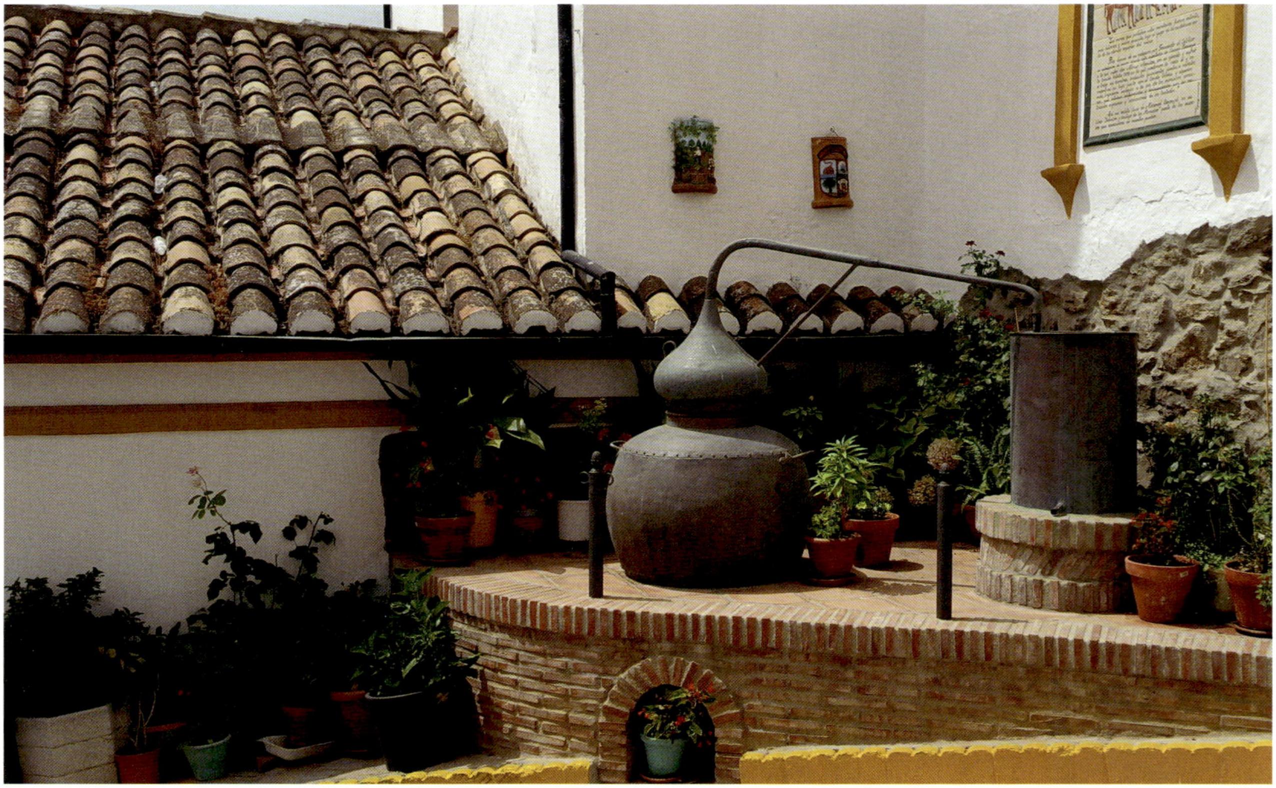

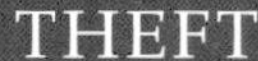

THEFT

INSIDE JOBS
Geoff Manaugh

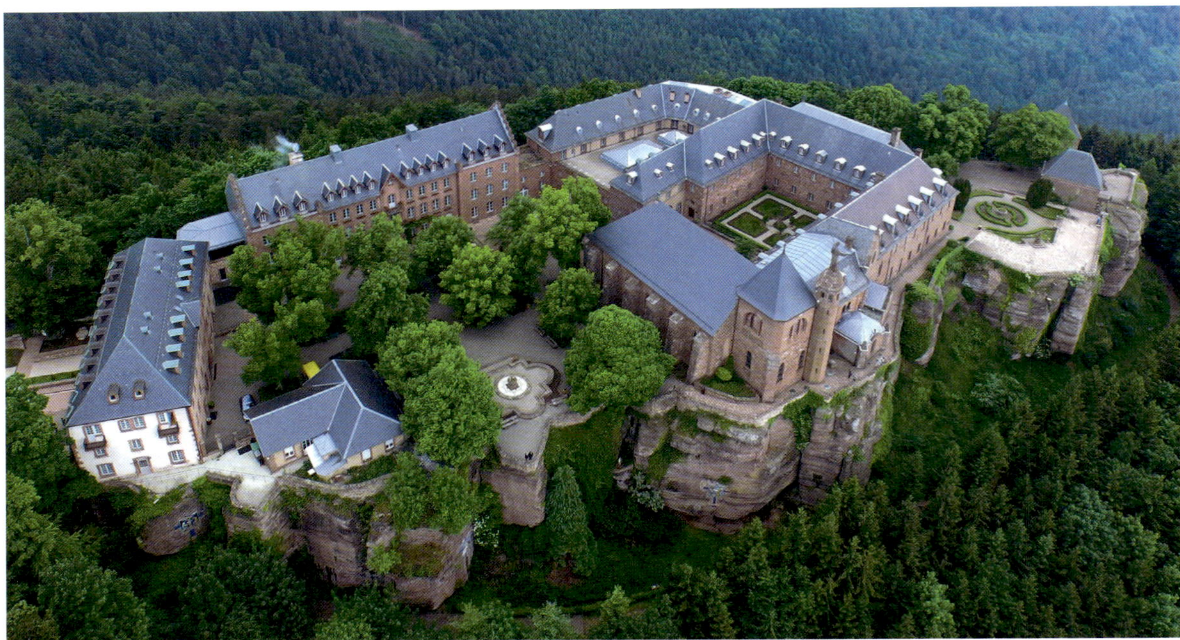

The books and manuscripts were disappearing from a room no one seemed to be entering. Its doors were almost never opened, the room itself closed to public view. There was no believable explanation for where the materials might be going, so the least believable reasoning soon took hold. It was the work of the devil, the residents said. A poltergeist. A symbolic act of God meant to communicate *something*, if only they could interpret the signs.

This was, after all, a monastery—indeed, one of the world's most picturesque, Mont Sainte-Odile, perched high in the mountains of France, nearly on the border with Germany—and its library was vanishing into thin air. A manuscript here, a bound volume there; five, six, a dozen, all quickly adding up to nearly a thousand key pieces of church scholarship missing from the shelves and tables.

When the police were finally notified, they chose not to perform an exorcism. Being a secular institution, they instead installed a hidden surveillance camera, and, in May 2002, the truth came to light. It was not a ghost at all, but an engineering teacher from Strasbourg. He had been entering the room through a long-forgotten secret passage, access to which was hidden inside one of the bookcases. Unseen—indeed

entirely unsuspected—he was able to remove the library's priceless collection piece by piece, emerging from the walls to take entire shelves of books at a time.

Perhaps more spectacular than the teacher's indirect method of approach was how he came to know the passage was there in the first place. According to the *Guardian*, this otherwise law-abiding engineer first learned about the route "after discovering a forgotten map in public archives" revealing how the monastery's attic was covertly joined to the library on a lower floor. This chance discovery of a discarded floor plan made him one of the very few people in the world who knew the architectural connection existed at all; it had long ago ceased being used by the monks themselves, having fallen into a state of neglect resembling spatial hibernation.

Bringing the passage back into service as a reliable form of internal circulation was not, in fact, easy. According to some newspaper accounts, doing so required scaling the outside walls of the monastery, then navigating a precipitous attic stairway. According to others, the man posed as an overnight guest staying in another part of the monastery that

Above: The monastery of Mont Sainte-Odile, Alsace, France.

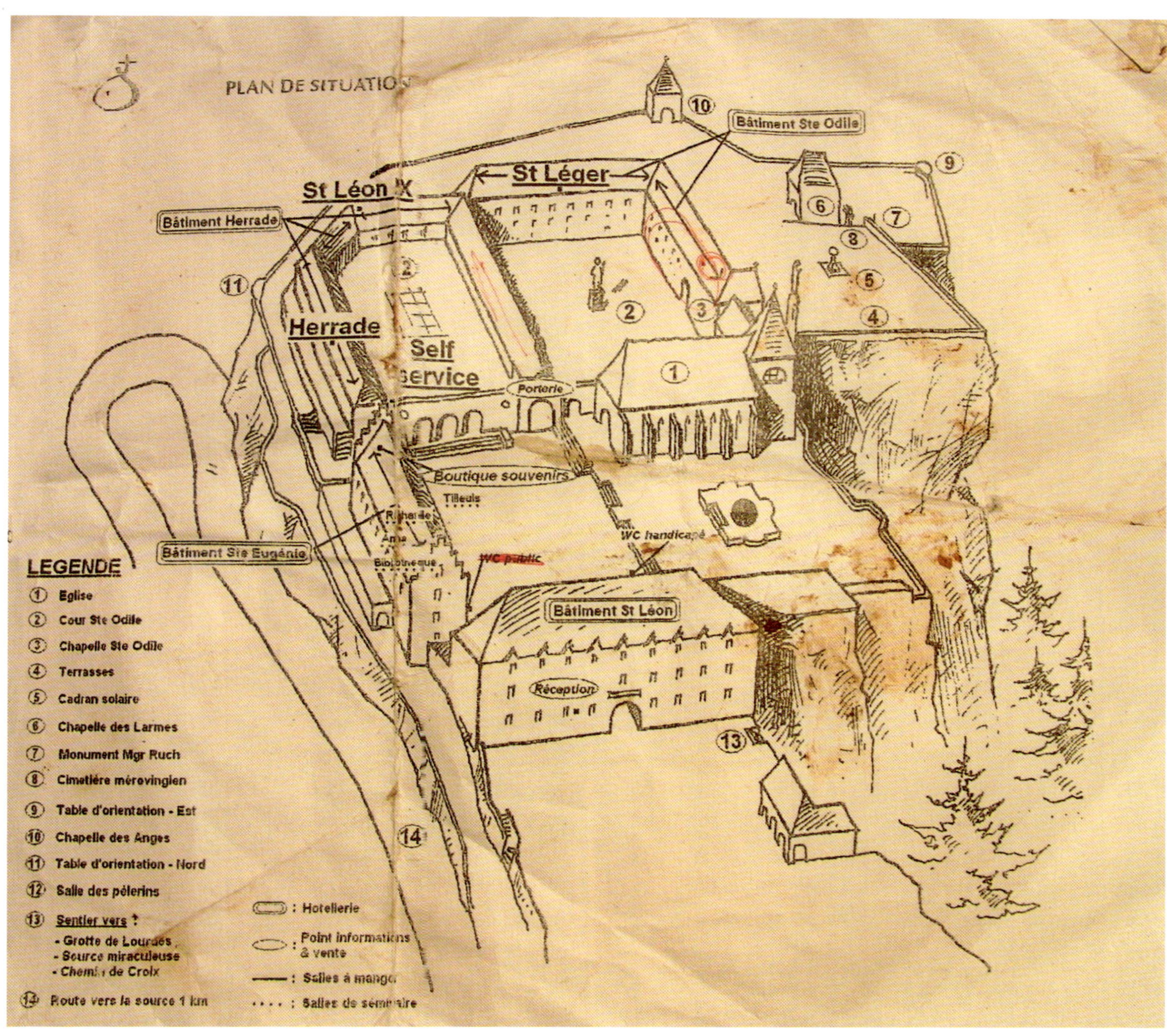

Map of monastery and adjoining hotel. This map was obtained and used by an amateur sleuth who visited the monastery in May 2011 looking for its secret passages. Courtesy <adventurecycletour.wordpress.com>.

had been converted into a hotel; carrying a suitcase, he would slip into a room with access to a hidden passageway, climb down a rope ladder, then enter the library through the trick bookcase. Some reports also claim that he had to locate "a hidden mechanism" tucked inside the wall that would cause the back of the bookcase to flip open, allowing entrance into the library. Regardless of how he ultimately gained access to the books, his actions transformed the confines of the monastery into a kind of three-dimensional puzzle. Indeed, the very fact that these accounts diverge suggests something of an epistemological uncertainty at the heart of such crimes: that a burglar can misuse a piece of architecture so radically it becomes almost impossible to narrate what actually took place there.

Half a world away, another prolific book thief found equally furtive ingress through similar spatial means. An avid lock picker, expert counterfeiter, and methodical planner committed to researching the targets of his heists, Stephen Blumberg stole an estimated twenty million dollars' worth of rare books and manuscripts from institutional archives and academic libraries around the United States. His plan for hitting the rare books collection of the University of Southern California in Los Angeles was characteristic: researching the history of the building, Blumberg had learned that a series of disused dumbwaiters had once functioned to deliver books between floors. The dumbwaiters were no longer active, but the shafts inside the walls of the library still offered a direct connection to book stacks that were otherwise inaccessible to the public.

Blumberg rightfully concluded that the shafts—like the M. C. Escher-like loop hidden inside the walls of Mont Sainte-Odile, connecting the monastery's attic to the back of a cabinet—were effectively an alternative circulation system hiding in plain sight. Moreover, he reasoned, the passageways themselves would receive little attention from the building's security team, which, in any case, most likely amounted to an underpaid student cramming for an exam at one of the exit doors. No alarms, no cameras, just narrow, chimney-like chutes invisible to outside view through which Blumberg could shimmy his way to treasure. And shimmy he did, successfully raiding the building from within. He got away with it, we might say, by going further inside, squeezing through the walls like a spider. Finally, having crawled back out through

the dumbwaiter system, he would simply conceal his chosen books beneath an overcoat and walk calmly out the library's front door.

Each of these crimes was made possible by the reawakening of a dormant interior, one disguised by and simultaneous with the buildings' visible rooms. There was another building *inside* each building, we might say, a deeper interior *within* the interior. Their burglaries thus both depended on and operated through an act of spatial revelation: bringing to light illicit connections between two internal points previously seen as separate.

Indeed, in both cases the actual theft of books seems strangely anti-climactic, even boring, merely a graduated form of shoplifting. Rather, it is *the way these crimes were committed* that bears such sustained consideration. The burglars' rehabilitation of a quiescent architectural space brings with it a much broader and more troubling implication that we ourselves do not fully understand the extent of the rooms and corridors around us, that the walls we rely on for solidity might in fact be hollow, and that there are ways of moving through any building, passing from one floor to another, that are so architecturally unexpected as to bear comparison to animal life or even the supernatural. In the end, burglars—dark figures burrowing along the periphery of the world—need not steal a thing to accomplish their most unsettling revelation.

GIVE AND TAKE
D. Graham Burnett

His name was Bradford. Or Bradley. Or Bradman. Maybe even Bradforth. He lived "a little more out that way." Up somewhat. Beyond 48th Street. The wave of his hand suggested north of Chestnut; even, perhaps, north of Market. Because he wanted to be a doctor, he needed to borrow the concentrated hydrochloric acid.

Things make sense if one does not suspect they don't. And suspicion must be learned. What follows is the story of how I learned mistrust. Also, there was theft.

. . .

It would have been the winter of 1983, making me twelve. My family lived in West Philadelphia at that time, in a row house between Pine and Osage on South 46th Street—number 409. This was the edge of "University City," a neighborhood defined by proximity to the University of Pennsylvania. My parents were academics—my father a dean, my mother a lecturer in the French department. We had only recently moved from grassier bits of the country: Indiana (where the backyard of our white clapboard Cape Cod gave onto the wide expanse of the neighboring cornfield); North Carolina (where the momentum of my soapbox racer down the long, steep driveway could almost carry me to the edge of a small pond, wherein lurked lunker largemouth and bluegill keen to rise to a spider with rubber legs). West Philadelphia was very different. I recall arriving at the end of the road trip up from the South, seated in the back of a red Pinto flashed with a *Starsky & Hutch* stripe that bent like a hasp across the hatchback. There was graffiti. A boy about my age, seated on a basketball at the corner of Baltimore Avenue, eyed me, unblinking, as the car idled at a light. Then he gave me the finger—slowly, deliberately, holding his hand as still as the rest of him. I was frankly shocked. And genuinely hurt.

. . .

Snow fell. A dump. No school. I suited up to shovel the sidewalk, steps, and stoop: long johns, sweatpants, corduroys tucked into rubber boots that closed with funny hooks—a metal tongue that could be folded

around one or another rung of the little ladder-clasp. Within the boots: thick socks, then a plastic bag, and then a second pair of tube socks over all that. And above: sweaters, parka, gloves, scarf, hat. Already by mid-morning, the two-toned gong of the doorbell chime had rung several times—men from the neighborhood presenting themselves as willing to do this work for a flat fee of ten dollars. My mother politely turned them away. Her son was upstairs, she explained sociably. He'd be down in a moment. He was getting his warm things on. And then (perhaps going a little further than was strictly necessary in the context of the racial and economic discontinuity convoked across the threshold of our sun porch at that moment) she took a brief turn into the importance of a young man learning to work—manual labor being essential to a proper upbringing, etc. Not that her feint in this direction was high-handed or preachy. My mother wasn't like that. It was rather that she was seeking the common ground. Awkward common ground, yes, in the face of the men whose cold work was less moral-ritual than subsistence-scramble. But her intentions were of the finest water.

Down the steps I came, shouldered the shovel, and made my way out into the snow. And I shoveled. I had been at it for a time when a young man approached, and asked if I needed any help. I said I didn't, but thanked him for the offer. I had to do it myself, I explained. My mother wanted me to do it. He understood; said that he had already done the same for his mother, and now was out making a little pocket change. He didn't say it quite like that. But that was the gist of it. I shoveled.

. . .

Twelve is a "between" sort of age. I was a boy. Yet when I looked in the mirror, I could see—now and again, depending on the light and my mood—the shape of a man. My arms were different than before. My chest too. But all this meant little, practically speaking. I had some downy hair on my nuts. I could ride my bike around by myself—but only on the sidewalk, and only within a three-block radius of the house. It was autonomy, of a sort, but extremely limited. I took a school bus to school, with my little sister—

and we wore uniforms (hers a blue polyester kilt, white shirt, gray sweater; mine gray slacks, navy blazer, and a rep tie of gold and blue). Sometimes we slept in the same bed, still, like children—but less and less, as I had begun to feel a bit odd about it. I had recently written away to a mail-order address in the back of a magazine, sending a check for $14 to secure a long-sleeved T-shirt emblazoned with the logo of the Canadian brewery called Moosehead, and featuring the racy slogan "The Moose is Loose" in cursive down one arm. I treasured it, because I felt it made me look very grown up.

The boy who watched me shovel was less of a boy than I. He said he was fifteen. And he may have been. He was physically taller and a good deal thicker, and the stuff of a mustache could be seen above his upper lip. He sat on the step. After a while, he stood up, and explained that since he didn't have any work to do right then, he'd help me out. Just for fun.

I saw no harm in that—nor can I quite imagine what I would have done if I had. So we shoveled together. For a while. The resonant scrape of the blade on the sidewalk. The arresting *whump* of that blade striking suddenly on a cleft or crack beneath the wet powder: the smooth push-and-plow slammed to a stop; the rounded butt of the shovel shaft striking the ribs; the sharp kick stunning cold hands. Thrown snow left delicate traces on the sycamore trunks, for all the world like a *bûche de Nöel* sprinkled with soft sugar.

· · ·

I know, now, what my mother thinks she was thinking when she brought us hot chocolate. Because I have asked her. She recalls how pleased she was by the idea that I might be making a friend. And it was not insignificant to her, then, that this was a *black* friend. Neither of my parents had ever lived in an actual city or in a racially diverse community of any kind, and they were both excited (and a little trepidatious) about their big decision to reject the leafy suburbs and move the family to Philadelphia proper. My mother had gone to great lengths, back in Indiana, to avoid letting us go to the nearby swim club in the summers (which was effectively white-only)—driving my sister and me to the YMCA closer to Indianapolis, as a show of her left-Catholic/progressive distaste for Midwestern semi-rural bigotry. So, looking out from the kitchen, what my mother saw mattered to her.

To me less so—or at least not in any conscious way that I can now recover. I didn't know many boys my age in the neighborhood. (We'd only moved in the year before.) Here was someone to play with. Bradford (or Bradley, or Bradman, or Bradforth) and I threw a football around in the snow after drinking our chocolates. After this brief interlude, we took up our shovels and tromped the radius of a few blocks, knocking on doors and volunteering to shovel walks. Ebony and ivory. Fresh-faced youths. We got quite a bit of work, split our gains fifty–fifty, and parted fast friends.

· · ·

I had hobbies at this time. I could do some elementary programming in BASIC on a RadioShack TRS-80 16k "Color Computer" wired to the RCA television in the family room. (I made a game in which you could bomb, from a spaceship-like aircraft, a glass-enclosed city; it was schematic.) Data storage consisted of an audio cassette player that plugged into the back of the computer. I had a microscope and a chemistry "lab" arranged on a pair of low tables in the basement laundry room. (I attempted to mutate paramecia by bubbling cigarette smoke through their small aquarium; I made gunpowder-impregnated coffee filters which burned in interesting ways; I wrested, by means of a makeshift still, a few drops of noxious liquor from a funk of yeast-fermented flour and sugar.) I possessed, and loved, a "150-in-1" electronics kit: a tray of electronic components (photoelectric cell; speaker; relay; various diodes and transistors) that could be linked by short wires strung between springy contact posts to create various simple devices (a doorbell; an AM radio tuner; a Morse-code transmitter).

What else? My sister's room was in the back of the house, and overlooked the alley. She played with dolls and stuffed animals. One day we made blowguns together, fletching straight pins with a tuft of orange thread and puffing them through a drinking straw. I could hit a grapefruit at four paces, the darts sticking fast in a perfect and satisfying silence. My mother had an office in the finished part of the basement, and she worked on a book that dealt with foreign language learning. One night, after my sister was asleep, she

---

Overleaf: The enlightenment project. The Tandy Corporation's 150-in-1 electronics kit, mid-1970s.

Science Fair ®

150 in 1

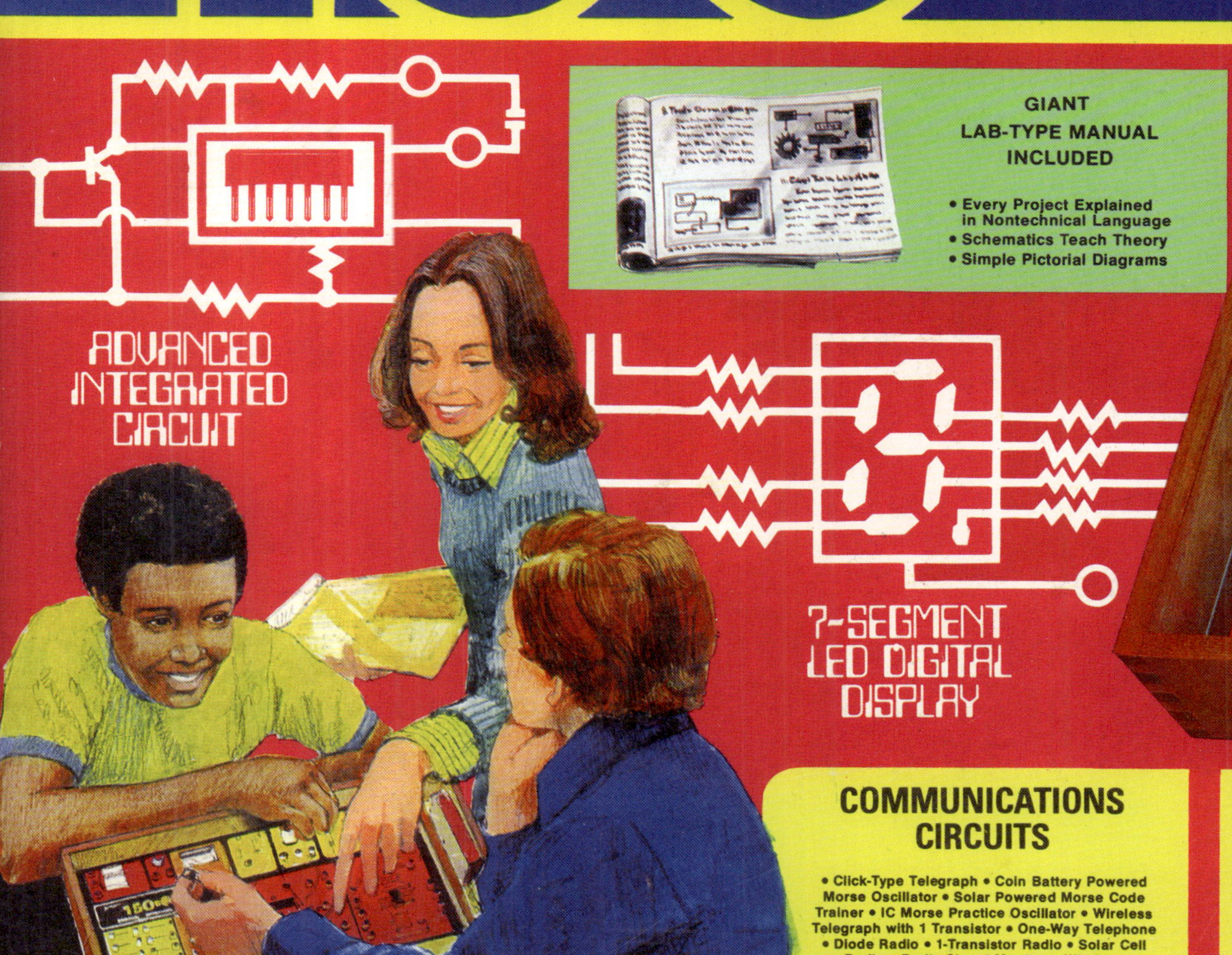

ELECTRONIC PROJECT KIT

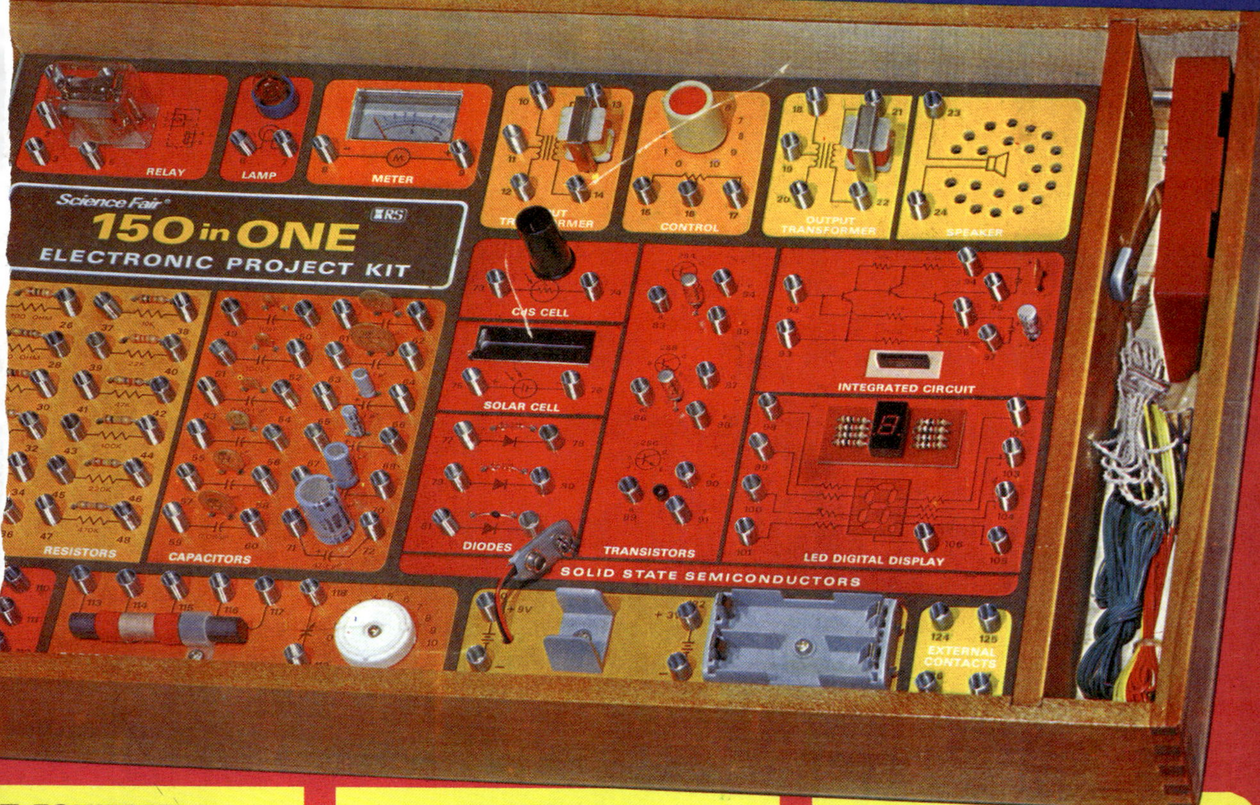

ST EQUIPMENT CIRCUITS

• ...ter with Indicator Lamp • Acoustic ... • Output Meter • Output Level Meter ...meter • AC-Galvanometer • High ...ance Ohmmeter • DC Voltmeter ...zed DC Voltmeter • Audio Meter with ...d Meter • AC Capacitor Bridge • Hum ...ector • Audio Signal Tracer • High ... Signal Tracer • IC Oscillator Tester ...al Generator • Acoustic Light Meter

ELECTRONIC SOUND EFFECTS

• Electronic Bird • Electronic Cat • Electronic Bird with CdS • 2-Way Electronic Bird • Chicken Peeping • Knocking Noise • Woodpecker Sound • Light-Controlled Electronic Harp • 1-Transistor Toy Organ • Wireless Electronic Organ • Light-Music Maker • Electronic Metronome • Electronic Motorcycle Noise • Machine Gun Sound Generator • Sound Effects Generator • Sleep Inducer

COMPUTER CIRCUITS

• AND Circuit • OR Circuit • AND Circuit with LED • Pulse Display • OR Circuit with LED • One Shot Multivibrator • NOR Circuit with Transistor • NOR Circuit with LED Display • Light Controlled NAND Circuit • "1" or "2" Alternating Automatic Display • Flip-Flop Lamp Flasher • Set/Reset Flip-Flop

read me most of the *Crito*, my head in her lap. My
father, on weekends, perused the *Philadelphia Inquirer*
under a green Tiffany lamp that hung in the breakfast
nook of the large kitchen. Sometimes we would play
floor hockey in the kitchen, with a balled-up pair of
his socks as the puck, my (deceased) grandfather's
cane as the stick, and me in "goal"—the doorway to
the back steps—making kick saves in my stocking
feet. In 1979, shortly after the death of Sid Vicious, my
father went to the record store and bought a vinyl of
Never Mind the Bollocks Here's the Sex Pistols, which he
placed with the other albums we owned in a rack with
sliding louver doors under the turntable. But only after
instructing me that I was never to open it. It was to
remain in its sealed plastic sheath forever, because
it was a collector's item. I opened it in 1984, and
listened to it. He was quite upset. I am not sure why
I did that. It was obviously the wrong thing to do.

· · ·

Obviously the wrong thing to do. My new friend came
over again the next day, a Saturday, and I showed him
my room. We played with my 150-in-1 kit, making a
siren sound. I showed him the unopened Sex Pistols'
album in its pristine sleeve. We went down to my
"laboratory" in the basement, and I displayed my rack
of chemicals, my cigarette-smoking device, my mutant
paramecia, which swam, I alleged, in an anomalous,
spiraling fashion. (I believed this then, but I do not
think, now, that it was so.) My mother served us homemade chocolate chip cookies in the breakfast nook. She
asked him about his family. His mother was a nurse,
he explained, and that was why he wanted to study
medicine.

Before he left, he asked me if he could borrow my
"Moose is Loose" shirt. He thought it was cool. I went
upstairs and got it for him. And could he also take, on
a temporary basis, my jar of hydrochloric acid? This
small, amber jar, which contained a slightly syrupy
pale yellow fluid, was, from my perspective, the most
sacred object in my lab. The holy of holies. The central
elixir. I had secured it from a colleague of my father's
at the university, and I had never used it for anything,
but rather simply held the vial at times, and thought
about power. This stuff could *melt gold*. It could *eat
your face*.

I hesitated. But only for a moment. What profits us
selfishness? And suspicion, I had none. I went down

to the basement and got it for him. We said goodbye at
the front door, having made plans for an after-school
playdate later that week. He would come over. I recall
his asking what time was best. I said around 4:30. And
I remember saying not before that, because no one
would be at home.

· · ·

I never saw him again. But on Tuesday of the
following week, my mother returned home from
teaching her afternoon class and, upon entering the
kitchen, found it decidedly cold—even frigid. It took
her only a moment to realize that the door at the top
of the basement steps (normally locked when we were
not at home) had been kicked open, shattering the
doorjamb, long sharp splinters of which lay about on
the linoleum floor. Startled, she left the house and
called the police from the neighbor's.

By the time my sister and I got home, my mother,
father, and a police officer were standing around in
the basement laundry-room-cum-laboratory looking
at how the window had been jimmied. A crowbar,
evidently, which had popped the small lock like a
bottle cap. I remember very clearly the look on the
cop's face when my mother asked if he intended to
fingerprint the window frame. No. That wasn't going
to happen. An investigation? Not to speak of. The
police were very busy. And what would really be
the point anyway? It wasn't as if they were going to
somehow track him down and catch him. The cop's
face said: "This isn't a Sherlock Holmes story, ma'am;
this is West Philadelphia."

It was about this time that the neighbor turned
up carrying our stereo amplifier. He had found it
in the pachysandra under his back porch in the alley.
Odd. But the man in blue didn't think so. "He just left
it there to come back for it later," he explained. "He'd
look pretty suspicious carrying a big stereo with a
cut cord around the streets in broad daylight." The
neighbor put the amp on the step. It had a case of
smooth-grained wood and a linear tuner dial which
I knew from experience glowed a warm orange when
it was on. But not now. The clipped cord had the
stubby, truncated air of a Doberman pinscher's tail.

It took time to figure out the other things that
had been stolen. It was not as if the house had been
ransacked, nor had any of the things that my parents
considered valuables—the sterling silverware they had

received on their wedding, a few pieces of family
heirloom jewelry my mother kept in a small box in
her closet—been touched. The things we gradually
discovered had been taken were idiosyncratic: a pair
of inexpensive cufflinks my father had left in an
ashtray by the front door; a battered suede bomber
jacket of my father's that had been in the front hall
closet, together with a leather trench coat my mother
had bought as a graduate student in Paris; a crumpled
wad of Italian lira banknotes that had been on top of
a small basket of pocket change my father kept on
his dresser. These latter became part of the lore of the
burglary: there were something like 1,400 lira to the
dollar in those days, and my parents surmised (perhaps
wrongly, and possibly merely for the reassurance of
comedy) that the thief, upon encountering bills with
so many zeros on them, no doubt accounted himself
instantly in possession of great wealth and hastened
to make his escape. What else could explain his
meager haul?

But who knows, really?

My father repaired the cord, stripping the wires,
twisting them back together where they'd been cut, and
taping the new joints with shiny, black electrical tape.
It looked like my garter snake after swallowing a good-
sized frog. Which is a little like the way I felt.

· · ·

In the wake of all this, we put a deadbolt lock on the
basement door. And I embarked on what I can now
understand as a strange exercise of traumatic techno-
parapraxis. I set to the task of making a burglar
alarm with my 150-in-1 kit. If a shadow darkened
the doorway, breaking a flashlight beam, it tripped a
switch that ran current through the solenoid of an old
doorbell that I took apart. The solenoid was positioned
in such a way that when the rod sprang from the coil,
it hit a small knife switch that had been wired into
the power cord of the audio cassette player (which I
removed from the TRS-80). Powered up, the cassette
player played a recording I had made. A voice—mine—
saying, in a whisper, "I think I hear someone in the
hall. Get my gun … There he is!"

Followed by a loud BANG.

· · ·

I slept with that alarm set up at my bedroom door for
a year or so. And about that time, I bought a Ruger .22
semiautomatic carbine, took the alarm down, and slept
with the gun, loaded, tucked under my bed.

· · ·

Every theft is, first, an act of betrayal. Unless this is
completely wrong. And here I remain fundamentally uncertain. On the one hand, to take what is not
one's own, in secret, is to turn on anyone who trusted
enough to fail to take the precautions that would have
stopped this occurrence. That would certainly seem to
be a betrayal. On the other hand, however, that whole
world of "trusts" can suddenly feel, under scrutiny, like
a charming little conjuration of the well-positioned—
like downtown Aspen, say, or parts of La Jolla. It is a
beautiful sort of place, but a strong odor of contingency
wafts through that air.

The gun under the bed said, "I feel betrayed by
this theft, and I am taking precautions." But even then
I also smelled the scent of the contingent. Lying in that
same bed, I once had a dream in which he wore my
shirt, showing it to his friends. And that made sense
to me.

I have always wondered what he did with the acid.

A PHONY CLAIM?
Margherita Peliti

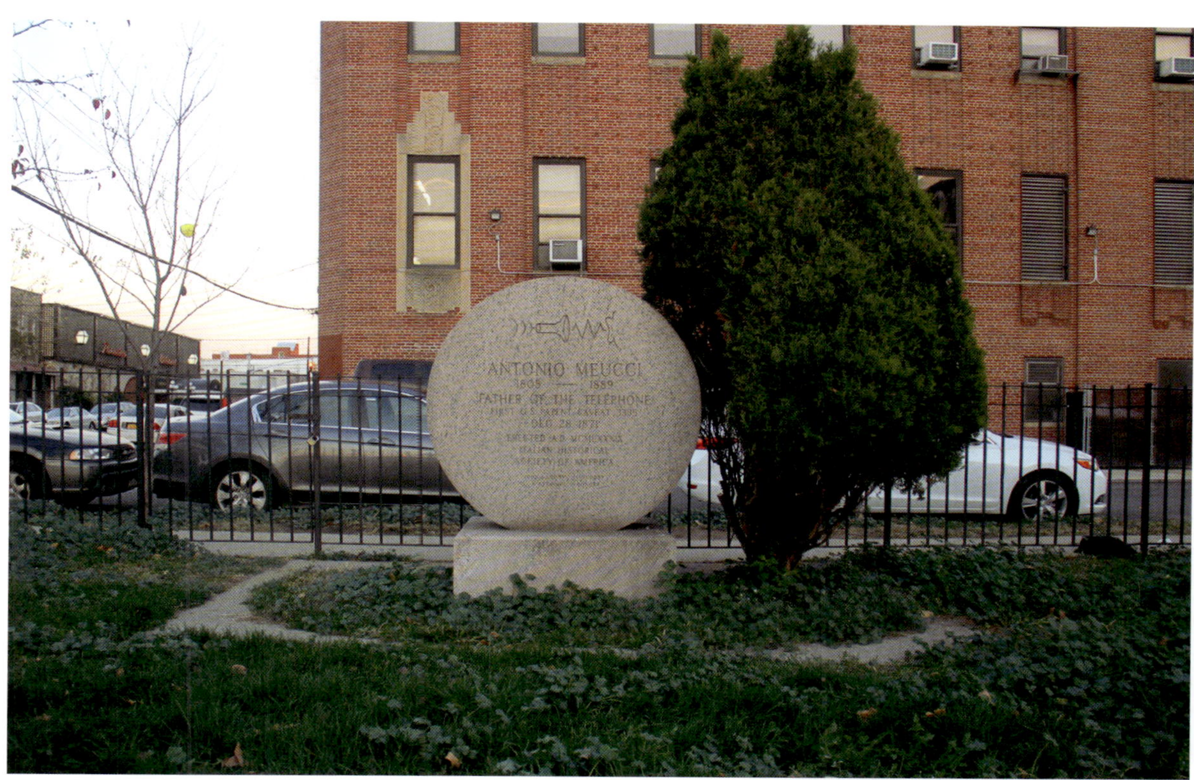

It is my heart-warm and world-embracing Christmas hope and aspiration that all of us—the high, the low. the rich, the poor, the admired, the despised, the loved, the hated, the civilized, the savage—may eventually be gathered together in a heaven of everlasting rest and peace and bliss—except the inventor of the telephone.

—Mark Twain, *New York World*, 1890

On 11 June 2002, the United States House of Representatives passed Resolution 269, sponsored by then-Congressman Vito Fossella, of Staten Island, New York. The resolution honors "the tragic and extraordinary career" of Italian-American inventor Antonio Meucci, and suggests that Alexander Graham Bell might have arrived at his most famous invention by less than scrupulous means. The parliament of Canada, where the Scottish-born inventor spent much of his adult life, responded just ten days later by passing a motion stating that "Alexander Graham Bell of Brantford, Ontario and Baddeck, Nova Scotia is the inventor of the telephone."

Born in 1808, Meucci studied mechanical engineering, chemistry, and physics in his native Florence. According to one biographer, already as a seventeen-year-old the inventor had been hired, along with others, to produce a pyrotechnic display in celebration of the grand duchess of Tuscany; the festivities quickly turned into mayhem, however, possibly due to a powerful new propellant that Meucci had devised. Out-of-control rockets landed among the crowd that had gathered in Piazza della Signoria, causing damage and injuring a few onlookers. Meucci was suspected of deliberately sabotaging the celebration, and only narrowly escaped a criminal conviction.

In the 1830s, more trials followed—for negligence as an employee and other minor offences, and for involvement in plots for the unification of Italy. This last accusation landed Meucci in jail for several months

Above: Not entirely forgotten. The memorial to Antonio Meucci, Meucci Triangle, south Brooklyn. Photo William Simpson.

during 1833 and 1834. The following year, the inventor was offered the job of chief stage engineer at the Tacón Theater in Havana, Cuba, and seized the opportunity to flee Italy.

During his tenure at the Tacón, Meucci delved deeply into the study of galvanism. He developed an interest in medical electricity theories, and repurposed part of the theater to serve as his laboratory. One day, while administering electrical shocks to an ailing employee, Meucci heard the man's screams as if they emanated directly from the wire—and understood immediately, as he himself was to recount several decades later, that speech could be transmitted electrically. One year later, in 1850, the inventor immigrated to Staten Island, where he planned to follow up on his discovery. Bell was then only three years old.

Over the course of the following decade, Meucci kept working at his *telettrofono*, and by 1860 he judged the results good enough to bring his invention to the public.[1] He published a description of his instrument in a New York–based Italian-language newspaper, *L'Eco d'Italia*, and attempted, unsuccessfully, to secure funds in order to start a telephone business. By this time, his own capital had dwindled after a series of ill-fated schemes that included a sausage plant, a candle factory, a brewery, and a business manufacturing celestas at his home; by the 1870s, Meucci was living on public assistance. In 1871, the inventor finally managed to scrape together enough funds to file a provisional patent (then called a caveat) on his invention—only to let it lapse three years later.

In 1876, Bell took out his historical patent no. 147765, which set the ground for the century-long monopoly on the telephone held by the American Bell Telephone Company and its successor AT&T. About a decade later, the telephone industry had grown into a profitable and steadily expanding business, and there soon followed a series of lawsuits between Bell and a disparate roster of companies that did not accept his claim to be the original inventor of the telephone. Among those was the Globe Telephone Company of New York, which had hired Meucci as a technical consultant, and which American Bell sued in 1885 for infringement.

At the trial, Meucci produced several drawings that showed how his devices, which predated Bell's patent by more than a decade, had all the features of a working electromagnetic phone. But the instruments themselves were missing, having been sold to pay for the inventor's hospital bills after an explosion on the Staten Island ferry had left him badly scalded. The issue of *L'Eco d'Italia* in which Meucci had described his *telettrofono* was missing, too: both the journal's archives and the inventor's own copy had been destroyed in fires. And the caveat, in place of a description of the device's innards, contained only an arcane reference to a "well-known conducting effect of continuous metallic conductors as a medium for sound." The judge on the circuit court decided that there was no evidence that Meucci had ever built anything more than a tin-can telephone, and Bell's patent was upheld.

Thus, Meucci's achievements, and his extraordinary and tragic life. As for Bell, biographers place him in New York, at Western Union's headquarters, over a few days in March 1875—that is, one year before being granted his patent. Did Bell draw the bulk of his inspiration from direct observation of Meucci's models stored at Western Union, as Congress seems to imply? This seems unlikely, as Meucci had entrusted them to a different company, the American District Telegraph, and there is no reason to believe that Bell had ever set foot there.

It's quite possible that Meucci might have invented the telephone before Bell did. His friend and fellow revolutionary Domenico Mariani recalled his many conversations with Meucci's ailing wife in the late 1850s—when he would joke with her about Meucci being the devil, because of what he had come up with. It is certainly true that Meucci's ebullient talent produced a diverse range of inventions, including improved methods for the manufacture of stearic candles and sparkling fruit drinks; he even patented a proprietary method for making and canning Bolognese sauce. But the recognition he most craved—for the creation of the telephone—eluded him.

---

1 Most sources render this word as *telettrofono*, although the resolution passed by the House of Representatives, as well as a later resolution passed by the Senate, spell it with only one *t*.

H. Res. 269

In the House of Representatives, U.S.,

June 11, 2002.

Whereas Antonio Meucci, the great Italian inventor, had a career that was both extraordinary and tragic;

Whereas, upon immigrating to New York, Meucci continued to work with ceaseless vigor on a project he had begun in Havana, Cuba, an invention he later called the "teletrofono", involving electronic communications;

Whereas Meucci set up a rudimentary communications link in his Staten Island home that connected the basement with the first floor, and later, when his wife began to suffer from crippling arthritis, he created a permanent link between his lab and his wife's second floor bedroom;

Whereas, having exhausted most of his life's savings in pursuing his work, Meucci was unable to commercialize his invention, though he demonstrated his invention in 1860 and had a description of it published in New York's Italian language newspaper;

Whereas Meucci never learned English well enough to navigate the complex American business community;

Whereas Meucci was unable to raise sufficient funds to pay his way through the patent application process, and thus had to settle for a caveat, a one year renewable notice of

an impending patent, which was first filed on December 28, 1871;

Whereas Meucci later learned that the Western Union affiliate laboratory reportedly lost his working models, and Meucci, who at this point was living on public assistance, was unable to renew the caveat after 1874;

Whereas in March 1876, Alexander Graham Bell, who conducted experiments in the same laboratory where Meucci's materials had been stored, was granted a patent and was thereafter credited with inventing the telephone;

Whereas on January 13, 1887, the Government of the United States moved to annul the patent issued to Bell on the grounds of fraud and misrepresentation, a case that the Supreme Court found viable and remanded for trial;

Whereas Meucci died in October 1889, the Bell patent expired in January 1893, and the case was discontinued as moot without ever reaching the underlying issue of the true inventor of the telephone entitled to the patent; and

Whereas if Meucci had been able to pay the $10 fee to maintain the caveat after 1874, no patent could have been issued to Bell: Now, therefore, be it

Resolved, That it is the sense of the House of Representatives that the life and achievements of Antonio Meucci should be recognized, and his work in the invention of the telephone should be acknowledged.

Attest:

Clerk.

THE ROBBER AND THE ROBBED
Jerry Toner

At night, the emperor Nero used to disguise himself as a slave and go wandering through the streets and taverns of Rome. This was before the Great Fire of 64 CE—which Nero was to be accused of starting himself—when the streets of the city were narrow, twisting, and dark. The emperor would lurk in the shadows until someone passed by and then leap out and violently assault him (although one victim fought back and pummeled the emperor to within an inch of his life, an act for which Nero later forced him to commit suicide). Nero would then break into shops and steal from them. Safely back at his palace, he would auction off his loot to the highest bidder. When it became well known that the emperor himself was indulging in such a wanton crime spree, many others began, not surprisingly, to copy his example. It was said there were so many marauding gangs that at night Rome became like a city that had been captured by the enemy.

What is remarkable about this story is that it shows that a man who was head of the Roman legal system and the ultimate judge and source of Roman law was happy to behave like a common thief. Now, the story may well be an invention designed to discredit an emperor who was unpopular with the literary class, but, true or not, the tale also highlights the major place that crime had in ancient Roman society. Most of us think of ancient Rome as a generally well-ordered and disciplined society, but the Roman Empire was rife with crime and theft. People at all levels of society, from the rich in their villas to the poor in their taverns, were affected by such antisocial behavior. Rome was not a safe place to keep hold of property.

The Roman world had no police force in the modern sense, only a group whose primary purpose was to put out fires in the city of Rome itself. Most people had to fend for themselves. If someone steals from us now, we know to head straight to the police to get them to investigate. If a thief stole from a Roman, the victim himself had to bring a civil court case against the accused. The cost and difficulty of this served to deter most. It took money and connections to get the law to look at your case. This personal nature of the accusation also highlights the minimal role that the state had to play in dealing with theft. The state provided the means to hear and judge the case and the means to punish the guilty, but it was up to the victims to collect the evidence and bring the case to court.

Another option was to petition the emperor to ask him to hear the case. One such petition from second-century CE Roman Egypt—given to the emperor's representative there, the local governor—provides us with a good idea of the kind of theft that affected ordinary life. Written on papyrus, it is from a man called Andromachus, a native of the town of Tebtunis, who complains that two men called Orsenouphis and Poueris had made a brazen attack upon his house in the village. They beat him up and then stole a variety of goods from him: a white tunic and robe, a cloak, a pair of scissors, some beer, and a quantity of salt. But the fact that a petition was sent did not mean it was given a hearing; the system could never cope with the demand. On a two-day visit to a single town in Egypt, one governor received 1,804 petitions, an impossibly large quantity to take on.

Other petitions make it clear that claimants did not always tell the truth. One dating from 193 CE was sent to the governor by a man who had a piglet stolen. He claimed it was worth 100 drachma, but this was about five times what piglets usually cost. Why lie to the governor? It might have been a way to exaggerate the size of the claim and so make it more noticeable. Or perhaps it was a way of leaving room for negotiation in any out-of-court settlement between the victim and the accused. The very act of sending off a petition was itself a way of making it known that the victim was taking steps to gain redress, even if there was no real belief that the case would be heard by the governor or that the victim would go to court. The victim could go to the thief and his neighbors and tell him or her that he had sent a petition. Give me my property back or else, in other words. But of course the thief might well decide to take the risk and gamble that the governor would do nothing and, most of the time, he would have been right.

The case of poor Andromachus also highlights the petty nature of much Roman theft. But theft also took place on a grand scale. The second-century emperor Commodus (he of the film *Gladiator*) is alleged to have charged wealthy senators with treason and then

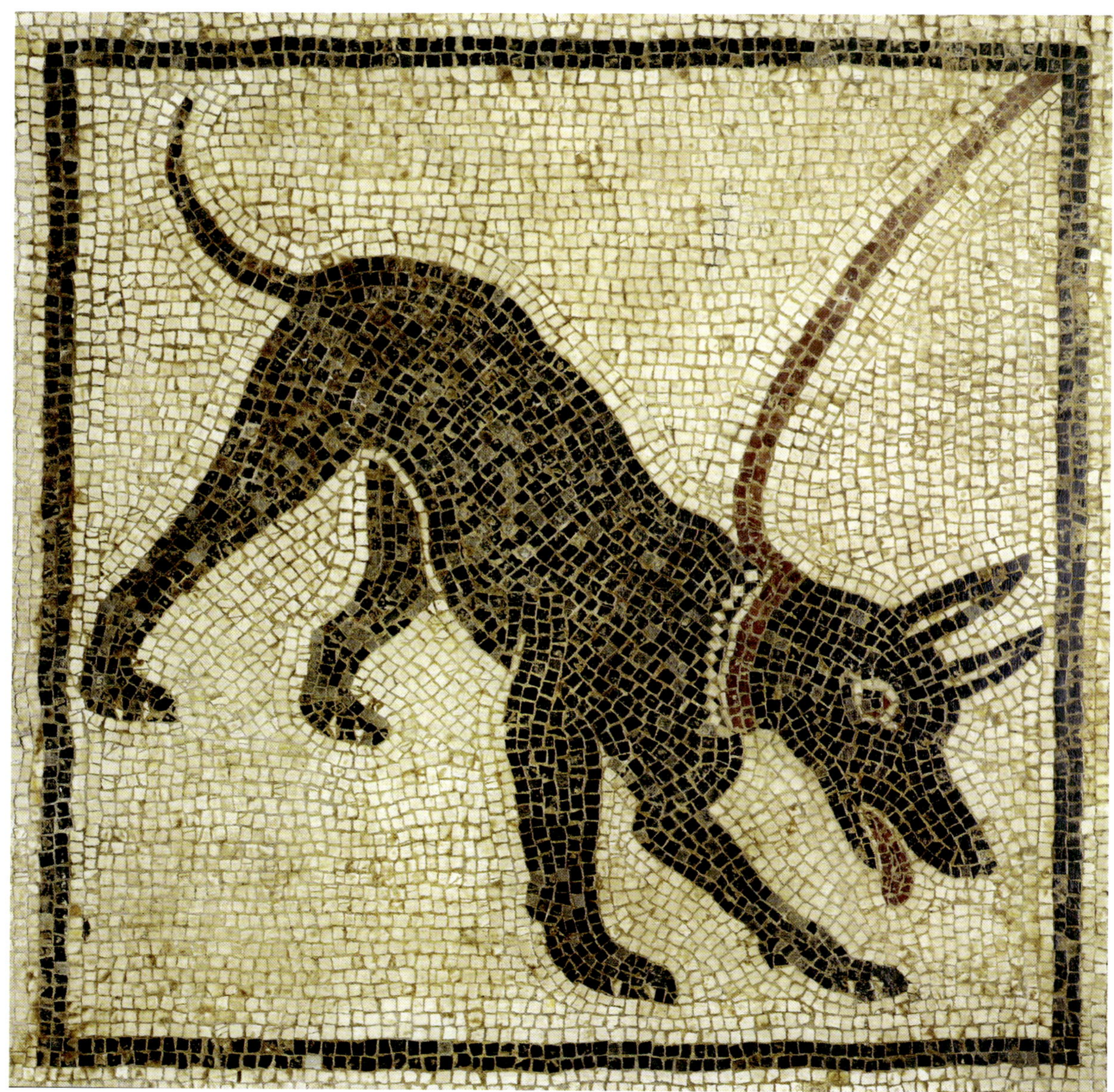

Mosaic from the "House of Orpheus" in Pompeii warning would-be thieves of the presence of a guard dog, first century CE.

executed them precisely so he could confiscate their property for the imperial treasury. Quasi-legal theft of this kind was an easy way for emperors who had no respect for their own laws to boost their incomes. Whether large or small, theft, as is also clear from these examples, often involved the use of violence, an act which we would today class as robbery. Theft with violence was endemic in the Roman world. One petition from a goldsmith describes how a female donkey-driver called Kofis bludgeoned the shopkeeper with many blows before stealing some earrings. Another from some farmers in North Africa pleads to the emperor Commodus for help against some soldiers who were intimidating them with abuse and beatings.

The cases looked at so far also emphasize that theft in the ancient world took place in a society where many of the victims and criminals knew each other. In Dorotheus of Sidon's book of astrology written in the first century CE, there are accounts of victims of theft who have paid to consult the astrologer about who the perpetrators might have been. The criminals are, Dorotheus counsels, either from within the household, or have visited the house and are known to the victims. He even goes so far as to offer other helpful pointers for identifying the person responsible, such as "thick is the hair on his hand," or he is "fat-cheeked and narrow in the forehead."

The astrologer's cases also give a sense of how easy it was to enter ancient houses. The Romans did develop locks and padlocks, some of which had sophisticated spring actions, and most archaeological digs of domestic Roman sites usually yield a good crop of these devices. Many door locks were made of wood, though, and would not have posed much of a deterrent to a determined thief. Dorotheus warns his clients that the thieves will simply break the locks or they will use their friendship with family members to make copies of the keys. The houses themselves were also not that sturdy. Great remains like the Colosseum can blind us to the reality that most Romans lived in buildings that were poorly constructed. Dorotheus says that burglars will gain entry after simply digging under the walls of the house or knocking holes through them.

The wealthiest members of society had to make extra provisions to ensure the safety of their belongings. The owners of villas would deploy a slave as a gatekeeper to make sure that undesirables were kept out during the day and that no one tried to scale the walls or force the locked gates during the night. Dogs were widely used to guard property and were sometimes depicted in mosaics, presumably as an extra warning to anyone thinking of entering the house uninvited. Valuable items would be kept under lock and key in strong rooms in the center of the house to prevent burglars simply knocking through an outside wall. The House of Menander in Pompeii, for example, has such a safe room underground, beneath the house baths, where a chest was discovered containing over a hundred pieces of fine silverware. Most people could not afford such strong rooms and instead had the option of storing their valuables in a temple for safekeeping. The temple at the north end of the forum in Pompeii has a crypt that may have served as a kind of municipal strong room in the same way that the vault under the Temple of Saturn did in Rome (although that did not prevent Julius Caesar from helping himself to its contents). These temples might have been safe from theft but they were still vulnerable to fire. When the Temple of Peace burned down in 238 CE, many of the richest people in Rome were, according to the historian Herodian, reduced to penury overnight, although in reality they probably also stored considerable assets in private strong rooms or held them in the form of property.

Goods that had been stolen were unlikely to be recovered. One question to the gods contained in a set of oracles asks, "Will I find what I have lost?" Of the possible answers, 70 percent of the responses were that the items would not be recovered. Only 30 percent were positive, with a third of those saying that such recovery would only happen after a time. The lack of police or other means of tracing petty criminals meant that the recovery of stolen property was extremely difficult. What counted in the victim's favor was that often, as Dorotheus warned, it was people within the household—family members or slaves—who had perpetrated the theft and so they were more likely to be found out.

If victims did turn to the law, they would have encountered legal precepts pertaining to theft very different from today's. The Romans did not use distinct terms for theft and burglary, the latter of which in its original Saxon meaning meant nocturnal housebreaking. But they did, as we shall see, treat theft from a house during the night more severely than if it had occurred during the day. The Romans'

primary distinction was between "manifest" and "non-manifest" theft, which meant whether the thief had been caught in the act or not, and therefore was more or less clearly guilty. This largely depended on how close to the scene of the crime the thief was caught, although exactly where the line could be drawn was a matter for debate among lawyers. Catching a thief with a stolen jug outside the owner's house would be "manifest," but finding the jug a mile away where the thief happened to be standing would not. We punish theft equally regardless of whether we catch a thief in the act or catch him three days later a hundred miles away, so long as we can prove beyond reasonable doubt that he did it. The Romans graded their punishment to correlate with the degree of certainty about the accused's guilt. Since there was no fingerprinting or the like to ensure guilt, circumstantial evidence must have played an important role in many cases of "non-manifest" theft. Roman law had a strange rite for the discovery of stolen goods, known as the "plate and loincloth search." The victim had to walk semi-naked through the suspect's premises while holding a plate in his hands. This was designed to prevent him from touching any evidence or indeed planting it in the house. It may also have represented an offering to the household gods. In theory, the victim would spot his stolen items and thereby prove the case. In reality, such a procedure would only have been useful in recovering large or living items such as a horse or a slave, not for coins or small valuables. But if the stolen goods were discovered, the theft became "manifest" and the criminal therefore liable to more severe punishment.

Theft did not only pertain to physical objects. One grim legal side effect of the widespread ownership of slaves was that, since they were treated as possessions, runaway slaves were effectively stealing themselves from their master. Financial theft was also a risk. According to one hostile account of the life of Pope Callistus, who was pontiff between ca. 217 and 222 CE, he was guilty of financial theft as a young man. Callistus had started life as a slave and was instructed by his owner, a wealthy friend of the emperor's, to set up a business as a banker in Rome's fish market. Before long, various investors had deposited substantial amounts of money with him, since he was backed by the financial might of an emperor's associate. But Callistus secretly spent it all. When his owner demanded that he present his accounts for inspection,

Callistus was so terrified that he tried to run away but was captured and put to work on a treadmill by his master. In the end, this fraudulent slave changed his ways, became an administrator in the Christian church, and, finally, ascended to the papacy itself.

The motivation for most theft was likely poverty. Columella, an important writer on agriculture in the first century CE, describes how country slaves would claim to have sown more seed than they had actually used, and steal, shirk, and fiddle the books. Seneca warns owners to guard against their slaves' "thieving hands." This kind of petty theft helped slaves to supplement their meager rations, while fixing the accounts could enable them to save more money, which could then be used to buy extra food or be put toward buying their freedom.

What kinds of punishment awaited those convicted of theft? In the early laws of Rome, known as the Twelve Tables, thieves were treated differently depending on whether or not they were caught in the act, the time of day in which it occurred, and their social status. Unarmed thieves who were freeborn and were caught in the act during the day were flogged and then made the slave of the victim. Slaves, armed or not, were whipped and then hurled from the Tarpeian rock to their deaths. The victim was legally permitted to kill the thief on the spot if he was caught in the act during the night or if the thief was armed during the day. However, in the case of an attempted armed theft during the day the victim could only kill the thief with impunity if he first shouted out a warning. The purpose of the shout is not expressly stated in the early laws but presumably was meant to give the thief a chance to surrender himself and to alert neighbors to what was going on, thereby ensuring that the killing was a more public act that could not be used as an underhand way of murdering someone. Cases where the thief had been caught in the act were not given a full trial, but simply heard by a magistrate.

By the time of the late republic and early empire, physical punishment had been abandoned for freeborn thieves, and in most cases victims were instead given compensation for their loss. Typically, this would be set at a multiple of the value of the thing stolen, generally four times. Being prosecuted as a thief meant that a freeborn person lost certain legal privileges, such as being able to appear as a witness in court and that, like slaves, they became liable to suffer physical

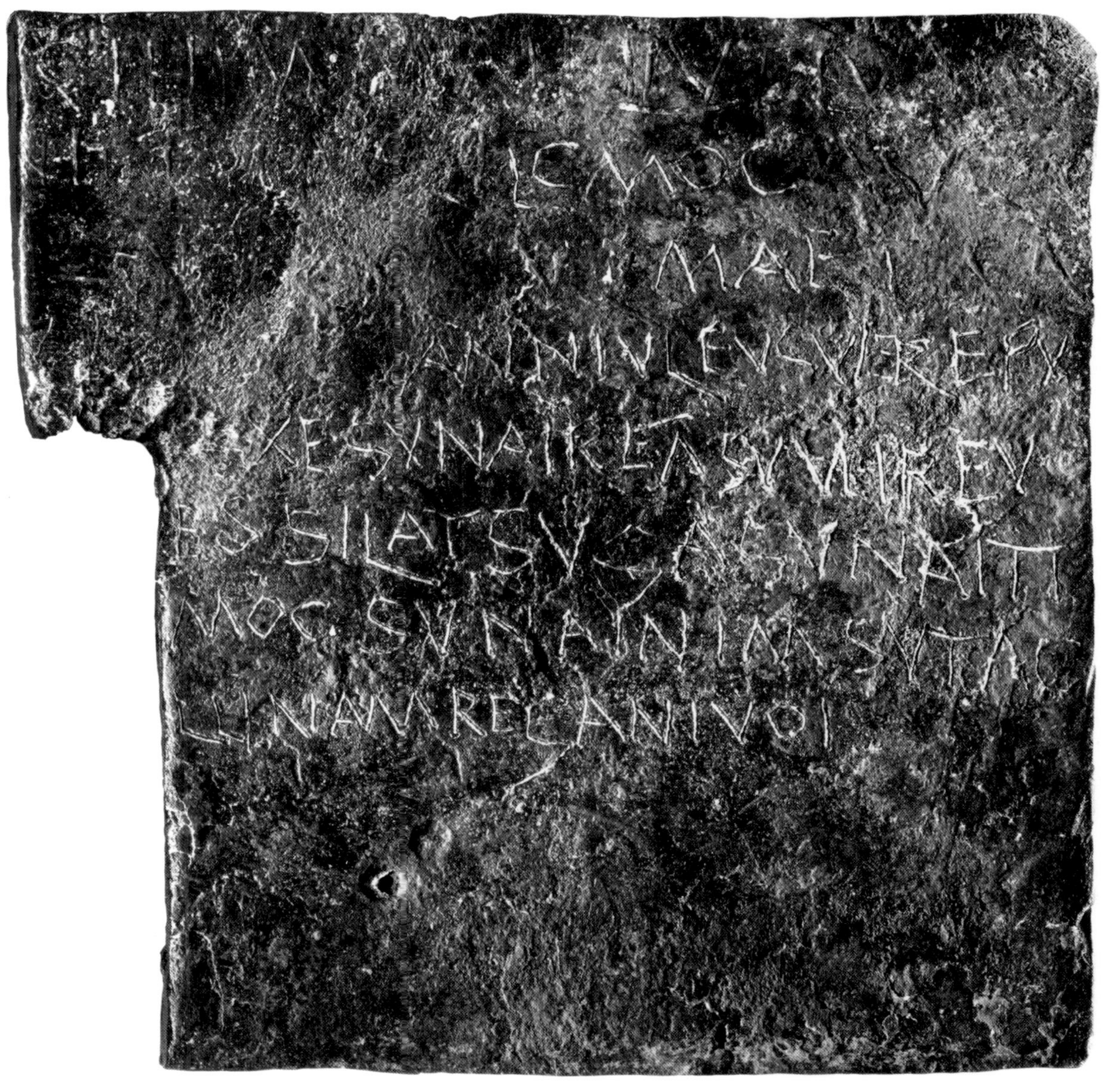

"Vilbia" curse tablet, found in Bath, England. The tablet,
each word of which is written in reverse, reads, "May he
who has stolen Vilbia from me become as liquid as water."
This is followed by ten names, which historians believe
are the possible culprits. Historians are uncertain whether
"Vilbia" is a proper name referring to a person, or a noun
designating an object. The artifact is thought to have
been made in Roman Britain between 43 CE and 410 CE.
Courtesy Bath and North East Somerset Council.

punishment for any further crimes they committed.

The punishments for thieves who were slaves were always brutal. Slaves had almost no legal rights and their owners were able to punish them as they saw fit. One particularly striking example of this lack of basic human rights is that if a slave appeared before a court, even as a witness, then he or she had to be tortured to ensure that the evidence they gave was truthful. They were, in the words of one source, merely "tools that can speak." Those convicted of theft could be flogged, crucified, or, if they had stolen themselves by running away, condemned to the mines or to be thrown to the beasts in the amphitheater. A sense of the shocking normality of domestic punishments can be gleaned from an inscription from Puteoli that lists the prices charged by a kind of municipal punishment service. Floggings cost four sesterces (about the price of a few loaves of bread), and included the gibbet to which the slave would be bound. Diodorus Siculus describes how slaves in the mines were physically destroyed, forced by the whiplashes of their overseers to endure the most dreadful hardships. They often prayed for death because of the magnitude of their suffering. Those thrown to the wild animals in the public shows in places like the Colosseum might find themselves facing a hungry lion, a bear, or a bull. Sometimes they would be given a wooden sword to prolong the entertainment; other times they would simply be tied to a stake so they could be mauled to death in full view of the crowd. Perhaps the most famous example of men being crucified by the Romans for theft were the two unknown robbers who were executed alongside Jesus, although in one gospel they are described in more general terms as criminals.

The severity of the law and the possibility of substantial compensation no doubt meant that many victims chose to pursue the legal route if they could. But there were many other ways to seek retribution for theft that lay outside the law. One method was to try to attack the reputation of the thief by means of gossip or graffiti. One piece of graffiti written on a wall in Pompeii states simply, "Ampliatus Pedania is a thief." We can see this text acting both to shame the perpetrator publicly but also to warn others about his misconduct. Even if literacy levels were low, it put the accusation out there in the public sphere where it could then be spread by verbal means. More direct acts of vengeance could include physical assault or even communal acts of stoning, but these all carried risks, above all of bringing in the law against the avengers.

But what action could be taken against an unknown thief? Here religion came to the fore. Magic in the form of curse tablets was a commonly used tactic to try to bring divine retribution against a thief who had made his or her escape. These curses were often scratched onto a lead surface and then dedicated to a particular god. One large group has been found in Bath, England, and survives because the lead tablets were thrown into the spring that supplied the water for the popular bathing complex. Where motives for the curses are specified, obtaining redress against a thief is the most common. Often the curses are trying to recover the lost items, which were mainly small, easily stolen items such as clothing, jewelry, and coins. Many of these items were probably taken from people who had come to bathe in the spring waters and had left their possessions unattended while they did so. In another find in the English village of Uley, a number of curses deal with stolen animals: "Honoratus to the holy god Mercury," says one. "I complain to your divinity that I have lost two wheels and four cows and many small belongings from my house." The curse then asks the god to strike down the thief with an illness: "Do not allow health to the person who has done me wrong, nor allow him to lie or sit or drink or eat, whether he is man or woman, whether boy or girl, whether slave or free, unless he brings my property to me and is reconciled with me." This is not so much a case of an eye for an eye as a serious illness for a cow. It gives some idea of how deeply the victims felt their loss and probably also how significant such losses could be for them financially. Most curses seem to have been written by professional curse-writers, who would obviously have charged for their services, which again reflects the importance that victims placed on the loss of their possessions. One common tactic in the curses is to give the stolen item to the god being petitioned. If the god now owns the stolen object, then it is the thief who has a problem, since he or she has, in effect, robbed a superhuman power.

There is evidence for people holding some sympathies with thieves and robbers. In one story dating from the start of the third century CE, a bandit called Bulla Felix, "the lucky one," lived in the woods with his band of men, robbing travelers and raiding towns, all the while successfully evading Roman capture. But,

like the later Robin Hood, he only stole from those rich
enough to afford it, gave rewards to captured artisans
who worked for him, and administered justice in a
way that the Roman courts seemed unable to do. He is
portrayed as the valiant opponent of an unjust government and social system and perhaps reflects wider
popular sentiments of this kind. Travel was habitually
dangerous within the Roman world, where armed
bandits—typically far less noble in their aims and
deeds than Bulla Felix—would rob any passing traveler who came their way. The biblical tale of the good
Samaritan who stopped to help the man wounded
in such an attack underlines how well known these
attacks were and probably also how rare it was to
receive any help. Very few people would likely have
harbored any sympathy for the more familiar kind of
bandit.

Theft affected the Romans just as much as, or even
more than, it affects contemporary society. Like us,
they took a variety of precautions to try and prevent
it. They sought to gain redress in the courts if they
could, but would also make use of a wide range of
alternative strategies to enable them to recover their
stolen goods and punish the thief. The punishments
the courts meted out could be incredibly severe but the
likelihood of being caught was low. We can see them
as occasional, exemplary punishments designed to
have the maximum deterrence through their brutality.
But perhaps this very brutality also revealed that the
state was unable to do much for the majority of those
affected by theft. All most of them could do was turn
to the gods and try to get their help in the search for
justice and retribution.

GIFT OF GENERAL DODDS
Julian Lucas

I was visiting Benin, taking pictures of a palace in Abomey, when a prince with a machete made a grab for my phone. He was shirtless, angry, and wearing a beautiful slumped cap, done in black velvet and embroidered with silver stars. He was speaking Fon, but I could tell that he was angry—not with me but with my guide, who paraphrased their argument in French. Seated just behind him on the motorcycle, two languages removed, I tried to make out the details of our lèse-majesté.

The prince was a groundskeeper—that's what the machete was for—but he was also accustomed to receiving royalties from visitors. This privilege, recently and without explanation revoked by the Bureau of Tourism, was an inheritance from his ancestor, King Tegbesu. Tegbesu had built the palace that crumbled behind us, now nothing more than a gate with walls, a blood-red heap under the sky's chalk-dusted blue. Photographing, even just looking at this heirloom, would cost money. So we gave him a few thousand francs and drove off. As he shrank with the walls, I watched him stuff the colorful bills down the front of his pants, leaving, on the sparkling hair below his navel, a smear of orange earth.

. . .

On 16 November 1892, French troops reached Abomey, then capital of the Kingdom of Dahomey. The city was in flames, burned by King Béhanzin when France refused his terms of surrender. He began with his own sprawling compounds, then set fire to the homes of his subjects, compelling everyone to follow his retreat. The blaze was three kilometers wide, and it scorched the city's sanguine walls to pitch. Guerrilla struggles would follow, but this was the formal conclusion of the Franco-Dahomean Wars, one front in the "scramble for Africa" which by 1914 would leave nearly the entire continent in European hands. The conflict began in 1890, when the French—already master of large swaths of West Africa—turned their pith helmets and howitzers on Dahomey, their partner for centuries in the slave and palm oil trades. Nine months of fighting won them rights to the port city of Cotonou. And in 1892, after a short truce, France came back to take the

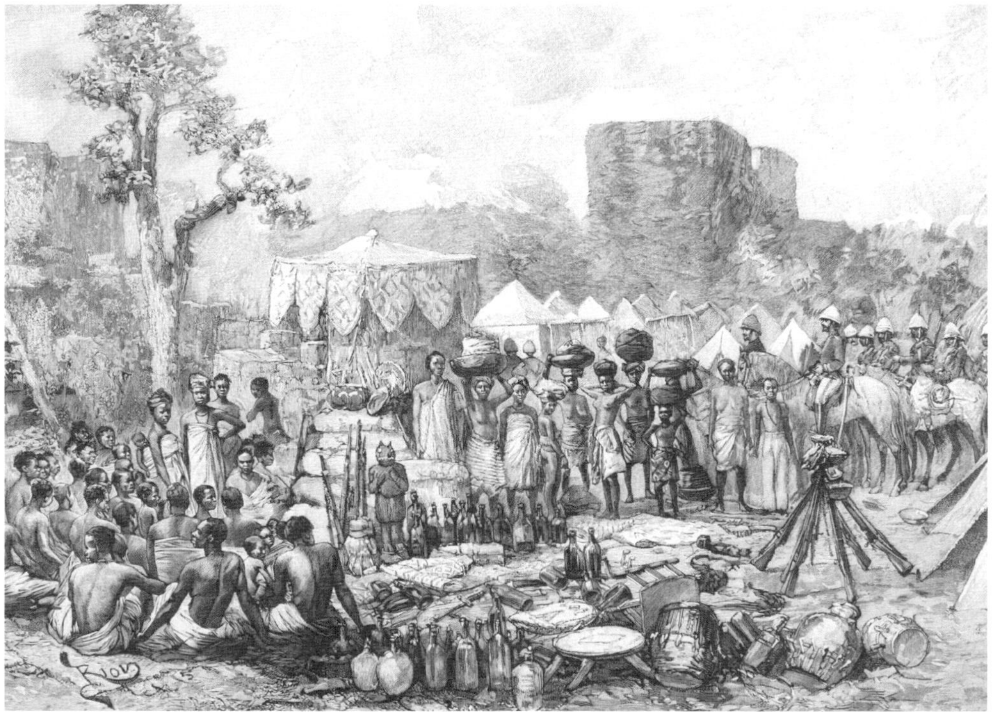

General Dodds's camp at Place Goho in Abomey. Illustration in Alexandre L. d'Albéca, *La France au Dahomey*, 1895.

whole kingdom. The press pitched in before this second war even began. Three months before the start of the campaign, *Le Petit Journal* printed a color lithograph of King Béhanzin, enthroned among skulls and guarded by a woman warrior. "He doesn't speak a single European language," the article remarks. "Our country will easily finish him."[1]

The man who did the finishing was Colonel Alfred-Amédée Dodds, a Senegalese métis and one of the most experienced officers in the French colonies. Dodds had put down riots on the Indian Ocean island of Réunion, led expeditions against the Serer and Fula in Senegal, and played a decisive role in the capture of what is now Hanoi, Vietnam.[2] Now in Dahomey, less than six months after his arrival, he had all but destroyed West Africa's most powerful independent state. His troops entered Abomey on the morning of 17 November, setting up their bivouac in the still-smoking ruins of Béhanzin's palace. They were a mixed bunch—pith-helmeted French marines, Senegalese cavalrymen, allied warriors from the nearby kingdom of Porto-Novo, and hundreds of local porters, two of whom carried Colonel Dodds to the city in a hammock.[3]

Looting began almost immediately after the French flag was hoisted over Béhanzin's palace. The invaders, primed by travelers' tales of Abomey's wealth, were quickly disappointed by the king's leavings—mostly alcohol, textiles, and half-functioning guns. But the mood of anticlimax quickly lifted. Soldiers, drunk on the king's Dutch gin, gamboled through the ruined courtyards in billowing Dahomean skirts, taking shade under the huge appliquéd parasols of courtiers. They turned over the soil, and found under it cannons, blunderbusses, statuettes, bracelets and necklaces of cowrie shell and coral—a city's worth of hurriedly hidden treasures. The clearing before the colonel's tent became "a veritable bazaar" of plunder.[4]

The ordinary soldiers took what they could, anxiously watching the bulging parcels of their officers, whom they suspected of requisitioning the best of the loot. They were right. Dodds, promoted by telegram to the rank of general, had amassed a collection of artifacts including silver scepters, ancestral altars, intricately carved palace doors, and King Béhanzin's golden throne. But the real prize was a set of three therianthropic statues, life-sized half-man, half-animal portraits of Dahomean kings. These were the royal *bocio*, magic battle standards hewn by the court carver,

Sosa Adede, from the trunks of trees. A sword in each hand, looming over the troops, the *bocio* were wheeled to the front lines of battles. They were expected, in urgent circumstances, to come alive and fight.[5]

Le Petit Journal had published lithographs of other "garish … painted gods," captured in an earlier battle, whose powers had failed to save them from "our heroic little soldiers." But it might be nice, an editorialist mused, if the marines brought "us back some of these spiteful guardians of the Dahomeans … they won't miss the wood."[6] The writer got his wish. In 1893, Dodds donated his finest finds, including the three *bocio*, to Paris's Musée d'Ethnographie du Trocadéro. Since then, the three royal *bocio* have been almost continuously on display in Paris—first as trophies, then as ethnographic curiosities, and finally as works of art. Millions of people have seen them, including Pablo Picasso and Guillaume Apollinaire, who visited them at the Trocadéro before it closed in 1935.[7] They were then moved to the ethnographic Musée de l'Homme.

Since 2006, they have been held by the Musée du quai Branly, a controversial rebranding of France's larcenous legacy as a broad-minded homage to non-Western art. The Dahomean *bocio* are mounted on three high cylinders in the main collections hall. Guezo, broad-chested and iron-colored, leaning back as though about to strike; Glele, the lion, his blunt snout snapping with tiny, filed teeth; and Béhanzin, the shark, green as a tank and missing a portion of his fearsome jaw. Frozen in the bent-legged, forearm-out posture of fencers, the statues stand back-to-back in a defensive huddle—staring, as though encircled, at the dimly lit expanse. At the base of each figure, a small plaque reads, "Gift of General Dodds."

. . .

The plunder of art is now recognized as a crime under international law. A latter-day Dodds would have to contend with more than half a century of treaties, the most important of which, the 1954 Hague Convention on the Protection of Cultural Property, was adopted after the looting of European museums and private collections during World War II.[8] This convention

<hr>

Opposite: French soldiers at Cana examine captured Dahomean *bocio*. Unlike the statues taken from Abomey, these were destroyed. Image from *Le Petit Journal: Supplément Illustré*, 26 November 1892. Courtesy Bibliothèque nationale de France.

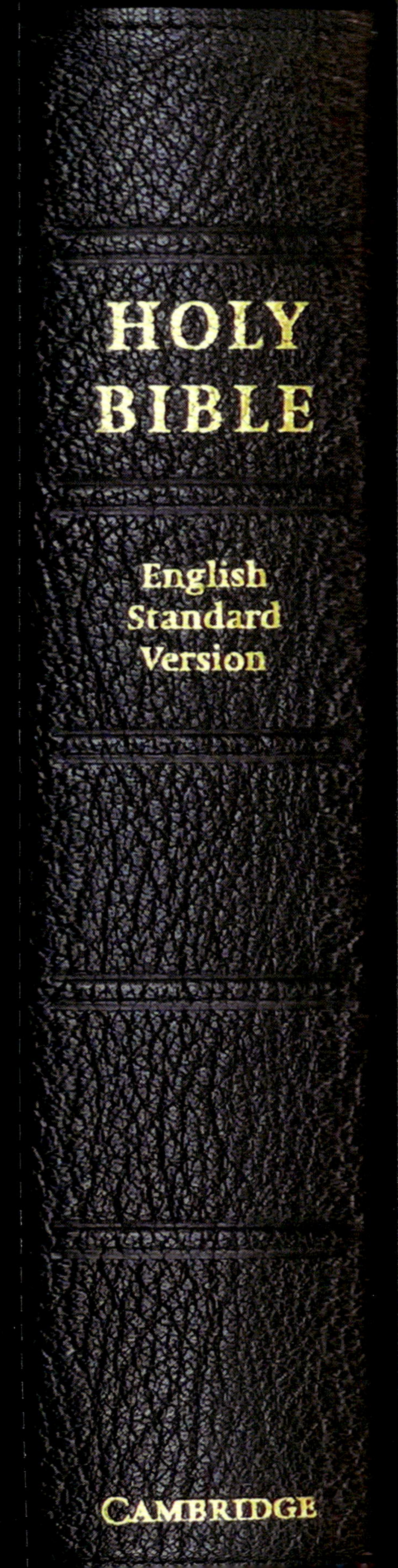

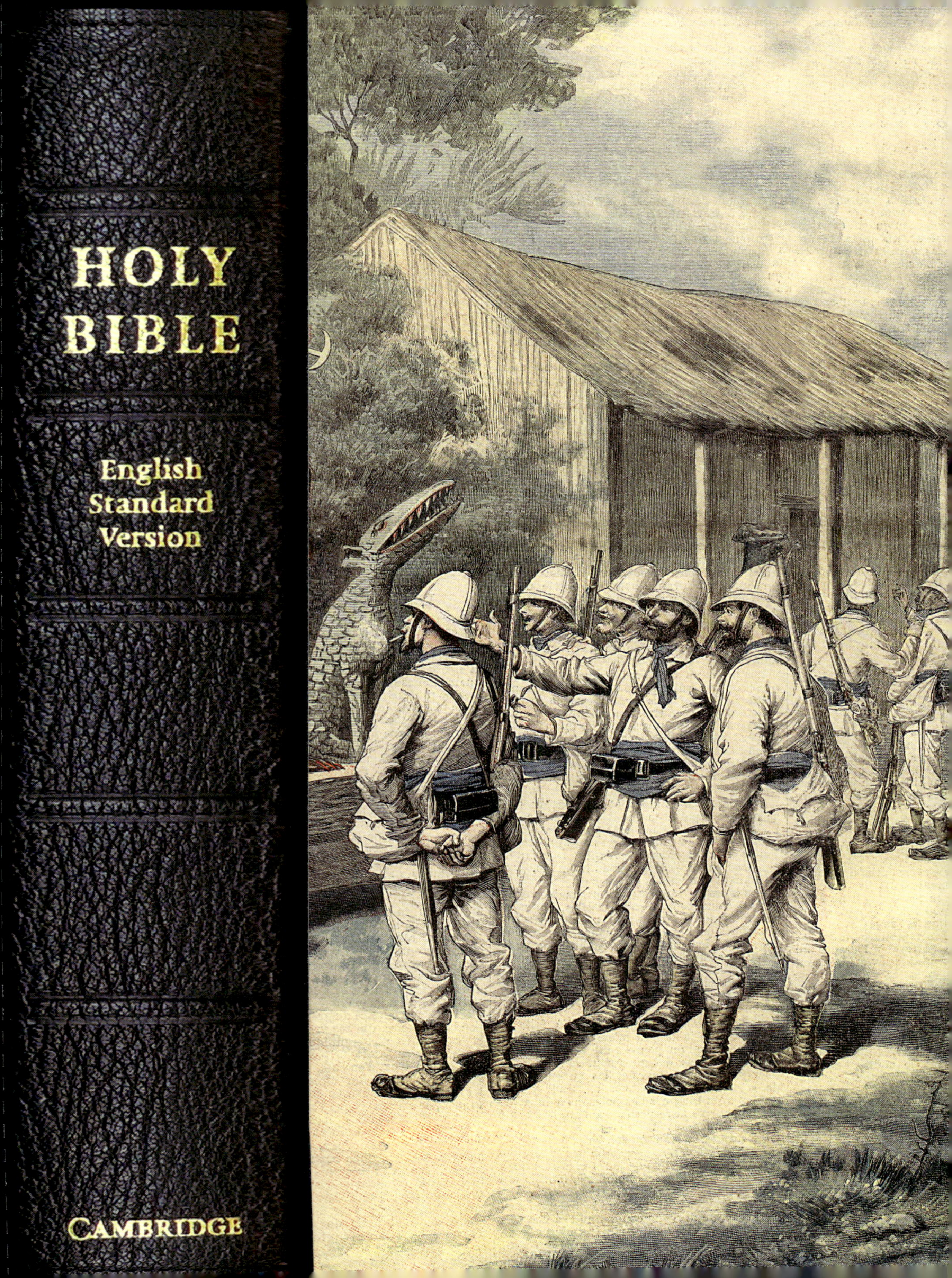

HOLY
BIBLE

English
Standard
Version

CAMBRIDGE

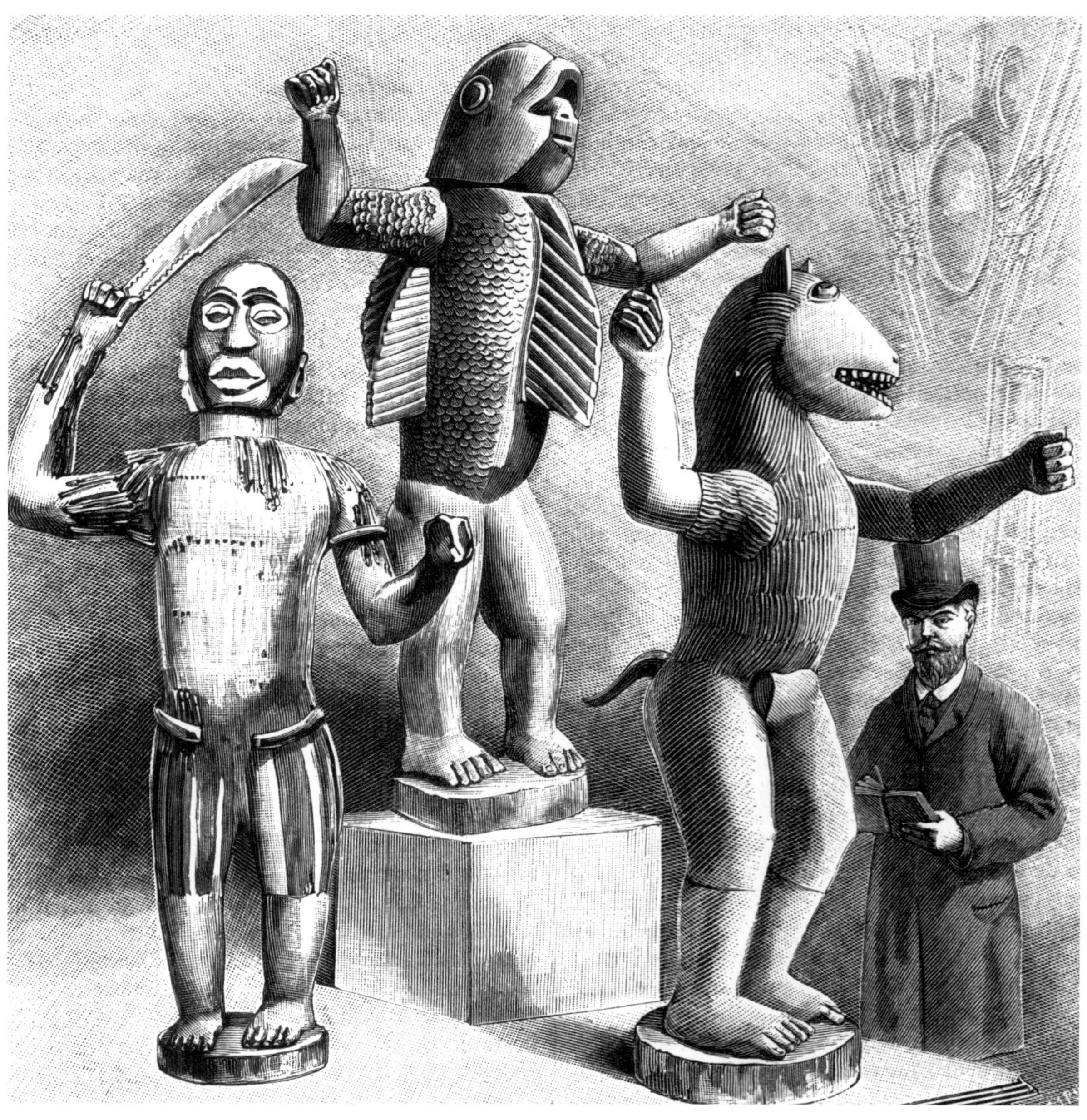

Bocio depicting the Dahomean kings Guezo,
Glele, and Béhanzin exhibited in Paris at the Musée
d'Ethnographie du Trocadéro. From *La Nature*, vol. 22,
no. 1086, 1894. Courtesy Conservatoire numérique
des arts et métiers.

and the treaties that followed it have frequently been observed, even by powerful occupiers with little incentive to do so.[9] But the treasures of Dahomey, stolen sixty years too early, are still subject to the "finders keepers" convention. Excepting the occasional "loan" of smaller pieces to museums in Benin, they seem likely to remain where they are, if not without objection.[10] In 2013, Nicéphore Soglo, former president of Benin, and Louis-George Tin, head of CRAN (the representative council of black associations in France), called for the return of France's "biens mal acquis" (ill-gotten gains) in a strident editorial for *Le Monde*.[11] It was about as effective as Béhanzin's *bocio* were on the battlefield—which is to say, not at all.

But one can dream. In Ishmael Reed's satirical novel *Mumbo Jumbo* (1972), a multinational cell of art thieves called the Mu'tafikah orchestrate an elaborate plan to liberate the "Ikons of aesthetically victimized civilizations" from "Centers of Art Detention" across Europe and America. The masterstroke in their worldwide effort is a heist at the Metropolitan Museum of Art, where they plan to seize a massive Olmec head from Mexico. Art world warriors from every continent,

the members of the Mu'tafikah plan not just to return what was stolen, but to create "renewed enthusiasms" for non-Western traditions.[12] Restoration is not merely a remedy for past injustice, but the beginning of new creation.

One Beninese artist who would make a good Mu'tafikah is Romuald Hazoumè, who recently exhibited an unusual *egungun* at the Fondation Zinsou gallery in Cotonou. This sacred Yoruba masquerade, a representative from ancestral spirits, is traditionally a sumptuous, sequined costume, veiled in a long fall of cowrie shells. But Hazoumè's, no less elaborate, is made of street trash, assembled from the kerosene canisters that litter every corner of motorcycle-choked Cotonou. Garishly red, blue, yellow, and black, it trails its greasy skirts before the reverent crowd—a gathering of canister faces arranged in a semicircle around it. These are only surrogates for the work's ultimate audience. Hazoumè has offered the mask, and others like it, in exchange for the real Yoruba *egungun* detained in Western museums. But he has received no answer. From the world's Centers of Art Detention has come only that sound so familiar to their visitors—silence.

---

1 See Jean Bayol, "Behanzin: Roi du Dahomey," *Le Petit Journal: Supplément Illustré*, 23 April 1892. The original reads: "Il ne parle aucune langue européene. … Notre pays viendra facilement à bout." The entire run of the newspaper is available online at <catalogue.bnf.fr/ark:/12148/cb32836564q>.

2 For biographical information about Alfred-Amédée Dodds, see François Desplantes, *Le général Dodds et l'expédition du Dahomey* (Rouen: Mégard et Cie, 1894).

3 Meanwhile, Béhanzin retreated to the Couffo river, where he became so distraught that he cut off his elderly mother's head. She was to bring the kingdom's pleas for help to her deceased husband, King Glele; the hoped-for ancestral intercession never arrived. Béhanzin would soon be captured and exiled to Martinique. See Edna Bay, *Wives of the Leopard: Gender, Politics, and Culture in the Kingdom of Dahomey* (Charlottesville: University of Virginia Press, 2012), p. 304.

4 Alexandre L. d'Albéca, *La France au Dahomey* (Paris: Librairie Hachette, 1895), p. 111.

The original reads: "Au bout de quelques jours, devant la tente du général, on a un véritable bazar." For other soldiers' accounts, see Jules Poirier, *Campagne du Dahomey* (Paris: Imprimerie Librairie Militaire, 1895); François Michel and Jacques Serre, *La campagne du Dahomey, 1893–1894: La réddition de Béhanzin* (Paris: L'Harmattan, 2001).

5 For an analysis of royal *bocio*, see Suzanne Preston Blier, "Power, Art, and the Mysteries of Rule," in *African Vodun: Art, Psychology, and Power* (Chicago: University of Chicago Press, 1995), pp. 315–346.

6 See "Au Dahomey," *Le Petit Journal: Supplément Illustré*, 26 November 1892. The original reads: "J'espère qu'ils nous rapporteront en revenant quelques-uns de ces mauvais protecteurs des Dahoméens; ceux-ci d'ailleurs seront quittes pour en tailler d'autres; le bois ne leur manque pas." Exhibiting more of the same venomous curiosity, the paper later published an engraving of their fallen enemies' incinerated corpses. The writer of "Crémation des cadavres

dahoméens" in the 3 December 1892 edition of *Le Petit Journal: Supplément Illustré* notes: "Curious detail: After their death, the skin of the Dahomeans flakes off and becomes less black." The original reads: "Détail curieux: Après leur mort, la peau des Dahoméens s'écaille et devient moins noire."

7 For the reception history of the *bocio*, see Julia Kelly, "'Dahomey!, Dahomey!': The Reception of Dahomean Art in France in the Late 19th and Early 20th Centuries," *Journal of Art Historiography*, no. 12 (June 2015), pp. 1–19; Gaëlle Beaujean-Baltzer, "Du trophée à l'œuvre: Parcours de cinq artefacts du royaume d'Abomey," *Gradhiva*, no. 6 (November 2007), pp. 70–85.

8 No similar outrage was occasioned by the expropriation of art from the overseas colonies of European countries, evidence for Martiniquan writer Aimé Césaire's claim that Hitler was unforgivable because he did to Europe what until then had only been done to Europe's colonial subjects. See Aimé Césaire, *Discourse on Colonialism*,

trans. Joan Pinkham (New York: Monthly Review Press, 2000), p. 36.

9 Carol A. Roehrenbeck, "Repatriation of Cultural Property—Who Owns the Past? An Introduction to Approaches and to Selected Statutory Instruments," *International Journal of Legal Information*, vol. 38, no. 2 (Summer 2010), p. 199. After the invasion of Afghanistan, coalition governments returned tens of thousands of stolen artifacts to Kabul's National Museum.

10 To commemorate the centennial of King Béhanzin's death, in 2006 the Musée du quai Branly loaned Beninese museums several small artifacts from its Benin collection. Béhanzin's throne and *bocio* were not among them.

11 Louis-Georges Tin and Nicéphore Soglo, "Appel concernant les biens mal acquis de la France," *Le Monde*, 10 December 2013.

12 All quotations from Ishmael Reed are from *Mumbo Jumbo* (New York: Scribner Paperback Fiction, 1996), p. 15.

INSIDE THE MECHANICAL TURK
The Editors

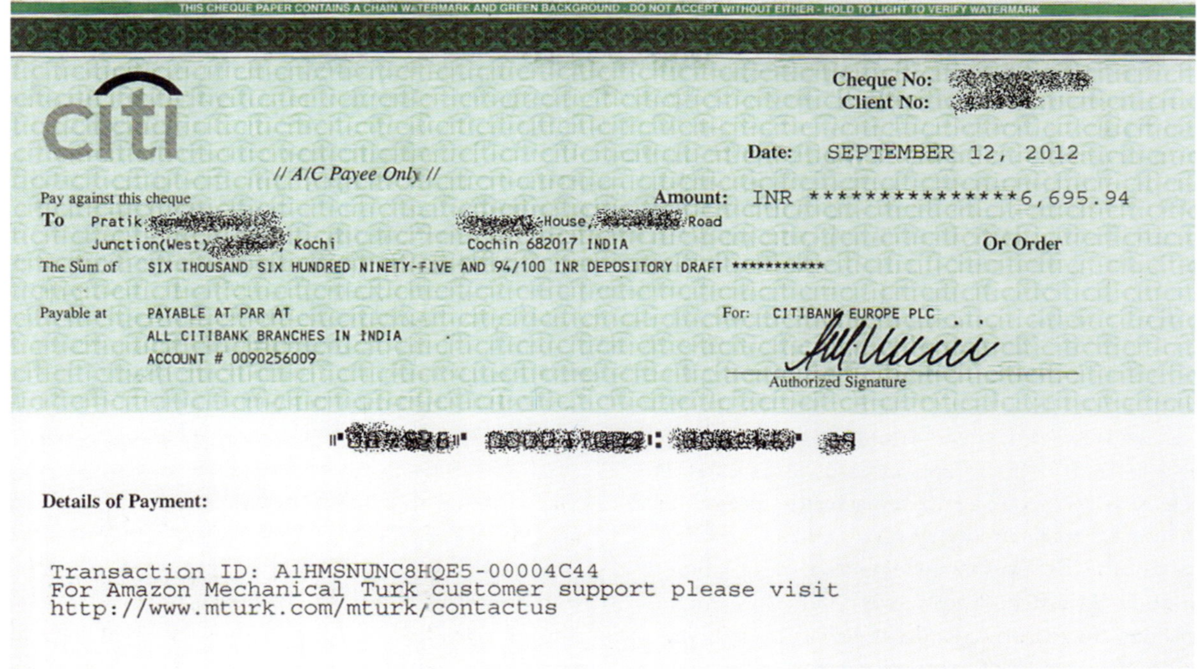

Amazon.com's Mechanical Turk platform is an online labor "exchange," debuted in 2005 by the Internet retailer, in which individuals contract to perform various tasks for others at an agreed-upon rate. Named, with an improbable amount of historical flair, for a celebrated eighteenth-century device—purportedly an extraordinarily skilled chess-playing automaton, it was later found to have in fact been operated by a human player secreted inside the cabinet behind which it sat—the modern-day Mechanical Turk is "a marketplace for work that requires human intelligence," according to Amazon. The platform "gives businesses access to a diverse, on-demand, scalable workforce and gives Workers a selection of thousands of tasks to complete whenever it's convenient." These tasks range from data entry, cataloguing, and transcription to identifying image details, serving as survey subjects, and the like: most are activities that humans do better than machines, most take between a few minutes and a few hours, and all are compensated at exceptionally low rates. The wages offered for the fifty most recently posted HITs—Human Intelligence Tasks, in Amazonian parlance—on the late November afternoon in 2015 on which we are writing this, for example,

range from a high of $2.50 (playing an online multiplayer game and then responding to a survey on it) to a low of $0.01 (more than a dozen tasks, from finding phone numbers and email addresses on a web page to copying down all the purchases on a printed receipt). Amazon charges "requesters," those with available jobs, an additional fee of 20 percent on each transaction. According to its website, there are more than half a million workers in over 190 countries standing ready to take on the 442,274 tasks currently on offer.

It's been roughly a decade since the widespread emergence of large-scale computer-supported work platforms, and labor scholars and policy analysts from bodies such as the Geneva-based International Labor Organization have increasingly begun to turn their research efforts toward the conditions of participants in so-called crowdsourced labor environments.[1] Interested to learn for ourselves what the men and women at work "inside the box" thought about the labor they were performing, *Cabinet* signed up

---

Above: Payment to an Indian Mechanical Turk worker, September 2012. The payment is roughly equivalent to 120 US dollars.

to become a requester and posted the following HIT (directed at US workers because tax laws here make it very complicated to employ foreign freelancers):

Please write an essay of 300–500 words about whether labor can be stolen or not. Do you feel that your labor has been stolen on occasion? Do you feel that this assignment is itself a form of theft, or does the fact that you have taken this assignment mean that it is, by definition, a fair, equitable exchange? Be honest. What we are offering is equivalent to the minimum US federal hourly wage. US workers only.

Enticed by the rate of \$7.25 per text, relatively generous in Mechanical Turkey, we quickly received the ten essays we had requested. Most did not accept that their work was being stolen through either their typical "MTurk" labor or (perhaps not surprisingly) by the essay they were then themselves writing. Many described the various problems encountered with the platform. The most frequent complaint was that requesters sometimes "reject" work, for which they do not pay, for reasons that the respondents felt were capricious—creators of academic surveys, who are apparently frequent users of the service, would seem to be particularly egregious offenders, scratching entire projects due to no fault of the workers. Others discussed attempts to organize *de facto* "unions" to argue for fair treatment and protection. (Amazon's policy is apparently not to intervene in disagreements between requesters and workers.) What follows is a representative sample of the responses, printed verbatim.

WORKER NUMBER: AT3C00TKZK13L
TIME OF SUBMISSION: NOV 20 2015, 09:35 AM PST

I have been on Mturk for about three years now. Theft of labor is one of risks here on the internet. I have been burned a few times when I wrote descriptions and the requester did not pay, and I forgot to check their reviews. Sometimes, the requester is new and does not have enough reputation to go by, and they disappear as soon as they get their work done. It truly is frustrating for workers to complete the work, and then do not get paid. In many occasions, I have seen my work published without my authorization, and it hurts because most of us do this for a living. Labor can definitely be stolen. At Mturk we do not have any rights or protection against abusive requesters. We provide our personal information for tax purposes, but we are effectively contractors. However, we do not know anything about our employers. They do not need to provide their contact information, or even a real name. We can send them an email, but most of the time our correspondence is ignored. Furthermore, according to Mturk, requesters do not have to provide a real reason to reject our work. Labor should also have a set price just like in the real world there are minimum wage laws. In addition, as contractors, we have to pay part of the taxes that a employer normally pays, and that cuts into our revenue even further. There have been movements to promote a fair payment for tasks on the platform, such as we are dynamo, and there have been some changes from big universities regarding academic studies to promote fair pay per minute. The marketplace is varied; some requesters pay extremely well, and others want hours of work for pennies. Part of the problem is that some workers still complete tasks for abysmal pay, which requesters take as that being the ideal pay they should offer. Labor on the internet should have protection for both parties. Workers should be compensated fairly for work completed correctly, and requesters should receive adequate responses to their requests. A balance should be in place to mediate any issues, and there must be accountability for unfair treatment of workers. As of now, there is still uncertainty when you accept a job, complete it correctly, and the requester decides they do not need to pay you for your time and effort. For example, this assignment is fair as long as I get the promised compensation for it. I followed the instructions, and completed the task with care. Once I submitted and I get the reward, the content of this text becomes yours to use as convenient. It is theft when the task is rejected, and the text is used anyway. US based worker. Omaha, Nebraska. 27yo. Male.

WORKER NUMBER: AIOF4ZQQ9UDZ4
TIME OF SUBMISSION: NOV 18 2015, 03:47 PM PST

Absolutely yes. Given the decision most people would tell Wal-Mart to go fuck themselves. Target, Toys'rUs. All of these people depend entirely on employees to exist, yet they pay their employees worse slavery wages. In fact, it would probably cost them more to keep and care for slaves. You have to consider that people are forced into the get money or get punished

status quo. There is no going to live off the land or living simple. You have to get money to pay for land, taxes, permit fees, water wells, well permits, etc. Essentially you are forced to participate and so long as you are being forced then I think it is a crime, and entirely wrong, to pay someone peanuts for work that is, calorie wise, probably greater than most of the investors and executives in the company spend. I think that a company that relies entirely on the efforts of their employees to exist as a company OWES the workers a fair share of the profits and that laws should actually be changed to ensure that this happens. If we were not forced to work I wouldn't think this, but we are, so if we are forced to participate then we are owed. Now, there is "the american dream" to consider. What about going on your own and building a company and become rich and...okay shut up right there. Who is going to do all the work in that company? Yeah, that's what I thought. So no, it's not a matter of people agreeing to work for a certain amount of money, we are forced to work for what is offered. Most college students who are highly skilled aren't even going to find a good job anymore. Don't even get me started on how illegal immigration is a serious theft of labor by driving up the employers supply of workers and driving down the wages they're willing to pay.

WORKER NUMBER: AK7LGB1QOGA1P
TIME OF SUBMISSION: NOV 19 2015, 10:22 AM PST

Labor can and has been stolen, but what most people consider as "stolen labor" today is nothing more than a failure to negotiate. An employer states what they want done and how much they will pay. A candidate for the position can decide if they believe that their labor is worth the amount, or more, than what is being offered. As long as they are free to make that decision, no laws are broken, and people are paid for their efforts, then no labor is being stolen. In fact, the opposite is happening. It's not labor that's being stolen, it's pay that is being stolen. The agreement was that the employee would do certain tasks for the employer for a certain amount. The employer has been following through on their end of the agreement, but in some cases, the employee is not by showing up late, going home early, taking long breaks, picking and choosing which tasks will be done, calling in sick, etc If the employee feels that they deserve more, then they need

to negotiate for more. If the employer refuses to negotiate, or the outcome is still not to the employee's liking, the employee has the choice to leave and find employment elsewhere. The employee is always free to leave. That's not to say that labor cannot be stolen, despite an agreement. An example of labor stolen is what happened in a company many years ago. The company had advised the workers that there was no over time pay for any of the hourly workers. The reason given was that, according to the company, they already paid a very good wage for all worked hours, so it "all evened out" in the end. A couple of years passed and a lawsuit was started against the company for not paying over time. As one may guess, just because a company pays a decent wage for all hours, it does not mean that a company does not have to pay over time hours for their hourly workers. It also does not matter if the employee agreed to the terms at the time they were hired. What the company did was against the law - and in that case, yes, the labor was stolen. If laws are being broken, it is absolutely possible that labor can and has been stolen. If pay is being withheld, despite a person's efforts, then yes, one could consider that stolen labor. However, low pay for a job does not equal stolen labor.

WORKER NUMBER: A2O5OJXCUFQ3FV
TIME OF SUBMISSION: NOV 19 2015, 09:30 AM PST

I believe labor is always going to be needed in our society. Thousands of years ago we dreamed of having unlimited labor force to accomplish anything and everything. Now in the twenty first century we have not only the huge massive human work force but also we have the machine work force too. This has created the supply of labor to be far more then the actual labor itself. Therefore we have to figure out how to evenly disperse these jobs. When we start picking out who gets this profession and who gets this education we start to lose focus on fairness and equitable exchange. When we decide some countries deserve more soldiers then others we hurt our human rights. The only way to be comfortable with this huge worf force we now have is we have to have a community of people who do not need to work and they just need to live their lives with their family. It is surprising how every one who who hits sixteen years old has to go out and start looking for a career. They are unsure about what they want and for our last generation to push this kind of need for work

on us is not going to help the overall equal economy. It is clear now that we must make peace with over-population and not force everyone to work to eat and sleep safely. If that does mean leaving a huge portion of citizens under no government law in a populated area that should be fine. As long as you are on that side you do not have to worry about fighting for labor or finding a career to pay the bill. Labor should be something we take pride in and not something we want to own and not share. WE have turned this view on labor to be our survival. All a human needs is water and some break to live. Why do why need 18 years of schooling to fight for the right type of labor that can assure my families stability?

WORKER NUMBER: A149ROBL26JWPJ
TIME OF SUBMISSION: NOV 19 2015, 10:54 AM PST

As an experienced MTurk worker who's reasonably curious about various ethical and economic elements of work and labor, I think it is interesting to consider the economic relationship between MTurk users and requesters. In an increasingly globalized economy, I can see this type of business relationship becoming more and more common, so I think it is important to analyze this kind of economic model. As someone with libertarian leanings, a mindset that I feel is often shared among a minority of Turkers (although some of the most successful users seem to lean this way), I find MTurk fascinating, yet as a user, I also find it somewhat frustrating. Amazon has a generally non-interventionist policy regarding MTurk, and, as a result, users really have no formal recourse when work is rejected. Workers who have work rejected some-times feel like they were wronged and that their labor was "stolen". More experienced users, more likely to hold above-mentioned non-interventionist/libertarian views, typically shrug off rejected work, as their more experienced accounts are not affected by the slight "rating" decrease, and they understand that their lost time and productivity are sunk costs. Newer workers, however, will often demand intervention from groups like academic IRBs and Amazon itself. They often bemoan the loss of their time and labor, especially when this is one of their first rejections. However, I do not agree with the assertion that individuals' labor is being "stolen" here, because I don't think this is some-thing that can happen in this economic arrangement.

I feel the only forms of economic relationships that constitute "stealing" labor involve outright slavery and extreme forms of indentured servitude - in most other cases, people are free to opt in and out of economic relationships. Even if one side is favored in "negotia-tions", the other party is not obligated to consent. Also, I feel like rejected work is not necessarily "stolen" anyway—work is typically not maliciously rejected by requesters. Many rejects stem from poor work quality/results due to ignorance of how the platform works, or miscommunication between parties, in terms of expectations, formatting, etc. Requesters sometimes have unrealistic expectations of the work that they will receive relative to their pay, and some scamming workers unfortunately essentially submit useless data - from the requesters' perspective, I can see not wanting to pay someone who has submitted cherry-picked "N/A" or "not found" answers, even if the information was technically unavailable. Ultimately, workers must develop "professional judgement" to help determine if their work will be rejected. I was able to use said judgement in determining whether or not to accept this assignment, and I felt confident doing so, so I wouldn't say my work is being "stolen" here (assuming it is accepted!). In summary, I feel it is fundamentally impossible for one's labor to be "stolen" on a platform like this - individuals have freedom to select work "contracts", even if they have little leverage in nego-tiating them—and workers that think otherwise are misinformed about the site's fundamental nature.

1 For a useful recent study that considers the working conditions of crowdsourced laborers, see David Martin, Benjamin V. Hanrahan, Jacki O'Neill, and Neha Gupta, "Being a Turker," in *Proceedings of the 17th ACM Conference on Computer-Supported Cooperative Work and Social Computing* (New York: Associat on for Computer Machinery, 2014), pp. 224–235. Available at <hci.cs.uwaterloo.ca/faculty/elaw/cs889/reading/p224-martin.pdf>.

While preparing the report on our recent visit to our Andalusian outpost (see "Jubrique Update"), we were thrilled to receive an email from our friends at *Lapham's Quarterly* inviting us to join them for "Coexistence of Cultures & Faiths: A Voyage to the Historic Cities of Morocco & Andalusia," a twelve-day intellectual holiday cruise aboard the luxury ship *L'Austral*. The chance to return to southern Spain, this time while engaged in "open-ended conversation with some of the leading public intellectuals of our generation," was, needless to say, enormously enticing. Alas, after outfitting the staff with the cravats and fountain pens appropriate to such an occasion, we found that *Cabinet*'s edutainment budget could no longer cover the $14,790 per person needed to participate in this adventure for "discerning travelers." But all is not lost. Inspired by the *Lapham* model, *Cabinet* is pleased to announce that it too will stage a cruise of sorts this coming spring—"Barely Staying Afloat: An Aquatic-Intellectual Voyage up the Gowanus." Stay tuned for more information.

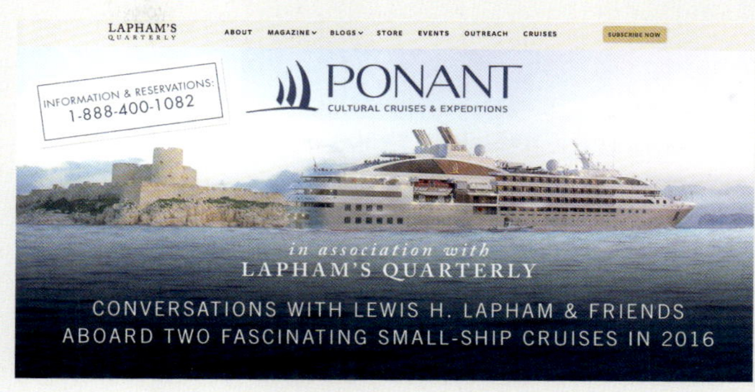

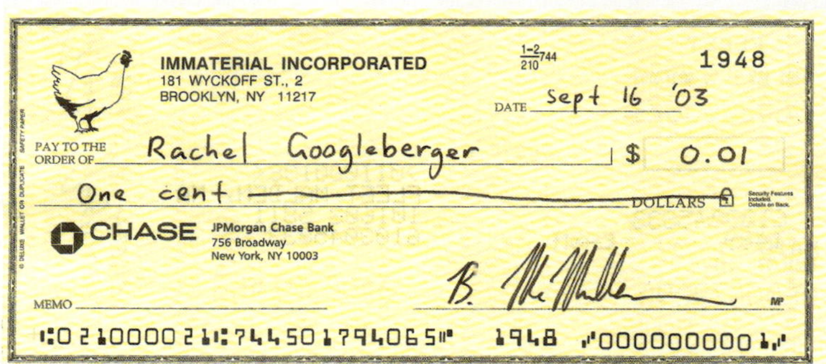

In addition to its obvious edificatory effects, our cruise will also hopefully serve as a fundraiser to help recover our losses from the fountain pen and cravat fiasco. However, we've also recently discovered an alternative fundraising strategy, namely, recashing previously cashed old checks. As ultra-veteran *Cabinet* readers may remember, in 2003 we met curator Rachel Gugelberger, whose improbably wonderful surname provided the occasion for us to issue her thirty checks—one a day, each in the amount of one cent, and each to an increasingly far-fetched misrendering of her family moniker (examples included Mrs. Web Utility Meat Sandwich, Emperor Ra'l Go'r, and May'Shel Kukenperker.) To our and Gugelberger's surprise, her bank cashed twenty-eight of the thirty checks. (One was refused because we had forgotten to write out the amount, and one was lost by Gugelberger.). We printed the fronts and backs of all the cashed checks in *Cabinet* no. 14 and also featured them on our website.

Imagine our bewilderment when a recent bank statement showed check number 1948, dated 16 September 2003, as recently deposited. Although only one cent, this return of the repressed prevented us from balancing our books for that month. Had the bank made an error? Had Gugelberger fallen on such hard times that upon discovering the long-lost check in some drawer she had decided to get her penny's worth? A quick glance at the old issue confirmed that the check in question had in fact long since been cashed, and as old-timers will remember, cashed checks in 2003 were physically returned to the issuer, which meant that the original check could not have been recashed, accidentally or otherwise. By looking online at our bank's scan of the front and back of the recashed check, it became clear that someone had in fact used the new-fangled "mobile deposit" option to redeposit a facsimile of the original check created by scanning its front from the magazine or our website, and pairing it with the pristine back of an unrelated check, which s/he then endorsed. As we go to press, we are reconciled to the prank (which is in the spirit of the original) but our books remain unreconciled. Our bank is eager to open an investigation because such an action, even if it concerns a negligible sum, nevertheless constitutes forgery of a financial instrument protected by federal law. We are not keen to follow our bank's advice. Although this has added to our administrative workload this month, we also have some admiration for the stunt in that it carries an element of genuine risk as well as demonstrating a certain level of artistry. A warning! We are old-fashioned and admire originality; anyone who copies this caper can expect a visit from the bunco squad.

The obvious criminal elements in our readership put us in mind of a recent discussion that occupied a good part of an afternoon here. While editing Jerry Toner's article, we learned that thieves in the Roman Empire were punished on a graduated scale of guilt based on whether or not they had been "caught in the act," a concept in Roman law that was largely a matter of proximity to the scene of the crime. Roman lawyers apparently could not agree what exactly the spatial parameters for "catching someone in the act" were. Ten feet from the victim's house? A hundred? As is often the case, we moderns first enjoyed a snicker at an archaic practice, one that apparently could not systematically establish at what distance from a crime one could be said to still be "caught in the act." And then we realized that we also have absolutely no idea what this apparently very familiar concept means in practice. If a criminal is in your apartment stealing your cravat and fountain pen and is interrupted by the police, we would certainly say that he has been caught in the act. Is the act over the minute he has left your private property? It would seem safe to say that the act has concluded when he has returned to his own apartment and stashed the loot for his spring trip to Andalusia and Morocco. If apprehended there, we would not say that he had been caught in the act, even if his apartment were next door to yours. But what if he lives in a different neighborhood; is he caught in the act if he is apprehended walking back to his home a mile away? Or does the thief in fact decide when the act is concluded? A nervous criminal might still feel himself to be "in the act" halfway across town, whereas the very cool customer might even celebrate at your neighborhood bar, content in the knowledge that the deed is done. The question finally lies at the intersection of spatial, temporal, and psychological considerations that give us new respect for the conundrum with which our Roman friends also wrestled.

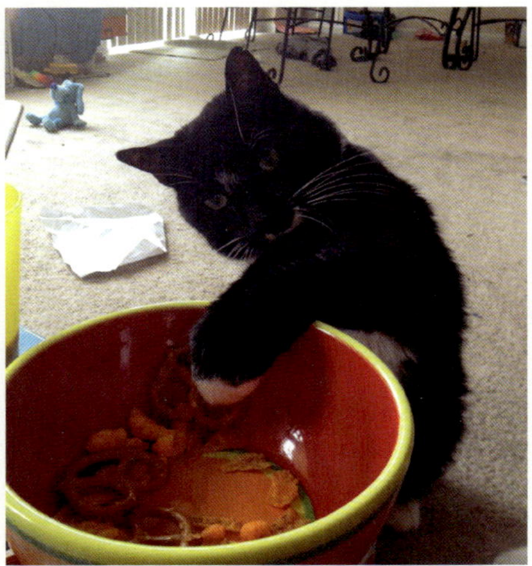

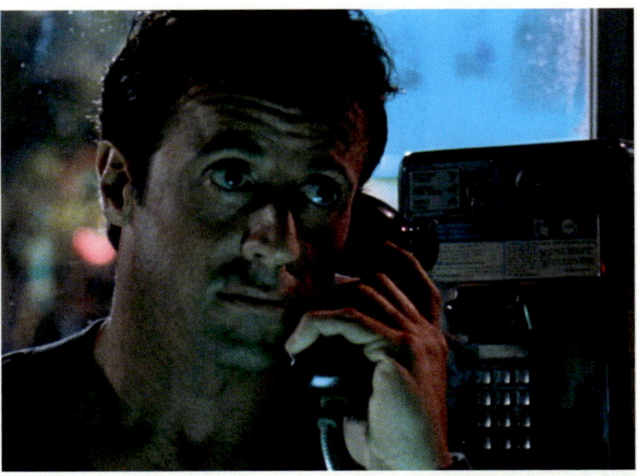

While researching this issue, we read a terrific article written by Ron Rosenbaum in 1971 on "phreaking," all the ways in which the US phone system could at that time be manipulated using various sounds. It included this quote from a dealer who is selling phreaking devices to the Mafia:

I wouldn't mind seeing them [the Bell telephone company] screwed. A telephone isn't private anymore. … And you know what else. You don't hear silences on the phone anymore. They've got this time-sharing thing on long-distance lines where you make a pause and they snip out that piece of time and use it to carry part of somebody else's conversation. Instead of a pause, where somebody's maybe breathing or sighing, you get this blank hole and you only start hearing again when someone says a word and even the beginning of the word is clipped off. Silences don't count—you're paying for them, but they take them away from you. It's not cool to talk, and you can't hear someone when they don't talk. What the hell good is the phone? I wouldn't mind seeing them totally screwed.

Makes one nostalgic for the days when one could be nostalgic that human silences were being stolen and replaced by automated machine silences.

Panorama of the City of New York, Queens Museum.
Photography: Spencer Lowell

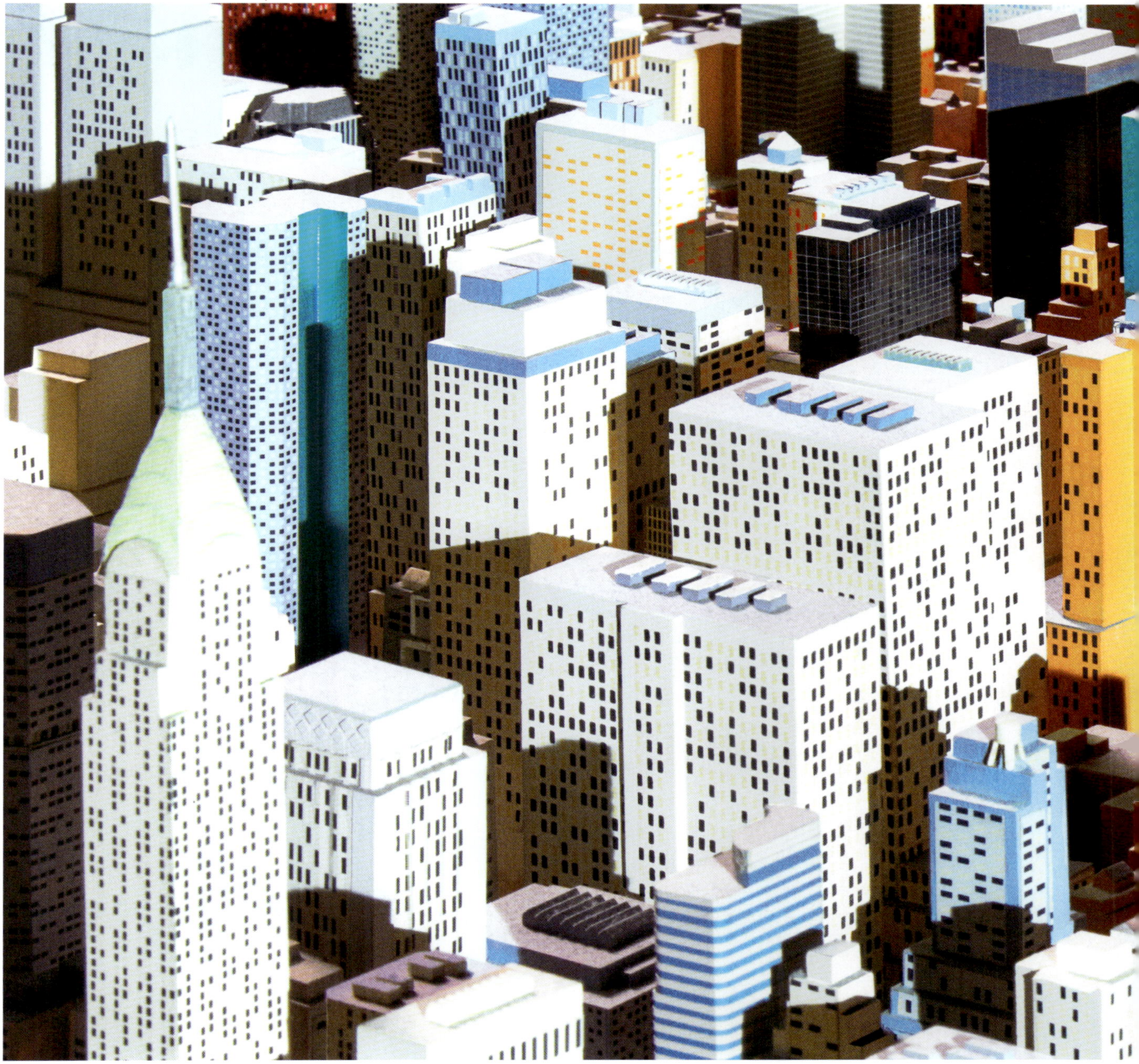

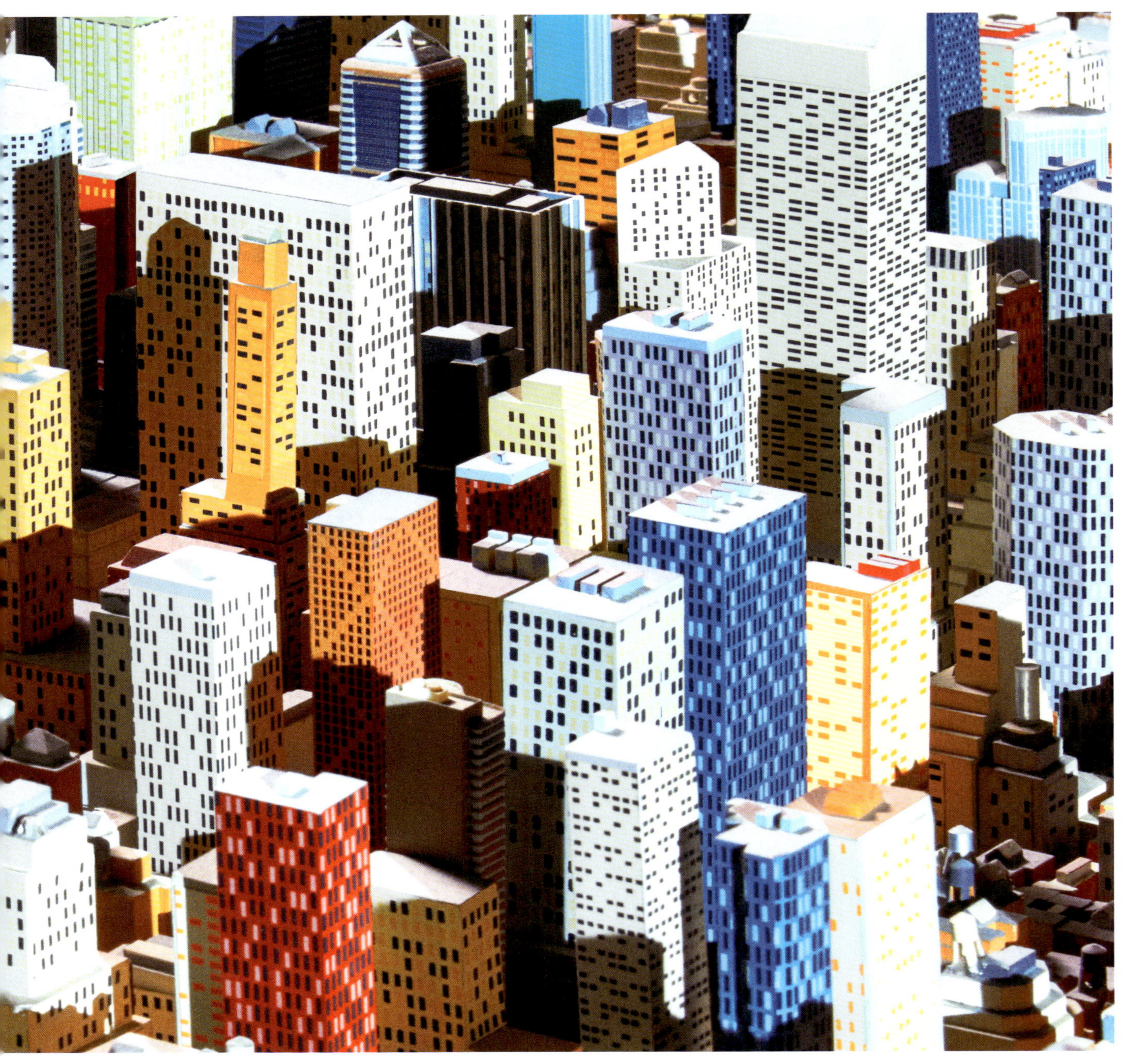
New York
Randall's Island Park
May 5–8, 2016
Preview Day
Wednesday, May 4
frieze.com

FRIEZE
ART
FAIR

Main sponsor
Deutsche Bank

Contemporary Art

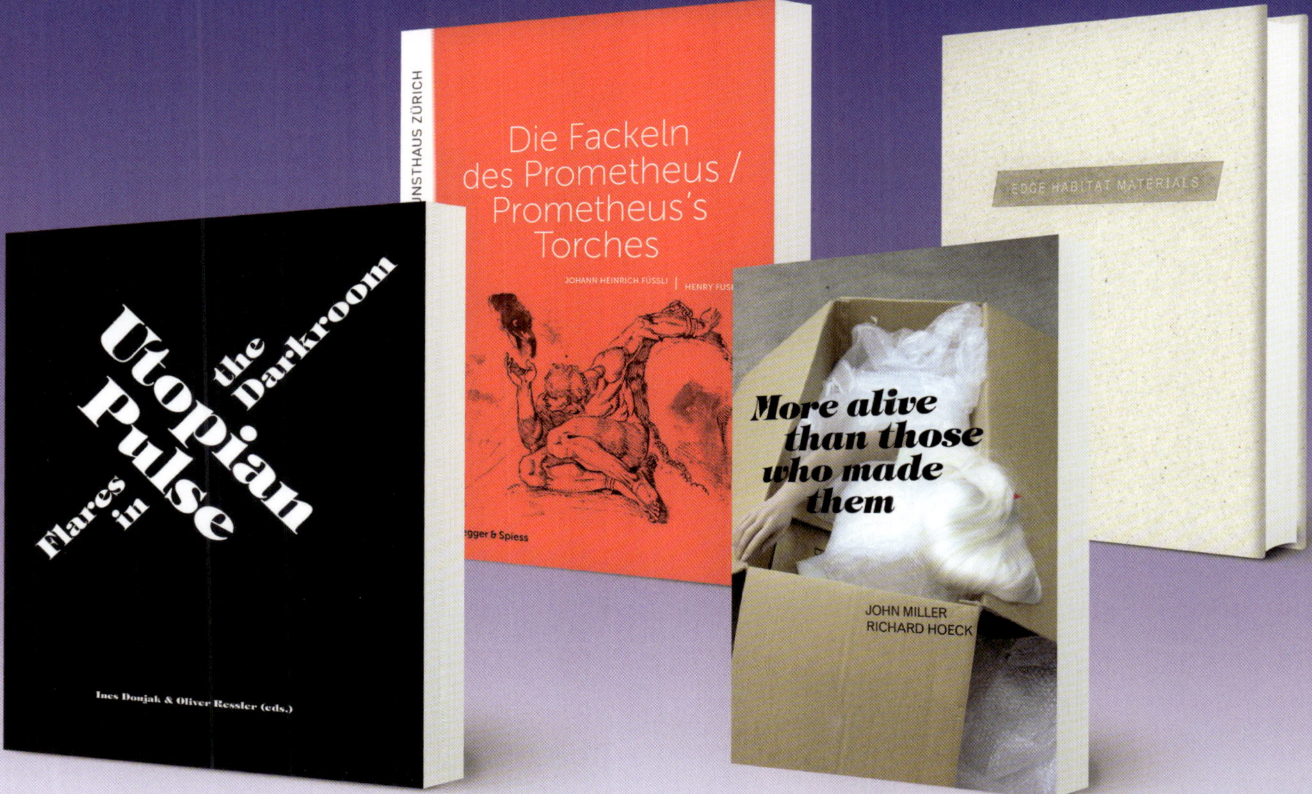

e-flux

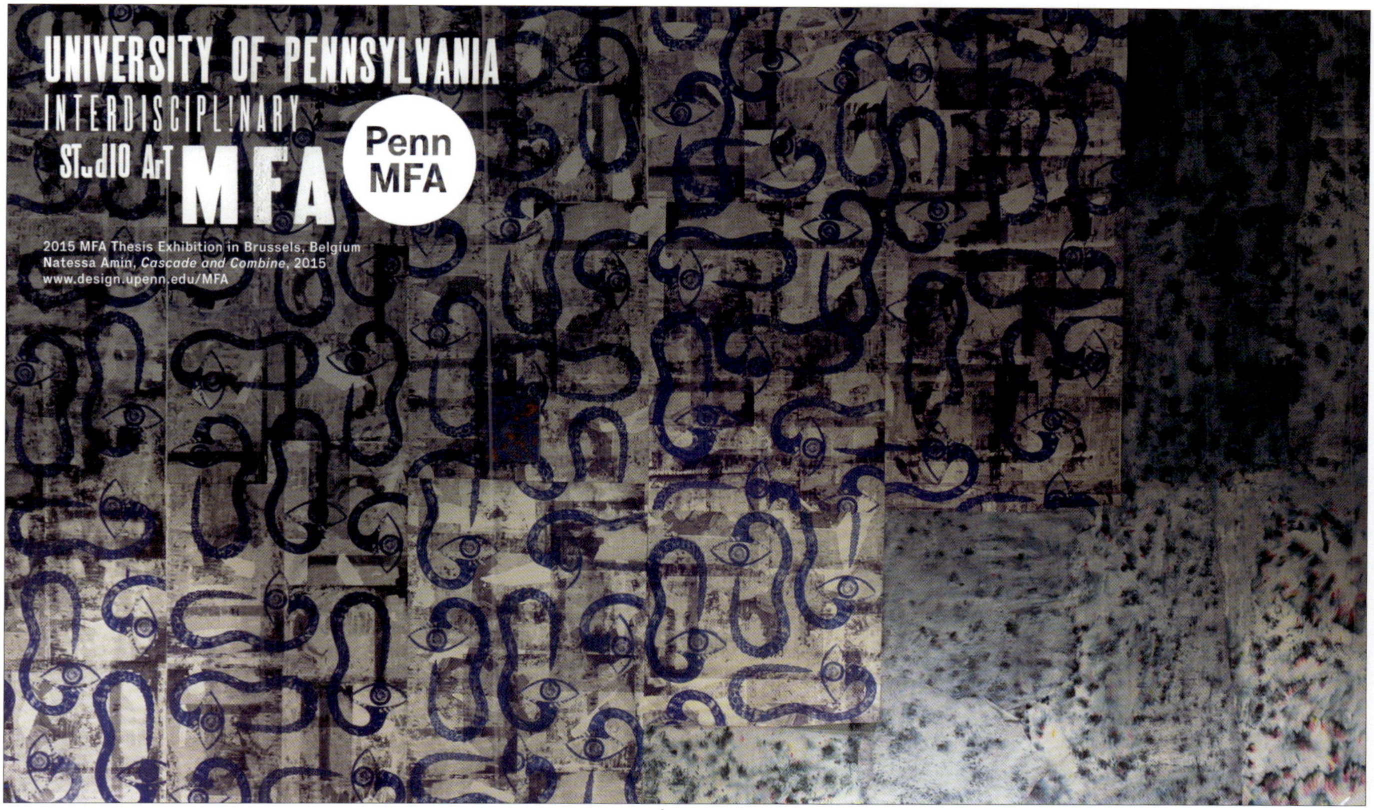

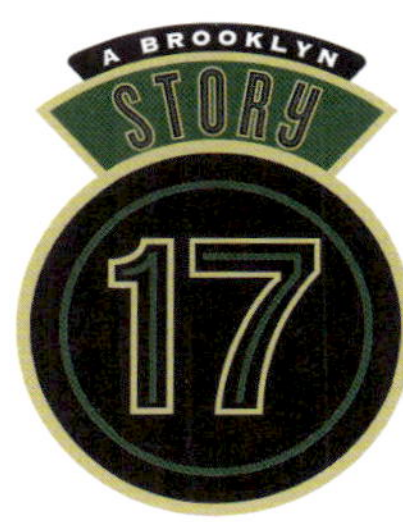

My first batch of homebrew was a disaster. The beer itself was passable, a well-balanced amber ale made with malt extract and cascade hops acquired at the only homebrew shop in New York City in 1984, Milan Laboratory on Spring Street in Soho. Milan was run by two brothers who inherited the business from their father who was reputedly a wizard at home winemaking. Beer brewing was a small part of their business. I took their advice on a few of my early beer making efforts, but, like many early craft brewers, I later came to rely on home brewing guru Charlie Papazian's "The Complete Joy of Homebrewing." Back to my first batch. The beer was fine. The problems began after I siphoned it into 12-ounce bottles and attempted to seal the bottles with tin bottle caps. The device for crimping the bottle caps around the lip of the bottle was called a hammer-capper. It was a circular steel collar that fit snugly over the bottle cap. The idea was to strike the collar with a hammer, forcing the bottle cap to crimp over the lip of the bottle. The first dozen or so bottles I attempted to cap shattered. At some point, I cut my hand on the broken glass. My temper flared. The kitchen was a mess. My wife Ellen herded the children out of the kitchen. I think I salvaged six bottles of a 48 bottle batch. Shortly after that, I purchased a lever capper that eased the caps onto the bottles. I was on my way to starting a brewery.

Steve Hindy
co-founder

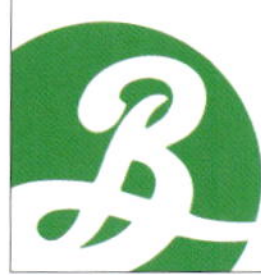

The James Gallery

centerforthehumanities.org/james-gallery

THE GRADUATE CENTER
CITY UNIVERSITY OF NEW YORK

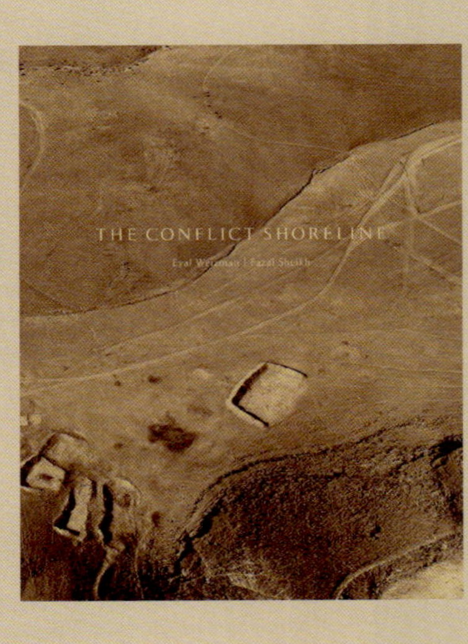

THE CONFLICT SHORELINE: COLONIZATION AS CLIMATE CHANGE IN THE NEGEV DESERT
Text by Eyal Weizman; photographs by Fazal Sheikh

Published by Steidl in association with Cabinet Books
$29 ($22 for subscribers)

Available now at cabinetmagazine.org / books

UNITED STATES POSTAL SERVICE ® — Statement of Ownership, Management, and Circulation (All Periodicals Publications Except Requester Publications)

1. Publication Title	2. Publication Number	3. Filing Date
Cabinet	0 2 0 – 3 4 8	10/23/2015

4. Issue Frequency	5. Number of Issues Published Annually	6. Annual Subscription Price
quarterly	4	$32

7. Complete Mailing Address of Known Office of Publication (Not printer) (Street, city, county, state, and ZIP+4®)
181 Wyckoff Street, Brooklyn NY 11217

Contact Person: Sina Najafi
Telephone (Include area code): 718 222 8434

8. Complete Mailing Address of Headquarters or General Business Office of Publisher (Not printer)
181 Wyckoff Street, Brooklyn NY 11217

9. Full Names and Complete Mailing Addresses of Publisher, Editor, and Managing Editor (Do not leave blank)

Publisher (Name and complete mailing address)
Immaterial Incorporated, 181 Wyckoff Street, Brooklyn NY 11217

Editor (Name and complete mailing address)
Sina Najafi, 181 Wyckoff Street, Brooklyn NY 11217

Managing Editor (Name and complete mailing address)
none

10. Owner (Do not leave blank. If the publication is owned by a corporation, give the name and address of the corporation immediately followed by the names and addresses of all stockholders owning or holding 1 percent or more of the total amount of stock. If not owned by a corporation, give the names and addresses of the individual owners. If owned by a partnership or other unincorporated firm, give its name and address as well as those of each individual owner. If the publication is published by a nonprofit organization, give its name and address.)

Full Name	Complete Mailing Address
Immaterial Incorporated	181 Wyckoff Street Brooklyn NY 11217

11. Known Bondholders, Mortgagees, and Other Security Holders Owning or Holding 1 Percent or More of Total Amount of Bonds, Mortgages, or Other Securities. If none, check box ▶ ☒ None

Full Name	Complete Mailing Address

12. Tax Status (For completion by nonprofit organizations authorized to mail at nonprofit rates) (Check one)
The purpose, function, and nonprofit status of this organization and the exempt status for federal income tax purposes
☒ Has Not Changed During Preceding 12 Months
☐ Has Changed During Preceding 12 Months (Publisher must submit explanation of change with this statement)

PS Form **3526**, July 2014 [Page 1 of 4 (see instructions page 4)] PSN: 7530-01-000-9931 **PRIVACY NOTICE:** See our privacy policy on www.usps.com

---

13. Publication Title	14. Issue Date for Circulation Data Below
Cabinet	2/15/2015

15. Extent and Nature of Circulation			Average No. Copies Each Issue During Preceding 12 Months	No. Copies of Single Issue Published Nearest to Filing Date
a. Total Number of Copies (Net press run)			9,709	9,500
b. Paid Circulation (By Mail and Outside the Mail)	(1)	Mailed Outside-County Paid Subscriptions Stated on PS Form 3541 (Include paid distribution above nominal rate, advertiser's proof copies, and exchange copies)	2,837	2,667
	(2)	Mailed In-County Paid Subscriptions Stated on PS Form 3541 (Include paid distribution above nominal rate, advertiser's proof copies, and exchange copies)	0	0
	(3)	Paid Distribution Outside the Mails Including Sales Through Dealers and Carriers, Street Vendors, Counter Sales, and Other Paid Distribution Outside USPS®	4,894	4,747
	(4)	Paid Distribution by Other Classes of Mail Through the USPS (e.g. First-Class Mail®)	481	354
c. Total Paid Distribution [Sum of 15b (1), (2), (3), and (4)] ▶			8,212	7,768
d. Free or Nominal Rate Distribution (By Mail and Outside the Mail)	(1)	Free or Nominal Rate Outside-County Copies included on PS Form 3541	0	0
	(2)	Free or Nominal Rate In-County Copies Included on PS Form 3541	0	0
	(3)	Free or Nominal Rate Copies Mailed at Other Classes Through the USPS (e.g. First-Class Mail)	17	15
	(4)	Free or Nominal Rate Distribution Outside the Mail (Carriers or other means)	124	105
e. Total Free or Nominal Rate Distribution (Sum of 15d (1), (2), (3) and (4))			141	120
f. Total Distribution (Sum of 15c and 15e) ▶			8,353	7,888
g. Copies not Distributed (See Instructions to Publishers #4 (page #3)) ▶			1,356	1,612
h. Total (Sum of 15f and g)			9,709	9,500
i. Percent Paid (15c divided by 15f times 100) ▶			98.31%	98.48%

17. Publication of Statement of Ownership

☒ If the publication is a general publication, publication of this statement is required. Will be printed in the **January 2016** issue of this publication.   ☐ Publication not required.

18. Signature and Title of Editor, Publisher, Business Manager, or Owner — Date

Sina Najafi, Editor-in-chief   10/23/2015

I certify that all information furnished on this form is true and complete. I understand that anyone who furnishes false or misleading information on this form or who omits material or information requested on the form may be subject to criminal sanctions (including fines and imprisonment) and/or civil sanctions (including civil penalties).

PS Form **3526**, July 2014 (Page 2 of 4)

HOW TO ORDER
1. Mail a check to Ca
   Brooklyn, NY 1121
2. Shop online at <ca
3. Call +1 718 222 8
4. Fax +1 718 222 3'

Checks, made out to
US bank. We also acc
(paypal@cabinetmaga
Visit <cabinetmagazir
editions, posters, and

See also www.cabinetmagazine.org

CABINET BOOKS
Prices include postag

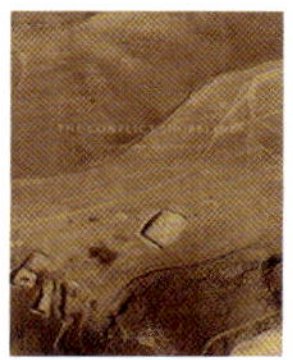

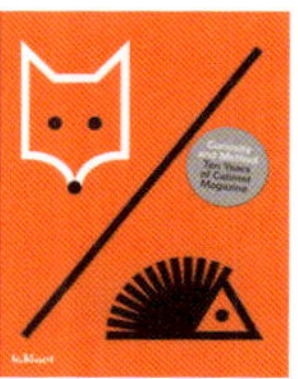

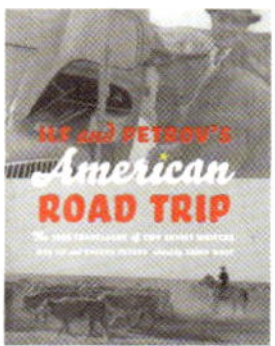

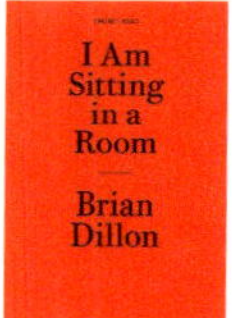

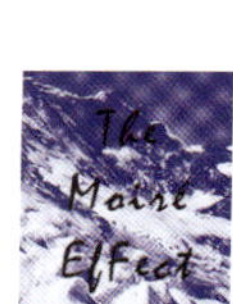

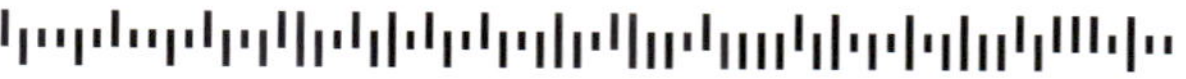

Bonus anecdote from *Cabinet* no. 58 ("Theft"):

In 1998, the recently formed country of Bosnia announced a competition for a new national anthem. The winning entry came courtesy of Dusan Sestic, a Serbian composer. For his trouble, he was promptly labeled a traitor by some fellow Serbs even as he incurred the wrath of Bosniaks unhappy that an ethnic Serb had written their national anthem. In 2009, Sestic ran into even more trouble. His anthem, it turned out, was curiously similar to the opening music of *National Lampoon's Animal House*. Sestic is adamant that he did not plagiarize the tune, suggesting that perhaps a repressed childhood memory of the film's theme influenced his composition.

Source: Alex Marshall, *Republic or Death! Travels in Search of National Anthems* (Random House, 2015).

CABINET
300 Nevins Street
Brooklyn, NY 11217 USA
phone + 1 718 222-8434
fax + 1 718 222-3700
info@cabinetmagazine.org
www.cabinetmagazine.org

Issue 64, Summer 2017

Cover: Cleaning Jefferson's nose. A team from Kärcher, a German company specializing in large-scale cleaning projects, uses pressure washers to blast lichen and other organic material off the presidents' faces at Mount Rushmore. The project began on 4 July 2005 and was completed in early August 2005.

Cabinet (ISSN 1531-1430, USPS # 020-348) is a quarterly magazine published by Immaterial Incorporated, 181 Wyckoff Street, Brooklyn, NY 11217. Periodicals Postage paid at Brooklyn, NY, and additional mailing offices.

POSTMASTER: Please send address changes to Cabinet, 300 Nevins Street, Brooklyn, NY 11217.

Printed in Belgium by Die Keure, whose printing plant smells the best.

ADVERTISING
phone + 1 718 222-8434
advertising@cabinetmagazine.org

DISTRIBUTION
Cabinet is available in the US and Canada through Disticor, which distributes both using its own network and through Ingram, Ubiquity, Small Changes, Cowley Distribution, Kent News, MSolutions, the News Group, Chris Stadler, and Don Olson Distribution.

To carry Cabinet through one of these distributors, contact Melanie Raucci at Disticor: phone + 1 631 587-1160, mraucci@disticor.com

Cabinet is available in Europe and elsewhere through Central Books, London: orders@centralbooks.com

Cabinet is available worldwide as a book, with an ISBN, through DAP: phone + 1 212 627-1999, dap@dapinc.com

For further information, contact: circulation@cabinetmagazine.org

INDIVIDUAL SUBSCRIPTIONS

1 year (4 issues):	2 years (8 issues):
US $32	US $60
Canada $38	Canada $72
Western Europe $40	Western Europe $76
Elsewhere $50	Elsewhere $96

Please send a check in US dollars made out to "Cabinet," or mail, fax, or email us your Visa/MC/AmEx/Discover info to:

300 Nevins Street
Brooklyn, NY 11217 USA
phone + 1 718 222-8434
fax + 1 718 222-3700
subscriptions@cabinetmagazine.org
www.cabinetmagazine.org/subscribe

INSTITUTIONAL SUBSCRIPTIONS
Institutional subscriptions are available through library agencies such as EBSCO, or directly from Cabinet:
www.cabinetmagazine.org/subscribe

SUBMISSIONS
We only accept submissions via email. Guidelines available at:
www.cabinetmagazine.org/information/submissions.php

Editor-in-chief
Sina Najafi

Senior editor
Jeffrey Kastner

Editors
D. Graham Burnett, Christopher Turner

UK editor
Brian Dillon

Associate director
Kelley Deane McKinney

Art director
Everything Studio

Associate editor
Julian Lucas

Image researcher
Evelyn Davis

Editorial assistant
Marko Gluhaich

Website directors
Ryan O'Toole, Luke Murphy

Editors-at-large
Saul Anton, Sasha Archibald, Mats Bigert, Brian Conley, Christoph Cox, Jeff Dolven, Leland de la Durantaye, Jesse Lerner, Jennifer Liese, Ryo Manabe, Alexander Nagel, Sally O'Reilly, George Prochnik, Frances Richard, Daniel Rosenberg, Aaron Schuster, David Serlin, Debra Singer, Justin E. H. Smith, Margaret Sundell, Allen S. Weiss, Eyal Weizman, Margaret Wertheim, Gregory Williams, Jay Worthington, Tirdad Zolghadr

Contributing editors
Molly Blieden, Eric Bunge, Pip Day, Charles Green, Adam Jasper, Srdjan Jovanovic Weiss, Lytle Shaw, Cecilia Sjöholm, Carl Michael von Hausswolff, Sven-Olov Wallenstein

Cabinet national librarian
Matthew Passmore

Cabinet is a non-profit 501(c)(3) magazine published by Immaterial Incorporated. Our survival depends on support from generous foundations and individuals. Please consider supporting us at whatever level you can. Donations are tax-deductible for those who deal with Uncle Sam. All gifts are acknowledged online. Contributions of $25 or more will be acknowledged in the next possible issue; those above $100 will be noted in four issues. Checks to "Cabinet" can be sent to our office; please write "Smelling salts to revive you!" on the envelope.

Cabinet wishes to thank the following visionary foundations and individuals for their support of our activities during 2017. Additionally, we will forever be indebted to the extraordinary contribution of the Flora Family Foundation from 1999 to 2004; without their support, this publication would not exist. We would also like to extend our enormous gratitude to the Orphiflamme Foundation and the Opaline Fund for their generous support.

$100,000
The Lambent Foundation

$50,000
The Warhol Foundation for Visual Arts

$15,000
The New York City Department of Cultural Affairs

$10,000
The National Endowment for the Arts

$6,000
Margaret Sundell & Reinaldo Laddaga

$3,000
The Danielson Foundation

$1,500–$2,500
Stina & Herant Katchadourian, Steven Rand & Nancy Wender, Terry Winters

$501–$1,000
Martha & Thomas G. Armstrong, Sara Clugage, Spencer Finch, Christian Scheidemann, Sandy Tait & Hal Foster, Elizabeth Merena, Edward C. Wilson and Hesu Coue Wilson Family Fund

$500 or under
Pamela Cederquist, David Hariton & Tod Lippy, Steven Igou, Lenore & Richard Niles, Debra Singer & Jay Worthington

$250 or under
Tauba Auerbach, Jeff Beall, In memory of Dr. Mark H. Beers, Mia Enell & Nicholas Fries, Ernest Fasanya, George Ganat, Alex Goodfriend, Cynthia Hansen, Peter Hapstak, Peter Jaszi, Craig Kalpakjian, James Katzenberger, Carin Kuoni & John Oakes, Scott LeBouef, Deborah Lovely, Meredith Martin & Joshua Siegel, Paul McConnell, Helen Mirra, Jason Olin, Jan Peacock, Andrew Pederson, Jocelyn Price & Christopher Leone, John Sargent, Eric Schmid, Pooja Shah & Rebecca Ward, John Sherburne, James Siena, Rod Stasick, Jude Tallichet & Matt Freedman, Volker Welter, Margaret Wertheim

$100 or under
Jesper Andersen, James Baker, Katherine Borkowski, Dennis Bruns, Donald Cameron, Graham Connell, Scott David, Judith Dolven, Cooper Downs, Jonathan Drori, Kate Flint, Mary Fobian, Burton Fox, Peter Jaszi, Richard Klein, Esben Krohn, Jim Martin, Michael Metzger, Charles Dee Mitchell, Jan Peuker, Beth Regardz, John Paul Ricco, Christopher Scavone, Laurel Schultz, Sharon Shanks, Austen Sofhauser, Vanessa Valenzuela, Peggy Wang, William Whaley, Daivid Will

CONTRIBUTORS

Elaine Ayers is a doctoral candidate in the Program for the History of Science at Princeton University. Her dissertation, "Strange Beauty," examines specimens situated between art and science in nineteenth-century collections. She is a visiting researcher at Stanford University's global digital humanities project "Natural Things: Ad Fontes Naturae," and curator of an exhibit, "Tropics of Flora," opening in spring 2018 at the Linda Hall Library, Kansas City.

Joshua Bauchner is a doctoral candidate in the Department of History at Princeton University. His dissertation considers everyday life and the sciences of mind and body in the nineteenth century.

D. Graham Burnett is an editor of *Cabinet* and co-author, most recently, of *Keywords;...Relevant to Academic Life*, &c. (Princeton University Press, 2018).

Brian Dillon is UK editor of *Cabinet* and teaches writing at the Royal College of Art, London. His books include *Essayism* (Fitzcarraldo Editions, 2017), *The Great Explosion* (Penguin, 2015), *Objects in This Mirror* (Sternberg Press, 2014), and *I Am Sitting in a Room* (Cabinet Books, 2012). *In Pieces: writings on art*, etc. will be published by Sternberg Press in 2018.

William Germano teaches literature and humanities at Cooper Union, New York. His books include *Eye Chart* (Bloomsbury, 2017), *The Tales of Hoffmann* (British Film Institute, 2013), *From Dissertation to Book* (University of Chicago Press, 2005), and *Getting It Published* (University of Chicago Press, 2001). His upcoming projects include a guide to revising academic writing and a history of operas based on Shakespeare's plays.

David B. Goldstein is a critic, poet, food writer, and associate professor at York University in Toronto. His publications include *Eating and Ethics in Shakespeare's England* (Cambridge University Press, 2013) and the poetry collection *Lost Originals* (BookThug, 2016). He is currently co-director of "Before 'Farm to Table': Early Modern Foodways and Cultures," a Mellon Foundation–funded research project at the Folger Shakespeare Library.

Julian Lucas is an associate editor of *Cabinet* and a contributing writer at the *New York Times Book Review*. His criticism has appeared in the *New Republic* and the *New York Review of Books*. He is working on a collection of essays about the representation of American history in computer games, literature, art, and reenactment culture, with an emphasis on slavery and colonial conquest.

Jacob Mikanowski is a writer and critic based in Berkeley, California. His work has appeared in publications including *Aeon*, the *Atlantic*, the *Guardian*, the *Los Angeles Review of Books*, the *New York Times*, and *Slate*. Previously, he studied and taught European history and anthropology at the University of California, Berkeley.

Justin Patch teaches music and media studies at Vassar College in Poughkeepsie, New York. His current book project, "Discordant Democracy: Noise, Affect, and Populism in the Presidential Campaign," is under contract with Routledge. His scholarly work has appeared in journals including *American Music*, *Americana*, *Soundings*, the *European Legacy*, and the *Journal of Popular Music Studies*.

Avinoam Shalem teaches the arts of Islam at Columbia University. He co-curated the 2010 exhibition "The Future of Tradition: The Tradition of Future" at Haus der Kunst, Munich, and directs the project "When Nature Becomes Ideology: Palestine after 1947." He recently co-edited *The Image of the Prophet between Ideal and Ideology:*

A Scholarly Investigation (De Gruyter, 2014) and *Gazing Otherwise: Modalities of Seeing in and beyond the Lands of Islam*, volume 32 of the journal *Muqarnas* published in October 2015. His most recent book is *The Chasuble of Thomas Becket: A Biography* (Hirmer, 2017).

Justin E. H. Smith writes from Paris. His next book is *Irrationality: A History*, to be published in 2018 by Princeton University Press.

Courtney Stephens is a filmmaker and writer based in Los Angeles, where she co-curates the film and lecture series Veggie Cloud. Her forthcoming film *The American Sector*, co-directed with Pacho Velez, explores the Cold War's legacy in the American landscape and imagination.

Christopher Turner is an editor of *Cabinet* and Keeper of Design, Architecture, and Digital at the Victoria and Albert Museum, London.

Pacho Velez is a filmmaker and a professor in the Culture and Media department at the New School. His films include *The American Sector* (forthcoming; co-directed with Courtney Stephens), *The Reagan Show* (2017), and *Manakamana* (2013).

AF328626

COLUMNS

LEFTOVERS / UP, UP, AND AROUND
Joshua Bauchner

"Leftovers" investigates the cultural significance of detritus.

———

The paternoster elevator deserves its name, which derives from rosary beads, the Our Father being the first of the cycle of prayers the beads accompany. The mechanism consists of a set of open elevator cars pegged to a chain or belt, running continuously in two side-by-side shafts over wheels located in both the basement and attic. As a car passes the turnaround wheel, it remains upright, shifting horizontally to the other shaft before continuing its journey. In the paternoster lobby, this appears as twinned shafts, each with a car passing by in opposite directions. The usual tempo of 0.3 to 0.4 meters per second is slow enough to allow for comfortable ingress and egress and fast enough to ensure a waiting time of no more than ten seconds. When the car traveling in the direction you want to go is level with the landing, you grab a handle and step in.

I first encountered the paternoster elevator during a recent stay in Vienna. Though Austria has only about a dozen remaining, it is part of the machine's primary habitat, which otherwise includes Hungary, Slovakia, Czechia, Germany, Denmark, the Netherlands, and the United Kingdom.[1] While the device originated in London—it was first developed and patented in 1878 and then marketed as Hart's Cyclic Elevator—it found its most receptive audience in Germany. There, it took root in Hamburg in 1885 and was a common component of that city's massive commercial development around the turn of the century. In 1905, each of the city's ninety-two paternoster installations delivered roughly 730 people each day to their

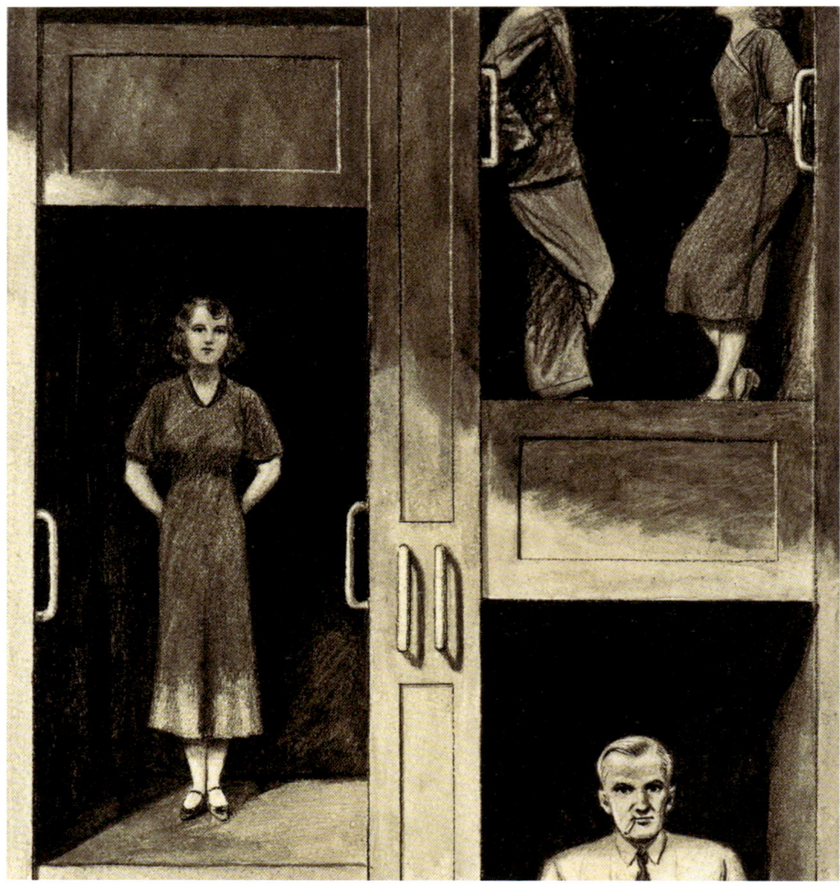

Willibald Krain, *Paternoster*, circa 1928. Courtesy Stadtmuseum Berlin.

floors, yielding over twenty million total rides for the year.[2] From there, it spread across the country and came in many ways to be identified with it. Though new installations in the Federal Republic were prohibited after 1972, there remain over two hundred in service, and nearly all contemporary writing on the topic, in English and German, deals in some manner with the device's relation to its adopted homeland.[3]

But is there anything specifically Germanic about the paternoster? Armchair sociology by enthusiasts and observers alike identifies the machine as an embodiment of the efficient and reliable Teutonic culture.[4] There seems indeed to be some resonance between a stilted and impersonal office culture and its automatic people conveyor. Heinrich

Böll deftly animates this in "Murke's Collected Silences," his 1958 satire of a particularly erudite version of this office culture, that of the radio broadcasting headquarters of a nameless West German city in the 1950s. "Every morning, as he entered the broadcasting headquarters," Böll writes, "Murke submitted himself to an existential gymnastic exercise"—he rode the paternoster elevator through the attic. Struck always with the same angst that something would happen, he would arrive safely back at the second floor, "cheerful and composed," ready for the sure-to-come inanities of the day. On this day, these include primarily slicing out the word "God" and splicing in the phrase "that higher Being Whom we revere" twenty-seven times in two half-hour recorded lectures on "the

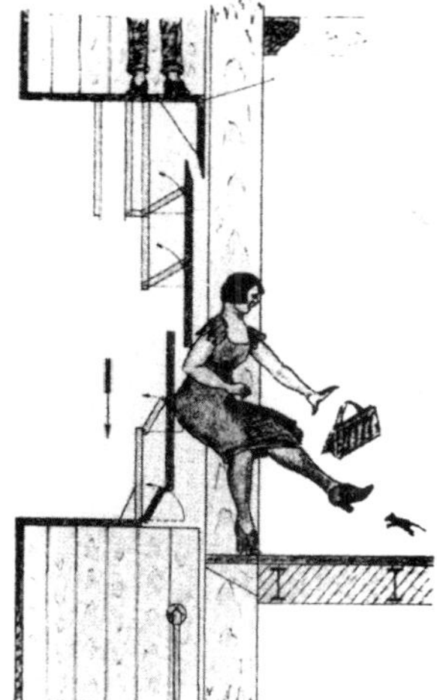

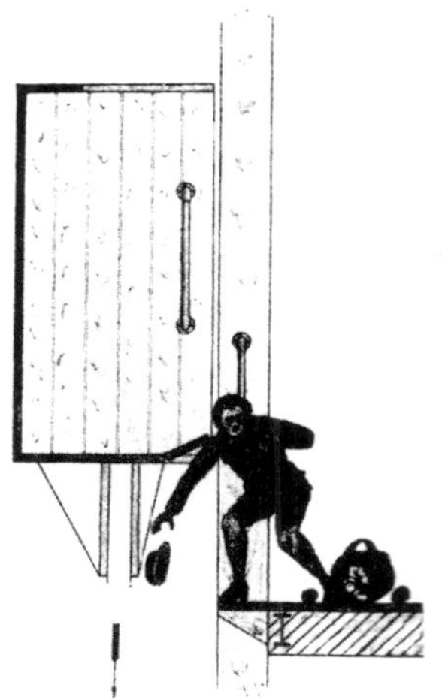

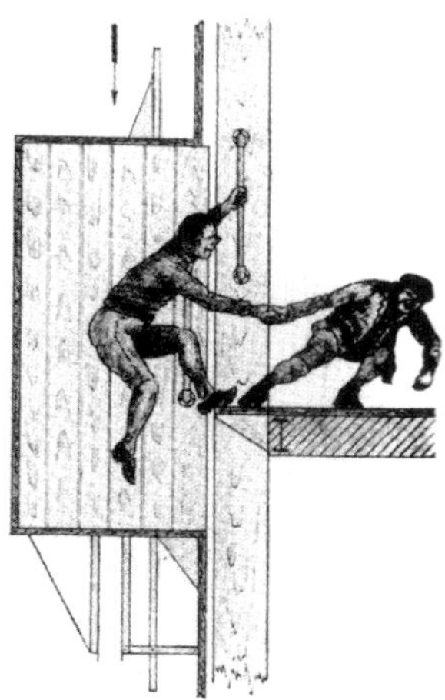

Swiss cartoons depicting a range of possible paternoster-related accidents, 1933.

essence of art" by the particularly noxious Professor Bur-Malottke, who has recently shed the religious mentality gained in his 1945 conversion. While the paternoster disappears after the story's opening gambit, its repetitive rhythm underlies, of course, the repetitive slicing and splicing that make up Murke's workday, as well as the everyday and seasonal rituals of the radio station itself.

On a larger scale, Günther Grass employs the elevator in the novel *Too Far Afield* (1995), his lengthy meditation on German reunification and its echoes of the first "unification" of 1871. In his review for *London Review of Books*, the literary scholar Frederic Jameson highlights Grass's use of the elevator motif, an image that moves, via repetition, from a merely "poetic conceit" to an unanticipated historical "reality" (Jameson's scare quotes): "Fonty's plea for the preservation of this characteristic piece of old-German technology is celebrated in terms of the 'eternal return,' while in the climactic history lesson of this endless reiteration of historical cycles, the masters of German destiny are caught, descending in the *Paternoster* feet first until the all too familiar features are reached."[5] I admit to not making it through this tome but must say I side with the then editor of *Der Spiegel*, Helmuth Karasek, who remarked during a televised roundtable discussion of the work, "Do you really find that a deep image, when someone says, life goes up and down?"

Such identifications of a national-cultural fundament with a technology ring generally quite hollow. One need only to read the letter sent by the Berlin building authorities rejecting a proposed paternoster in 1904. They explain the ability of Hamburg residents to seamlessly use such a device by referencing the "care and skill" gained in that port city through familiarity with ships and navigation.[6] Berliners were too uncertain at sea to be trusted with such a device.

Or further, turn one's attention to the series of letters that followed Jameson's review, which highlight various English instances of the paternoster, mostly in universities. Here, some of the same bureaucratic traits that could plausibly animate the relation between the paternoster and the German office appear again, only in a donnish context: collegial pettiness and a prevailing monotony, both of which are soothed by the minor distraction afforded by the machine.[7] Indeed, at the time of a fatal accident in the paternoster of Claremont Tower of the University of Newcastle in 1975, installed only eight years before, there were around seventy such elevators in the country.[8] A fatal accident due to mechanical and not user failure of course makes more sense than any cultural affinities as the reason for the decline of the machine in the United Kingdom.[9]

Yet a 1980 analysis of the accident highlights another aspect of the paternoster, seemingly beyond the national question. Its conclusion opens with an at once nonchalant and yet deeply alarming observation: "The design of the paternoster appears to have remained largely unchanged for many years and since machines have, on the whole, performed their functions satisfactorily until this time, there has not been any incentive to carry out a comprehensive study of lift safety. It is now clear that the present system, which generally has been viewed as a simple machine, is in fact highly complex and suffers from the following fundamental weaknesses."[10] Setting aside the weaknesses, what about the paternoster distorts and excites our perception of it? From the engineer's perspective, this results in taking something "highly complex" for "a simple machine"; from that of the lay public, this produces something else. But what exactly?

To answer, I turn back to the paternoster with which I am most familiar, in Vienna's City Hall, and the building's resonance in its slightly different

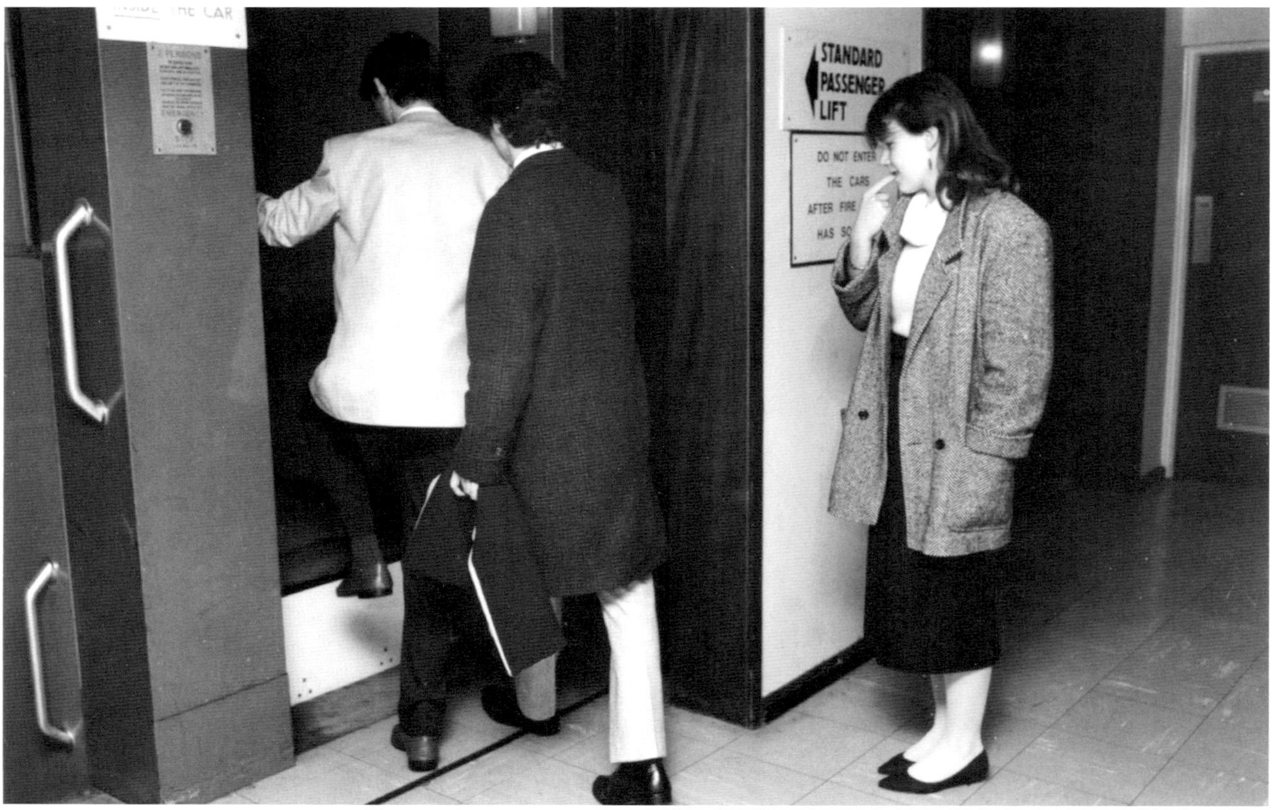

Paternoster lift in the Chemistry Tower, University of Salford, Manchester, 1986. The building was demolished in 1993. Courtesy University of Salford Library Archive.

national context. I have spent count-less weeks in the library in City Hall, arriving always via the paternoster elevator that leads directly there. The building is magnificent and massive, five floors over twenty thousand square meters of ground, includ-ing seven interior courts. The large windows and finely appointed high vaults, especially on the *bel étage* with the library, give the entire build-ing a levity and quickness without tipping into the cavernous.[11] And with the many courts, nearly all corridors are windowed, avoiding any sem-blance of a cramped administrative maze. Finished in 1883, the build-ing—the most significant neo-Gothic structure in Vienna—was one of the works that resulted from the massive mid-century reconstruction of the old city walls and glacis into a ring boulevard (the Ringstraße) that also became home to countless palatial

apartments, and a number of major public works, such as the university, the Burgtheater, the Art History Museum, and the Natural History Museum.

At a time prior to political unity in Germany, the Gothic Revival of the late eighteenth and early nineteenth centuries was a major aspect of the aesthetic fashioning of a culturally unified German nation. (Goethe pro-claimed it *the* German architecture.) But the style had a different status in the lands of the Habsburg empire. And indeed, Friedrich Schmidt's building is only Gothic at first glance. The complexity and enormity of the project demanded a number of practical considerations that over-rode its supposed style. The city's political annexation of its immedi-ate suburbs in 1850 increased the population nearly tenfold overnight, to just under half a million; it had grown

by another two hundred thousand by the time the design competi-tion for City Hall was announced in 1868. These administrative demands necessitated a turn toward the more pragmatic English version of the Gothic Revival, even if the project was finally also guided by a critical historicism that drew from a number of past styles beyond the Gothic. But it was the task of bringing all of the quickly growing city's administrative functions under one roof—while also providing space for a representative body, the proper pomp and circum-stance required for interacting with the court, and facilities to support all of this—that made the building the functional work it is. This is most obvious in the balance between the building's administrative sectors, situ-ated along the streets to afford the public easy access, and the celebra-tory and ceremonial ones, accessed

via grand stairwells from the interior courts. While the Gothic adornment is unmistakable, it is the balance and purpose with which Schmidt housed the workings of a massive modern bureaucracy that drive the building. When asked in which style the building was, he replied, "I must candidly admit that I don't know! … If anything is characteristic of the style of the building, then it may be the spirit of the modern age, in the proper sense of the word, which is fully expressed in it. I can only say what I strove for."[12]

From the beginning, then, Vienna's City Hall was a modern machine of sorts. Its embodiment of the uncontrollable and even inhuman mechanical aspects of state administration are evidenced in its extended and complex construction process, which, beset by financial difficulties and constant structural challenges, lasted fifteen years. And beyond this, its birth was intertwined with the major technical advances of the day, made clear in the city administration reports from the first years after its opening. The building was almost immediately fitted for electric lighting, a telephone center and network, and elevators, none of which were of course included in the original plans of 1868. At the same time, despite the massive amount of new space, there were crowding issues from the beginning, requiring the consideration of new construction in the adjacent area.[13] It was only with the erection of a new administrative building on the neighboring tract, started in 1913, that the paternoster came to be. In light of the continuous movement of people between City Hall and its new twin, there was a call for better dispersal of traffic.[14] As highlighted by the engineer Adolf Ernst's promotion of the device against the resistant Berlin authorities, the paternoster was perfectly suited for such a task in the modern city-machine: "The pressure and tumult of people busily hurrying through the streets is

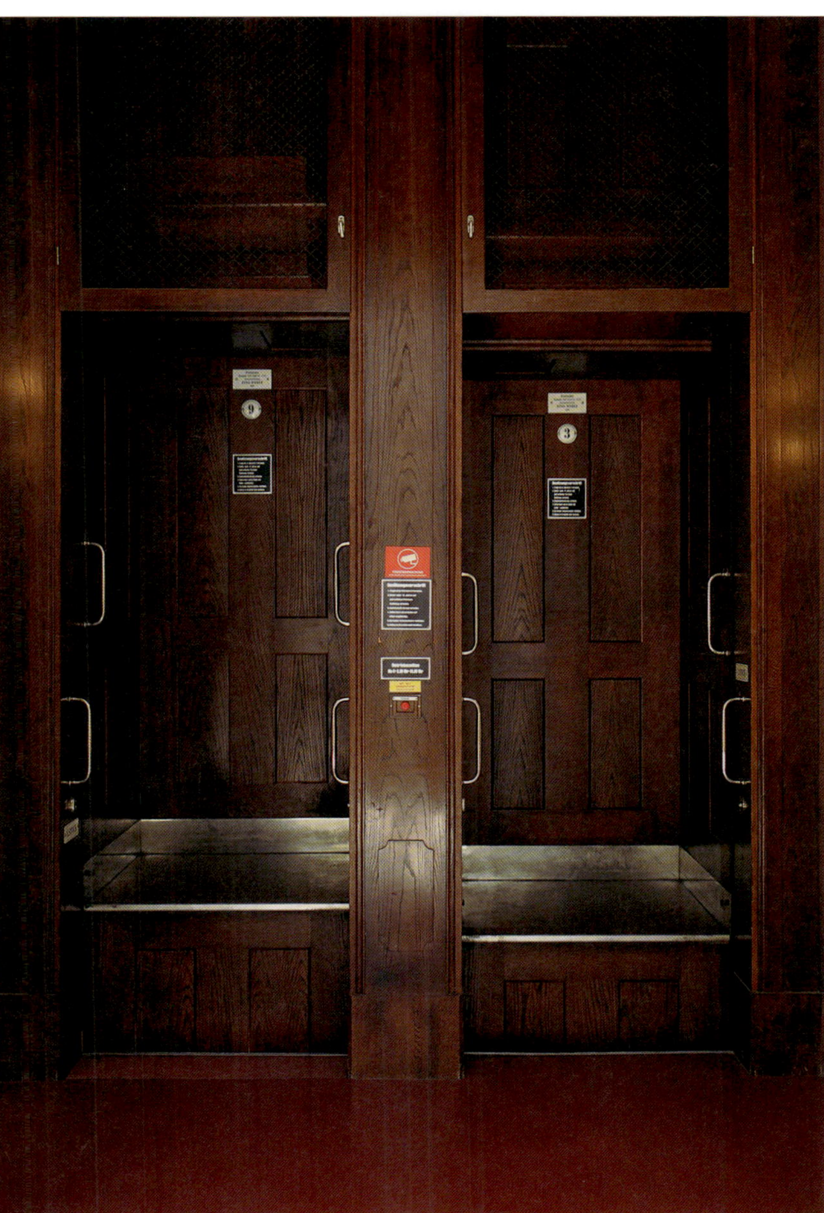

Paternoster elevator in Vienna's City Hall. Photo Joshua Bauchner.

growing persistently; from there, the tangle of ants floods inexorably into office buildings, where the throb of business life emanates and then again returns."[15] In Vienna, this throb was administrative. A paternoster, one in each of the buildings, was the solution.[16]

What is most notable in the reports about the paternoster elevator in City Hall is the complete lack of distinction around the technology. There is nothing in them about moving people autonomously and the danger it might pose; it was merely another new technology necessary for the larger machinery of the building. And here, I think, is why the paternoster so excites present-day riders, especially those new to the device: it confronts us with the bald truth that most machines function

perfectly well without humans. In German, *Paternosterwerk* (paternoster works) had already for hundreds of years denoted a hydraulically powered endless bucket chain for lifting water; the apparatus worked by having the container tip over at the apex of its circuit to empty its contents. And this same principle had been put to use in the mechanized hoisting and conveying of excavated materials other than water for nearly a hundred years before it was used to move people. The only innovation that separates these older technologies from the one that moved humans was a platform that remained upright as it went over the top, though even this stable platform design was first developed for the transportation of goods before it was adapted a few years later for transporting people.[17] What we feel when we walk up to a paternoster and see it already moving is precisely this historical reality: an entire mechanical world humming along outside of our purview, humans largely unnecessary to its being.

A particularly Viennese expression of this feeling was captured by the banker-cum-writer Paul Schütz, writing under his pseudonym Konrad Paulis, in the poem "Before the Paternoster Elevator," which he deposited in the archives of the City Hall library some time before he died in 1955. After describing the sounds and sights he observes as he stands before the machine, the faces as they rise and fall in the "continuous perpendicular round dance," he notes:

Only sometimes, something goes
through the machinery
very eerily, like
a shivering, shuttering quake
effected by cautious ur-energy …
I see it and think of life.[18]

The poem's otherwise hackneyed approach to the machine and its "eternal human round dance" is pierced by this penultimate stanza.

For a moment, Paulis apprehends the machine as it is, unconcerned with its occasional passengers and overtaken by its deeper mechanical identity.

Two generations earlier, the irascible critic Karl Kraus also stood before a paternoster, but he turned his attention to the other side of the autonomous machine: how the elevator was integrated into the larger machinery of the modern administrative city. Here, his loathing of the so-called Austrian spirit, at once officially religious and expressly punitive, combines with his usual critique of language to analyze the ostensible contradiction between the machine's earthly nature and heavenly name. On the occasion of the opening of one of Austria's first paternoster elevators in Vienna's regional court in 1906, he wrote: "A paternoster-lift! Two worlds in one word. The spirit of Austria makes the connection explicable. One would like to believe that the denomination was dreamed up in a 'cell for the condemned.' But paternoster-elevators really exist. … The word does not sound precisely pacifying. An elevator, upon entering which it is recommended to offer an Our Father. And when one has reached the fourth floor of the court, one feels obligated to say a Gloria in excelsis Deo."[19]

<hr>

1 These are the countries with at least eight remaining running paternoster elevators, according to "Liste laufender paternoster," 10 November 2017. Available at <www.flemming-hamburg.de/patlist.htm>.

2 Adolf Ernst, "Die gefahrfrage der paternosteraufzüge für personen und die schutzmittel zur verhütung von unglücksfällen," *Zeitschrift des Vereines deutscher Ingenieure*, vol. 51, no. 11 (1907), p. 411.

3 The most complete history of the device is Jeannot Simmen and Uwe Drepper, "Der paternoster: Die endlose zirkulations-mechanik der gründerjahre," in *Der fahrstuhl: Die geschichte der vertikalen eroberung* (Munich: Prestel, 1984).

4 See, for example, Bertrand Benoit, "Is It Time for Germany's Doorless Elevators to Move On?," *The Wall Street Journal*, 25 June 2015; and Kate Connolly, "Lovin' Their Elevator: Why Germans Are Loopy about Their Revolving Lifts," *The Guardian*, 14 August 2015, available at <www.theguardian.com/world/2015/

aug/14/elevator-germans-loopy-revolving-lifts-paternosters>.

5 Fredric Jameson, "Prussian Blues," *London Review of Books*, vol. 18, no. 20 (17 October 1996). Available at <www.lrb.co.uk/v18/n20/fredric-jameson/prussian-blues>.

6 Adolf Ernst, "Die gefahrfrage der paternosteraufzüge," p. 414.

7 Letters sent in response to Jameson's "Prussian Blues." Available at <www.lrb.co.uk/v18/n20/fredric-jameson/prussian-blues>.

8 V. Knight, "The Paternoster Lift," *Proceedings of the Institution of Mechanical Engineers*, vol. 194, no. 1 (June 1980), p. 131. A short version of the accident: One cabin's bracket failed during the horizontal transfer from up to down, leading to its subsequent misalignment and blocking of the following car, which was then propelled by a third car into the attic machinery.

9 And if one were to be quantitatively earnest about it, neither the UK (where it was born) nor Germany (where it first spread) would be the first place to look for contemporary cultural resonances of the paternoster. Czechia boasts by far the highest number of paternoster elevators per capita, with fifty-eight for just over ten million inhabitants, or one for roughly every 180,000 people, nearly twice as many per capita as Germany.

10 V. Knight, "The Paternoster Lift," pp. 137–138.

11 The library is on the what the building calls its first floor, which is in fact the third floor (fourth by American count) and roughly double the height of the four other above-ground floors.

12 Quoted in Felix Czeike et al., *Wiener rathausbuch* (Vienna: Jugend und Volk, 1983), p. 37. My translation.

13 "Das neue rathaus," in *Die gemeinderverwaltung der stadt Wien in der zeit vom 1. Jänner 1914 bis 30. Juni 1919* (Vienna: Wiener Magistrat, 1923), pp. 255–256.

14 "Stadtrats-Sitzung vom 29. April 1915 (P. Z. 4816, M. A. 22, 10990)," *Amtsblatt der stadt Wien*, vol. 24, no. 36 (4 May 1915), p. 634.

15 Adolf Ernst, "Die gefahrfrage der paternosteraufzüge," p. 453. My translation.

16 "Stadtrats-Sitzung vom 29. April 1915 (P. Z. 4816, M. A. 22, 10990)."

17 Jeannot Simmen and Uwe Drepper, "Der paternoster," pp. 230–231. A *Paternosterwerk* was already invoked as the model for the elevator in an article about the first Hamburg installation. The specific term *Paternosteraufzug* (paternoster elevator) was in use by 1895 at the latest. "Fahrstuhl-anlage im Dovenhof zu Hamburg," *Deutsche Bauzeitung*, vol. 21, no. 20 (9 March 1887), pp. 117–118; and Adolf Ernst, *Die hebezeuge: Theorie und kritik ausgeführter konstruktionen*, 2nd ed. (Berlin: Julius Springer, 1895), p. 322. It made its way into English only after the turn of the century.

18 Konrad Paulis [Paul Schütz], "Vor dem paternoster-aufzug," *Lebendige stadt: Literarischer almanach*, vol. 1 (1954), p. 68 (ellipses in original). My translation.

19 Karl Kraus, "Antworten des herausgebers: Österreicher," *Die Fackel*, vol. 8, no. 207 (17 July 1906), pp. 24–25. My translation.

SENTENCES / A HISTORY OF THE LIGHTS AND SHADOWS
Brian Dillon

"Sentences" is a column by Brian Dillon each installment of which examines the mechanics and style of a single sentence chosen by the author.

———

"Our moods are apt to bring with them images which succeed each other like the magic-lantern pictures of a doze; and in certain states of dull forlornness Dorothea all her life continued to see the vastness of St. Peter's, the huge bronze canopy, the excited intention in the attitudes and garments of the prophets and evangelists in the mosaics above, and the red drapery which was being hung for Christmas spreading itself everywhere like a disease of the retina."
—George Eliot

The sentence—how else to say it?—embarrasses me, and not only because I could never hope to match its wisdom and its rhythms and that weird image at the end. In the spring of 1991, I was in the final year of a degree in English literature at University College Dublin. In a fit of enthusiasm at the start of the first term, I had gotten myself elected as student representative at departmental meetings. I was twenty-one years old, and all ardent for the months ahead, which I hoped would lead on to graduate school. For the first time in my life I was primed for some hard work, eager for academic success. I took a class on "Narrative and Interpretation" in the nineteenth century, and flung myself at novels and stories by the Brontës, James Hogg, Edgar Allan Poe, and Henry James. I had not yet opened *Middlemarch* (1872) when a group of fellow students came up to me after a lecture and broached the subject of Eliot's novel.

Unlike the rest of the course, *Middlemarch* was being taught by a visiting professor from Texas, and word had gone around that this character was attached to the Great Books program back in Austin. Knowing nothing about the pedagogical history of these programs in the United States, my friends and I delighted in mocking a naïve allegiance to the sturdy canon. We imagined this dude and his pals all sitting around in Stetsons, occasionally slamming a meaty palm on some classic volume and declaring: "It's a great book!" And so I didn't balk when my classmates asked that I go see our professor and inquire, because they had grown afraid of its heft: Do we have to read all of *Middlemarch*? Might we not sample instead a few chapters that touched on our theme? I don't recall much about this shameful interview in his office, except the gales of laughter and an assurance that *Middlemarch* was nothing but narrative and interpretation.

Of course, it is something else too: a novel about sympathy in more than one sense. As a portrait—better, a panorama—of provincial life in England around 1830, *Middlemarch* is intimately concerned with how much its characters know about one another, the extent to which they can credit each other's interior lives, the capacities they own for understanding and indulgence. I'd been prepared for all of this—stock moral stuff in Victorian realism—but not for the way Eliot speaks of sympathy, or its absence: in strange and complex metaphors such as open and close our sentence. I was not expecting language like this, in which sympathy is physical or chemical as well as spiritual, moral, and aesthetic. Here is a sentence whose art as well as import demanded I become a more sympathetic reader—and person.

The twentieth chapter of *Middlemarch*, in which the sentence appears, finds Eliot's enthusiastic but limited young heroine Dorothea Brooke weeping alone in Rome. She has married the clergyman and scholar Edward Casaubon and discovered too late that her much older husband's intellectual inwardness, so attractive at first, disallows the learned and literary union she had anticipated. (Casaubon is also likely impotent, and incapable of completing his life's work, a "Key to All Mythologies.") They have come to Italy on honeymoon, and in her state of matrimonial defeat, Dorothea finds the sights pass in front of her eyes like a funeral procession. The spectacles of classical civilization and Catholic culture are enervating when they are not irritating: "her mind was continually sliding into inward fits of anger or repulsion, or else into forlorn weariness." And so Dorothea wanders alone through palaces and basilicas, amid colossal statues and crumbling ruins—all glowing with "the monotonous light of an alien world."

It might have been the light that struck me first in the sentence. The magic-lantern slides in the long opening clause: they recall dream images that loomed in the drugged brain of Thomas De Quincey half a century before. The unconscious mind, says the author of *Confessions of an English Opium-Eater*, is like the splendid mechanism of a phantasmagoria, projecting its horrors into the black-box theater of the eye. And shouldn't we think also of Proust? Little Marcel sent to bed in the afternoon with a magic lantern to entertain him, watching on his bedroom wall the medieval romance of Genevieve of Brabant, whose betrayer Golo wears a red cloak. And what about Virginia Woolf, who wrote in "Modern Fiction" (1925):

Opposite: Illustration by Annette Smith Burgess (detail) for William Holland Wilmer's *Atlas Fundus Oculi*, 1934.

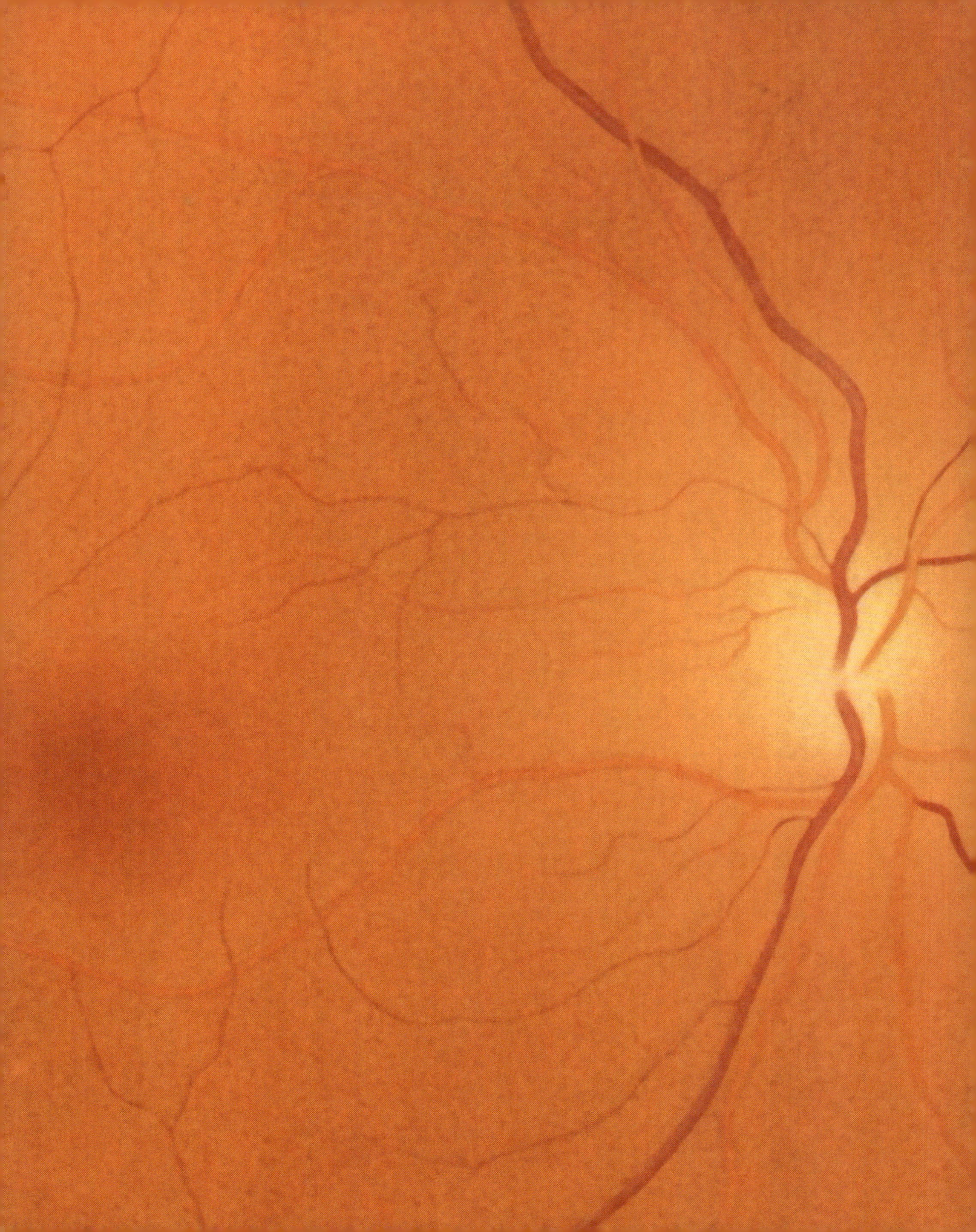

"Life is not a series of gig lamps symmetrically arranged; life is a luminous halo, a semi-transparent envelope surrounding us from the beginning of consciousness to the end." How odd (I should not have thought) to find George Eliot in this lineage of illuminating metaphors for mental life under modernity and modernism.

But wait, it's all much more complicated. Because even before we get to the semicolon—more on that creaky little hinge in a while—Eliot, or her nameless and all-seeing narrator, is already mixing her metaphors. The frieze of images in a distraught and distracted mind like Dorothea's: what is it like, exactly? A magic-lantern-show, for sure, but not only or not quite. The pictures are products of "a doze," which is to say that a mood is like a dream—they both make pictures, like a magic lantern. As J. Hillis Miller, one of her most astute scholarly readers, points out, this is typical of Eliot: her descriptions of one thing in terms of another will often suggest some further metaphorical turn or metonymic swerve. The milieu of *Middlemarch* is like a flowing body of water. Or it is like a web. Or perhaps a minutely scratched steel mirror or pier glass, to which narrator and reader alike must bring the weak light of understanding and sympathy—the scratches will seem to encircle our limited perspective on individuals and events. Maybe the world of the novel—and maybe the world—is like a densely woven fabric, and the best we can do is pick at its pattern in one place, hoping thereby to comprehend the whole.

Dorothea knows little of this; she simply stares and sobs. It is one of the arguments—if that is the word—of the novel: we all live according to guiding (and misguiding) metaphors, but we do not fully know it, let alone understand where they may take us. And the novelist herself? Eliot had borrowed the architectural and anatomical imagery for Dorothea's oppressed mind from her own travels in Italy in 1860. Here she is in her journal of that year, describing St. Peter's: "The exterior of the cathedral itself is even ugly; it causes a constant irritation by its partial concealment of the dome. The first impression from the interior was perhaps at a higher pitch than any subsequent impression either of its beauty or vastness; but then, on later visits, the lovely marble, which has a tone at once subdued and warm, was half-covered with hideous red crapery."

In reality, the drapery was for Holy Week and not for Christmas, but there it is: the source of the real shock in Eliot's sentence. *Like a disease of the retina.* You could say of this medical metaphor, which may have grown over years in the writer's mind or presented itself to her in a flash on considering her journal of 1860, that it is quite of a piece with other aspects of the novel. Eliot's idealistic young physician Tertius Lydgate devotes himself—until his researches are derailed by his own unhappy marriage—to a quest for the fundamental matter of which human organs are made. Optical metaphors are everywhere in *Middlemarch*, but dominate especially Lydgate's thoughts. Like the novel's narrator, he believes that authentic knowledge demands a constant movement between the panoramic and the microscopic view, between concentration and expansion: "There must be a systole and diastole in all inquiry." Readers of the novel get used to—perhaps many do not even notice—the way such metaphors migrate between the minds of the narrator and her characters.

How have we arrived at this image? Via, in that first clause, the generalizing and sententious tone that Eliot's narrator so often adopts. "Our moods are apt to bring with them," she tells us, and we must be brought with her, into the hall of mirrors that her metaphors make. There's a turn at the end of the first corridor, marked by the semicolon and the somewhat presumptuous, eliding "and," which demands that we keep on following, unquestioning, because we are now face to face with a concrete instance of the sentence's opening generalization. Except, except: all is now dreamlike and phantasmagorical. "Dull" and "forlorn" are favorite words of Eliot's—the latter is a reminder of Keats's "Ode to a Nightingale": "the very word is like a bell"—and they're attached precisely to the state Lydgate describes of moving between broad and narrow views. A kind of stupefaction or stupidity brings with it an alarming and even monstrous clarity, vividity. Real and mental objects loom, and look like other objects.

Aged twenty-one, I thought I'd found the whole of George Eliot in this single sentence: a conviction almost as wrongheaded as Casaubon's belief in a key to mythologies or Lydgate's in his organic universal. But my mistake was also a lesson. I learned not to judge any writer by the broad categories—"Victorian," "realist"—too easily applied to their books. And I learned not to judge other readers, such as our professor with his beloved Great Books, and other humans in general, for their apparently conventional attitudes, when in fact they had done the hard work, the adventurous work, that I had not. But it was years later, when I had to teach *Middlemarch* myself, that I fully grasped the eccentricity of Eliot's "like a disease of the retina." Because the question is: whose retina? Eliot's? The narrator's? Dorothea's? The reader's? It's unclear where and when the spreading in question takes place: in St. Peter's or in the memories of Dorothea and her inventor? Still, the image creeps into the mind, and its blindness and insight belong to all of us who convene in this capacious and mad sentence.

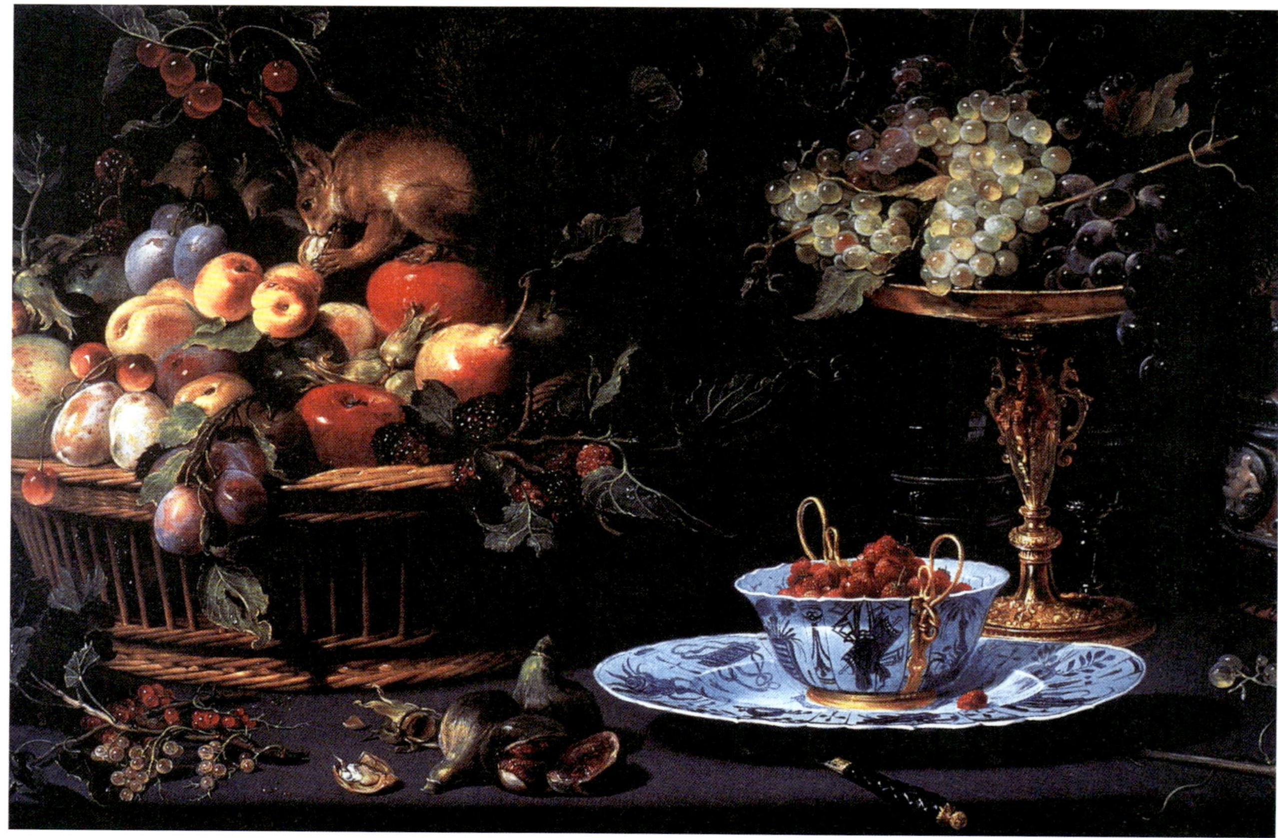

A fluffy guest. Frans Snyders's 1616 *Still Life with Fruit, Wan-Li Porcelain, and Squirrel.* Courtesy Museum of Fine Arts, Boston.

INGESTION / SQUIRRELS AND SPIDERS
David B. Goldstein

"Ingestion" is a column that explores its topic within a framework informed by history, aesthetics, and philosophy.

———

We are sitting motionless in a room lit only by the light of its windows at the moment before dawn, or perhaps by the kind of cloudy afternoon that all too frequently washes the city of Antwerp. We have returned to a scene at once primal and urbane—a scene of overflowing fruit, spilling out over expensive Chinese porcelain and Venetian glassware. The fruit looks sweet, and is perhaps forbidden to us because of its sweetness, though who can really say what is forbidden and why. All we know is that the fruit acknowledges and solicits our frank hunger. The silent table groans with a careless wealth now rendered useless and forgotten. So still is this room that an opportunistic squirrel has gained entrance and is making a meal of this bounty. If we can't eat it, the squirrel is more than happy to oblige. At the end of our long gaze is only this: the reclamation of our agricultural toil by our inadvertent animal "messmates."[1] A vacant room, a table set, a wild animal, and us, invisible, peering, perhaps screwing up our courage to snatch a fig or currant, to feast upon the void.

Frans Snyders, the first great Flemish master of the still life, undertook *Still Life with Fruit, Wan-Li Porcelain, and Squirrel* in the first flush of his mastery. At the age of thirty-seven, following a productive apprenticeship with Pieter Brueghel the Younger and a long Italian sojourn, he was establishing himself as a renowned painter of fruits, game, and markets. The son of a wine merchant who, along with Snyder's mother, also ran a busy Antwerp inn, the painter grew up steeped in a bustling world of urban cuisine. Throughout his life he remained fascinated by the ecological relationship between humans and their food and how both shape a complex culture. He died at age seventy-eight, in 1657, a wealthy man, possessed of a reputation that has not dimmed. "Even the least imaginative historian," writes Walter Liedtke, "might be tempted to call [him] the Rubens of still life painting."[2]

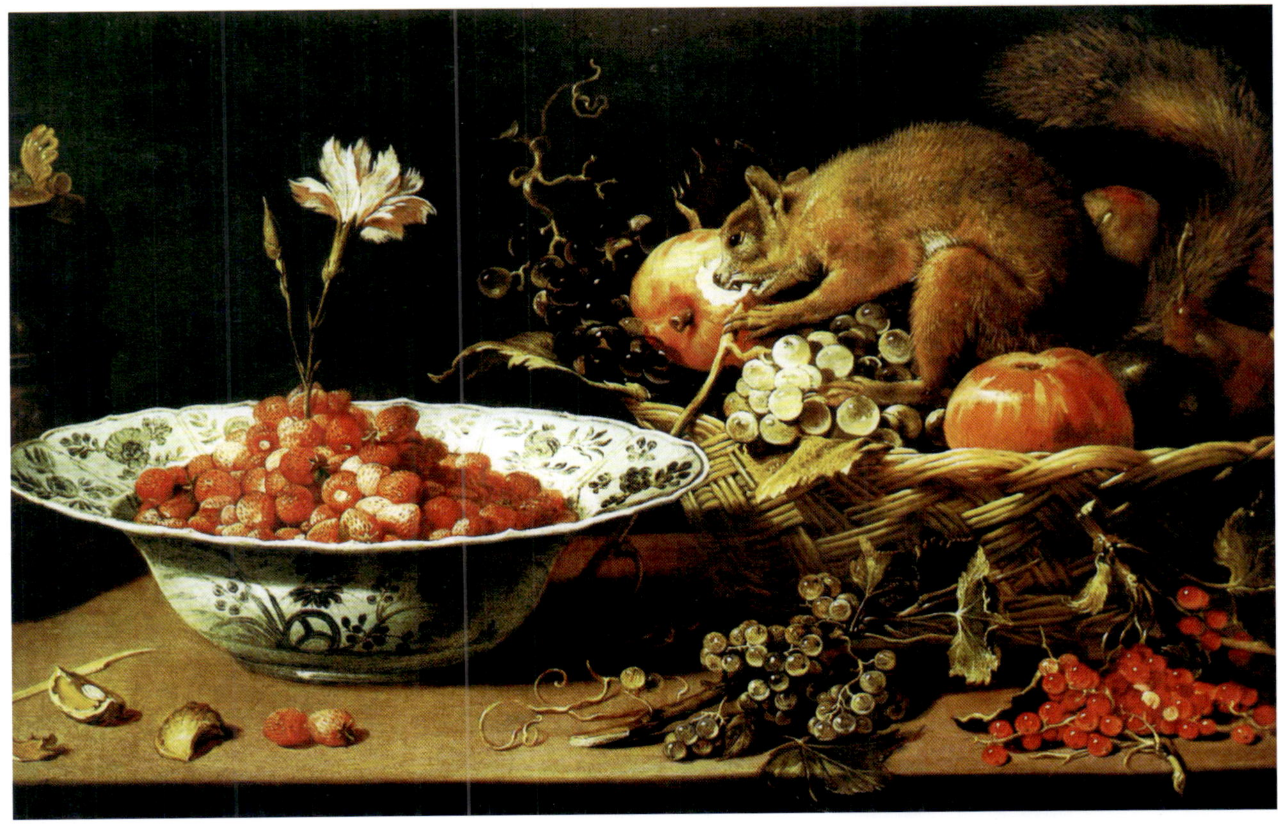

An unfluffy interloper. Frans Snyders's 1615 *Fruit Piece with Squirrel*.

Snyders had painted the first of what was to become a subgenre of squirrels perched atop fruit a year earlier, in 1615. *Fruit Piece with Squirrel*, with its contracted focus upon squirrel, fruit, and porcelain bowl, seems like a study for the later painting or an epitome of it. But Snyders's narrowed lens produces a different effect. In the 1615 painting, Snyders has the offending squirrel crouched over an apple it is actively consuming. Meanwhile, broken walnuts and fallen strawberries—evidence that the squirrel has been at work for some time—litter the table. The painting presents a grotesque display of competing species, with the squirrel's teeth and possibly even its saliva marking the fruit as a contested prize. Once the creature has bitten into it, we're less eager to take it for ourselves. Rather than a scene of bounty, it is manifestly one of decay and waste. The squirrel echoes the viewers' own rapacious appetites, our teeth tearing uninvited at fruits our host has strictly forbidden us to touch. We too have transgressed, and are transgressing still.

In Shakespeare's *The Winter's Tale*, first performed in London four years before Snyders started painting squirrels in Flanders, King Leontes suddenly feels his stomach churn with jealousy at the (false) realization that what he imagined was a scene of perfect domestic harmony is stained by the presence of an interloper. It's not the squirrel Leontes thinks on, however, but the spider, creature of stealth and venom. "There may be in the cup / A spider steeped," he conjectures, "and one may drink, depart, / And yet partake no venom, for his knowledge / Is not infected." But if one knows the spider is there, the poison suddenly bursts forth, "crack[ing] his gorge, his sides, / With violent hefts."[3] If a squirrel eats your fruit and no one is there to see it, does it make a mark? As with the proverbial tree in the forest, Leontes would say it does not. But if you are

sitting and watching it gnaw your apple, revulsion ensues; the beauty of the scene turns to disgust.

The rawness of the earlier *Fruit Piece with Squirrel* might cause us to reevaluate the later *Still Life with Fruit*, which in hindsight takes on a more restrained character. This reevaluation starts with the squirrel itself. Then, as now, squirrels were the subject of conflicting attitudes. For some medieval and Renaissance commentators, they symbolized voraciousness, infidelity, or sinfulness more generally. But a tradition stretching back to the Romans associates squirrels with moderation and simplicity. Pliny the Elder considered the squirrel an emblem of good husbandry, "provid[ing] victuals against winter" and resisting excess.[4] The German Protestant theologian Wolfgang Franz, in his *Historia animalium sacra* (1612), characterized squirrels as "a fit resemblance of a frugal man … securing himself against all mischances of fortune, providing suitable remedies against them … all his life long."[5] In addition to these humble qualities, squirrels had been widely embraced as pets in European middle and upper-class families since the Middle Ages.[6] Rather than a feral, spidery interloper, Snyders's squirrel may thus be a denizen, one whose very presence connotes wealth and leisure in the Netherlandish Golden Age. Like the ubiquitous dog in *When Species Meet*, Donna Haraway's meditation on interspecies companionship, the squirrel is not just a parasite but also a guest, the messmate invited to further mess the meal. Given the squirrel's role in the early modern household imaginary, Snyders's *Still Life with Fruit, Wan-Li Porcelain, and Squirrel* begins to look less like a descent into undifferentiated ecological collapse than a celebration of human virtue and ingenuity in concert with its environment.

The reciprocity between human ingenuity and nonhuman beauty in

Snyders's later painting extends to the reciprocity of global networks. Those circuits included the exchange of culinary commodities in a period fraught with developments in trade, colonization, and conspicuous consumption. Cosmopolitanism functioned as both squirrel and spider to its Dutch practitioners—as an engine of economic and cultural fluidity (and, of course, imperialism) and a constant threat, real or imagined, to moral and social stability. *Still Life with Fruit* foregrounds the cosmopolitan nature of its bounty through its recognizably foreign tableware. The Wanli porcelain bowl, a common feature of the genre and a favorite of Snyders's, a most certainly arrived from China on a ship of the Dutch East India Company, whose trade routes had made such rare china available to the middle class for the first time.[7] Like the Venetian tazza and the succulent Levantine currants and figs laid on the table, the Chinese bowl indicates less an absorption of the foreign than a display of it, transforming a domestic scene into a global one.[8] The grapes piled magnificently in the upper right-hand corner of the painting were probably also imported, but speak in an overdetermined way of more metaphysical pleasures—the intoxication of wine, the spiritual intensity of communion, and even the pleasure of art for its own sake, since "Titian's grapes" were a famous shorthand for the virtuosic play of light and shadow in Renaissance painting.[9] The materials of the painting itself declare a complex opulence—*Still Life with Fruit* is done on copper instead of canvas, one of the largest such paintings of the period.[10] In this painting, the global and the local become host and guest to each other. The central question behind the picture is whether those we let into our houses enrich or threaten us. Is cosmopolitanism a spider, a squirrel, or a spider-squirrel? Snyders gives us a table-sized allegory for the

metaphysics of global commodity culture.

The difference between the earlier *Fruit Piece with Squirrel* and the later *Still Life with Fruit, Wan-Li Porcelain, and Squirrel* is the difference between, say, *Romeo and Juliet* and *The Winter's Tale*. The ingredients are similar: in Snyders's paintings, fruit, porcelain, table, squirrel; in Shakespeare's plays, young lovers, warring families, angrily self-righteous parents, an escape into the unknown—but the effect and outcome are completely different. In *Romeo and Juliet*, Juliet sees the spider, and it is Romeo's family name, the name of her enemy. Perhaps without that revelation, the cup would have been drained and none the wiser. Instead, the spider infects all the ways in which the lovers' families act, with cruelty and much splitting of gorges and sides. No remedy is ever produced for the spider's venom: after the lovers' deaths, neither Capulets nor Montagues can agree on much more than a monument which is essentially a way of making the spider eternally visible. In *The Winter's Tale*, by contrast, Leontes comes to see that what he presumed was a venomous spider is actually something more like a squirrel, a pastoral figure of frugality and good hospitality. Likewise, in the earlier painting, decay, strife, and corruption weigh upon life's apparently most comfortable and noble aspects. In the later one, those dark impulses still express themselves, but are contained by a kind of easy natural-ness, somewhat the way Leontes's lost daughter Perdita presides over her sheep-shearing festival in Act 4 by casually acknowledging death and change in the flowers she distributes to her guests: "These are flowers/ Of middle summer, and I think they are given/ To men of middle age."

The genre of still life was viewed by early modern art theorists as a kind of palate cleanser in the banquet of high art. Blaise de Vigenère, in his

sixteenth-century French translation of the major ancient Greek text on still life painting, *Eikones*, described still life as an *entremet*, a side dish, to "insure continual surprise throughout a feast," in Susan Koslow's words.[11] As such, still life functioned in a way akin to the dessert or banquet course of Renaissance culture—as a pause, a clearing, a space in which relation-ship unfolds anew. It was a moment of both rest and discovery, like a slightly overstuffed essay or a squirrel hiding nuts in its cheeks. At the close of *The Winter's Tale*, Shakespeare plants a literal still life for us: the statue of Hermione, the wife Leontes spurned in his spidery jealousy and assumed he had killed with his hatred, who now stands before him motionless. Yet "the fixture of her eye has motion in't, / As we are mocked with art," observes Leontes. The magic of still life is that it is both still and life—it shows us the stillness at the heart of life and the liveliness of what seems a frozen object. Leontes is viewing an actual person disguised as a statue. Snyders shows us a painting disguised as a living ecol-ogy. When the statue of Hermione moves, Leontes exclaims, "If this be magic, let it be an art / Lawful as eating." Snyders paints a prospect onto our own stillness, the stillness of a squirrel opening its little kernel of meaning to reveal an art as lawful as it is furtive.

1 The term "messmates" is from Donna J. Haraway, *When Species Meet* (Minneapolis: University of Minnesota Press, 2008), p. 4.

2 Walter A. Liedtke, foreword to Susan Koslow, *Frans Snyders: The Noble Estate: Seventeenth-Century Still-Life and Animal Painting in the Southern Netherlands* (Antwerp: Fonds Mercator Paribas, 1995), p. 7.

3 William Shakespeare, *The Winter's Tale* ed. Frances E. Dolan (New York: Penguin Books, 1999). All references are from this edition.

4 Pliny the Elder, *The Historie of the World Commonly Called, the Naturall Historie of C. Plinius Secundus. Translated into English by Philemon Holland Doctor in Physicke. The First Tome*, trans. Philemon Holland (London: Printed by Adam Islip, 1601), p. 218.

5 My citation comes from the English

translation of the book. See Wolfgang Franz, *The History of Brutes; Or, a Description of Living Creatures. Wherein the Nature and Properties of Four-Footed Beasts Are at Large Described*, trans. N. W. (London: Printed by E. Okes for Francis Haley, 1670), p. 212.

6 Kathleen Walker-Meikle, *Medieval Pets* (Woodbridge, UK: Boydell Press, 2012), p. 5; Susan Koslow, *Frans Snyders*, p. 109.

7 On Wanli porcelain in Netherlandish Art, see Julie Hochstrasser, *Still Life and Trade in the Dutch Golden Age* (New Haven: Yale University Press, 2007), p. 122; *Dawn of the Golden Age: Northern Netherlandish Art, 1580–1620*, ed. Ger Luijten et al. (Amsterdam: Rijksmuseum; Zwolle: Waanders Uitgevers), p. 604.

8 On the Levantine source of currants and figs in paintings of the period, see Julie Hochstrasser, *Still Life*, p. 81.

9 Susan Koslow, *Frans Snyders*, p. 54. On the symbolism of grapes, see Eddy de Jongh, "Grape Symbolism in Paintings of the 16th and 17th Centuries," *Simiolus: Netherlands Quarterly for the History of Art*, vol. 7, no. 4 (1974).

10 Susan Koslow, *Frans Snyders*, p. 80.

11 Ibid., p. 49.

INVENTORY / CONCRETE POLITICS
Courtney Stephens and Pacho Velez

"Inventory" examines or presents a list, catalogue, or register.

———

In one sense, the Berlin Wall fell on 9 November 1989. But in another, it still stands, with a number of its concrete panels left in place around the city as monuments. Berlin is not the only site, however, for such acts of commemoration. In the United States, we have identified more than seventy large sections of the wall that are on public display in places ranging from Ripley's Believe It or Not! to the Ronald Reagan Presidential Library. But what exactly do these artifacts commemorate? For all their sturdiness—a typical panel weighs around three tons— these portions of the wall are unstable symbols, variously billed as historical artifacts, decommissioned weapons, war trophies, and even artworks. Over the past year, we've traveled across the country documenting more than fifty of these installations.

In the early 1990s, as the wall was being disassembled in Berlin, American collectors of all stripes— entrepreneurs, educators, politicians, and military officers—looked into acquiring their own "fragments of history." To meet the demand, German logistics firms began offering large sections for foreign export. Within a year, eight panels had migrated to Fulton, Missouri. They mark the spot where, in 1946, Winston Churchill conjured the wall in a speech that warned of an "iron curtain descending over Europe." It would be another fifteen years until the East German state connected various physical barriers into a true border, crafting Churchill's metaphor out of concrete and rebar, guard towers and orders to "shoot on sight." In Spartanburg,

South Carolina, two panels decorate the front lawn of Menzel LP, a company founded by German immigrant Gerhard Menzel in 1965. His son imported the panels in the 1990s, and adorned each with a plaque facing the nearby highway. One reads "Ich bin ein Berliner," and the other, "Tear down this wall." When viewed from a distance, the two panels look like a brutalist petrol station.

What does this obsolete German barrier represent in the American landscape? "Tear down this wall," either written on a plaque or played as an audio loop, accompanies many fragments, as though these words, uttered by an American president, were the spell that collapsed the wall, though it was actually two years between Reagan's speech and the chain of events we now call the "fall" of the Berlin Wall. Encountering the quote beside three wall panels at the US military's Defense Language Institute in Monterey, California, as student soldiers file out of a building bearing the words "Near Eastern Languages," it is hard to see the wall as anything other than symbolic justification for the United States' next foreign intervention.

These wall sections have also become integral pieces of the myth-making project undertaken by every presidential library. The libraries of Franklin Roosevelt, John Kennedy, Richard Nixon, Gerald Ford, and Ronald Reagan each acquired a panel, eager to cement their namesake's legacy within the narrative of the Cold War. George H. W. Bush, the sitting president when the wall came down, also procured a section. In addition, a colossal sculpture in front of his library shows a replica segment of the wall over which five Wild West–style bronze horses are leaping to freedom—or at least attempting to. Perhaps as a result of engineering requirements, the legs of two of the three lead horses have been placed in positions that bode ill for their escape plans. The CIA

awarded the artist, Veryl Goodnight, the Agency Seal Medallion for "Best Artistic Expression of the End of the Cold War." For its part, Bill Clinton's library was supposed to include a panel too, but it disappeared from a storage unit in New Jersey, and has yet to resurface.

Almost immediately after the events of November 1989, the complicated narrative needed to understand what forces brought the wall down was reduced to a set of iconic photos of the wall cracking under the blows of sledgehammers; as though all the state's power had been temporarily embodied in this concrete form, and then demolished by the people. The drama of those images, transmitted around the world, invested these concrete slabs with a deeper resonance. The wall became an open symbol, a charm applicable to all sorts of struggles. In front of the Underground Railroad Freedom Center in Cincinnati, it stands for escape. At the Christ of the Ozarks Statue in Eureka Springs, Arkansas, a section emblazoned with a line from Psalm 23 (in German) acts as a biblical tablet dedicated to religious freedom. At the massive Hilton Anatole hotel in Dallas, two panels live alongside the fifteen-ton propeller from the RMS *Lusitania*, whose sinking helped launch the United States into World War I. Like the mysterious black monolith in *2001: A Space Odyssey*, it's possible that these fragments of the wall are less monuments than predictive artifacts, thrusting their observers into particular political futures; they are talismans that must be encountered collectively for their true purpose to be revealed. The plaques that accompany these sections of the wall repeatedly dedicate them to the idea of the free world, to freedom of speech, to freedom itself, implicitly offering the United States as the incarnation of the ideal. Perhaps these Americanized fragments are, finally, only Rorschachs for the country's self-image—a dense gray mirror.

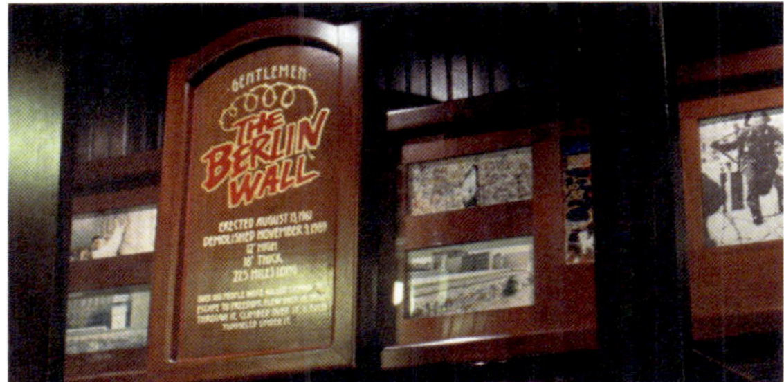

Main Street Station Casino, Las Vegas, Nevada

At this casino, visitors may piss on a piece of the wall installed behind a plexiglass barrier in the men's bathroom. The party responsible for this memorial to America's regard for East Germany has been lost to history. Boyd Gaming Corporation, which owns the casino, told CNN that the fragment was already installed when they bought the property. All photos Courtney Stephens and Pacho Velez.

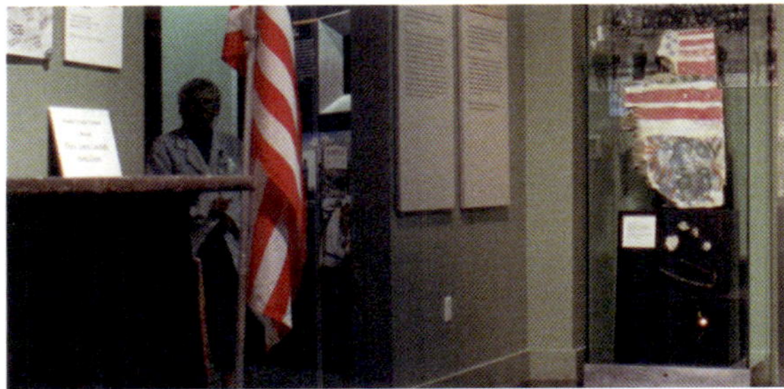

The National Atomic Testing Museum, Las Vegas, Nevada

The museum "tells the story of America's nuclear weapons testing program at the Nevada Test Site." Walking through its rooms—the Atmospheric Testing Gallery, the Ground Zero Theater, and Control Point—mimics a journey through nuclear history that leads to a final display: the Berlin Wall, presumably representing the end of the nuclear era. The museum recently shoehorned another exhibit between the wall and the gift shop—an I-beam from the Twin Towers.

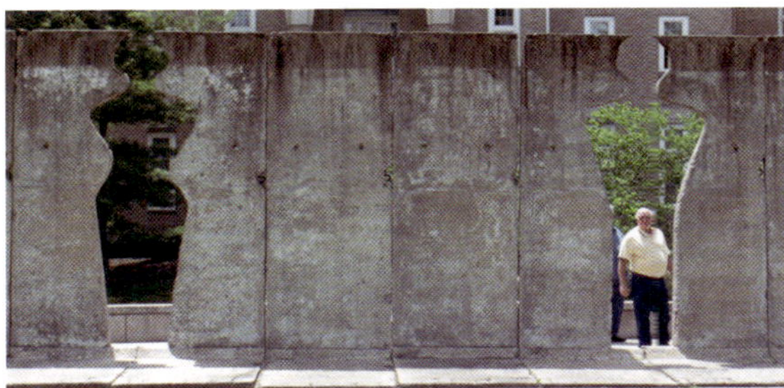

The National Churchill Museum, Fulton, Missouri

On 5 March 1946, Winston Churchill delivered his "iron curtain" speech from this spot on the Westminster College campus. On 9 November 1990, on the first anniversary of the fall of the wall, the school unveiled *Breakthrough*, a sculpture by Churchill's granddaughter Edwina Sandys. The two excised figures are installed at Franklin D. Roosevelt's Presidential Library and Museum in Hyde Park, New York.

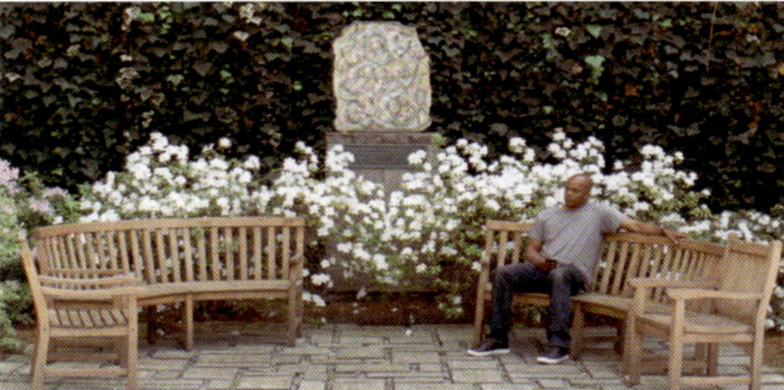

Warner Bros. lot, Los Angeles, California

There's a modest chunk on the Warner Bros. studio lot, near the gift shop. Beneath it is a plaque that reads: "This is a remnant of the Berlin Wall, which stood as a barrier against the free exchange of ideas, information, and culture." A longtime employee told us that one year, as a Christmas gift, the studio handed out small pieces of the wall, i.e., rubble, to their employees.

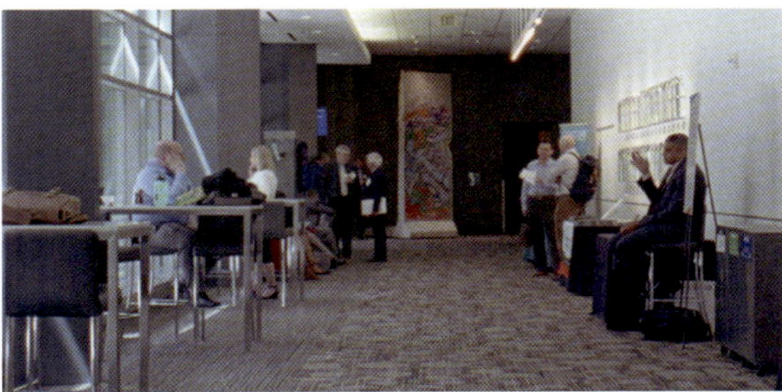

Microsoft headquarters, Redmond, Washington

In 1996, the Daimler-Benz corporation gifted this fragment of the wall to Bill Gates. Now displayed on the ground floor of their Executive Briefing Center, it is considered one of Microsoft's nearly five thousand pieces of art, the largest corporate collection in the country. Within this collection, the wall holds the distinction of being the only piece produced by "unknown artists"—the East German state itself?

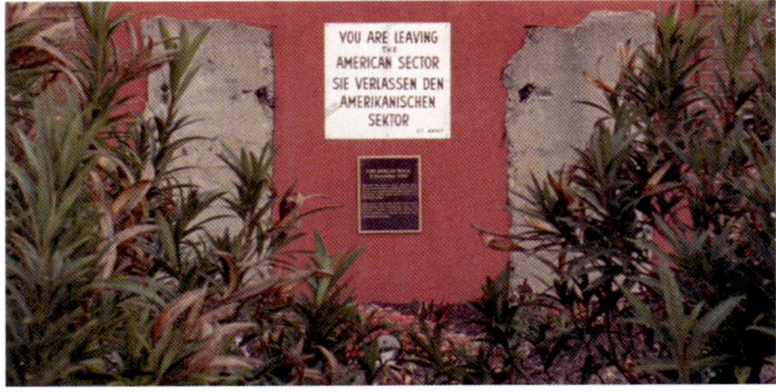

Freedom Park, Fort Gordon, Georgia

During our visit, we expected the curators of the fort's US Army Signal Corps Museum, to whose collection the wall sections belong, to say that they symbolized the destruction of a barrier to open communication. But as an employee of the museum explained, "It has nothing to do with the base being Signal Corps." Their museum displays it on the grounds of the fort because part of the army's mission is to "preserve artifacts related to army missions, ... like I'm sure they're collecting stuff over there in the Middle East."

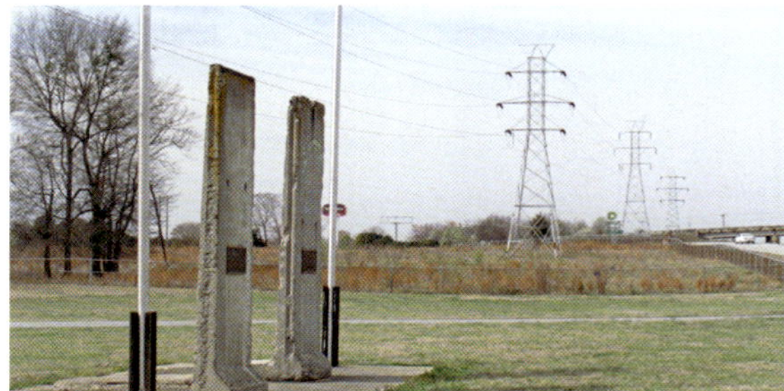

Menzel LP, Spartanburg, South Carolina

Shortly after the wall fell, the German-American CEO of Menzel LP had these two fragments loaded into a shipping container and sent across the Atlantic. Installed in a field beside the company's factory, these monuments to the power of capitalist industry are mostly visible to passing motorists.

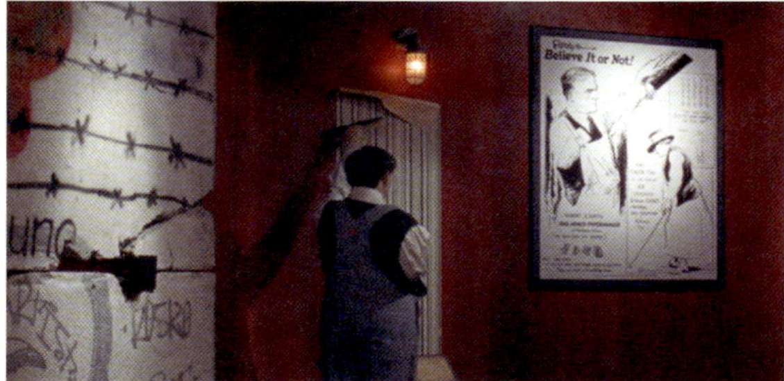

Ripley's Believe It or Not!, San Antonio, Texas

A large panel of the wall is installed next to a mannequin of a one-armed wallpaper hanger at Ripley's Odditorium, directly across the street from the Alamo. As is the case with a number of other venues, the sections on view at the various Ripley's locations come from the *hinterlandmauer*, a second wall built to the east of the first and separated from it by a no-man's-land.

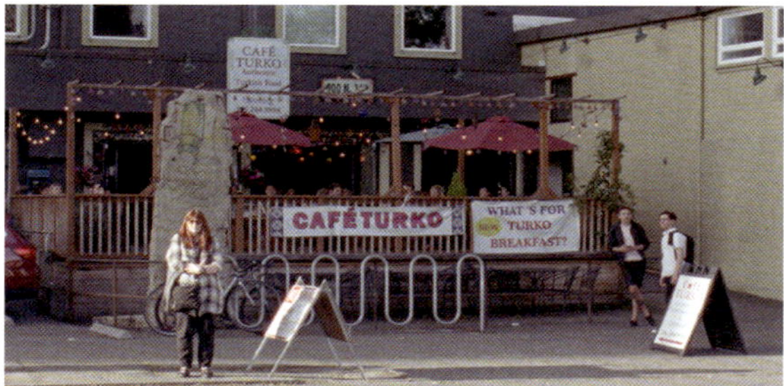

Café Turko, Seattle, Washington

What does the wall symbolize at a Turkish café? Is it a comment on Germany's fraught relationship with its Turkish population? It turns out that the piece used to belong to the History House, a neighborhood museum, now defunct. When they closed their doors, and were obliged to clear out the premises, the hefty piece ended up next door at the café.

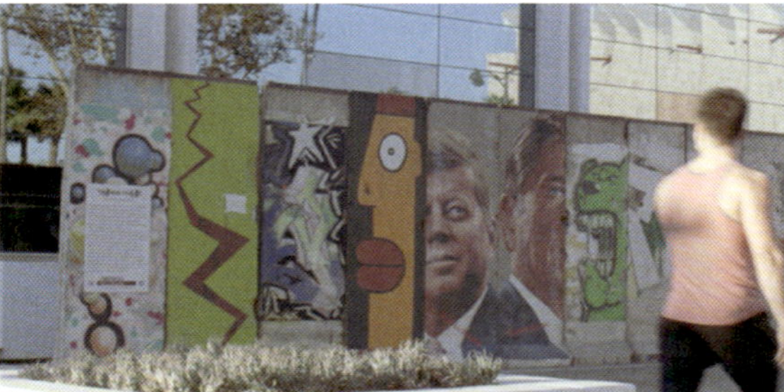

5900 Wilshire, Los Angeles, California

The largest section of the wall outside of Berlin sits on one of the city's major east-west avenues—five displaying original graffiti, and five painted by commissioned artists. To mark the twentieth anniversary of the dismantling of the wall, LA's Wende Museum, which imported the sections, created a sixty-foot-long synthetic board structure that blocked traffic on Wilshire Boulevard the night of 8 November 2009. The museum invited the public to paint on it, and then help knock it down.

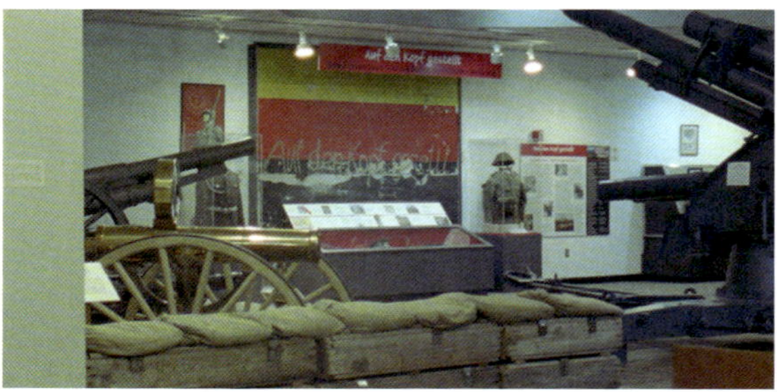

The Virginia War Museum, Newport News, Virginia

Here, a section of the wall—another obsolete weapon?—is installed in a room with a variety of machine guns, tanks, sabers, and other military artifacts from earlier conflicts.

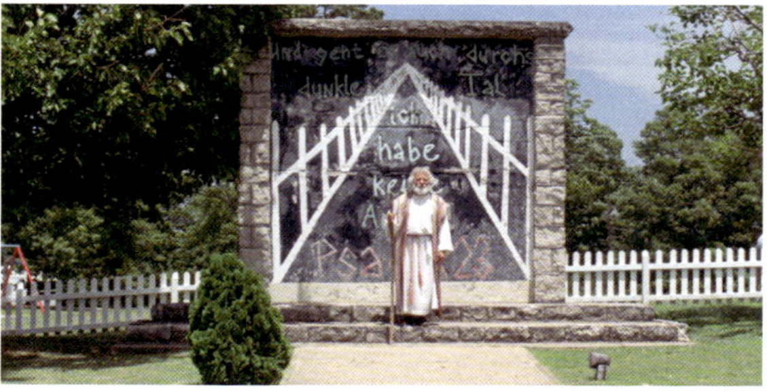

The Great Passion Play, Eureka Springs, Arkansas

This piece stands on the grounds of a venue for a theatrical performance—featuring sheep, horses, donkeys, and 150 actors—that tells the story of the last week in the life of Jesus Christ. It has been running in Eureka Springs every summer since 1968. The grounds feature a number of other attractions, including the Holy Land Tour, Noah's Ark Park Petting Zoo, and, most notably, The Christ of the Ozarks, a 67-foot-high, 340-ton statue of Christ that looks out over the town of Eureka Springs.

The following is an inventory of all known sections of the Berlin Wall on public display in the United States as of October 2017. Access to certain sections is limited because of the nature of the institution in which they are exhibited; see the Notes field for details. Also note that the sections on view at certain locations are in fact pieces of the so-called *hinterlandmauer*, an inner wall built by the East Germans in order to create an empty "no-man's-land" that could be easily guarded. Large parts of this inner wall were composed of horizontally oriented concrete slabs.

SITE	LOCATION	NOTES
Northern Arizona University	Flagstaff, Arizona	The minder assigned to us by the university said that she'd walked past this fragment for years and never realized what it was.
Military Intelligence Heritage Museum	Fort Huachuca, Arizona	The sign next to the wall dates it to 1961–1990 the wall fell on 9 Nov 1989.
Matson Money West	Scottsdale, Arizona	This display inside the financial institution's building is accessible to the general public only by special appointment.
The Great Passion Play	Eureka Springs, Arkansas	
The Wende Museum	Culver City, California	This section bears graffiti by Thierry Noir, who claims to be the first street artist to have painted the Berlin Wall.
5900 Wilshire	Los Angeles, California	These ten sections of the wall are in fact owned by the Wende Museum.
Loyola Marymount University	Los Angeles, California	
Warner Bros. lot	Los Angeles, California	Passing employees made jokes about our film camera: "Film? We don't shoot that around here anymore." The lot is not accessible to the general public.
Rosenthal Vineyard	Malibu, California	
US Army Defense Language Institute Foreign Language Center	Monterey, California	Seagulls use these pieces as a perch.
Mountain View Public Library	Mountain View, California	The graffiti on the wall reads, "Wir lieben dich." A guy passing on his bike asked us, "Does that mean 'freedom'?" We explained that it means "We love you."
Chapman University	Orange, California	A professor was teaching on the lawn in front of this piece, using it as a backdrop for a lecture on entrepreneurialism.
Norton Air Force Base Museum	San Bernardino, California	
Ronald Reagan Park	San Bernardino, California	
Reagan Ranch Center	Santa Barbara, California	The center has been run by the Young America's Foundation since the late 1990s. This was the only site that denied us permission to film.
Ronald Reagan Presidential Library and Museum	Simi Valley, California	At the local library, a mural depicting notable landmarks in the area includes this panel, recognizable for its graffiti of butterflies and flowers.
Richard Nixon Presidential Library and Museum	Yorba Linda, California	
Mizel Museum	Denver, Colorado	
Miami Dade College	Miami, Florida	
Miami Ironside	Miami, Florida	
Ripley's Believe It or Not!	Orlando, Florida	
Universal City Walk	Orlando, Florida	
Atlanta International School	Atlanta, Georgia	The accompanying plaque reads: "Together we cultivate a spirited sense of hope in human potential."
National Infantry Museum	Fort Benning, Georgia	This was the only location where our camera bags were searched for weapons.
Freedom Park	Fort Gordon, Georgia	
Kennesaw State University	Kennesaw, Georgia	
Friends Suwanee Grill	Suwanee, Georgia	
Honolulu Community College	Honolulu, Hawai'i	
Brown Line Western Ave CTA Station	Chicago, Illinois	A store near this metro station had a display of dirndls and lederhosen in its window.
Eureka College	Eureka, Illinois	Each year in early November, the school conducts a "fall of the wall" ceremony, where students parade through campus carrying the flags of former Soviet bloc nations.
	Fort Leavenworth, Kansas	Our guide told us stories about Chelsea Manning, who had recently been released from the Midwest Joint Regional Correctional Facility, which is located on the base.
Museum of World Treasures	Wichita, Kansas	
Long Wharf	Portland, Maine	The accompanying sign, which reads "The Berlin Wall," uses the font of Pink Floyd's *The Wall*.
Ripley's Believe It or Not!	Ocean City, Maryland	
John F. Kennedy Presidential Library and Museum	Boston, Massachusetts	The museum also has on display the piece of paper on which Kennedy wrote out, "Ich bin ein Berliner."
Hult International Business School	Cambridge, Massachusetts	
Grand Valley State University	Allendale, Michigan	
Gerald R. Ford Presidential Museum	Grand Rapids, Michigan	
Grand Rapids Public Museum	Grand Rapids, Michigan	The day we visited, a man came in with a Soviet military uniform he'd acquired from an estate sale, hoping the museum might want to acquire it.

SITE	LOCATION	NOTES
	Fort Leonard Wood, Missouri	Our request was kicked up the chain of command so many times we ultimately never accessed this piece.
The National Churchill Museum, Westminster College	Fulton, Missouri	The gift shop sells chunks of verified rubble from the wall for $5.99 a piece.
Main Street Station Casino	Las Vegas, Nevada	
The National Atomic Testing Museum	Las Vegas, Nevada	A docent here recounted telling her son about the piece in the casino urinal across town. His response: "Mom, I pissed on the Berlin Wall *in Berlin*."
Colgate University	Hamilton, New York	
Franklin D. Roosevelt Presidential Library and Museum	Hyde Park, New York	
520 Madison Avenue	New York City, New York	
Battery Park City	New York City, New York	
Ripley's Believe It or Not!	New York City, New York	
United Nations	New York City, New York	This segment is located in the UN's Peace Garden, overlooking the East River.
Stony Point Justice Court	Stony Point, New York	This piece was placed on its site by a troop of Boy Scouts.
Milton J. Rubenstein Museum of Science and Technology	Syracuse, New York	In their gift shop, a small fragment of the wall costs only $1. Our museum guide told us that they make the fragments in-house, chipping them off two panels in the basement.
The Research Triangle Park	Durham, North Carolina	
Capital University	Columbus, Ohio	
National Underground Railroad Freedom Center Museum	Cincinnati, Ohio	
National Museum of the United States Air Force	Wright-Patterson Air Force Base, Ohio	
US Army Artillery Museum	Fort Sill, Oklahoma	
German Society of Pennsylvania	Philadelphia, Pennsylvania	The wall is located inside their private garden, but is visible from the street.
Vereinigung Erzgebirge	Warminster, Pennsylvania	
Menzel LP	Spartanburg, South Carolina	
Memorial Park	Rapid City, South Dakota	
George H. W. Bush Presidential Library Center	College Station, Texas	
Hilton Anatole Hotel	Dallas, Texas	Over the two days that we shot here, the wall pieces were intermittently blocked by large vertical banners directing MetroPCS conference attendees to their correct banquet rooms.
Rice University	Houston, Texas	A utility worker at the school pulled over when he saw us filming, and recalled to us having seen Roger Waters play in the former "death zone" between Potsdamer Platz and the Brandenburg Gate in 1990.
Ripley's Believe It or Not!	San Antonio, Texas	While we were filming, a man had his daughter photograph him doing a handstand up against the panel of the wall for his Crossfit Instagram account.
University of Virginia	Charlottesville, Virginia	These pieces, known as the Kings of Freedom murals, are part of the Robert and MeiLi Hefner Collection. Prior to their current installation, they were on display at venues including the Kirkpatrick Center in Oklahoma City; the Aspen Art Museum in Aspen, Colorado; the Oklahoma City Omniplex; and Bedok Reservoir, Singapore.
Central Intelligence Agency	Langley, Virginia	Installed next to their parking lot, the piece is not accessible to the general public.
The Virginia War Museum	Newport News, Virginia	
German Armed Forces Command	Reston, Virginia	
Microsoft headquarters	Redmond, Washington	This section is located in a conference center on the Microsoft campus and is not accessible to the general public.
Café Turko	Seattle, Washington	
Seattle Center	Seattle, Washington	While we were visiting, the Seattle Center was hosting Pagdiriwang, an event celebrating the anniversary of Philippine independence. Given the United States' imperial ambitions in the Philippines, the wall's presence felt like an ironic counterpoint.
Embassy of the Federal Republic of Germany	Washington, DC	
Johns Hopkins University, School of Advanced International Studies	Washington, DC	
National Museum of American History	Washington, DC	
Newseum	Washington, DC	In addition to several sections of the wall, the museum features the only intact guard tower that we've seen in the United States.
Ronald Reagan Building and International Trade Center	Washington, DC	The piece stands right next to metal detector at the rear entrance.
United States Diplomacy Center	Washington, DC	The center is in the final stages of construction and is currently open only for educational programs and special functions. It is scheduled to open to the general public by early 2019.

MAIN

LANGUAGE AT THE END OF THE WORLD
Jacob Mikanowski

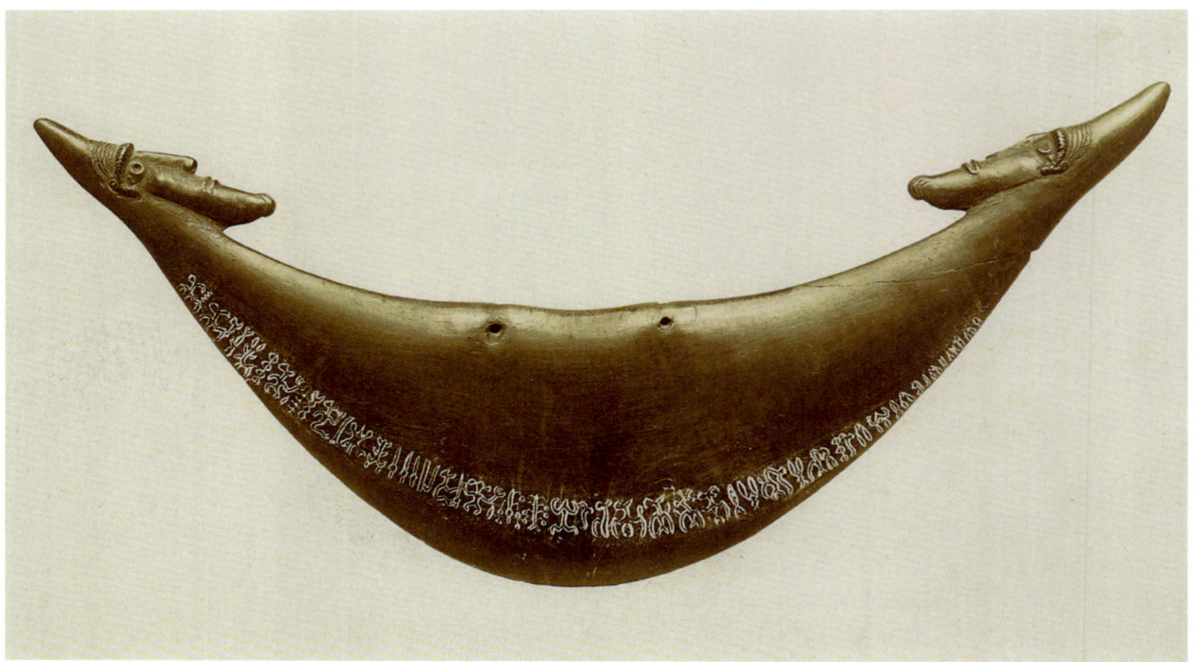

Of all the literatures in the world, the smallest and most enigmatic belongs without question to the people of Easter Island. It is written in a script—rongorongo—that no one can decipher. Experts cannot even agree whether it is an alphabet, a syllabary, a mnemonic, or a rebus. Its entire corpus consists of two dozen texts. The longest, consisting of a few thousand signs, winds its way around a magnificent ceremonial staff. The shortest texts—if they can even be called that—consist of barely more than a single sign. One took the form of a tattoo on a man's back. Another was carved onto a human skull.

Where did the rongorongo script come from? What do its texts communicate? No one knows for sure. The last Easter Islanders (or Rapanui) familiar with rong-orongo died in the nineteenth century. They didn't live long enough to pass on the secret of their writing system, but they did leave a few tantalizing clues. The island's spoken language, also called Rapanui, lives on, but today it is written in a Latin script and its relation-ship to rongorongo is unclear. So far at least, no one has successfully connected one with the other. To this day, rongorongo remains a puzzle, an enigma, and a mirror for the folly of those who try to solve it.

Rongorongo is the only script native to the Pacific. Like so much else, it makes Easter Island unique. It is the most isolated inhabited place in the world; an old name for it, Te Pito 'o te Henua, means either "navel of the world" or "end of the world."[1] It is over a thousand miles from the nearest speck of land. The prevailing winds could make a sea voyage to central Polynesia a journey of over ten thousand miles. Only sixty-three square miles, the tiny island is a triangle with a base of fourteen miles and a height of eight. It can be circum-ambulated in a day. To the people of Easter Island, the universe was an ocean, and the earth a speck of land on top of it. From somewhere to the west came the canoes of the ancestors. From the north and south came great flocks of migrating birds.

The stillness of this isolation was shattered on Easter Day, 1722, when the island was spotted by the

---

Above: A crescent-shaped, wooden neck ornament from Easter Island made some time in the first half of the nineteenth century. The artifact, decorated with two bearded male heads on either end, contains a line of rongorongo glyphs along its bottom edge. Courtesy British Museum.

Dutch explorer Jacob Roggeveen. He and his crew came ashore for one day, traded their cloth for chickens, and shot a dozen islanders, including the emissary who had arrived on their ship to welcome them the day before. After five days they set sail. No other Europeans visited for the next forty-eight years, when a Spanish ship under the command of the viceroy of Peru made a reconnaissance. The Spanish named the island San Carlos, and claimed it in the name of their king, Carlos III. To make the transfer official, the Spanish commander, Felipe González de Haedo, asked the island chiefs to put their mark on a document of cession. The Spaniards surrounded the event with great pomp: drums, fifes, flags. The Rapanui chiefs signed the document as best they could, with sketches of vulvas and frigate birds, signs familiar from the island's abundant rock art.

Then the Spanish left. Their claim, and the name San Carlos, were both swiftly forgotten. But their short stay left a profound impression on the Rapanui. After the visits of the Europeans, they began to construct "earth ships," mounds the size and shape of a boat, surrounded by a ditch that, when filled with water, gave the impression of a ship floating at sea. Katherine Routledge, a pioneering ethnographer of Easter Island life, was told by her informants that the Rapanui would use these earth ships to "gather and act the part of a European crew, one taking the lead and giving orders to the other."[2] In this way, they communed with "the men who came from far away" who "had pink cheeks and said they were gods."[3]

The earth ships appear to have been an attempt by the Easter Islanders to duplicate foreign technology in the form of magic. Something similar may have happened with rongorongo. The Rapanui seem to have intuited the concept of writing, and the power of literacy that came with it, and then set about creating a system of their own. When they did so, they began entirely afresh, building it from first principles and local materials. As a consequence, it resembles no other writing system on Earth. The signs they chose come largely from items familiar to the island. Some come from animal life: fish, squid, sea turtles, crayfish, frigate birds, caterpillars. A few seem to represent plants or human figures, sitting and eating. Others are simple geometric forms: a circle, a cross, stacks of lozenges.

The glyphs of rongorongo are unique. So is the manner in which it was written and read. In fact, it was not written, but carved. Its scribes used shark's teeth to inscribe its symbols on wooden tablets. Wood is scarce on Easter Island, and most of these inscriptions were made on pieces of driftwood. One decorated an oar. A second, a beam. A third, a statue of a bird. However, most of the surviving examples of rongorongo decorate square tablets. These appear to have been written from bottom to top, and were read following a pattern called the reverse boustrophedon. Boustrophedon is a Greek word meaning "in the manner of an ox," and scripts written in it move like an ox plowing a field, reversing direction with each line.

How did the Rapanui go from signing their names to a bogus document of annexation with simple drawings to creating a complex writing system incorporating hundreds of signs? We will most likely never know. First contact with Europeans was a trauma, one to which the Rapanui responded with incredible creativity and cultural ferment. But peering into the history of how this happened is unfortunately almost impossible, for it means looking through the scrim drawn by a holocaust.

The trouble began in 1861, when a Dubliner named Joseph Charles Byrne arrived in Peru with a proposal to cure that country's labor shortage. He suggested that instead of searching the world for willing immigrants, they trade in indentures, and use the vast pool of humanity on their doorstep. What this really meant was the wholesale enslavement of Pacific islanders. In 1862, the first of the large-scale slave raids arrived. Within the span of a few years, most of the island's population was deported and enslaved. Some of the surviving Rapanui ended up on Tahiti, where they succumbed to disease and starvation. By 1871, approximately 94 percent of Easter Island's population had been forced to move elsewhere or had died. Only a little over a hundred people remained, the majority

---

Opposite: Page of diagrams of various motifs and glyphs observed by Katherine and Scoresby Routledge on their 1913–1915 Mana Expedition to Easter Island, during which they also visited Chile and the Juan Fernandez Islands. The bottom two rows depict sixteen glyphs from rongorongo boards. The page is signed by Henry Balfour, an archaeologist who accompanied them on their voyage; it is believed that the drawings are his. Courtesy British Museum.

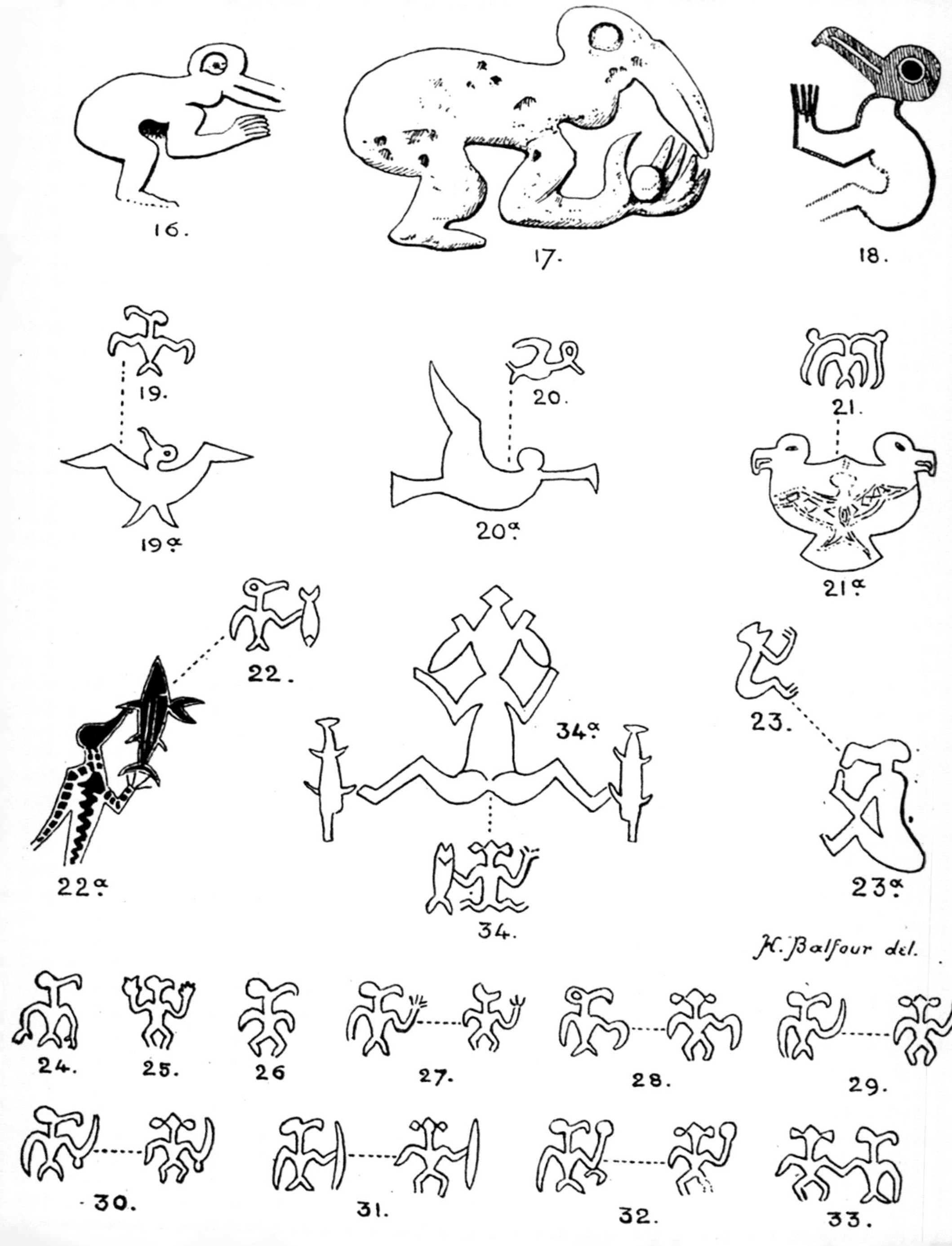

16.

17.

18.

19.

19ª.

20.

20ª.

21.

21ª.

22.

22ª.

34ª.

34.

23.

23ª.

H. Balfour del.

24.   25.   26   27.   28.   29.

30.   31.   32.   33.

of whom had been forced to work on sheep farms. It was, in the words of one historian, "one of the greatest human losses registered anywhere in the Pacific at this time."[4]

Buzzards came to feast on what remained. In the 1870s, a French rancher, Jean-Baptiste Doutrou-Bornier, attempted to purchase the entire island. A megalomaniac and a sadist, he nearly succeeded. He drove off Catholic missionaries with fire, surrounded himself with kidnapped consorts, and declared himself a king. After a few years, he owned 80 percent of the island's land and over four thousand sheep. A year later, he was killed in an ambush. Other pirates came to take his place. Easter Island became a prison, a work camp for the few people who hadn't been kidnapped or driven away. The old ways, and especially the arts of literacy, held by a narrow elite, all vanished. However small as a speck of land, the island had been home to a full-fledged civilization, with its own architecture, myths, rulers, and rites. Now all was in ruins.

It was in the midst of this disaster that the world became aware of rongorongo. In 1864, Joseph-Eugène Eyraud, a member of the Catholic mission on the island, noticed in all the houses tablets and staffs inscribed in an unknown script. He did not succeed in learning what it expressed. Curiously, no previous visitor to the island had ever observed them, perhaps because of a taboo. Four years later, the bishop of Tahiti, Florentin-Étienne Jaussen, received a piece of polished rosewood, wrapped in human hair, from one of his parishioners, a Rapanui convert. He was amazed to discover that it was covered in an unknown form of hieroglyphs. He immediately wrote to the Catholic mission on the island, asking them to search for more examples of the unknown script. They were only able to turn up a few. One man questioned by the bishop confessed "that there was nobody left on the island who knew how to read the characters since the Peruvians had brought about the deaths of all the wise men."[5] The tablets had thus lost all their potency. In the absence of literacy, the tablets, once objects of sacred power, became simply pieces of wood. They were burned for heat and used as reels for fishing lines. According to rumor, one Rapanui man even cobbled together a canoe out of them.

For the next two decades, little more was learned about rongorongo script. One potential breakthrough came in 1886, when Ure Va'e Iko, a steward of the last paramount chief of Easter Island, "read" one of the tablets for a visiting American naval officer, William Judah Thompson. Ure took some convincing. Now Christian, and not wanting to do something forbidden by the priests, he initially refused payment and fled to the hills. Eventually, though, he was made to comply.

It isn't clear whether Ure was reading from the tablet, or whether he even knew the rongorongo script. It seems he may have known it at one point, but had forgotten it by the time he met with Thompson. One of the chants he delivered, a "procreation chant," details a series of paradoxical and, indeed, baffling couplings: "Itchiness copulated with Badness: There issued forth the *kape* taro"; "Parental God copulated with the Slimy Vagina of God: There issued forth the deep sea"; "God Parent copulated with Compacted Sand: There issued forth the tree"; "The fish Rat-Tail copulated with Maggoty Hina: There issued forth the whale."[6]

Ure's words appear to be unconnected to any specific tablet. Instead, they are the words of a traditional chant, the first thing students in rongorongo schools memorized before they proceeded to master the script. Still, it gives some sense of the flavor of what the tablets might contain. (Indeed, according to the leading modern scholar of rongorongo, it is the key to deciphering them all). But in the 130 years since Ure delivered his recitation, very little progress has been made in decoding rongorongo. Undeciphered scripts work like Rorschach blots. Lacking a defined meaning, their inscrutability allows their would-be interpreters to project all their fantasies, wishes, and desires onto the blank space they hope to fill in. This was the case with Egyptian hieroglyphics before Champollion, and with Mayan glyphs before Knorozov. It remains the case with rongorongo.

The process of fantastical translation began early, with one Dr. Allen Carroll, a Sydney physician who may have been the illegitimate son of the Duke of Norfolk and who believed the tablets to be the work of pre-Inca South Americans. Carroll's translations take the form of fulsome paeans to unnamed gods, and sound a bit like bowdlerized versions of the *rubaiyat* of Omar Khayyam: "To those who are our Guardians, oh give ear to us in your temple. You are our protectors. … Ye gods."[7]

Carroll was the father of the so-called "rongorongo fringe." Many more followed in his footsteps. Most share a single, driving idea: the conviction that the Rapanui could not have invented their script on their

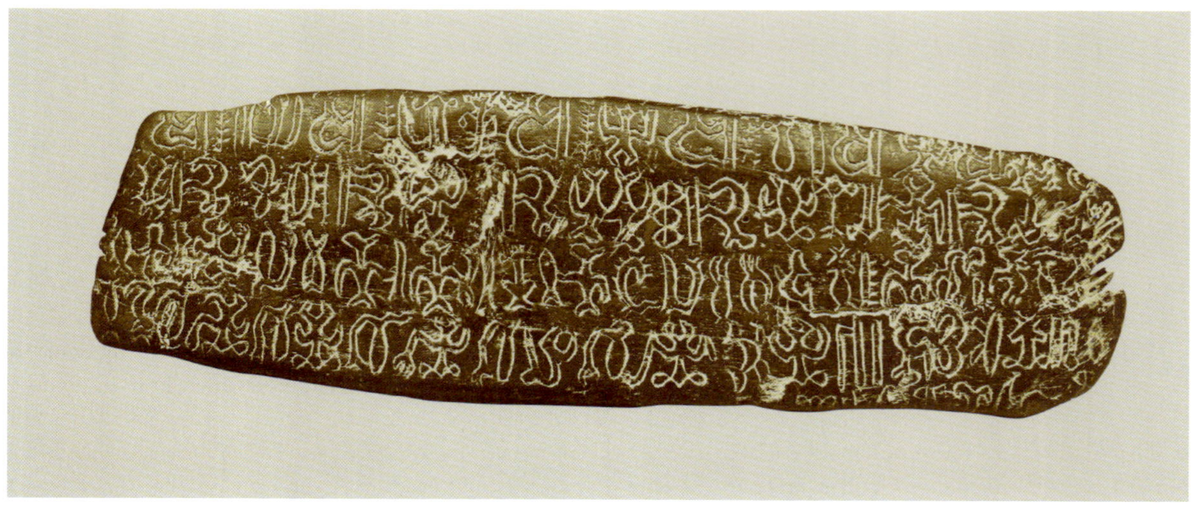

own. The islanders' writing was necessarily the mark of an older, greater civilization, they believed. All agreed it must have come from somewhere else. Where exactly it came from was the only thing left to debate.

Erich von Hornbostel saw connections with the pictographs of the Panamanian Cuña and the unintelligible signs of the *Yü Pei*.[8] Guillaume de Hevesy, a Hungarian engineer resident in Paris, sparked an uproar in the 1930s when he discerned a genetic link between rongorongo and the equally undecipherable Indus script found at Mohenjo Daro. An industrious, though confused, Argentine professor tried to fit it into a graphic system spanning the entire Indo-Pacific. A German paleontologist found traces of rongorongo glyphs in the patterns of Sumatran ship fabrics. Peter Lanyon-Orgill, a polyglot and possibly insane Cornishman, found hints of them everywhere from Land's End to Zimbabwe, and created his own journal to publicize his findings. One Swiss scholar believed they represented the remains of a Pacific empire that had sunk into the sea. A psychologist at Bard was convinced it arrived in Easter Island from Egypt, via the "Asiatic Script Bridge." The Polish folklorist Henryka Romanska discerned in one of the tablets a hymn to the sun god Ra. In her rendering, it sounds strangely like a pastoral composed by an Edwardian author with repetition compulsion: "The bird gladly with the flower flies / The bird gladly with the fruit flies."[9]

The members of this group, with their errant but earnest efforts to link rongorongo to real events in human antiquity, seem positively levelheaded compared with what came next: fifty years of speculation about aliens, giant tidal waves, shipwrecked Spaniards, and the lost continent of Mu.

But while the fantasists were at work, a body of rongorongo-related scholarship more grounded in reality arose as well.

In the 1940s, Alfred Métraux proved conclusively that the Easter Island script had no connection to the civilizations of the Indus. A querulous, foul-tempered Frenchman, he stepped in to lead a scientific expedition to the island when its original leader died of pneumonia off Cape Horn. Some twenty years later, his body was found near the Château de la Madeleine in the Vallée de Chevreuse. In his journal, he wrote that he died "like Socrates."[10] The true culprit appears to have been a love affair gone awry.

The most sustained effort to decipher rongorongo rooted in professional linguistics took place in St. Petersburg. The dogged work of the Russian school helped to sort the script into a clear inventory of signs. Through the use of internal analysis and statistical comparison, its members hoped to place the study of the script on a firm scientific basis. But their careful analysis yields results that nonetheless sound insane— in Irina Fedorova's translation, one text ends: "yam, yam, taro, taro, he cut a tuber of yam, he took a tuber of taro, a tuber, a tuber, he dug up, he cut, he cut, taro, turi sugar-cane."[11]

Above: A tablet with rongorongo inscription. The British Museum, which owns the object, dates it to the eighteenth or early nineteenth century. Courtesy British Museum.

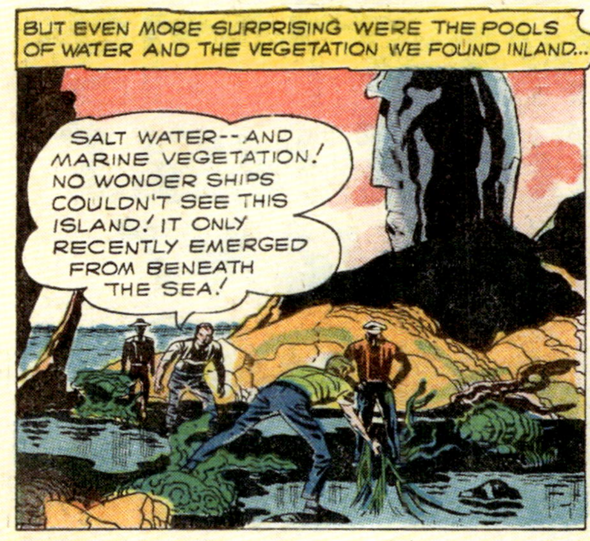

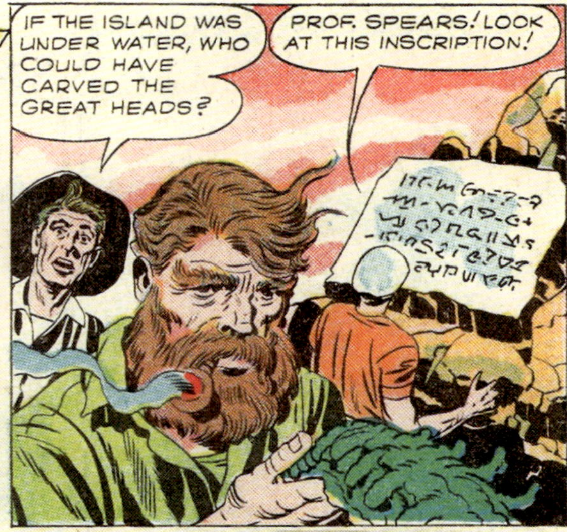

For all the effort that has gone into them, none of the translations done so far provides a reliable guide to what the rongorongo tablets actually contained. Ure Va'e Iko's recitation to Thompson offers a possible thread, but it may say more about the Rapanui oral tradition than the written one. We do know that the oral tradition was vast, and varied. Most of it was sung. According to one early commentator, Rapanui songs expressed "the surprise of being alive and also the sadness of life."[12] Whether the tablets do the same remains to be seem. Our best indication of what the rongorongo script was used for comes, however, not from songs or attempts at deciphering, but from ethnographic data, especially that gathered by Katherine Routledge in 1914 from some of the few Rapanui elders who survived the holocaust of the 1860s.

Routledge was a remarkable woman, who has been unjustly forgotten. She was the daughter of a wealthy Quaker family, which made a fortune manufacturing brick in northern England. She showed an independent streak early on, graduating from Oxford with a degree in modern history and traveling to South Africa as part of an investigative committee after the Second Boer War. In 1906, she married an Australian adventurer named William Scoresby Routledge. Together, they settled in Kenya, where Katherine studied the customs of the Kikuyu and Scoresby quarreled with everyone he met. In 1910, they decided to head to Easter Island to learn what they could about its monumental statues. They had a yacht specially built for this

purpose, and hired a crew of eager young Englishmen, most of whom quit during the year it took to sail to Easter Island. They arrived in 1914, in the midst of a diplomatic crisis caused by the outbreak of World War I. While German cruisers rendezvoused offshore, Katherine immersed herself in the culture of the island. Together with her husband, she explored caves and documented fallen statues. Her most valuable work, though, came from speaking with the few old people who remembered life on the island before the arrival of the Peruvian slavers. Her best informants were two elders, Kirimuti and Tomenika, confined to a leper colony in the north of the island.

Their memories reached back to the 1850s, when the island was still ruled by Nga'ara, an *'ariki mau*, or paramount chief. King Nga'ara, as he is sometimes called, reigned from sometime in the mid-1830s to the time of his death in 1859. During this time, he elevated literacy to almost the status of a religion. He seems to have considered the teaching and learning of rongorongo as one of his most important tasks. He spent his days traveling around the island, visiting the various rongorongo schools and interrogating their

Above: "Prof. Spears! Look at this inscription!" Rongorongo makes an appearance in "The Stone Sentinels of Giant Island," which initially appeared in April 1959 in the "House of Mystery" series published by DC Comics. In the comic, seen here in its 1971 reissue, Spears solves the riddle of rongorongo and saves the day.

pupils about their progress in the script. He would hold a tablet up and make a student read it. If they did well, he would clap loudly and give rongorongo artifacts to their teacher. If they did poorly, he would blame the teacher and confiscate their tablets.

The cult of literacy culminated every year at the annual 'Anakena festival. Held on a sacred beach, said to be the first place the original migrants to the island put to shore, the festival drew hundreds of people in a celebration of reading and recitation. All day, rongorongo experts would read their tablets in front of a crowd waiting to applaud their successes and jeer their failures. At the end of the day, the king would mount a platform held aloft by eight men and lecture the bards on their duty to perform well. Then he would give each man a chicken.

Later in life, Katherine Routledge went mad. Her family blamed the malign influence of a Rapanui prophetess named Angata, with whom she was close. More likely, she succumbed to the paranoid schizophrenia that afflicted her brother. She spent her last days in an asylum, and her notes were left in the archive of the Royal Geographic Society, where they were mostly forgotten.[13] Combined with testimonies gathered by a few other researchers, they allow us to piece together a rough inventory of the various uses to which rongorongo tablets were put. Some were hymns in praise of chiefs. Some listed the names of people killed in battle. A great many of the inscriptions were charms. The written word was a conduit of magical power, which could be harnessed for various ends. Some tablets could save people from danger. Others dealt with vengeance: a *timo* tablet had the power to kill a murderer. A *pure* tablet could enhance fertility. Songs incised on artifacts could increase the harvest or the size of a catch. This may explain why they went unseen before Joseph-Eugène Eyraud's arrival in 1864. The most significant piece of information, though, from Routledge's informants might be the detail about the schools. It took pupils only a few months to master rongorongo. As Steven Fischer, the current leading student of the script writes, "If the little Rapanui children could learn it," then "so can we."[14]

Fischer thinks he has the rongorongo problem scotched. In his reading, the various tablets are all procreation texts—endless series of begats and begettings, tying living Easter Islanders to their mythical ancestors. As is usual in the tiny, querulous world of rongorongo studies, his opponents disagree, accusing him of misreadings, false assumptions, and other methodological inadequacies. Fischer remains convinced that he is right, but one thing does give the self-proclaimed "glyphbreaker" (the title of his autobiography) pause. As he notes in his vast scholarly tome on the script, one of Routledge's informants told her that her husband used to stay up at night reading his cache of rongorongo tablets. She used to hear him reading, and when he did so, he would periodically "stop in the middle and chuckle."[15]

What was he laughing at? It seems unlikely to have been a ritual formula. Whatever the rongorongo texts really say, they upend all our expectations of the nature of literacy. It was created in a place without cities, or even, really, commerce. Its inscriptions had the force of magic, but their meanings were not in themselves sacred. It is an unbreakable cipher, yet it could be mastered by children. Best of all, by refusing to be decoded, rongorongo mocks the primacy of Western reason. May it forever remain a riddle we can't parse, a joke whose punchline is forever slipping from our grasp.

1 Terry Hunt and Carl Lipo, *The Statues That Walked: Unraveling the Mystery of Easter Island* (New York: Free Press, 2011), p. 4.

2 Ibid., p. 154.

3 Ibid., p. 155.

4 Steven Roger Fischer, *Island at the End of the World* (London: Reaktion Books, 2005), p. 86.

5 Stéphen-Chauvet, *L'île de Pâques et ses mystères* (Paris: Éditions Tel, 1935), p. 381.

6 Steven Roger Fischer, *Rongorongo: The Easter Island Script* (Oxford: Clarendon Press, 1997), pp. 97–99.

7 Ibid., p. 111.

8 Ibid., p. 144.

9 Ibid., p. 241.

10 Ibid., p. 171.

11 Cited in Igor Pozdniakov and Konstantin Pozdniakov, "Rapanui Writing and the Rapanui Language: Preliminary Results of a Statistical Analysis," *Forum for Anthropology and Culture*, no. 3 (2006), p. 96. A PDF of this article, albeit with different pagination, is available at <pozdniakov.free.fr/publications/2007_Rapanui_Writing_and_the_Rapanui_Language.pdf>. In this document, the quotation appears on page 10.

12 Steven Roger Fischer, *Rongorongo*, p. 303.

13 Most of the information in this paragraph and the one above is derived from Jo Anne Van Tilburg, *Among Stone Giants: The Life of Katherine Routledge and Her Remarkable Expedition to Easter Island* (New York: Scribner, 2003).

14 Steven Roger Fischer, *Rongorongo*, p. 347.

15 Ibid., p. 282.

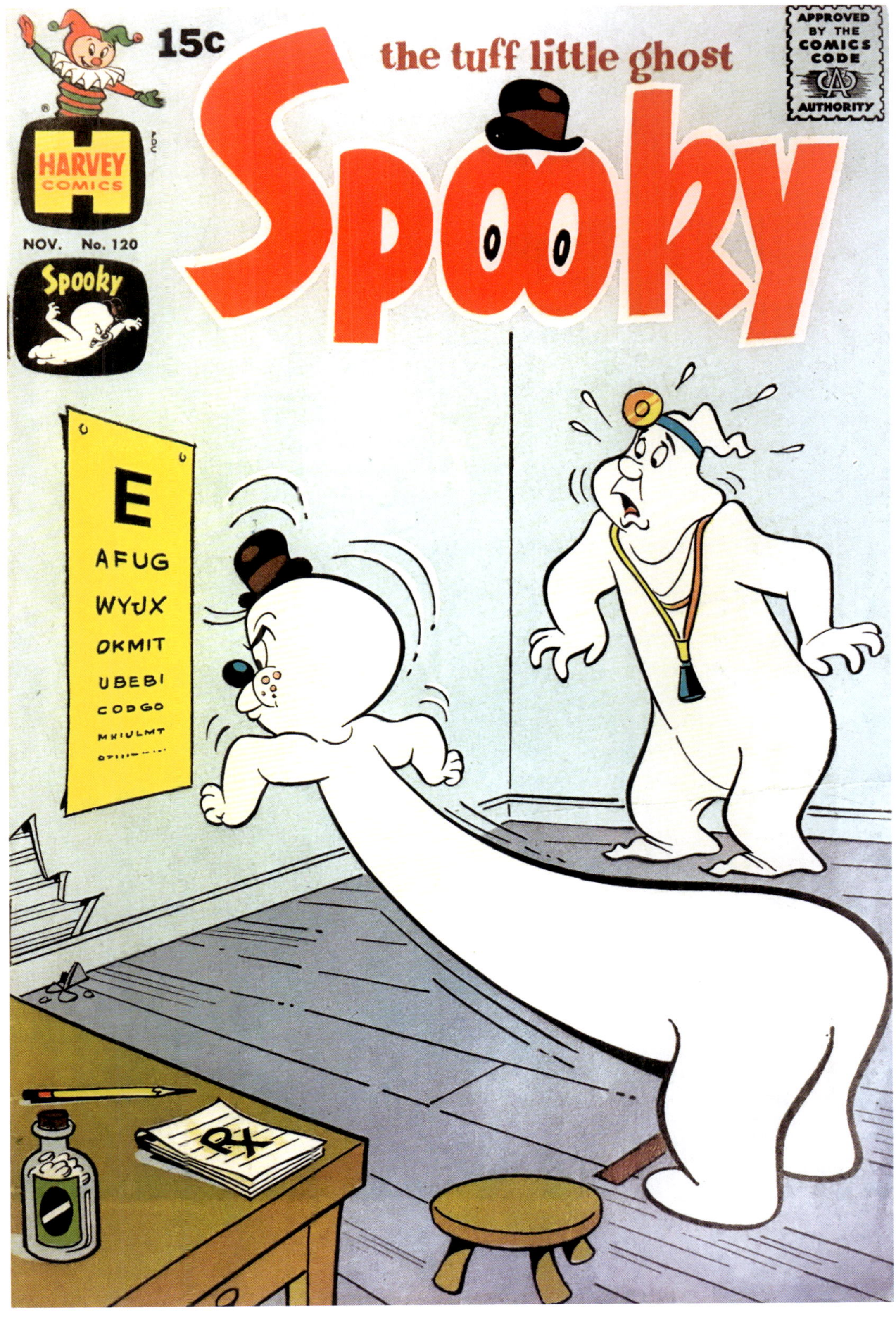
15c
the tuff little ghost
Spooky
HARVEY COMICS
NOV. No. 120
Spooky
APPROVED BY THE COMICS CODE AUTHORITY
E
AFUG
WYJX
OKMIT
UBEBI
CODGO
MKIULMT
RX

VISION QUEST
William Germano

The eye chart we all know is a visual display of letters arranged top to bottom, from largest to smallest. The invention of Dutch ophthalmologist Herman Snellen (1834–1908), it's universally recognized as a diagnostic tool for assessing the acuity of a person's vision. (Snellen's carte de visite included a tiny version of his chart as his signature). For a hundred and fifty years, the modern eye chart—in any of its increasingly sophisticated variations—has provided a means of calibrating visual acuity so that the findings could be shared among vision care professionals, the ophthalmologist or optometrist who examines you, or the optician who grinds your lenses and fits your frames.

There have been eye tests since antiquity—anybody can set up a means of deciding who has sharper sight—but an eye chart is a graphic tool built on principles of precision and reproducibility. The first real eye chart we have arrives on schedule, at the beginning of ocular modernity, in the era of Galileo, when the human eye became a space traveler. In 1623, the same year that Shakespeare's colleagues created a posthumous collection of his plays in one large folio volume, Benito Daza de Valdés published *Uso de los antojos para todo genero de vistas* (The use of eyeglasses for all types of vision), a vernacular guide to lenses and spectacles—how they worked, the different conditions they corrected, and how using them might change your life.[1]

We don't know much about Daza; he was born in Córdoba in 1591, became a Dominican friar and minor functionary of the Spanish Inquisition, and died in Seville in 1634.[2] The *Uso* is a surprisingly breezy little volume, and rare enough to be referred to as the Holy Grail of ophthalmology. There wasn't a second edition or even a translation into Latin, but if there were ophthalmological justice, Daza's book would be on a world tour of its own.

The *Uso*'s title page carries an extraordinary device: a pair of eyeglasses, radiant with energy. In place of the user's right lens is a brilliant anthropomorphic sun, and in the user's left lens sits the man in the moon. Lozenges with stylized concave and convex lenses bracket the image; light seems to stream outward to four eyes placed in the corners of the rectangular plate. These eyes watch and are watched. Divine light is present (he's a cleric, after all, and the book is dedicated to Our Lady), but the source of the radiance seems to be coming from the spectacles, as if to say that the illumination just might be within us. In the great age of the telescope and the microscope, a good pair of eyeglasses makes discoverers of us all.

Daza provides scales and diagrams that are functionally the earliest graphic tools for measuring visual acuity. They're crude by modern standards—a quick glance suggests a rain gauge or the device a shoe salesman uses on your foot—but Daza's testing scheme aims to maintain a transferable datum about a person's sight that itself becomes a tool for matching user to lens.

Much of the *Uso* is given over to dialogues in which gentlemen discuss their eye conditions with experts. In one, we're introduced to travelers Jorge and Esteban, *dos caballeros indianos*—two gentlemen from the Indies. At home, they've seen a pair of eyeglasses of Spanish manufacture, and they've traveled across the ocean to have their eyes checked by a famous specialist.

The travelers become the premise for a dialogue concerning ways in which eyes are imperfect and how lenses can be crafted to compensate. Jorge, nearsighted since early childhood, has struggled with glasses in what are for us quite recognizable ways: his embarrassment at needing them, his wife's advice that he shouldn't wear them because they make him look old, the frustration of arriving at the theater and, having forgotten his glasses, being unable to see the performance.

In early modernity, visual aids perform an important social function, a point Daza gamely makes through the introduction of Marcelo, another optometric straw man. Marcelo can see up close, but his distance vision is so bad that he salutes everyone he passes. This courteousness, he explains, has its drawbacks:

As I was walking down a street, I took off my cap to a lady who was at her window, and as I saw that my servants began to laugh at me, I asked them who that person was, and they

---

Opposite: Little ghost, big test. Spooky gets his eyes examined in the November 1970 edition of his eponymous Harvey Comics series.

VSO

DE LOS ANTOIOS

PARA TODO GENERO DE VISTAS:

En que se enseña a conocer los grados que a cada vno le
faltan de su vista, y los que tienen qualef-
quier antojos.

Y ASSI MISMO A QVE TIEMPO SE AN
de vsar, y como se pediran en ausencia, con otros auisos impor-
tantes, a la vtilidad y conseruacion de la vista.

POR EL L. BENITO DAÇA DE VALDES,
Notario de el Santo Oficio de la Ciudad de Sevilla.

DEDICADO A NVESTRA SEÑORA
de la Fuensanta de la Ciudad de Cordoua.

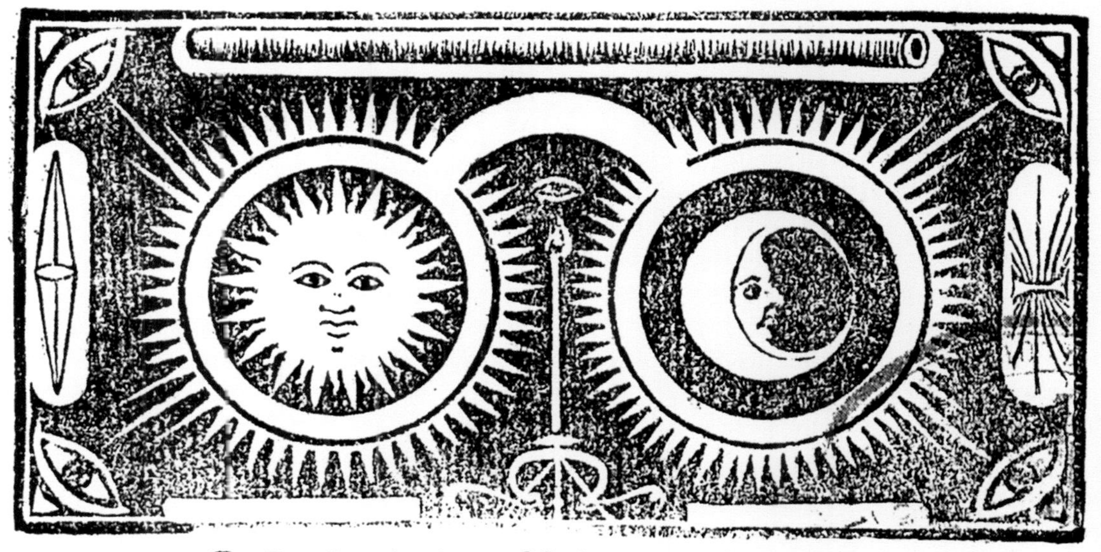

CON PRIVILEGIO.

Impresso en Seuilla, por Diego Perez. Año de 1623.

answered that it was a side of mutton that had been hung up. I blessed myself and made a thousand signs of the cross, for I would have sworn that I'd seen her, with all her veils and all her features.[3]

By the early seventeenth century, one could argue that eyeglasses were becoming *socially* necessary because it's impossible to behave properly if you can't see properly. Poor Marcelo is "pervirtiendo las cortesias"—perverting the order of courtesies—undermining the social order and the ideologies that protect it through sumptuary laws and other ritual displays of status. He needs eyeglasses so that he can tell a *doña* from a *criada*, a lady from her servant (or from a side of mutton). It's about more than watching the actors on stage. Vision correction morphs into a mechanism for social correction, which in turn is about self-development and social mastery.

. . .

Eighteenth-century work on optics, more concerned with physics than the physical, advanced our understanding of the workings of refraction, paying special attention to the operation of telescopes. Eyeglasses became both appliances and metaphors. One preacher, seizing an opportunity to moralize ocular anxiety, likens Scripture to a pair of spectacles useful for spotting sin.[4]

As a visual aid, eyeglasses were controversial, with authorities like George Adams (1750–1795) arguing that spectacles weakened eyes. Others, perhaps drawn to the market potential of spectacles in an increasingly literate society, promoted what the optician Benjamin Martin called "visual glasses," appliances touted for their capacity to refine and strengthen vision.[5] (Martin used colored glass, with the lenses set at an unusual tilt.) Missing in the arguments over whether eyeglasses were in fact a good thing was a systematic analysis of visual acuity and the connection, through a reproducible graphic, from the wearer to the maker of lenses.

In the 1830s, German ophthalmologist Hermann Küchler proposed a chart to test his patient's eyes, using images of common things he had cut out of calendars and other ephemera. In finding his materials in random printed sources, Küchler was doing what would become a principle of European avant-garde art almost a century later. Cutting out pictures and, later on, words from newspapers, Küchler's diagnostic project feels like a forerunner of modernism: Dada's

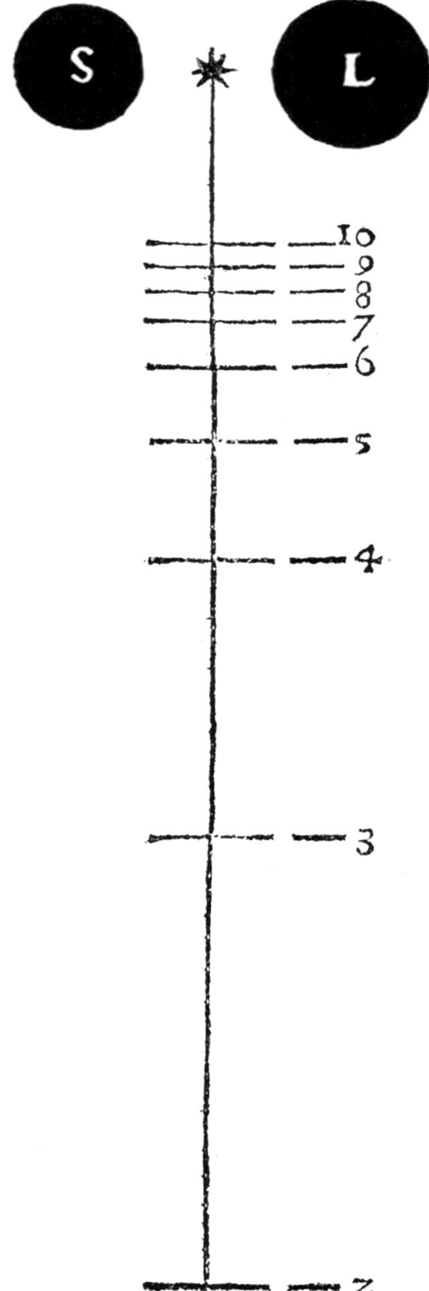

Above: An eye chart from Daza's *Uso.*
Opposite: Title page of Daza de Valdés's *Uso de los antojos para todo genero de vistas*, published in Seville in 1623.

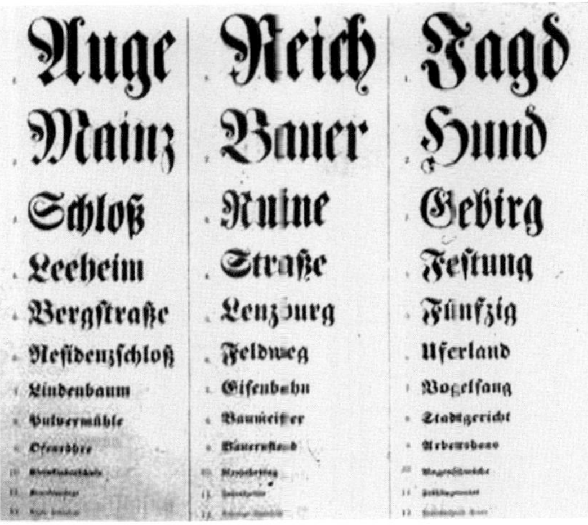

Abandoning objects for words. Hermann Küchler eye test from 1843.

language games, Duchamp's celebration of the ready-made, Hannah Höch's bouquet of eyes, and the dueling collages of Braque and Picasso.

Recognizing the limitations of a pictorial eye chart, Küchler adjusted his model, giving it a linguistic turn. His diagnostic objects became words, stacked one on top of the other, in descending order of size. There's something strangely compelling about the Küchler charts, with their singular nouns and German place names—*eye, Mainz, castle, empire, farmer, ruin, hunt, dog, mountain*—as if they're a word-association test derived from Romantic painting. In the descent from large type to small—the strong, clear figure at the top, and then the infinity fade—Küchler's model prepared the ground for the crucial unidirectional mechanism of the Snellen chart.

Building on German and Dutch ophthalmological work, Herman Snellen devised a graphic in 1862 that was ingeniously efficient: eleven lines, clear type, nine alphabetic forms distributed in an apparently random fashion, reduction in type size from top to bottom. Snellen called them *optotypes*.

By eliminating words, Snellen was able to counteract our quite useful ability to complete a familiar string of letters based on our knowledge of a language. It's how we read, drawing on our archive to fill the gaps. In Snellen's model, the sequences of letters are meaningless, so gaps don't really exist. He also proposed that the strokes of each letter be of equal weight, so that the eye would receive, through even tone, equal information concerning each element in

a letter (what graphic designers mean by "color"). Snellen's most important innovation, however, was in standardizing the perceived size of a letter as a function of visual angle: you live in 360 degrees, your horizontal field of vision is around 114 degrees, your little finger held sideways at arm's length is about 1 degree of arc. Each degree is further divisible into 60 minutes.

Snellen represented the relationship of viewer, distance, and eyesight in this formula:

$$v = \frac{d}{D}$$

It's often referred to as the "Snellen fraction": V is the acuity of vision, d is the distance from the eye chart, and D is the distance at which the viewer can read an object at 5 minutes of arc. To be able to do that at twenty feet is, in lay shorthand, to have 20/20 vision. To be able to see just the top line—only the giant E—is to have 20/200 vision, in which case you are legally blind, here meaning you can see at twenty feet what someone with "standard" vision can see at ten times the distance.

The reproducibility of Snellen's exam protocol was critical to its immediate success. Soon after the chart's appearance, the British army took up the test to evaluate its recruits throughout Her Majesty's vast empire.[6] Dutch invention and British imperialism converged, merging the graphic and the geographic, helping to make Snellen's chart the most influential and widely used diagnostic graphic in the world, both in its original form and in its variations and refinements.

The syntax of the Snellen chart would soon become the theme of endless variations. There are charts in Cyrillic and Chinese and Hebrew, charts with simple pictograms for children, sometimes referred to as "Snellen's garden." The Tumbling E chart consists only of the capital letter E in each of its ninety-degree rotations. The physician only needs to ask: which way does the E point? Left? Down? Up? Right? It's not what you would really call "tumbling," a verb you might associate with clowns or drunks; the "tumbling" E moves with military precision. There's also the Landolt C, a fat ring with a cut into it, like a letter C but much weightier, each cut pointing in one of eight directions. Like the Tumbling E, it's especially useful for the patient who cannot name, or distinguish, the letters of the Roman alphabet.

These Snellen variants begin crowding in on one another. An eye chart published by George Mayerle

in San Francisco in 1907 is a compendium of Snellen graphology. At the center is a column of symbols for the unlettered, its bottom three lines consisting of an American flag, an eye, and, finally, a simple black dot. To the right are columns of Chinese, Russian and Hebrew; to the left, English, German (in Fraktur type), and Japanese. It's a snapshot of a practicing optician's clientele around 1907, the year of the earthquake, in a vigorously polyglot San Francisco.

· · ·

While Snellen's name has become synonymous with diagnosing visual acuity, his chart is only a means of determining the clarity of distant vision. When it comes to testing close-up vision, we have to thank a different ophthalmological pioneer.

When you sit in your doctor's office, you are handed a small card, told to hold it at the distance you would a book or a newspaper, and to read what you can. This card is a descendant of the other, less celebrated eye chart, one conceived by Snellen's Austrian contemporary Eduard Jäger, Ritter von Jaxtthal, also known less formally as Eduard Jäger.[7] The reclusive physician was a tireless observer and recorder of the eye's anatomy, a proponent of the ophthalmoscope, and the developer of a vision test administered at reading distance.[8] Working with Vienna's Imperial Royal Printers, Jäger developed a test of graduated reading samples. The first of these tests was published in 1854, eight years before Snellen's eye chart.

Jäger wanted to understand how well people

Below: George Mayerle's eye test, San Francisco, 1907. Courtesy US National Library of Medicine.

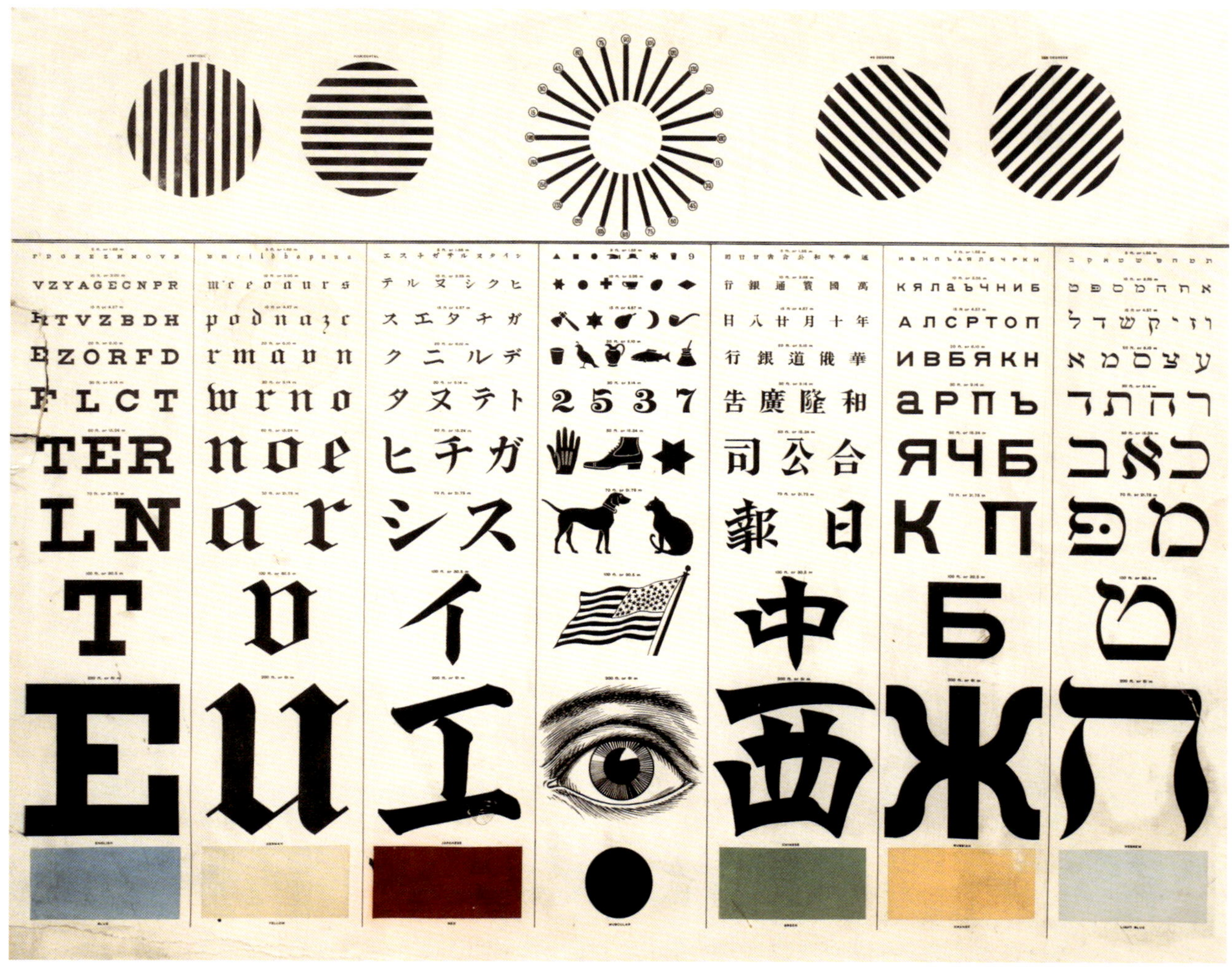

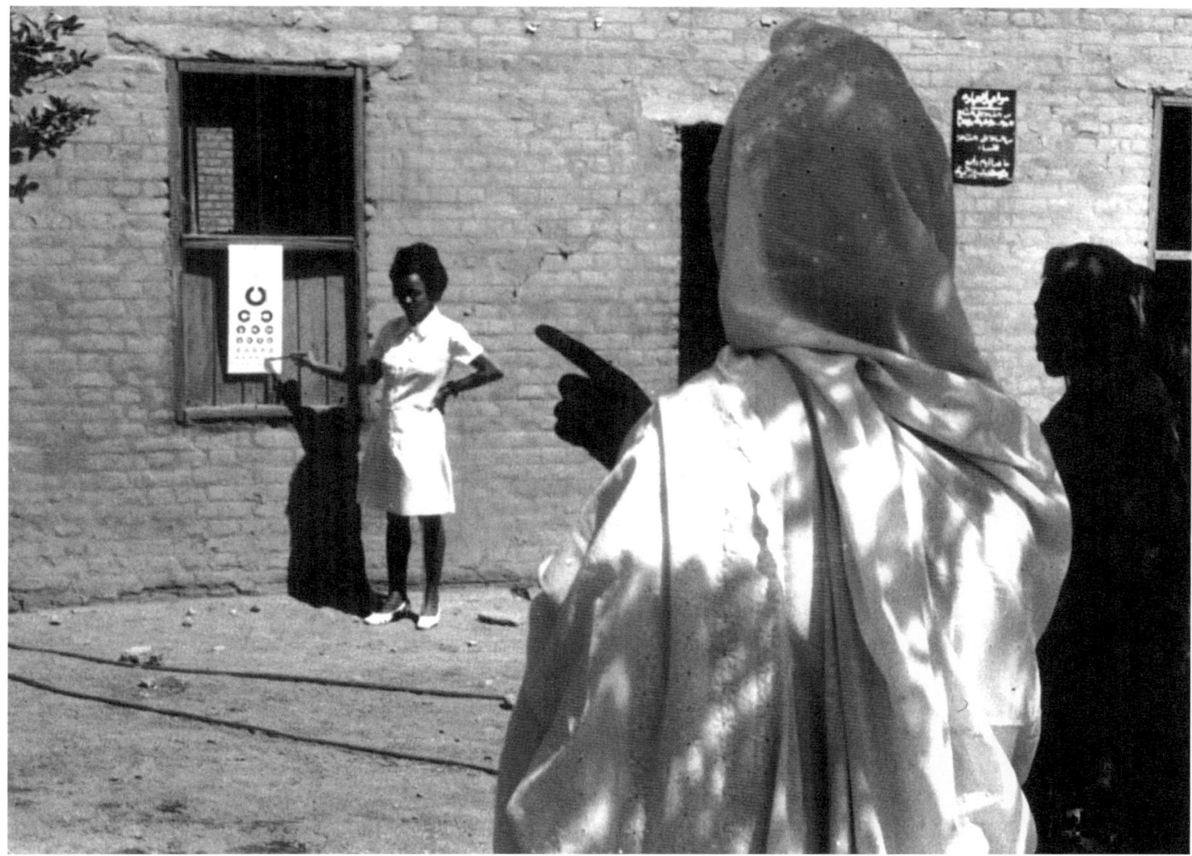

Above: A woman in a Sudanese village takes an eye test using a Landolt C chart, probably 1981. Photo Didier Henrioud. Courtesy World Health Organization.

read—a book, a letter, the newspaper—and created a tool intended to bring exactly that information to the surface. Jäger called his diagnostic *Schrift-scalen*, or, in English, test types. Unlike Snellen's optotype chart, which arranged graduated *letters* in a vertical pattern in order to test distance, Jäger arranged graduated *text*—excerpts of prose, typically such German greats as Goethe and Schiller—to be held in the hand at what is referred to as "a comfortable distance."

Printings of Jäger's test types survive in variant forms, but the most striking examples present the reader with a continuous narrative in graduated sizes—the first pages in the tiniest type and subsequent passages growing larger and larger, with each ending abruptly, as if in a visual fortissimo. Jäger never knew Calvino's *If on a Winter's Night a Traveler*, but there's something familiarly postmodern about

the Jäger nineteenth-century test types and their cool, abrupt incompleteness.

• • •

Snellen *plus* Jäger: testing for visual acuity involves determining it in two modes, far and near, working through the distinctions between letter and text, the instant and the current, and finally between symbol and narrative. In retrospect, we can see the graduated sizes of Snellen's optotypes and Jäger's test types as part of modernity's visual regime.

We've lived by Snellen's rules for more than a century. His eye chart format turned up in the 1920s in inexpensive optometers. You look through a little lens and move a tiny Snellen target along a balsa wood strip until you can see it clearly. The spot where the target lands is marked with a number corresponding to a lens strength. Almost a century later, there are quick self-test charts in your neighborhood drug store, where you can pick up cheap reading glasses, which might do in a pinch.

The most familiar descendants of Snellen's work, though, survive in T-shirts and posters and what might be called ophthalmological-themed tchotchkes, the progeny of designers who recognized in Snellen's syntax the dance of a visual grammar. Once you start noticing Snellen-based graphic design, you'll see it everywhere—on clothing, objects, and shop signs—pyramids of information with large letters or objects at top and often a satirical takeaway in the final, barely readable bottom line.

Part oracular pronouncement, part hieroglyph, sometimes poem, always picture, the eye chart is that ordinary object that tells us what we think normal looks like. How many other ways of getting that reassurance are there? Your vital signs are within an appropriate range, you live a middle-class life, are of average intelligence, you dream dreams you hope are like everyone else's. But the eye chart promises something else: the precision of the right answer, and the idea of the normal. Which it does by becoming an object that's all about lessons—lessons in reading, lessons in discrimination between shapes, in the threshold of diagnosis, in the borders between the machine and the body and between the organic and the appliance. It's a message that finally reaches us when, despite our best efforts, it slips out of sight.

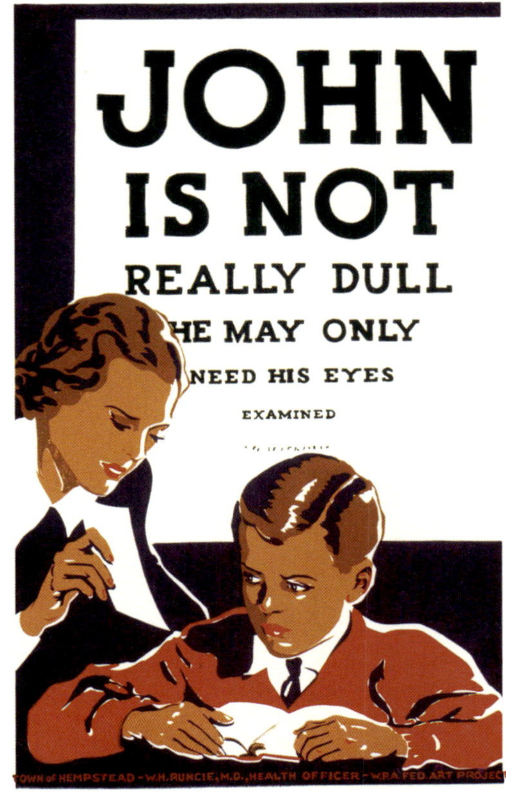

Works Progress Administration poster made at the request of the health officer of the town of Hempstead, New York, ca. 1936–1937. Courtesy Library of Congress.

1 Benito Daza de Valdés, *Uso de los antojos para todo genero de vistas: En que se enseña a conocer los grados que a cada uno le faltan de su vista, y los que tienen quales-quier antojos* (Seville: Printed for Diego Perez, 1623).

2 Madrid's Instituto de Óptica "Daza de Valdés" was established in 1946. A Spanish postage stamp honoring Daza was issued in 1966.

3 Benito Daza de Valdés, *Uso*, p. 33. My translation.

4 J. G., Vicar of Barton, *A Discovery of the Snake in the Grass: Or a Spectacle for Weak Eyes; Being a Sermon Preach'd at the Arch-Deacon's Visitation at Caster, in the County of Lincoln, May the 14th, 1716* (Nottingham: Printed by W. Ascough, 1716).

5 Benjamin Martin, *An Essay on Visual Glasses (Vulgarly Called Spectacles), wherein It Is Shewn from the Principles of Optics, and the Nature of the Eye, that the Common Structure of Those Glasses Is Contrary to the Rules of Art, to the Nature of Things, etc. and Very Prejudicial to the Eyes; The Nature of Vision in the Eye Explained, and Glasses of a New Construction Proposed* (London: printed for the author, 1756).

6 Despite military claims to rigor, standards for visual acuity in the armed forces have probably always been flexible. In 1914, a report by C. Devereux Marshall, F.R.C.S., could declare that "candidates for naval cadetships must possess full normal vision as determined by Snellen's tests, each eye being separately examined," while in the case of other branches of the Royal Navy "full normal vision is not required." Normal vision here is uncorrected vision, which is to say that Navy recruits could wear corrective lenses but would be ineligible for cadetships. The report goes on to offer, in elaborate detail, the levels of visual impairment permissible—and to which degree—for which positions throughout the empire. For each, the military machine of the Edwardian era specified how well you would have to be able to see to get and keep that particular appointment. A special emphasis is placed on color-blindness, and which positions would be unavailable to the color-blind candidate. There is even something called the Colour-Ignorance Test: "The object of this test is simply to ascertain whether the candidate knows the names of the three colours, red, green and white, and the test is to be confined to the naming of colours." No positions are specified for which being "colour-aware" would be a requirement. See C. Devereux Marshall, *Diseases of the Eyes* (New York: William Wood & Company, 1914), pp. 294ff.

7 The essential analysis is in Paul E. Runge, "Eduard Jaeger's Test-Types (Schrift-Scalen) and the Historical Development of Vision Tests," *Transactions of the American Ophthalmological Society*, vol. 98 (2000). I am indebted here to his rigorous research.

8 Paul E. Runge, "Eduard Jaeger's Test-Types," p. 403.

WELCOME TO ARMAGEDDON!
Julian Lucas

The beauty of sand, in other words, belonged to death.
— Kobo Abe, *The Woman in the Dunes*

When we say, "It's just a game," what we mean is that there are no consequences. Everything can be erased and done over, the pieces swept off the board and reset. Repetition invites impunity, and so players murder bystanders in Grand Theft Auto, crash airplanes in Flight Simulator, or make suicidal charges on the beaches of Normandy in Call of Duty. "We who are about to die reboot you," is the battle cry of the armchair gladiator. There is no reason to act with character in a world of experiment.

How far this seems from the truth of play, the pull of Thanatos expressed, for example, in the phrase "roll them bones." Or the underworld gravity of senet, one of the earliest recorded board games, often placed as a funerary talisman in ancient Egyptian tombs. Senet was not only about death but intended for the dead, who played against invisible opponents for the stake of their souls. Winning conferred a chance for eternal life in Aaru, the heavenly reed fields; the punishment for losing was oblivion.[1]

There are no resurrections in Armageddon MUD, a text-based role-playing game (RPG) set on the harsh desert planet Zalanthas. One of the Internet's oldest extant virtual worlds, it is an amoral fairytale about dune traders and bandits, assassins and sorcerer-kings, collaboratively written by thousands of players over a period of twenty-six years.[2] Created in 1991 by a thirteen-year-old coder named Dan Brumleve, the kernel of the story was cribbed from a Dungeons and Dragons campaign setting called "Dark Sun," source of the game's fantasy races (elves, dwarves, muls, halflings, half-giants), its *kaiju*-sized insects, and the foundational conceit of a once-verdant world desiccated by "defiling" magic.[3]

From there, the staff of "immortals" invented, raising from the wastes two autocratic city-states (blunt Allanak and subtle Tuluk, ruled by the Highlord Tektolnes and the Sun King Muk Utep, respectively); four great merchant clans (Stone Age multinationals with huge reptile-drawn caravans); dozens of noble houses, mercenary companies, gangs, and tribes; languages and accents; weapons, recipes, spells;

cultivars of imaginary fruit, each tagged with a taste and smell; and, at the very bottom of the world, a wind-tossed sea of silt upon which one might float, or drown.

The exact scope of the game is unknowable. Even if the notoriously secretive immortals were to release the map of "rooms" (delimited areas of play including everything from wind-swept ergs to cramped wagon cockpits, and numbering over thirty thousand), the catalogue of items, and the roster of characters (still growing at a Malthusian clip), decades of events, residing only in the memories of players, would remain undisclosed. Because Armageddon MUD is not a static or deterministic fiction but a book written in sand—a constantly moving, sentient flux of story in silicate. If Percy Shelley had built an RPG, he might have come up with something like this singular game, a vast, unmerciful "Ozymandias Online."

. . .

In the phylogeny of gaming, the multiuser dungeon (MUD) is the gingko tree, the fern, the horseshoe crab, an unlikely survivor that despite the Oculus Rifts and the Pokémon Gos still holds fast to its evolutionary niche. Ancestor of all online virtual worlds, MUDs are real-time interactive realities, entirely textual and accessible from the command-line via "telnet."[4] Their forms differ widely from game to game, but all share a general frame of organization—an ontology, epistemology, and ethics. "Being" in the MUD is divided into rooms, items, and mobiles, which are further divided into player characters (PCs) and non-player characters (NPCs). Knowledge is narrowly perspectival—*look east, sniff shirt, taste ginka*—and there are no walkthroughs, mini-maps, or god's-eye views. Action follows a grammar of possible commands (*eat tuber* but not *eat sword*) and a complex etiquette of playing conventions. All three come together in a representation that looks something like this:

```
> look
Amid the Dunes [NESW]
Smooth, undulating dunes of fine ochre sand
extend in all directions, stretching as far
as the eye can see. A leather waterskin is
here.
```

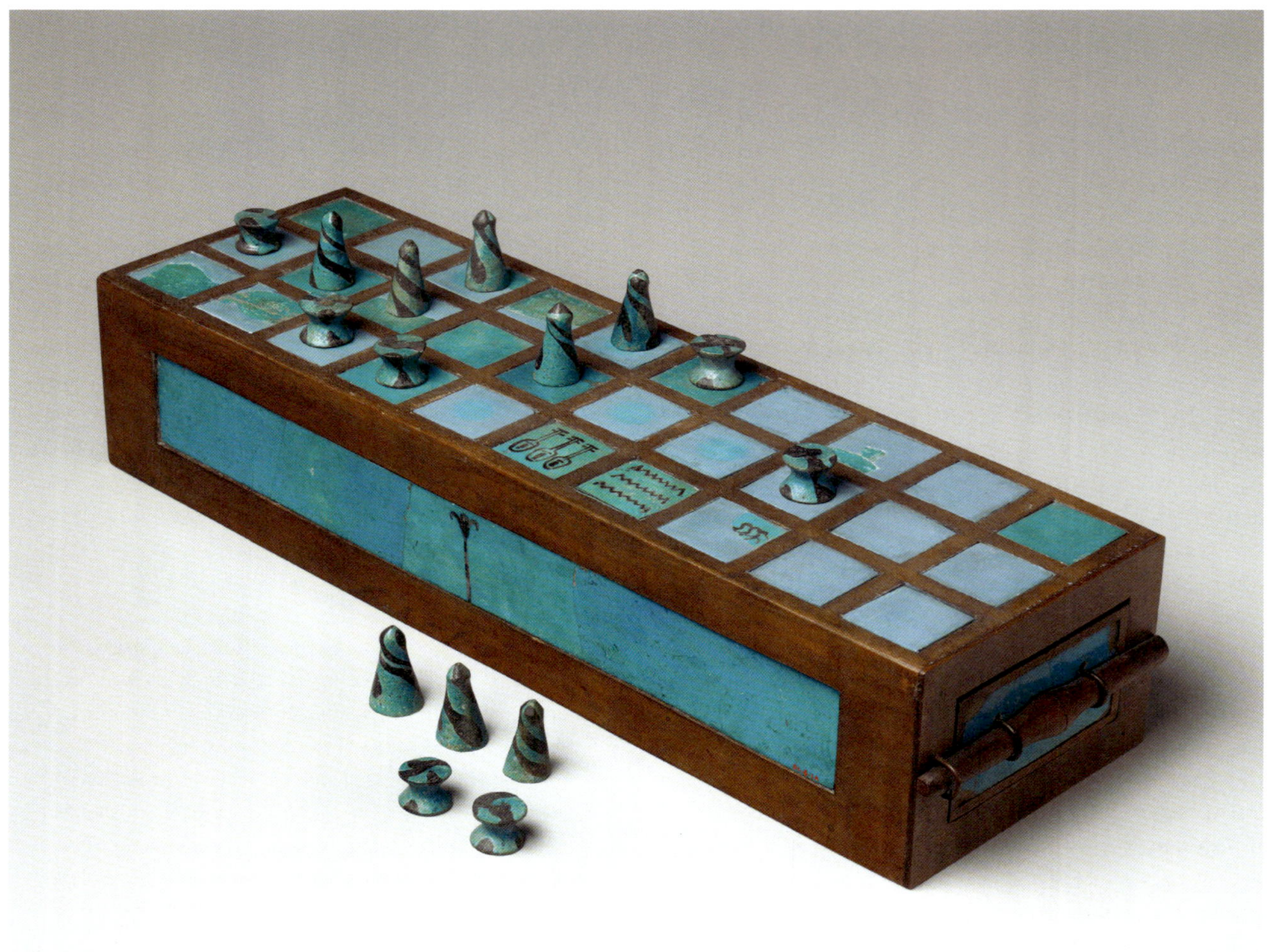

The ancient Egyptian game of senet. The faience inlays and playing pieces of this game box were discovered in a tomb at Abydos. The Metropolitan Museum of Art estimates that these artifacts were made between 1550 BC and 1295 BC; the box itself is a reconstruction. Courtesy The Metropolitan Museum of Art.

```
The corpse of the tall, muscular man is here.
  > get waterskin
You pick up a leather waterskin. It is empty.
```

A great-grandchild of the original MUD1 created by Roy Trubshaw in 1978, Armageddon MUD belongs to one of the first great waves of virtual-world proliferation. It began as a variant of DikuMUD, a codebase created in 1990 at the University of Copenhagen that gave rise to the genre called "hack and slash."[5] The main trunk of this genre's legacy is represented by graphical Massively Multiplayer Online Role-playing Games (MMORPGS) like EverQuest and World of Warcraft, where the "H&S' ethos of slaying beasts, leveling up, and collecting cool equipment still thrives. But Armageddon MUD evolved in a different direction—not beyond words, but deeper within them.

Two years after it was founded, it became "role-play intensive" (RPI), the first MUD to declare itself so, and that meant narrative rather than hack-and-slash competition was the central component of the experience.[6] Characters required approval by application, with short biographies befitting the larger story, and all play was mandated to be "in-character," without reference to the out-of-character world. The DikuMUD code was modified to facilitate complexity of expression; a system of negotiation and staff governance was created to ensure a coherent, immersive story; and a stark condition was imposed to solder the players to their new universe—"permanent death." It was a successful formula for a persistent virtual reality: more than forty thousand player-characters have lived and died since *Armageddon* launched, with a sum in-game time of over eight hundred and thirty-eight years.[7]

. . .

Armageddon MUD's Cartesian credo is, "I play, therefore I do not know"—which is to say that its vision of role-playing requires the suppression of knowledge and intention beyond one's character's ken. Player-characters, like jurors, are expected to act only on the basis of admissible evidence; that which comes directly from playing the game as that character. If you know, for example, that a conspiracy is underway in the city of Tuluk (whether from previous play as an involved character or an illicit tip from another player), your character must remain unaware. This form of sequestration is one facet of the in-character (IC) /

out-of-character (OOC) divide, a handy binary that is nothing less than the prime directive of Armageddon's immersive virtual world. Like the curtain in *The Wizard of Oz*, it separates the story's participants from its architects, even when these turn out to be the same people in different roles.

The MUD is structured as a simultaneous multidimensional novel, a feat enabled by a powerful and highly nuanced vocabulary of expressive tools. While the most essential command in a hack-and-slash MUD is *kill*, in Armageddon it is *emote*, an action that exists in most MUDs but which on Zalanthas approaches Jamesian levels of syntactic sophistication. Simply put, it is a command that allows characters to describe an expressive action, which is then "echoed" to every other player in the room. *emote smiles, emote scoffs, emote draws a line in the sand*. But also, *emote Turning a page of ~cabinet, @ furrows ^me brows and mumbles to &me.*, which would echo, "Turning a page of his issue of Cabinet magazine, the tall, muscular man furrows his brow and mumbles to himself."

The intricately punctuated syntax ensures that every player-character sees the action in question from the proper perspective. *&me* will echo "yourself" to the character emoting, but "herself" to everyone else in the room. Other commands, like *whisper* or *hemote* ("hidden emote"—only someone *watch*-ing carefully will see), are only perceptible to certain individuals, while other commands, like *think* and *feel*, only echo to the player who enters them, staff observers, and the rare clairvoyant "mindbender."[8] Each character has distinct vantage point, perceives a different set of details, and moves less according to any narrative planning than by their individualized relationship to an incompletely visible board.

Zalanthas, the "board" of Armageddon MUD, is defined by one major characteristic: it is a desert. This is not just a backdrop but the terrain of story, no more separable from the form of the game than is the drawing room from *Pride and Prejudice*. The hard-coded dangers of the Zalanthan wastes—sandstorms, giant insects, orc-like "gith" wielding obsidian swords—shape the narratives that characters end up living. Game mechanics (thought by some purists to interfere with the freedom of the imagination) encourage narratives with a material basis in the facts of the world, infusing role-play with a concreteness it would otherwise lack.[9]

Take water, a scarce resource in Zalanthas. On the level of code, it is represented by thirst. *You are thirsty. You are very thirsty. You are parched.* This companionable echo isn't simply inconvenient; without water, your character—no matter how well-written, no matter how integral—will die. So player-characters are forced to adopt one of a number of strategies: risk everything to seek water (or money for water) in the wilderness, deceive or steal from other characters, or align themselves with powerful clans that can provide, in exchange for obedience, an unlimited supply. These behaviors happen to be the very ones prescribed by the documentation describing Zalanthas, marked by autocratic monopoly, nomadic survivalism, and manipulative opportunism. Beginning with a super-structure, the game implements a (code)base to organically reproduce it.

The ideal behind this structure is a fully emergent narrative—a single, seamless world, inter-nally coherent and without limits, shaped from player-character decisions and carefully concealed mechanics by an invisible hand. To some extent, this world already exists. Most of the stories that unfold every day in Zalanthas require nothing beyond the imaginative cooperation of two players—or even just one player, their own mind, and the code. If you want to mine obsidian in the quarry west of Allanak, all you have to do is buy a pickaxe from an NPC shop-keeper and go. Find a player-character companion for some extra narrative interest; emote setting up camp together; start a romantic relationship or develop a murderous grudge. No special assistance required. But there are positive and negative limits to what the code enables, actions that should be possible, but are not, as well as actions that should not be possible, but are. In either case, the gap is closed by "immortal intervention."

. . .

If the dungeon master of a traditional dice game is a monarch, the immortals of Armageddon are the government of a liberal state.[10] Responsible for guiding a large narrative economy, their mission is to promote the growth and stability of story, which they prefer to encourage through indirect means. These include shaping the code and culture of the Zalanthan environ-ment, regulating the terms of role-play, "animating" NPCs ordinarily controlled by simple scripts, and

overseeing the progress of plotlines on a global scale.

Immortals guide history by choosing players for "special roles"—nobles, templar-priests, powerful merchants, military personnel, and the like, who are loosely overseen by immortal-"animated" NPC superiors—and by moderating HRPTs, highly recommended role-playing times: festivals, battles, catastrophes, riots, and other large-scale events that make a sizable impact on the game-world.[11] They also act for the silent majority of "virtual" Zalanthans, who are represented neither by players nor by scripted NPCs.[12] In a war, staff might be called upon to rewrite the rooms of a city after a general sets fire to its market quarter, or to rule on what portion of the virtual populace expires from hunger in a siege. At a bardic competition, immortals might act as the audience, improvising cheers and jeers from bystanders. No situation is too large or too small for their intercession.

Games are infamous for their invisible walls, boundaries where movement stops and a distant landscape reveals itself to be nothing more than wall-paper. These obstacles are a synecdoche for the larger limitations of the genre, which thrives on creating an illusory sense of completeness.[13] The immortals lift Zalanthas above this condition by acting (in a way that is only truly possible for text-based games) as "gods of the gaps," improvising the *terra incognita* beyond the world's edge.

No player-characters live in the remote village of Cenyr, thinly glossed by Armageddon's publicly avail-able documentation. But when one of my characters arrived there after a risky journey through the Red Desert, the NPCs in the marketplace began to speak. I asked questions and learned an incredible wealth of information: the date of the town's foundation, the rituals of the local wind cult, and the qualities of Cenyri music—free use of syncopation, rudimentary phrasing, a diatonic scale with blue fourth and fifth notes. What I had thought to be a small collection of rooms, fewer than a dozen among more than thirty thousand, turned out to contain an encyclopedic wealth of background—secret lore that might have been written by the immortals, lived out by players in prior years and recorded, or written on the spot by a staff member for me. Part of Armageddon's seeming limitlessness is the impossibility of telling the differ-ence between the three.

Armageddon's immortals imbue Zalanthas with a marvelous plasticity, an alternative to "procedural generation" that is creative and human rather than algorithmic. Their primary role, however, is not revealing the world to players, but enabling them to create it, in both its largest and smallest aspects. Of countless objects in the Armageddon universe, some few thousand are "mastercrafts," designed by characters who after attaining a certain level of skill (and, of course, *roleplaying* that attainment, emoting each painstaking step of whittling, flint knapping, chiseling, or leather-curing) are allowed to make their permanent mark on the game.[14] In three years of playing, I created one: *a carved ivory pipe*. Like most special items, it exists primarily as a simple string, difficult to tell from any other equipment in a busy shop's inventory or the description of a room. But a further command, *look pipe*, reveals it at a deeper level of granularity:

```
> A beautifully polished ivory horn has
been carved smoothly into a slender pipe
with a wide, deep bowl. Just over a cord in
length, it is long and thin from the mouth-
piece, curving gently downwards and growing
thicker towards the base. At bottom, the
ivory widens suddenly and curves up into a
wide, deep bowl. Etched across the shaft is
a rough and impressionistic map of Zalanthas,
from Gol Krathu to Vrun Driath, backgrounded
by a repeating pattern of dunes. Subtle and
detailed carvings of caravans, gith, argo-
sies, and other figures are set against the
material, as well as square, fingernail-sized
etchings of all the major settlements of the
Known World. At the very middle of the pipe-
stem sits a small image of Luir's Outpost,
complete with horn-crested walls. A dark,
nearly black sapphire, tumbled to a rough
polish, is set above the gates. A leather
strap allows the pipe to be worn around
the neck.
```

Seti, my merchant-carver, carried this pipe with him for months. For a while it was his signature accessory, the peacock feather he used to accentuate his presence and a distillation of the world as he knew it. But ultimately I gave it away, not knowing where it would end up—my errant contribution to the mosaic of Zalanthas.

• • •

With luck, daring, and imagination, characters in Armageddon MUD can redraw the world's map. The building and conquest of cities, the discovery of new regions, the extinction of species and clans: all have been effected by the careful planning and dramatic missteps of players, some of whom stay alive for years. Playing the long game requires fidelity (since only one character is permitted at a time), but also spontaneity, a force of intention that never loses its sense of stakes. "Permadeath," the impossibility of returning to a character once he or she has died, is the center of this narrative gravity, the mechanism that elevates Armageddon MUD from glorified digital Dungeons and Dragons to the level of art.

Imagine the draft of a novella burning up in your hands, a magnet denaturing your hard drive, the sudden and inexplicable end of a friendship. That is how players feel when they lose their characters—a hurt that at its worst spills over into out-of-character resentments but at best is transmuted into grief-stricken sublimity, the samurai's savor for an honorable end.

What it comes down to in the moment of danger is the simultaneous reconciliation of three perspectives. The player is at once a gamer, who must assess probabilities, marshal reflexes, master anxieties, and sift through very swiftly scrolling text; a character, who might be courageous or cowardly, empathic or coldly pragmatic; and a writer, who for roleplaying to succeed must always supersede the other two. Sometimes, this means accepting death, a demise that is more perfect than survival. Playing Armageddon MUD, like studying philosophy, is learning how to die.

A lonesome hunter I played befriended a stranger in the scrublands. We chased game together until we were thirsty, and the man offered to show the way to a secret spring. When we arrived at where it should have been, he improvised a fairytale about searching for water, which developed an edge of menace as it unwound. It was a Cain and Abel parable, and I realized midway that, as in *1001 Nights*, its ending would coincide with my own. It would have been easy to escape, but I stayed put and listened, never quite sure whether it was I or my doomed hunter who was too enamored with the tale to arrest it.

Other deaths were a surprise. *The rotund, plump-lipped* man, an unsavory spice merchant, was killed for smuggling company goods to a fence in the Labyrinth,

an Allanaki slum. His superiors threw a banquet to celebrate the syndicate's profits, and at its conclusion, gave him the key to a lavish new suite of apartments in reward for his good work. There, his supervisor gutted him with a *translucent, crystalline longknife*. The body, I discovered months later, was dumped in the Sea of Eternal Dust—Armageddon MUD's answer to the New Jersey Pine Barrens.

No matter how your character expires, whether of thirst in a cave or a spear wound in the arena, the server gives notice with a single sentence: "Welcome to Armageddon!" Immediately the connection is severed. Dominated by the huge ASCII head of a mantis, the main menu descends like a curtain and unceremoniously returns you to Earth.[15] The moment of ejection only confirms the game's reality. It is not the story that has ended, but only your participation in it. Back in Zalanthas, another player is already plundering your corpse.

. . .

Computers are often accused of disenchanting reality, of diminishing that salutary darkness necessary to discovery, creativity, even moral courage. Algorithms, according to the common wisdom, prevent us from encountering strangeness; safe within the "walled gardens" of our chosen platforms, guided by software to exhaustively vetted destinations, we achieve a kind of pyrrhic victory over the unknown. Art suffers, its aura diminished by every new mediation: screens that wash out particular hues of ink and paint, social networks that grind our individual preferences into a mulch of profitable groupthink; countless data-driven imagination-inhibiting overlays filming the space between us and messy, mysterious, intuitive "life."

But there are mysteries that properly belong to digital art, among them the special blend of choice and chance, compulsory ignorance and providential discovery, that is only possible in games. No medium is better suited to marking the limits of our knowledge, the contingent nature of events, the artifice and fragility of creation, because they are not texts but living environments, landscapes across which entities migrate and transform. Which is perhaps why so many iconic representatives of the genre take place on war-torn frontiers, deep in abandoned space stations, just after the apocalypse—in short, everywhere that

new worlds rise from catastrophe's detritus. Playing becomes a matter of deciphering remains, a poetics and hermeneutics of the artifact.

My last real character in Zalanthas was a traveling bard named Adjo Irofel. The virtual expression (and testing ground) of my desire to become a writer, I pieced him together from the personae of my adolescent reading. He was a Malian griot from the *Epic of Sundiata*, a *poète maudit* like Baudelaire or Rimbaud, a Renaissance courtier in the mold of Baltasar Graciàn's *The Art of Worldly Wisdom*. And, of course, he was me as I dreamed of becoming on the cusp of adulthood: erudite, well-traveled, wise, eccentric, loved. He played the mandolin and sang or recited lyrics, which I composed in Notepad with the assistance of my English teacher's handouts on prosody and www.rhymezone.com. The songs were about Zalanthas, its hidden histories and secret lore—and, toward the end, its nature: a metaphysical inquiry for Adjo, but an aesthetic one for me. More than anything, I was interested in the emergence and ephemerality of Armageddon's narrative, the way characters' actions persisted in the world even when unseen.

One afternoon, Adjo's noble benefactor Lord Raleris sat down beside him at a tavern and began smoking *a carved ivory pipe*. It had been more than two years since I'd seen it: the one object in the game's inventory of more than twenty-five thousand that I had designed. Raleris said that he had found it among the trophies of a wild mantis, slain after a killing spree near the city that had lasted for days. He speculated that the pipe must have belonged to one of the beast's victims, and Adjo, ignorant of this brush with a previous incarnation, joined him in wondering about its origin and make.[16]

A garden of forking paths connected Adjo to the object's creation—an untraceable sequence of human and algorithmic decisions that extended over two years. And, though I no longer play Armageddon, it comforts me to think that *a carved ivory pipe* is still at large, figuring, somehow, in the grand story of Zalanthas, of whose many authors I only ever spoke

---

Overleaf: "The rotund, plump-lipped man" was assassinated by his employers at the great merchant house of Kurac after selling company spice without permission. This log, captured by the author in August 2008, records his unsuccessful attempt to plead for his life.

Welcome to Armageddon!

You may:
(N) Create a new account
(C) Connect to your account
(V) Toggle ANSI/VT100 mode
(B) Toggle 'brief' menus
(D) Documentation menu
(X) Exit Armageddon
(?) Read menu options

Read the documentation
menu before creating your
character, please.

Armageddon is OPEN.
Choose thy fate:

You think:
    "She's going to kill me."

A Small Room [E Quit Save]
   This small, square room is constructed from a variety of different
types of wood, giving the walls and ceiling a haphazard appearance. The
floor is made of crude chunks of sandstone. A solid looking door takes up
part of the eastern wall. A window looks out over the street to the south.
A red jasper urn sits here.
A small, sun-patterned yellow rug lies here.
A rough hide sleeping mat lies beside the western wall, covered in a ragged blanket.
A simple grill, made of tile and blackened bone, sits here.
A black stone pickaxe sits here.
The sylphlike, streak-shorn woman is standing here.

The sylphlike, streak-shorn woman draws a glossy black bone dragon's pick.
The sylphlike, streak-shorn woman draws a translucent, crystalline longknife.
The sylphlike, streak-shorn woman says, in sirihish:
    "C'mon.... tell me a story."

The sylphlike, streak-shorn woman turns her glossy black bone dragon's pick slowly in
her hand.

Calmly, you say, in sirihish:
    "A few weeks ago, before I worked for Kurac..."

The sylphlike, streak-shorn woman rolls her eyes.

You say, in sirihish:
    "...I found a pouch of spice in the streets of Tuluk."

The sylphlike, streak-shorn woman says, in sirihish:
    "Ahh Tuluk. How you seem to revel in that shithole."

You say, in sirihish:
    "I thought I'd sell it in Luirs, but I forgot I had left it in my backpack.
Foolishly, I entered the city. Got arrested."

Snarling, you say, in sirihish:
    "I hate Tuluk."

The sylphlike, streak-shorn woman says, in sirihish:
    "Right."

You say, in sirihish:
    "When I was released, there was still some in my pack. I suppose it fell out or
    something."

The sylphlike, streak-shorn woman says to you, in sirihish:
    "You know, I think this is really an exercise in futility."

You say, in sirihish:
    "Just wait."

You say, in sirihish:
    "So I brought it to my apartment."

The sylphlike, streak-shorn woman says to you, in sirihish:
    "You'll lie whenever it suits you, with no apparent desire to do right by this
    group."

You shout in sirihish:
    "It's the truth!"

You shout in sirihish:
    "I swear, this is the truth!"

The sylphlike, streak-shorn woman says to you, in sirihish:
    "Alright, lay it out there."

The sylphlike, streak-shorn woman flips her glossy black bone dragon's pick in her
hand, pointing it down.

("out of character") to a few. A married couple from
Virginia, who played Bonnie and Clyde–style roles; a
teenage Christian rocker from Ohio, whose characters
were tormented by the temptation of evil; a graduate
student whose personae were adapted from Balzac's
Comèdie humaine. The rest remain behind the masks
of their characters, innominate ghosts in the server's
folkloric machine, giving life to those corners of the
internet where the MUD—long thought to be permanently defunct—enjoys a flourishing obsolescence.

1 See *Ancient Egyptians at Play: Board Games Across Borders,* ed. Alex De Voogt, Walter Crist, and Anne-Elizabeth Dunn-Vaturi (London: Bloomsbury UK, 2016), p. 55.

2 Top Mud Sites lists 1,929 MUDs as of June 2017, several dozen of which predate Armageddon by one, two, or three years. But with a few exceptions, most of them are small and nearly defunct. Armageddon is the oldest role-playing intensive MUD in existence.

3 No single person "created" Armageddon MUD. Brumleve was the original coder, but generations of builders and players are responsible for the game's present shape. One of the more famous among them is the writer Cat Rambo, known to Armageddon MUD as Sanvean. She is now president of Science Fiction and Fantasy Writers of America, a writers' guild that also gives out the annual Nebula Award.

4 You can play Armageddon MUD by clicking "Play!" at <armageddonmud.org> or by typing "telnet ginka.armageddon.org 4050" into the command line of any Internet-connected computer. Ginka, the sweet and spiky Zalanthan fruit for which the server is named, recalls the apple of Eden—beginning to play is a kind of Fall.

5 Armageddon MUD is based on the code of DikuMUD, which was derived from AberMUD, which was inspired by MUD1. See Richard A. Bartle's *Designing Virtual Worlds* (Indianapolis, IN: New Riders, 2004) for a detailed history of the genre.

6 Dan Brumleve credits "brutal enforcement of the role-playing standards," as well as the concealment of the game's coded mechanics, for Armageddon MUD's effective evolution into a world of story.

7 Statistics provided by staff administrator Nathvaan, forum message to author, 18 February 2017.

8 The think command, introduced in 1999, is one of Armageddon MUD's most distinctive features. See Cat Rambo, "I Think, Therefore I Role-play," *Imaginary Realities*, vol. 3, no. 1 (January 2000). Available at <imaginary-realities.disinterest. org/volume3/issue1/i_think. html>.

9 "D&D is a fantasy world governed by numbers. Numbers add the flavor of reality to fantasy," writes Michael Clune in his memoir *Gamelife* (New York: Farrar, Straus & Giroux, 2015), p. 30. Armageddon MUD heightens this reality effect by concealing its mechanics—the server quietly handles the character-sheets and dice.

10 The immortals are volunteers, selected from among players who submit applications. They are divided into builders, who design objects and regions; storytellers, who facilitate narratives; highlords and overlords, who oversee Zalanthas at the global scale; and coders.

11 As with any government, the immortals have their critics. Narrative librarians object to their behind-the-scenes orchestration of the game, and resent

their exclusive right to violate the OOC/IC divide—an exception quite like the state's monopoly on violence in political theory. Staff members know who plays whom, the hidden mechanics of the code, the secrets of various plots—and yet still keep mortal avatars of their own. Responding to the perceived unfairness of this, dissident Armageddon players have set up online forums where maps, craft recipes, spell formulae, plot secrets, and other "sensitive IC information" is freely shared. In turn, the staff persecutes these leakers, banning their accounts when they can be identified and urging players to stay away from their websites. Acting, one might say, in the interest of "narrative security," their goal is to preserve the mystery—and the reality—of Zalanthas.

12 The vast majority of Zalanthans are neither player-characters nor coded non-player-characters but rather *virtual non-player-characters* (VNPCs)—an implied population that has no coded existence (beyond the description-paragraphs of some rooms) but must be taken into account.

13 There are workarounds, like the procedural scenery generation that powers the infinite universe of No Man's Sky, or the widespread practice of facilitating player modifications, but both of these diminish the sense of reality. The former is inevitably repetitive (the diversity of features in automatically generated scenery is algorithmic and superficial), while the latter destroys the

sense of exploration (it isn't quite another world if you've created it yourself).

14 Armageddon players have been known to study real jewelers, leatherworkers, and carvers on YouTube in order to approximate their processes in-game. When this artisanal roleplaying is done well enough, admiring staff members, grateful for the accentuated realism, will sometimes give the character in question a skill bump, bringing them closer to the coveted opportunity to mastercraft.

15 The mantis, a human-sized insect, is one of the leading causes of death in Zalanthas—and, in the game's out-of-character community, a synecdoche for it. Death is referred to as "the mantis-head" in the game's official forums, and is also the *de facto* logo of Armageddon MUD.

16 The fourth rule of Armageddon MUD is as follows: "Your living character may not have any connection to your dead or stored characters. This includes relationships, looting your dead character's corpse, or possessing intimate knowledge that your past character had. We will reject an application that attempts to establish a link between the applying character and a dead character. We will store your character if we find, after approval, that you are establishing a connection to your dead characters."

ONFIM THE ARTIST
Justin E. H. Smith

It was not until the fortuitous discovery, well into the Soviet era, of troves of manuscripts in Novgorod that the modern world learned of medieval Slavonic literacy.[1] They are composed on *beresty*, thin pieces of birch bark that possess most of the virtues of wood-pulp paper, while requiring nothing for their manufacture. What is written on the *beresty* are, generally but not always, *gramoty*, texts or letters, usually in the Novgorodian dialect of Old Slavonic, but also, occasionally, in Karelian, German, or scattered other regional languages. A project of the Russian nonprofit organization Rukopisnye Pamiatniki Drevneï Rusi (Manuscript Monuments of Old Rus'), entitled Drevnerusskie Berestianye Gramoty (Old-Russian Birch Bark Gramoty), has catalogued and made available online a great number of medieval *gramoty*, searchable by year, by place of origin, by archeological dig, by condition of preservation, and by genre.[2]

There are around 956 catalogued *gramoty* from the period between 1050 and 1500 AD. Only eleven of these have been identified as having a literary or folkloric content, while most of the rest describe commercial transactions or legal disputes, or consist of transcriptions of biblical passages. It does not take much to earn the designation of literature. One Novgorod fragment classified as literary, No. 837, composed sometime in the mid-twelfth century and including a partial drawing of a bird, says simply:

… ОУАМЫШЬЛИШ[Ь]ЛИЖЄ…

Which gives us, when we add spaces between words:

… ОУ А МЫ ШЬЛИ Ш[Ь]ЛИ ЖЄ…

Which is to say, in modern Russian (dropping the initial word fragment): "А мы шли да шли," that is, "And we went and went," or, "And we went on and on," or, "We just kept on going."

If No. 837 is the *Odyssey* of the birch bark *gramoty*, No. 521 is the *Kama Sutra* and the *Song of Songs*, a truly beautiful fragmentary poem, composed in Novgorod in the early fifteenth century. It is catalogued as a "love spell," and when properly spaced, it translates roughly as: "May your heart burn and your body and soul burn [with desire] for me and for my body and for my face."

We are not drawn to these texts for their rich, living detail, any more than we are impressed with Neolithic stone tools in view of their horsepower. Their rough and fragmentary quality is their virtue and their poetry. This is what Anne Carson, most notably, understood in her faithful rendering of the fragments of Sappho, and it is what the human past has to most compellingly recommend it: its initial rudimentary form and subsequent further corruption.[3]

Alongside the hundreds of transaction records and complaints of theft or wrongdoing, we also find a handful of works produced by a boy by the name of Onfim—the Slavonic version of the Greek name Anthimos, borrowed, like literacy itself, from the Byzantine world. Some of Onfim's *beresty* are not *gramoty* at all and are not included in the database, since they contain no writings, but only drawings. Others are evidently homework exercises for which the boy has written out the Slavonic alphabet, or has composed basic words or rote sentences. Others still are a combination of words and drawings.

Onfim produced the entire body of his work around 1260 in Novgorod. There are twelve surviving *gramoty* (Nos. 199–210), six of which are adorned with illustrations (Nos. 199, 200, 202, 203, 206, and 210). Three of the works feature Onfim's name (Nos. 199, 200, 203), either standing alone as a signature or figuring in a sentence. No. 205 has an incomplete drawing and an incomplete signature. It is the combination of the illustration and the name that lend a handful of Onfim's surviving works what looks to us, today, like artistic genius: the power of the name added to the rough vision of the world, reproduced in scratchings on bark.

Onfim's human figures are stereotyped and instantly recognizable. Their faces feature two dots, and, often, a sort of capital *I*, a vertical line with long bars at the top and the bottom, which together form a single eyebrow, a long nose, and a purse-lipped mouth. (They make me think of Alice the Goon of Popeye fame, who, in turn, has long made me think of Vladimir Putin.) Human hands are represented as what look like pitchforks, with anywhere from three to eight fingers sticking

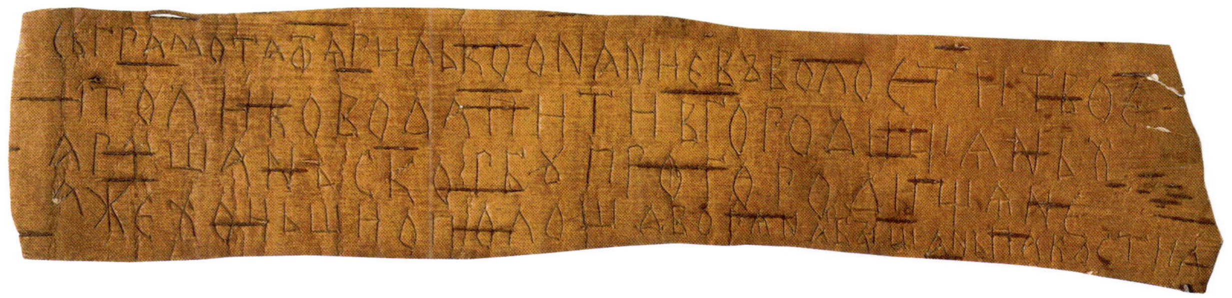

up as straight lines directly out of a perpendicular base line. There are generally no bodies, but only legs that go straight up to the base of the head. Or perhaps there are only torsos that do not terminate in a groin, but just keep going, somehow, until they become feet. Onfim's favorite themes are men, horses, weapons, and mythical beasts.

Gramota No. 200 has all the signature elements of a work by Onfim: the alphabet exercises, the horse, the weapon, the defeated enemy, and, finally, the signature. In the upper right corner, we have the beginning of the Cyrillic alphabet:

А Б В Г Д Є Ж …

Immediately below these traces of rote exercise, the artist has written an inflected form of his name:

ОНѲИМЄ

Onfim is, we may presume, the rider on horseback, slaying the man on the ground like St. George slaying the dragon. His signature is at once the mark of handwriting practice, of proud authorship of a work of art, and, finally, a projection of himself into a fantasy scene.

Though this work may be his most representative, it is not his most compelling. No. 206 gives us the most impressive assembly of pitchfork-handed men, underneath a text in which the author seems to have started out copying a passage of scripture (with a contracted Jesus: as in Byzantine Greek, all the charged and powerful words are shortened, as if by a sort of orthographic taboo), but to have shifted after just a few words to a syllabary exercise.

Gramota No. 203, in turn, depicts a remarkable fantasy scene, and represents a perfect fusion of image and text. With the words properly spaced, we obtain:

ГИ ПОМОЗИ РАБУ СВОЄМУ ОНѲИМУ

Which is to say: "Lord, help your servant Onfim!"

What exactly is happening in this scene? According to the Soviet philologist Artemii Vladimirovich Artsikhovskii, the words at the top of the *gramota* are a conventional and very common phrase in the period.[4] He describes the figure at the left as a boy, and implicitly as Onfim himself, while characterizing the figure on the right as indeterminate, as perhaps a man with his hands raised, or even a tree. Most importantly, he determines that the figure on the right is incomplete, evidently abandoned as the artist lost interest. But it may be that Artsikhovskii's presumption of the "schematic" character of the figures, and the conventional character of the text, prevented him from giving the dramatis personae more than a casual glance. If we study them attentively, we will notice what appears to be a third person lying on the ground, with his legs sticking up in the air and three toes sticking out from the one visible foot. There is a man or a creature on top of the man on the ground, with wild hair waving on his head. He may be clutching a snake or venomous asp, or he may have the serpent wrapped in his hair, and he may have just killed the man on the ground by means of it. Though it may not be clear what Onfim intended, it is at least clear he has not abandoned this drawing for lack of interest, and, in this light, however conventional the phrase at the top of the *gramota* may be, when he adds his name to it, as the servant of the Lord to be helped, and places it together with the violent scene born not of convention but of his imagination, the phrase becomes anything but rote. The artist is

Above: Old Slavonic writing on birch bark, ca. 1160–1180. Opposite: Renderings of three of Onfim's *gramoty*. Courtesy Drevnerusskie Berestianye Gramoty.

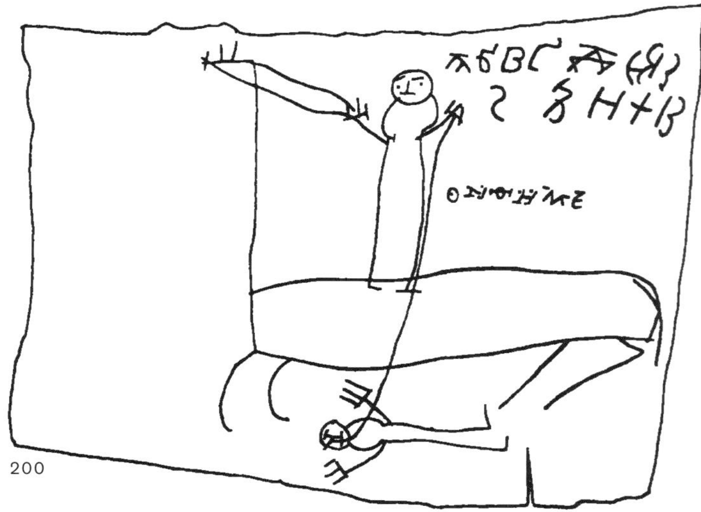

200

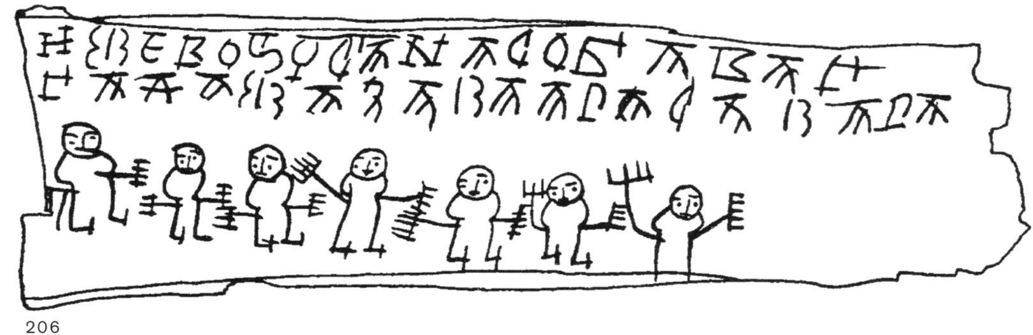

206

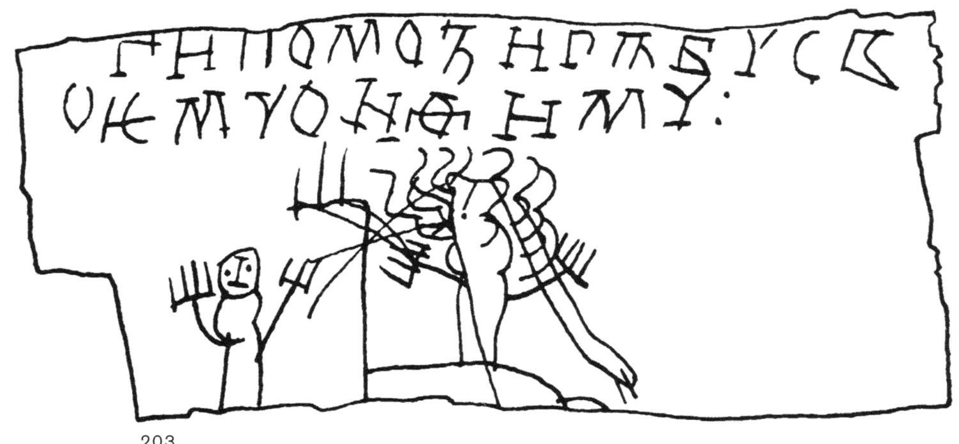

203

52 JUSTIN E. H. SMITH

imploring the Lord to help *him* in particular, Onfim, the subject and hero of this oeuvre.

But we still do not know which figure represents him. If he is the boy on the left, then why should the Lord help this calm and passive onlooker? We might be tempted to imagine a comic-book succession of images, where the left figure is the first panel, and the boy who was initially passive is drawn into the action on the right. Such spatial representation of temporal succession has been identified in art as early as the parietal drawings of the Paleolithic period. There is no reason to suppose it must have been absent in medieval Novgorod.

But if Onfim is in the "panel" on the right, is he the victim on the ground, or is he the monstrous assailant? Does he want the Lord to save him from attack, or to give him even more beastly power? Here we might look to *gramota* No. 199 for interpretive assistance. In this image, we know who Onfim is because he tells us. Speaking in the first person, the quadruped with the flayed tongue announces:

А ЗВѢРЬ

Which is to say: "I am a beast." In the text inside the box next to the beast, we find a dedication: "Greetings from Onfim to Daniel." There appears to be another figure, a human figure, on the ground in front of the beast. But it is not Onfim. Perhaps it is Daniel, Onfim's sidekick, being put in his place yet again, we might imagine, in the hierarchical order of their boyhood amity. Looking back to *gramota* No. 203 (they are not numbered in chronological order), it is hard not to see Onfim as the beast, subduing the man on the ground, so full of pride in his own power that he imagines the Lord himself will help him.

· · ·

The standard line in the scholarship has been to trivialize Onfim's achievement. Artsikhovskii's preferred adjective is "infantile" (ребяческий), while in English-language commentary, authors have often drawn facile comparisons with "refrigerator doodles."[5] Onfim is said to have been bored, to have been letting off steam, and to provide an illustration of the timeless truth that "boys will be boys."

In its corrupted and fragmentary forms, what the past gives us is strange and powerful. Attempts to

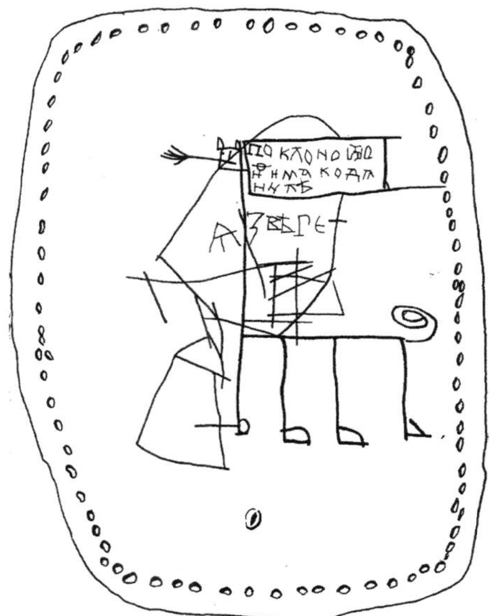

The marks of the beast. *Gramota* number 199.

assimilate Onfim to the present, the everyday, and the familiar serve, consciously or unconsciously, to remove this strangeness. *The Epic of Gilgamesh*, too, is the work of schoolboys doing rote exercises, scattered writings that were statistically collated and made to seem as though they came from a single author. We praise the epic, whose author has been elevated by posterity to the rank of genius, for taking on the most difficult and enduring themes of literature: life and death, love, fallenness. The fact that they endure from ancient Mesopotamia to the present day does not license us to assimilate them, but rather opens up the possibility of perceiving depth, antiquity, and perennity in what we can ordinarily only grasp as our trivial and fleeting everyday life. It is not that the loves and losses of the ancients are merely like our trivial frustrations in online dating, but that these very trivial frustrations are inscribed within the long golden chain of human experience, and it is only art and literature that can reveal the length of that chain to us. It is not that ancient images of dragons and battle are merely like our refrigerator doodles, but that our doodles, or our children's, inscribe us into the life of the imagination, whose recording in material traces it is the business of art and literature to continue.

It is easy to judge that Onfim's body of work is no *Gilgamesh*, but here one might reply that what makes

it less is also what makes it much more, namely, that it is the work of one person, and cannot be understood except in relation to that person: Onfim. *Gilgamesh* is no less anonymous than the Paleolithic stone tools produced millennia before it. Onfim's work is not only autographic; it is the autograph itself that is the subject of the work. The signing of the name is the insertion of the artist as the subject of the work.

This self-insertion is remarkable particularly in the context of the Slavonic middle ages. As scholars such as Alain Besançon have shown, the Eastern Orthodox artistic tradition only appears to lag behind the supposed advances made in the visual arts in the Western European Renaissance so long as we fail to take into account the deep difference of its spiritual ends.[6] The Orthodox icon in particular does a "worse" job of representing the world, in the sense of duplicating what we perceive in our visual field, than does Italian perspectival painting, but only because it is not the purpose of the icon to represent the content of our visual field at all, but rather to schematically— to return to a word Artsikhovskii had found suitable for his interpretation of Onfim—epitomize various tenets of religious dogma. Icons are not primitive or rudimentary attempts to duplicate the physical world; they are nuanced and complex attempts to embody the spiritual world.

But if this feature of Orthodox religious art seems to invite a comparison to Onfim and to other supposed primitives, there is another sense in which our boy artist has decidedly nothing to do with the icon painters. In the Eastern spiritual tradition, icons are painted for God, not for the artist, though of course in practice reputations were made by great work and ruined by poor work. As in the case of the eponymous Andrei Rublev and his envious adversary Kirill in the great 1966 film by Andrei Tarkovsky, we may be sure that men in medieval Russia, as everywhere else, were driven by a desire for acclaim.

Yet the ideal was one of selflessness, and the practice of signing one's name to a work never came into question. This only became widespread, in fact, with the rise of artworks as commercial objects in the burgeoning capitalist era of the late Renaissance in Western Europe: just one of many emerging techniques in sixteenth-century Florence and Flanders for keeping record of what belongs to whom. And yet, like Rembrandt, like Picasso, like George W. Bush, but like no icon painter in the vast surrounding territories in the surrounding centuries, like no Akkadian cuneiform copyist or Paleolithic flint-knapper, Onfim signed his name.

This touch is modern, but is also rooted in the ancestral practices of writing that straddle the boundary between documentation and magical ritual, incantation, or spell. *Gramota* No. 521, as we have seen, by an anonymous author, sought to cause some love object's heart to burn with desire through the simple act of writing this wish upon a *beresta*. Writing, on a certain lost understanding, had the power to change the world, even if it was never subsequently read by human eyes, like the prayers inserted in the Wailing Wall, or the Sanskrit inscriptions written into the tops of Southeast Asian temples, to be seen only from the sky.[7] It is difficult, now, to know whether Onfim's autograph belongs to the world of incantatory ritual, as in the writing out of love spells, or to that of proprietary documentation, as in the signing of a canvas whose loss one might otherwise risk in failing to record its provenance. Either way it is a powerful thing to write one's name: Onfim. He was a beast. Lord help him.

---

1 For a descriptive overview of Novgorod literacy in its historical context, see Valentin Lavrentevich Ianin, *Ia poslal tebe berestu …*, 3rd ed. (Moscow: Iazyki Russkoï Kultury, 1998). A partial but by no means exhautive list of scholarly resources that have been useful for the present author includes Artemii Vladimirovich Artsikhovskii and V. I. Borkovskii, *Novgorodskie gramoty na bereste (iz razkopok 1956–57)* (Moscow: Izdatel'stvo Akademii Nauk SSSR, 1963); Dietrich Frey-dank, *Auf gottes geheiss sollen wir einander briefe schreiben: Altrussische epistolographie* (Harrassowitz Verlag: Wiesbaden, 1999); Jos Schaeken, *Stemmen op berkenbast: Berichten uit mid-deleeuws Rusland: dagelijks leven en communicatie* (Leiden: Leiden University Press, 2012); Adelaida Anatolievna Svanidze, "People's Literacy, Education and Schools in Russian Towns, 13th–17th Centuries," in *Studien zur geschichte des ostseeraumes, II: Die städte des ostseeraumes als vermittler von kultur, 1240–1720*, ed. Julia-K. Büthe and Thomas Riis (Odense: Odense University Press, 1997), pp. 14–20; Wladimir Vodoff, "Les documents sur écorce de bouleau de Novgorod: découvertes et travaux récents," *Bibliologia*, no. 12 (1992).

2 See <gramoty.ru>.

3 Anne Carson, *If Not, Winter: Fragments of Sappho* (New York: Vintage, 2003).

4 See Artemii Vladimirovich Artsikhovskii, "Berestianye gramoty mal'chika Onfima," *Sovetskaia Arkheologiia*, no. 3 (1957).

5 See, for example, Paul Wick-enden of Thanet, "The Art of Onfim: Medieval Novgorod through the Eyes of a Child." Available at <gold-schp.net/SIG/onfim/onfim.html>.

6 See Alain Besançon, *The Forbidden Image: An Intellectual History of Iconoclasm* (Chicago: The University of Chicago Press, 2000).

7 See Sheldon Pollock, *The Language of the Gods in the World of Men: Sanskrit, Culture, and Power in Premodern India* (Berkeley: University of California Press, 2009).

AGAINST GRAVITY
Avinoam Shalem

*If we live in a "horizontal" world that suppresses the vertical,
it is nonetheless a world that is susceptible to verticality …
it is a world into which the vertical erupts.*[1]
— Anthony J. Steinbock, *Phenomenology and
Mysticism* (2007)

The 31 August 2015 issue of the *New Yorker* included a
long article by Elif Batuman titled "The Big Dig."[2] In it,
the American writer discusses the politics of power in
Turkey in relation to access to knowledge of the past.
The focus of the article is the debate about the large
archaeological area at Yenikapi, the very site on the
European shore of the Bosporus where the main station
of the Marmaray (the Marmara Rail) was constructed.
The huge infrastructural project involved building the
first tunnel to connect Asia and Europe, which established a long-needed railway link for the roughly two
million people who cross the Bosporus daily. Modern
solutions for addressing the rapid metamorphosis
of Istanbul into a megacity seem to clash with our
intellectual desire to survey and document the past.
Archaeology delays progress. From 2005 to 2013,
the construction of the aboveground rail and metro
stations was halted and an archaeological "Big Dig"
began. And, as it turned out, remains of a Neolithic
settlement dating from around 6000 BC were discovered, in addition to a fourth-century marble Apollo, a
carved ivory panel with the image of the Virgin Mary,
a ninth-century wooden box with a tablet for storing
weights for a portable assay balance, and dozens of
Byzantine shipwrecks. Batuman describes the two
faces, so to speak, of this site in 2013, at a time when
modern construction and archaeological excavation
were running in parallel:

*When I first visited the Yenikapi excavation site, in July,
2013, the Marmaray station was already nearly completed—
a concrete colossus topped by a flat, glass-enclosed rotunda—
but the metro station was still an archeological dig. The total
site was fifty-eight thousand square metres, about the size of
eleven football fields. Workers on the Marmaray side wore
fluorescent hard hats with matching vests. On the metro side,
they wore faded caps or white shirts tied around their heads,
against the blazing sun. They were constructing an edifice
of their own, as striking, in its way, as the station: a fortress*

*of plastic milk crates, ten crates high, stretching farther than
the eye could see, packed with broken amphorae, horse bones,
anchors, ceramic lamps, hewn limestone, mining refuse—
anything that had been left there, accidentally or on purpose,
by human hands. It was as if you were watching, in real time,
the ancient harbor being replaced by a modern station.*[3]

The contrast between the building of the modern
stations in Yanikapi and the digging at the archaeological site can be imagined as a graph with two
antagonistic vectors bound to each other: one vector
aims at digging deep into the ground while the other
rises above. Standing on the very spot that today
discloses the depths of Marmaray all the way to its
Neolithic layer, one might imagine, like Batuman
contemplating the twenty-story escalator of Sirkeci
Station, that the history of a specific place might look
like a huge building with dozens of floors and that
we, if we wanted to, could use an elevator to travel in
time, collecting knowledge about different periods and
civilizations. Archaeology certainly reveals to us that,
metaphorically speaking, each building, like a tree,
might have further "roots," structures that were built
beneath it; if skyscrapers are about desires, "earth-
scrapers" are about histories. The large archaeological
area—comprising the Forum Romanum and Trajan's
Forum—at the heart of Rome just behind the Altare
della Patria, the imposing monument completed in
1925, appears like a huge open wound in the urban
structure of Rome. But it also discloses that the urban
palimpsest of Rome's architecture cannot be restricted
to the view at and above eye level but is to be found
below the asphalt pavements too. Similarly, the city of
Amman is unique in its urban concept of exhibiting its
archaeological past, the old Roman city of Philadelphia,
in the very center of the town. The second-century
Roman theater at its heart appears like a massive
volcanic crater, whose floor marks what appears to be
the ground level of the Roman city, while the newly

Opposite above: The Roman *cardo maximus* running
through center of modern-day Jerusalem.
Opposite below: The second-century Roman theater in
Amman, which was known at the time as Philadelphia.
Photo Chang Ju Wu.

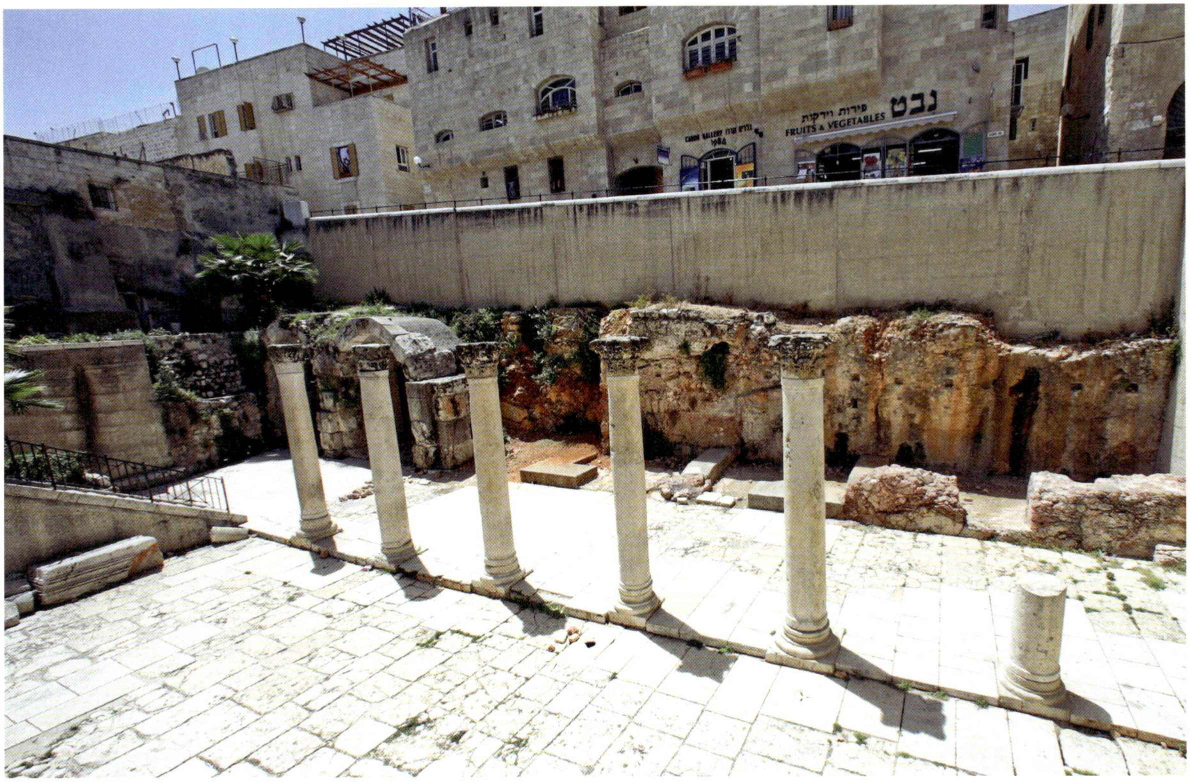

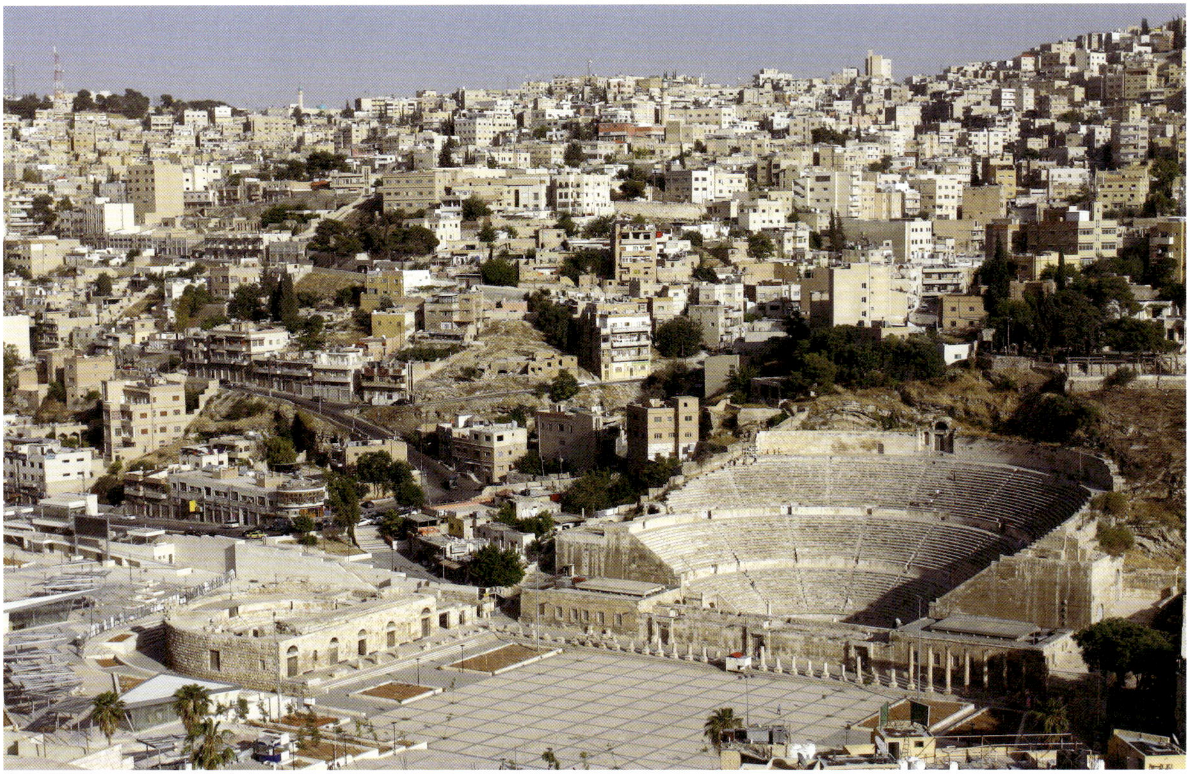

reconstructed dome over the eighth-century Umayyad palace located on the hill above signifies another great moment in the urban history of this site. An invisible vertical line stretches from the hill to the valley and marks the history of this space—a vertical emblem symbolizing Amman as a *chronotopos*. The *cardo maximus* at the very heart of the Roman city of Aelia Capitolina (Jerusalem), which has been exposed and remains visible under the present street level of the city, appears, as the Latin term clearly specifies, like a long scar on the city's chest. Although these abysses in the urban plan make transportation difficult, and sometimes even impossible, they offer a glimpse into the ancient history of the city. It is true that many cities all over the world are proud to call our attention to their ancient and even recent histories by exposing the ruins and remains of their "previous" architectural achievements. These sites are put on display like objects in vitrines in a museum—in these cases, an open one with no walls or roof. And yet, the decision to designate a large space at the very center of a metropolis in order to expose *underground* archaeological strata revealing different urban histories is a revolutionary plan. It suggests that the quest for knowledge might follow vertical search patterns.

Verticality is both a position and a motion. It designates a specific state or move usually described as perpendicular to the plane of the horizon. This means that this term is usually defined as opposed, or in contrast, to the horizontal. From a physical point of view, verticality is a motion governed by the natural phenomenon of the earth's gravity. But our discussion of verticality here is not concerned with its physical manifestation, but with figuring verticality as a pattern of thinking and a method of gathering and presenting knowledge.[4] When used as an adjective describing a mode of knowledge, the word "vertical" should be understood as beyond metaphor, and its use here goes beyond its figurative appeal, because verticality suggests a principle by which phenomena can be experienced, classified, and interpreted. And yet, as far as the gathering of knowledge is concerned, one cannot avoid its definitional relationship to the horizontal. Indeed, gaining knowledge by moving horizontally, namely conquering new territories and traveling to distant places situated beyond one's horizon, is quite common praxis. Hence, "expanding one's horizons" clearly refers to our ability to travel and think beyond

the limit of our sight and, metaphorically speaking, our immediate experienced knowledge. And, since the horizon is a dividing line into which all visibility vanishes, going toward and beyond it can present us with new sights and wisdom. Thus, cosmography is perhaps the best field for illustrating how knowledge is produced through the conquest of space. Opening and spreading out are vital activities for this particular method of acquiring knowledge, which depends on gaining and arranging information. For this, an encyclopedic mind is essential. Vertical knowledge, by contrast, concerns time rather than space, and its major objective involves the disclosure of essence, the *sui generis* of any entity, thing, or idea. The "Big Dig" in Yanikapi reveals the varied layers of time at the ancient harbor on the Bosporus. Like the concentric rings on a tree's trunk marking its annual growth, vertical knowledge aims at organizing information in a chronological order, keeping the sequence of time, from birth to death, initial to final, ancient to present.[5]

The exceptionality of the age of the Renaissance, and perhaps of each great age that can be termed a *renaissance*, was predicated on the mobilization of both spatial and chronological vectors of knowledge in tandem. On the one hand, the fourteenth century and the age of early humanism witnessed the rediscovery and rebirth of antiquity, a process that resulted in a greater consciousness of historical perspective and a better sense of the chronology of time.[6] As Erich Auerbach explains in his influential book *Mimesis*, first published in 1946 in Istanbul: "Humanism with its program of renewal of antique forms of life and expression creates a historical perspective in depth such as no previous epoch known to us possessed."[7] And, on the other hand, the discovery of the New World during the Renaissance was a sort of new outlook and perception, forcing any thinker of the Old World to revise and review her or his former standpoint. This new constellation of the cosmos, which had now been expanded temporally and spatially, required a new constellation of philosophical inquiries. In fact, as Enrique Dussel says, the discovery of the Americas forms the constitutive moment of modernity, in which Spain and Portugal played the major role.[8] He adds: "The birthday of modernity is 1492, even though its gestation, like that of the fetus, required a period of intrauterine growth."[9] Thus, the classical geography, which, just a century

earlier, was rediscovered and passionately restudied, was now shown to be inadequate, and the moral habits and the rituals of the "other" civilizations encountered disturbed the old monotheistic Christian order of the cosmos.[10]

But, of course, the chronological and the spatial, and in turn the vertical and horizontal, do not always work in tandem. Moreover, constructed and defined vis-à-vis each other, they have developed distinct characters, attributions, and values that aim at distinguishing between the two rather than emphasizing points of conjunction. The dialectic built between these conditions, emanating from the clear division we make between time and space, sometimes results in a black-and-white picture of the vertical and the horizontal. Whereas verticality is associated with duration, progress, and linear evolution, horizontality is usually linked to space, measurement, and growth. The elementary lens through which vertical phenomena are examined is the one that aims at finding similarity in habits of behavior, production, materials, and forms. Therefore vertical similarity is always situated within the precincts of the term "variation," and these "similarities" resemble in one way or another the originary prototype. Horizontal study seeks resemblance across rather than resemblance within, and variations are immediately translated into differences. Yes, the likeness and authenticity so much related to verticality stand in contrast to the diversity and pluralism associated with the horizontal. This is why theories associated with the vertical habitus of inquiry that posit originary sources as dictating all subsequent development should be compared with concepts such as center and periphery operational in "the horizontal mode of inquiry." It seems as if the local and the global are unpacked while thinking through these two veins of acquiring knowledge.[11]

The best example for illustrating vertical knowledge in writing is the use of the footnote system in scholarly essays. This system assures the transparency of the origin of our thoughts. In other words, it presents our vertical transmission of knowledge. Ideas expressed in the main body of the text display their earlier sources. Academic writings appear then as a procedure that involves following earlier writings, which could be best defined as chronographia. Moreover, new ideas are constructed on previous intellectual foundations and established propositions. (Or

should one say pre-positions?) The legal term *taqlid* in Arabic, meaning "to follow, or to hang" refers exactly to this habitus. Moreover, as far as *fiqh* (comprehension) is concerned, *taqlid* means "clothing with authority" and therefore indicates that the validity of knowledge is based on former authoritative voices. Similarly, the Arabic word *silsila* (meaning "chain" or "link") refers to the genealogy of any account or saying, and an author typically mentioned the genealogy of the transmission of his text at the beginning of his writing or speaking. Thus, the authenticity of the text is affirmed before the text is presented. The *silsila* is the archaeology of text. Like an archaeological site, the text with its added footnotes, namely its "underground" text, presents to the readers its history, or, one could say, its long biography. Moving from the text to the footnotes is in fact moving back in time. This form of vertical thinking and writing that turns backward in order to reveal the past makes the text seem as if it has gone through hypnosis or psychoanalysis. In fact, as Lars von Trier reveals in his film *Europa* (1991, the third film of his "Europa Trilogy"), any storytelling of the past starts with hypnotic induction.[12] The different excavated levels of the archaeology of Rome, Amman, and Jerusalem on display tell us that the past psychic records of these cities were translated into forms.

Diagrams that recall or are based on the idea of chains and ladders (see, for example, genealogy diagrams), or those visibly adopting the image of the tree of knowledge, dominate our pattern of thinking about the acquisition of vertical wisdom. For example, the thirteenth-century cosmographer Abu Yahya Zakariya ibn Muhammad al Qazwini in his *Wonder of Creation* ('Aja'ib al-Makhluqat wa-Ghara'ib al-Mawjudat), probably completed in 1276, organizes his description of the whole cosmos as if traveling from heaven all the way down to the surface of the earth. The planets, God's throne, and the divine creatures that surround and aid Almighty God are minutely described by Qazwini before he turns to reporting on the earth, its substances, rivers and seas, plants and animals. Moreover, while describing the earth's important and famous water sources, Qazwini dives, so to speak, into the depth of the seas and rivers and provides us with a full description of the underwater creatures of this fluid sphere.[13] In contrast to the *Mi'raj* (heavenly travel) of Muhammad, which preceded from the ground to the different heavenly spheres, Qazwini, like Dante,

travels downward. But both Qazwini and the Prophet Muhammad are moving downward or upward, respectively, as if on an invisible ladder or escalator.[14]

The well-known drawing of the "Tree of Architecture" that illustrates Sir Banister Fletcher's *A History of Architecture* (1896) clearly demonstrates how the whole history of architecture can be vertically organized, while suggesting "natural" growth and evolution. Having its foundations, namely its roots, in six personifications—geography, geology, climate, religion, the social, and history—the Tree of Architecture grows from the architecture of the ancient world and culminates in the age of modernity in the United States, of which the Flatiron Building in New York is the crown.[15] In fact, like the famous image of the Tree of Jesse, the Tree of Architecture in particular, and any diagram of the "Tree of Evolution" in general, suggest a schematic representation of the genealogy of things, as if order is solely based on chronology.[16]

The spiral skeleton and core structure of the Solomon R. Guggenheim Museum in New York, designed by Frank Lloyd Wright and inaugurated in 1959, dictates, whether intentionally or not, the vertical exhibition of knowledge. Though Wright wanted visitors to view the art by descending down the spiral gallery, from top to bottom, today's visitors travel up its ramp gallery, from the ground to the summit. In both scenarios, they collect knowledge in a continuous spiral and vertical line. Moreover, exhibitions in this space are usually organized in a chronological order, with the curator starting the narration on the ground floor and moving forward in time as the show ascends. This museum is therefore one of the best examples for the exhibition of the vertical order of things and ideas.

And yet, vertical knowledge should not be restricted to the systematization of things, to linear classification on an axis whose direction is described as "perpendicular to the plane of the horizon." I would like to expand the idea of vertical knowledge and apply it to any attempt at discerning the temporal by studying the morphology of things. It is *chronographia*, or rather *chronotopia*, that I am aiming at defining—the configuration of time as it is "reflected" in materials and spaces.

Time leaves its marks on each substance. It shapes and forms things, literally and metaphorically. And, we, the beholders can, if we wish, read these marks. We can learn from any surface—be it the stones of

an architectural structure, the body of a vase, or the painted marks on the surface of a picture—the histories of the object's existence. Our reading of these marks and textures relates to the archaeology of the object's course of production, the alterations it underwent at the hands of its owners, or simply the "natural" marks of time, such as its specific patina.[17] Unlike archaeology and geology, in which this inquiry goes in a literally vertical direction, the detection of time on art objects, for example, can take other directions. It can move from the upper surface of an illustrated manuscript's page to the lower surface of its parchment support, thus encoding the chronology of the production of the manuscript's illustrations. In other cases, such as a carved ivory panel, our inquiry can travel from the upper carved surface to its lower carved level. But our inquiry can also move from the center of the object to its peripheral areas, or from the artifact's front to its rear, because usually, though not necessarily, marks predating the panel's carving might be found on its reverse.[18] In short, it is the palimpsest character of things—the formations and transformations of objects across time—to which I am calling attention.[19] These "vertical" investigations are not necessarily illustrative of the desire to disclose the origin or source of things but rather to detect the object's multi-synchronic character, the morphological changes that took place at various stages of the object's life.

But this multi-synchronicity is not always simply the result of traces left on the object by its historical transit. In some cases, it—and the notion of vertical knowledge with which it is associated—has been actively mobilized at the outset as a powerful aesthetic strategy. An example of this can be found in the inner architectural décor of the Dome of the Rock in Jerusalem, which was erected around 691 AD (71 After Hijra) under the reign of the caliph ʿAbd al-Malik and marks a specific moment in the crystallization of the aesthetic language of late antiquity in Bilād al-Shām (Greater Syria). The most striking aesthetic impact of the building is perhaps its textural tension, which is due to the contrast between the rock's crude surface and the fine-cut marble slabs, with their natural veining and polychrome designs, arranged to create symmetric shapes and patterns. It seems as

------

Opposite: The "Tree of Architecture" from Banister Fletcher's *History of Architecture*, 1896.

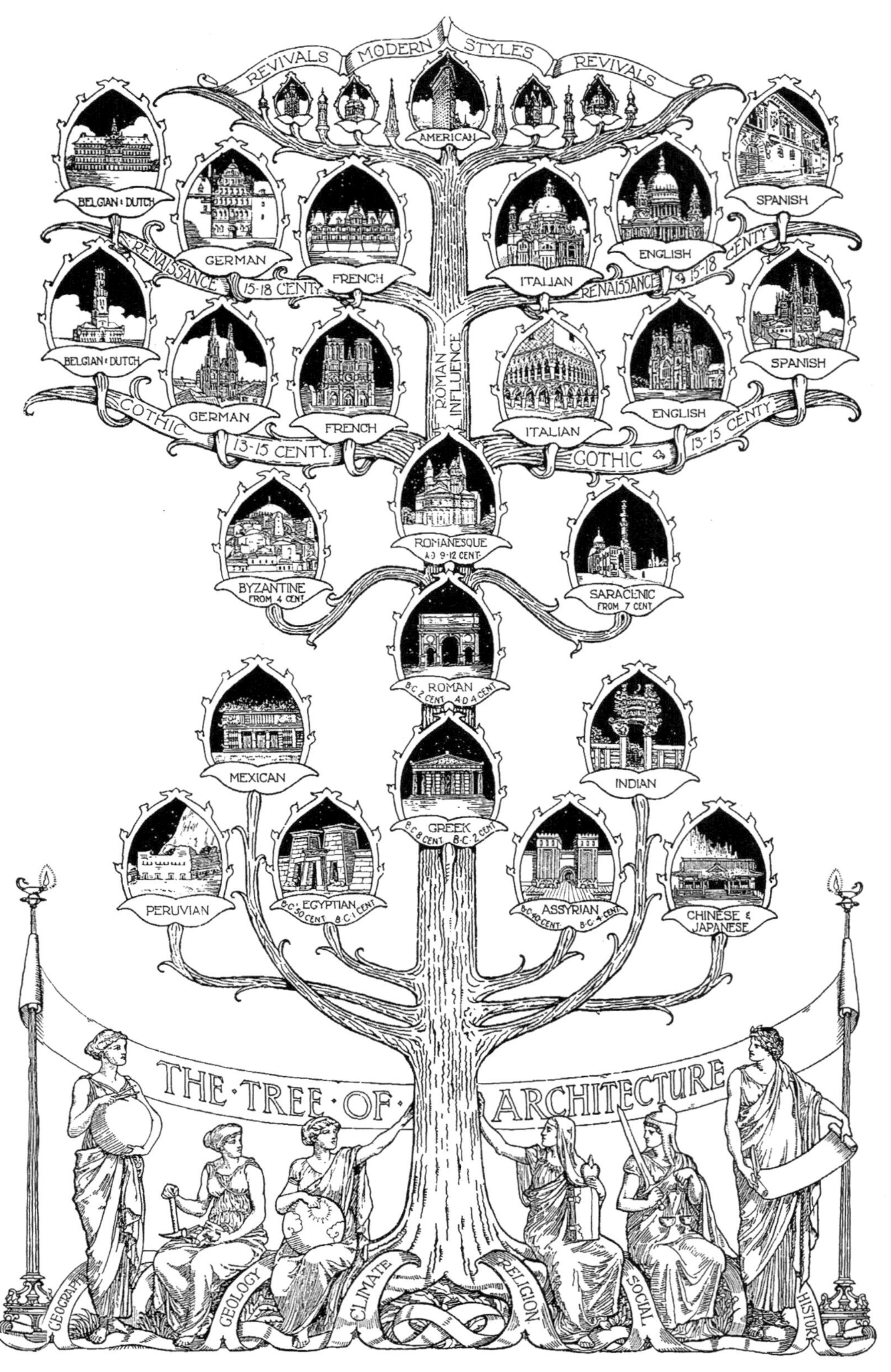
REVIVALS
MODERN STYLES
REVIVALS
AMERICAN
BELGIAN & DUTCH
GERMAN
FRENCH
ITALIAN
ENGLISH
SPANISH
RENAISSANCE 15-18 CENT.
RENAISSANCE 15-18 CENTY.
BELGIAN & DUTCH
GERMAN
FRENCH
ITALIAN
ENGLISH
SPANISH
ROMAN INFLUENCE
GOTHIC 13-15 CENTY.
GOTHIC 13-15 CENTY.
BYZANTINE FROM 4 CENT.
ROMANESQUE A.D 9-12 CENT.
SARACENIC FROM 7 CENT.
ROMAN B.C 2 CENT. A.D 4 CENT.
MEXICAN
INDIAN
GREEK B.C 8 CENT. B.C 2 CENT.
PERUVIAN
EGYPTIAN B.C 30 CENT. B.C 1 CENT.
ASSYRIAN B.C 30 CENT. B.C 4 CENT.
CHINESE & JAPANESE
THE · TREE · OF · ARCHITECTURE
GEOGRAPHY
GEOLOGY
CLIMATE
RELIGION
SOCIAL
HISTORY

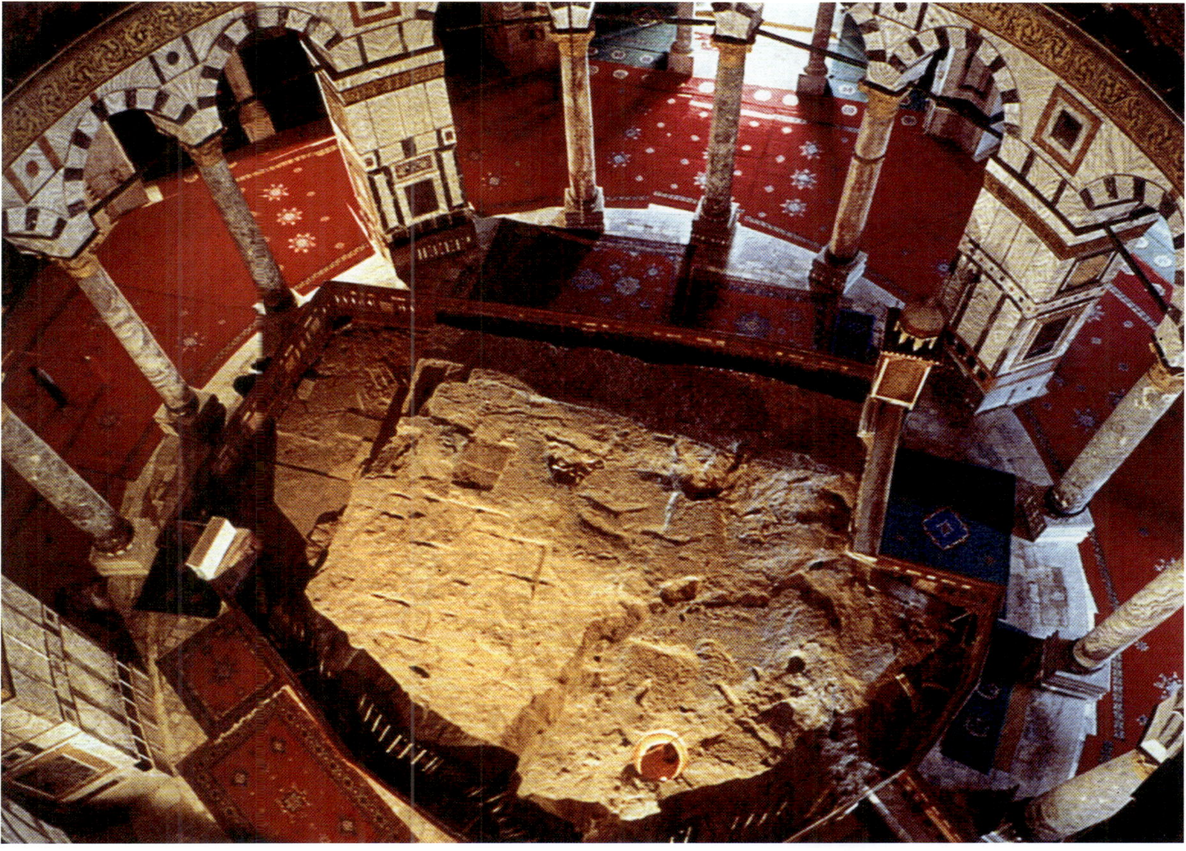

if the natural qualities of the stone were deliberately
exploited to achieve ornamental effects. Moreover, the
rock with its irregular and raw outline is enclosed and
guarded by the regular and well-planned circular and
octagonal arcades, and the rock's raw surface appears
as if tamed, or at least moderated, by the smooth
marble surface and the meticulous, minute mosaics.
As a whole, the Dome of the Rock displays stages in
the cultivation of stone, from the natural and crude to
the cut and polished, from the unfinished to the highly
sophisticated and refined. Calling the beholder's attention to the extraordinary amount of time spent creating
the artful aesthetic of stones at this site, it alludes
therefore to duration. Such durational aesthetics can
also be seen in early medieval glass objects. Numerous
glass containers datable to between the eighth and the
tenth centuries and assigned to either Syria or Iran
were decorated with fluid-like drippings in the form of
applied glass trails, loops, and even handles.

It might seem that the apparent softness of these
glass ornamentations—which give the impression of
dripping water—contradicts the hard, solid, if still
fragile, character of their material. But this juxtaposition in fact suggests that the glass object is telling us
of its former condition, before it hardened. It is as if
vertical knowledge of the warm, soft state of the object
as it was being formed is still inscribed in the final,
solid artifact. The dripping glass loops and flowing
handles are like aide-mémoire through which one can
delve into the vertical knowledge of the former state
of things. As Gaston Bachelard, in a passage cited by
Steinbock while discussing the relationship between
the essence of religious experience and "real verticality," writes: "This verticality is no empty metaphor;
it is a principle of order, a law governing filiation, a
scale along which someone can experience the different
degrees of sensibility."[20]

____

Above: A study in contrasts. The Dome of the Rock in
Jerusalem.

1 Anthony J. Steinbock, *Phenomenology and Mysticism: The Verticality of Religious Experience* (Bloomington and Indianapolis: Indiana University Press 2007), p. 14.

2 Elif Batuman, "The Big Dig," *The New Yorker*, 31 August 2015. Available at <newyorker.com/magazine/2015/08/31/the-big-dig>.

3 Ibid.

4 Though Steinbock takes another path in discussing the verticality of religious experience, and especially of the epiphany, his introduction discusses the usage of the idea of verticality beyond its metaphoric use. See Anthony J. Steinbock, *Phenomenology and Mysticism*, especially pp. 12–19.

5 There are several publications that discuss verticality as a structure of knowledge, notably Barry Schwartz, *Vertical Classification: A Study in Structuralism and the Sociology of Knowledge* (Chicago: The University of Chicago Press, 1981); see especially his discussion of vertical classification as related to the vertical order of the human body, pp. 34–78. See also Anthony J. Steinbock, *Phenomenology and Mysticism*; Gaston Bachelard, *The Poetics of Space*, trans. Maria Jolas (New York: Orion Press, 1964), pp. 17ff. Verticality has recently become a topic of discussion in architectural studies, mainly in the context of power and power display. See Eyal Weizman, "Introduction to the Politics of Verticality," available at <opendemocracy.net/ecology-politicsverticality/article_802.jsp>; Nina Rappaport's project Vertical Urban Factory at <verticalurbanfactory.org>; Peter Adey, "Vertical Security in the Megacity: Legibility, Mobility and Aerial Politics," *Theory, Culture and Society*, vol. 27, no. 6 (November 2010); Kevin Lewis O'Neill and Benjamin Fogarty-Valenzuela, "Verticality," *The Journal of the Royal Anthropological Institute* (N.S.), vol. 19, no. 2 (June 2013): Lucy Hewitt and Stephen Graham, "Vertical Cities: Representations of Urban Verticality in 20th-Century Science Fiction Literature," *Urban Studies*, vol. 52, no. 5 (April 2015).

6 Alexander Nagel and Christopher S. Wood, *Anachronic Renaissance* (New York: Zone Books, 2010); Alexander Nagel and Christopher S. Wood, "Interventions: Toward a New Model of Renaissance Anachronism," *Art Bulletin*, vol. 87, no. 3 (September 2005); and Christopher S. Wood, *Forgery, Replica, Fiction: Temporalities of German Renaissance Art* (Chicago: The University of Chicago Press, 2008).

7 Erich Auerbach, *Mimesis: The Representation of Reality in Western Literature*, trans. Willard R. Trask (Garden City, NY: Doubleday Anchor, 1957), p. 282.

8 Enrique Dussel, *The Invention of the Americas* (New York: Continuum, 1995), p. 26.

9 Ibid., p. 13.

10 For a discussion of the complication of the world of knowledge during the age of Spanish expansion, see Anthony Grafton, *New Worlds, Ancient Texts: The Power of Tradition and the Shock of Discovery* (Cambridge, MA: Harvard University Press, 1992).

11 See John Barrell, *The Idea of Landscape and the Sense of Place 1730–1840: An Approach to the Poetry of John Clare* (Cambridge: Cambridge University Press, 1972), in which he argues that linearity is related to the movement and mobility of humans, and circularity to stasis and to being bound to a place. See also Franco Moretti, *Graphs, Maps, Trees: Abstract Models for Literary History* (London: Verso, 2007), pp. 38–39.

12 See the seemingly enigmatic scene of hypnosis with which the film begins and the metaphor of the train in a tunnel symbolizing the vertical vector of travel in time.

13 See Persis Berlekamp, *Wonder, Image, & Cosmos in Medieval Islam* (New Haven: Yale University Press, 2011).

14 For these vertical visions of the cosmos in Islam, see the image of the Prophet ascending the celestial spheres, constellations, and signs of the zodiac in the illustrated manuscript of Nizami's "Khamsa" (Five Poems) produced in Isfahan between 1665 and 1667 (British Library, Add. 6613, folio 3v.).

15 Banister Fletcher, *A History of Architecture* (London and New York: Butterworths, 1896). See also the discussion of Fletcher's "Tree of Architecture" in Sandy Isenstadt and Kishwar Rizvi, "Modern Architecture and the Middle East: The Burden of Representation," in Isenstadt and Rizvi, eds., *Modernism and the Middle East: Architecture and Politics in the Twentieth Century* (Seattle: University of Washington Press, 2008), pp. 11–13, fig. I. 3.

16 Horst Bredekamp, *Darwins korallen: Die frühen evolutionsmodelle und die tradition der naturgeschichte* (Berlin: Wagenbach, 2005). See also Julia Voss, *Darwin's Pictures: Views of Evolutionary Theory, 1837–1874* (New Haven: Yale University Press, 2010): Alexander Demandt, *Über allen wipfeln: Der baum in der kulturgeschichte* (Cologne: Böhlau, 2002); and Peter Burke, *A Social History of Knowledge: From Gutenberg to Diderot* (Cambridge: Polity Press, 2000), pp. 81–115.

17 See the excellent discussion in Shannon Lee Dawdy, *Patina: A Profane Archaeology* (Chicago: The University of Chicago Press, 2016), especially her chapter "Conclusion: Patina, Chronotopia, Mana."

18 For more on the methods of ivory craftsmanship, see Anthony Cutler, *The Hand of the Master: Craftsmanship, Ivory, and Society in Byzantium (9th–11th Centuries)* (Princeton: Princeton University Press, 1994).

19 Nebahat Avcioğlu, "Istanbul: The Palimpsest City in Search of Its Architext," *Res*, no. 53/54 (Spring/Autumn 2008).

20 Cited by Anthony J. Steinbock, in his introduction to *Phenomenology and Mysticism*, p. 13. The Bachelard passage can be found in his *Air and Dreams: An Essay on the Imagination of Movement*, trans. Edith R. Farrell and C. Frederick Farrell (Dallas: The Dallas Institute, 1988), p. 10.

POLITICAL OVERTURES
Justin Patch

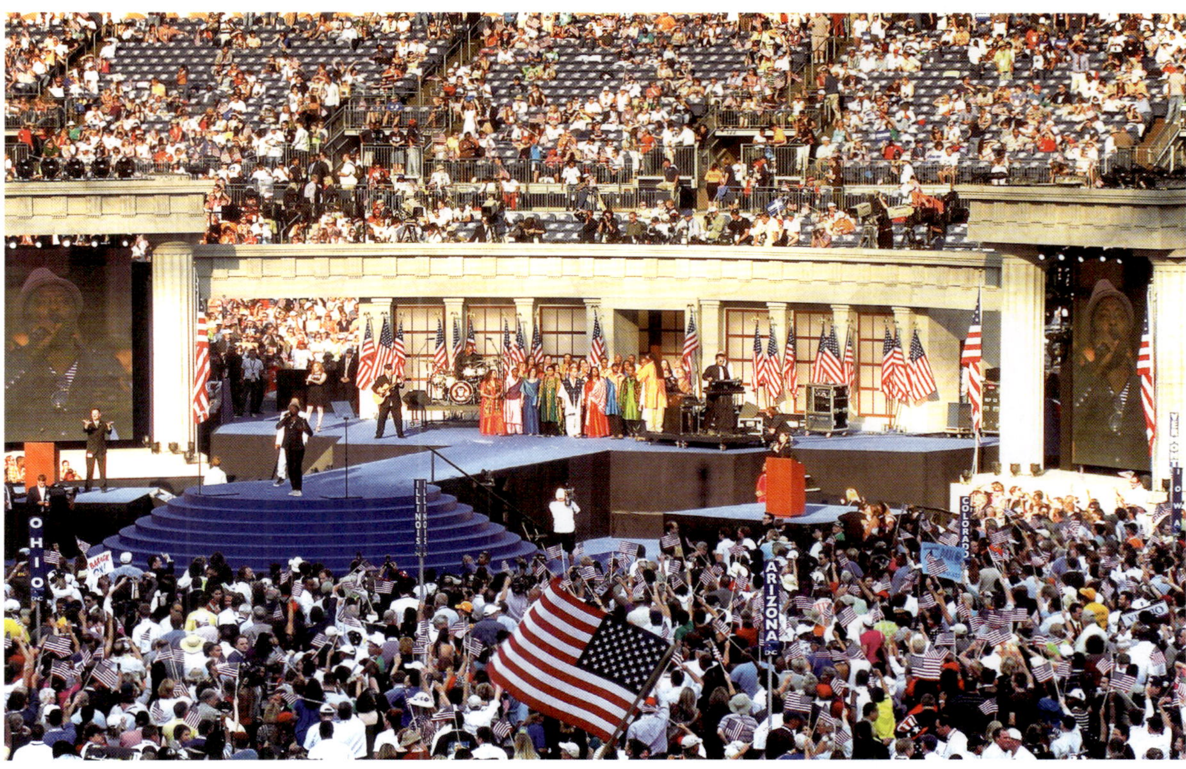

Above: Singer will.I.am performing at the 2008 Democratic National Convention in Denver, Colorado.

It is often said that politics makes strange bedfellows, but in the United States, political campaigns and music have always been natural allies. Both music and campaigns alter moods, transform atmospheres, change perceptions of time and space, and exert influence over emotion and intellect. Like campaigns, music can invoke nationhood and patriotism, and the national anthems, jingoistic tunes, and martial compositions that accompany them can move people to tears, or to violence. From urban pavement to rural grange halls, songs have unified labor movements, educated populist gatherings, and steeled the nerves of civil rights and anti-war protesters as they confronted hostility. When people challenge entrenched power, seek collective solace, celebrate victory, or project authority, music is their constant companion. Music forms identity, rewrites history, forges coalitions, and cultivates emotional connections, and its history on the campaign trail shows that candidates are fully aware of this potential. Music is also an empty signifier, open to wildly different interpretations, and when effectively deployed, it can serve the ventriloquist's hand, sometimes in counterintuitive ways. It can accommodate the state and the resistance with equal efficacy.

In an election campaign, music is an instrument of power; it provides an aura of sovereignty, aurally reinforcing the legitimacy of incumbent and challenger alike. It is this singular ability to reach the hearts and minds of voters that has made music an essential part of American presidential campaigns from the nation's infancy. Even as campaigns and voters have changed—as women and minorities fought and won the right to vote, as campaigns moved from the streets to the airwaves and onto digital platforms—music has remained a constant accompaniment. And as we slowly brace ourselves for the next presidential election, it is imperative that we understand the role that music has had in campaigns in order to better grasp the complex interplays of culture and the democratic process.

EARLY MUSIC

The use of music in presidential campaigns dates back to George Washington. A hero of the revolution, Washington was the clear favorite and went on to win elections in 1789 and 1792, the only unanimous electoral college victories in US history. A number of songs that had been written in praise of the leading role he played during the revolution were used in his honor while he campaigned. One such song, entitled "God Save Great Washington," was printed in the *Philadelphia Continental Journal* in 1786 and used in his campaign three years later. It was sardonically set to the tune of "God Save the King," England's national anthem, and opened with the words:

God save great Washington
His worth from ev'ry tongue
Demands applause;
Ye tuneful pow'rs combine,
And each true Whig now join
Whose heart did ne'r resign
The glorious cause.[1]

When Washington campaigned for re-election, his arrival and departure from the stage were consistently accompanied by a rendition of the "President's March," an instrumental written by Philip Phile in honor of Washington's first inauguration in 1789—the first instance of a campaign adopting such a strategy. The tune would go on to have a long life in American political history. In 1798, during a naval conflict with France, it was given patriotic lyrics by Joseph Hopkinson, who rechristened it "Favorite New Federal Song Adapted to the President's March." Better known as "Hail Columbia," it served as one of several *de facto* national anthems until "The Star-Spangled Banner" was officially selected in 1931, and is now the vice presidential anthem. Like many patriotic songs, the lyrics of "Hail Columbia" extol the virtues of freedom, liberty, love of country, and national defense.

Following Washington's lead, presidential candidates continued to enter and exit rallies to the strains of familiar patriotic tunes. Nationalist musical backdrops served the fledgling United States by bringing together an electorate divided by identity, geography, ideology, and loyalty. During a period in which publishing was limited, communication primitive, and a national identity still emerging and contested, referencing love of country and revolutionary glory was politically expedient. These patriotic songs, generally well-known popular tunes supplied with new lyrics, also engaged the public in collective singing.[2] This activity served to superimpose the candidate's identity on aurally familiar, affectively powerful sonic and textual material that celebrated a new nation, its people, and its leaders alongside the virtues of heroism, valor, and brotherly love.

One beneficiary of this was Washington's vice president, John Adams, a Massachusetts statesman who campaigned to "Adams and Liberty."[3] Also known as "The Boston Patriotic Song," its nine verses celebrate the virtues of the United States while emphasizing the differences between the fledgling nation and old Europe; predictably, it also heaped praise on Washington and Adams. The melody was borrowed from "To Anacreon in Heaven," originally a drinking song written for a gentleman's club in London by British organist John Stafford Smith. In 1814, Francis Scott Key would go on to use the well-known melody for "The Star-Spangled Banner," thus relegating its role as a paean to Washington and Adams to a historical footnote.

As campaigning evolved and both the country and voting rights expanded, candidates sought better methods to reach the public, create name recognition, foster party loyalty, and form emotional bonds with voters. By the mid-nineteenth century, the Democrats and Whigs, which had emerged as the two dominant parties, were experimenting with an approach that mobilized music in the form of "songsters," a word that referred both to the pocket-sized partisan songbooks formatted for easy distribution, and to the people, often young men, hired to sing these political jingles on busy street corners and markets. This practice attracted attention and spread the word about candidates and parties through spontaneous rallies and sing-alongs. Songsters continued the tradition of setting newly composed political lyrics to popular melodies. This allowed for easy crowd participation and proxy campaigning by singers who may or may not have been familiar with the candidate's policy platform. Public singing could foment positive feelings toward a candidate without his needing to explain his position on the issues of the day. But songsters also ushered in the age of negative campaigning, offering satires and lampoons of their patrons' opponents.

Throughout the nineteenth century, songsters dominated political campaigning as inexpensive printing presses made the songbooks they needed to pass on their political messages widely available. The mode of campaign outreach used, collective singing, was a common pastime widely practiced in sacred, secular, and political spaces. At a time of low literacy rates, people learned songs by ear, or from those who could read broadsides—single sheets of cheap paper with music and lyrics printed on one side, a common way of disseminating popular music before phonographs, radios, and player pianos. In churches, the practice of "lining out" or "deaconing," where a singer intones a line and the congregation responds, was a common practice.[4] For the labor movements of the nineteenth and early twentieth centuries, song was essential in spreading critical talking points, telling stories, and creating a shared identity. The Industrial Workers of the World, founded in Chicago in 1905, produced songbooks, had in their ranks famed singer Joe Hill, and made collective singing part of meetings and protests.[5]

Perhaps the most iconic early exemplar of the songster's art was "Tippecanoe and Tyler Too!," a song written for the 1840 campaign of William Henry Harrison (who earned the nickname Tippecanoe for his role in the 1811 battle of the same name) and his running mate John Tyler. In 1884, critic Helen Kendrick Johnson wrote: "'Tippecanoe and Tyler, too,' was to the

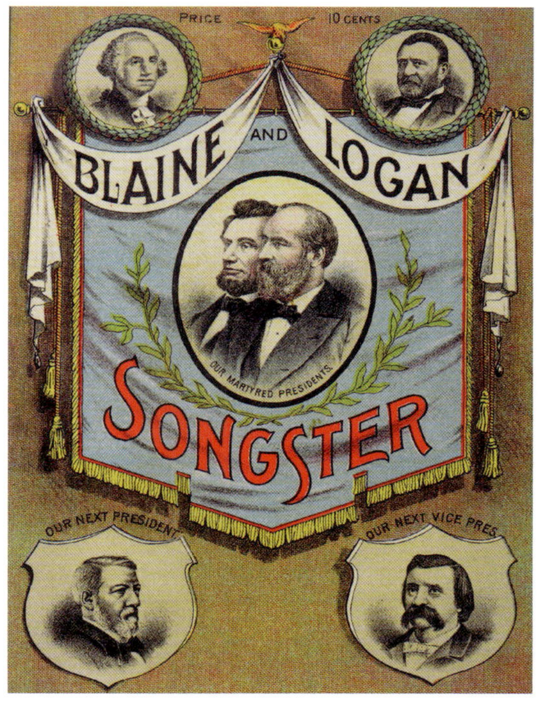

Sixty-four-page "songster" booklet featuring campaign songs for James G. Blaine and John A. Logan, the Republican candidates in the 1884 presidential election. The pair narrowly lost to Democrats Grover Cleveland and Thomas A. Hendricks.

The lyrics of "Tippecanoe and Tyler Too!," a song for the 1840 presidential campaign of William Henry Harrison and John Tyler, referred to a "ball a-rolling on." This metaphor was made real in the form of an enormous ball, emblazoned with the candidates' campaign issues, that their supporters would roll through the streets. Courtesy Library of Congress.

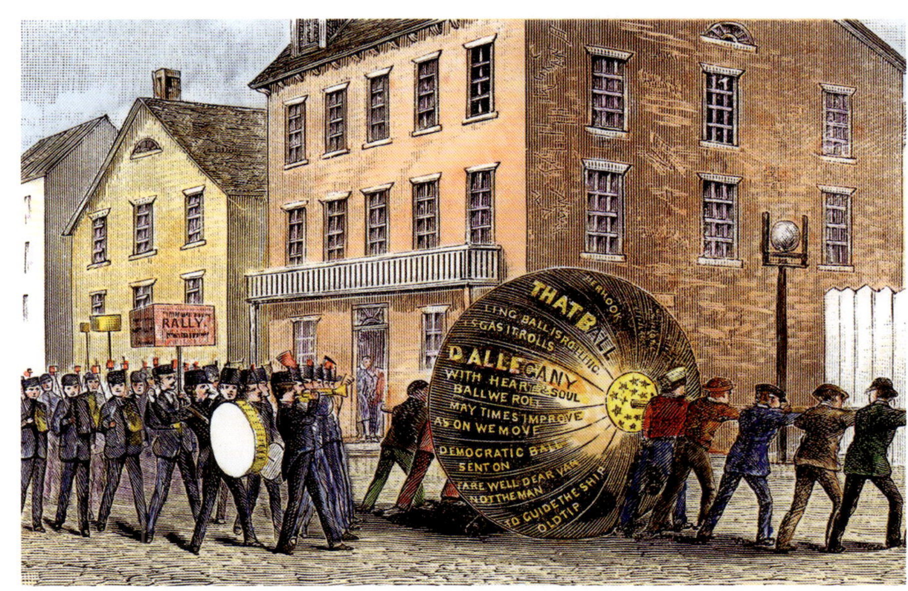

political canvass of 1840 what the Marseillaise was to the French Revolution."[6] Set to the tune of "Little Pigs," a simple, jaunty 6/8 melody, the eleven-verse song lauded Harrison and Tyler and disparaged the incumbent Martin Van Buren, deriding him as "little Van" and featuring a chorus with the line, "Van is a used up man." The song also did something that would become a mainstay of the modern campaign: it engendered feelings of inevitable victory. With lyrics like "Now you hear the Van-Jacks talking, talking, talking / Things

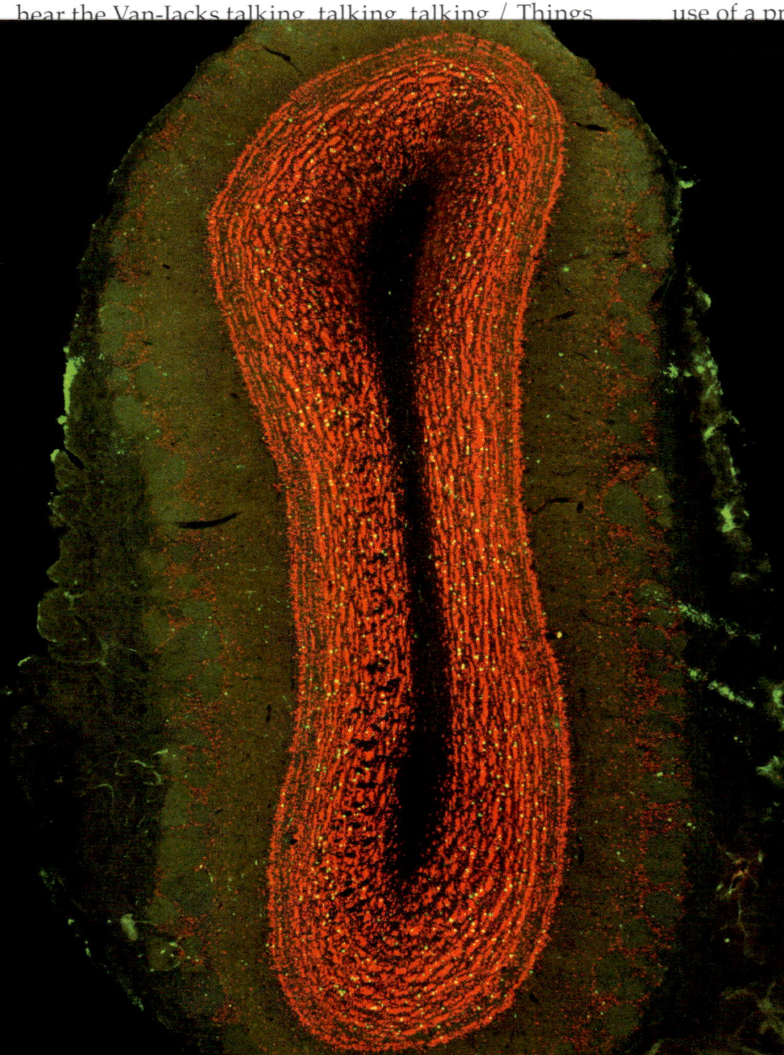

NEW MEDIA, NEW SOUNDS

The era of the songsters lasted through the early twentieth century. Even though collective singing is still used at campaign rallies, by the 1920s, radio and film had transformed the way candidates portrayed themselves to their audiences, a shift that would be repeated with the rise of television and social media. As cinema newsreels began to show the candidate's visage and the radio to carry their voice, there was less need for songsters as political bards. With mass media, voters could hear from a candidate directly, and often. Far from being abandoned, however, campaign music moved in two different directions. One was the creation of campaign jingles—short, original songs, written for the airwaves, that imitated advertising. The other was the use of a pre-existing piece of music, without alteration, theme song. Even the role of the songster ated: political songs were now recorded broadcast by PA-equipped trucks rather ired musicians.

media of film, radio, and, later, television, ties whose voices, images, and person- household names. At first, campaigns ar songs drawn from popular films, idates began to associate themselves elebrities to gain name recognition and n funds. Eventually, the mechanisms oduction of celebrity became campaign their own right, with rallies focused on dates into stars.

example of the use of pre-existing occurred in 1932 when Franklin Delano d as his campaign song "Happy Days n," which had been featured in *Chasing* m from two years earlier about a struggle troupe. Although 1932 was one of l years in US economic history, "Happy d the optimistic tenor of Roosevelt's successor, Harry Truman, used "I'm ut Harry," a popular love song from nd Eubie Blake's 1921 musical *Shuffle* ly, the first Broadway show to feature American cast). The lyrics feature such altz as "The heav'nly blisses of his kisses stasy / He's sweet like choc'late candy, he honey from a bee," and introduce t campaigns continue to wrestle with: popular songs are not written as campaign jingles and often contain lyrics that are inappropriate, embarrassing, or otherwise not politically expedient.

The American postwar boom ushered in a new era of production and consumption, which necessitated sophisticated strategies of advertising and marketing. Admen created captivating images, narratives,

and songs to pique customer interest and to create emotional attachments between consumers and products, skills that are still sought after by campaigns. Radio jingles were designed to promote affective brand recognition, not necessarily to pass meaningful information to the listener. War hero Dwight Eisenhower's 1952 campaign jingle and television ad "I like Ike" exemplified this new trend. The song repeats the slogan over a bouncy, almost childish march that makes no mention of policy, Eisenhower's character, or his proper name. The song even omits Eisenhower's war-hero status, which was part of his popular appeal. The text is hortatory, with the repeated couplet: "You like Ike, I like Ike, everybody likes Ike for president. / Bring out the banners, beat the drums, we'll take Ike to Washington." Confusingly, Irving Berlin penned a different song with an identical title for the same campaign. His version showcases his signature lyrical qualities, but is more politically didactic than the catchy, though textually unsubstantial, campaign jingle. According to historian Stuart Schimler, Berlin's song may have been the last well-known election song (as opposed to a jingle), although will.i.am's "Yes We Can" is also a candidate for that distinction.[9]

The year 1960 heralded the first modern campaign, one that was intensely media- and celebrity-driven. In a prescient move, John F. Kennedy's campaign employed a television specialist, an advantage that played out in the first ever nationally televised presidential debate. Radio listeners thought the debate was a draw or even a win for Richard Nixon, while television viewers overwhelmingly favored Kennedy, the upstart from Massachusetts whose image invoked youth, power, style, and romance. Musically, his campaign drew on star power. Frank Sinatra re-recorded his hit "High Hopes"—a song made famous by the popular 1959 film *A Hole in the Head*, and nominated for Grammy and Academy Awards—with lyrics altered to plump for Kennedy. While there was no formal attribution and the Kennedy campaign never used Sinatra's name on the recording or promotional materials, many listeners recognized Sinatra's signature voice and his endorsement was implicit, even for those who did not know that the singer helped raise money for Kennedy.[10] Despite being a media-driven campaign that emphasized youth and fresh ideas, it also tapped into earlier modes of political promotion. A recording of "High Hopes" and copies of the sheet music were distributed

to local Democratic Party offices before rallies, so that campaign staffers could learn the song. At rallies, staffers would pass out the sheet music and lead audiences in singing Kennedy onstage.

In making civil rights a cornerstone of his platform, Kennedy also reached out to performers from the African-American community. One of Kennedy's ads featured Harry Belafonte addressing the audience on the candidate's behalf. Belafonte explicitly identifies himself as an artist and not a politician, and cedes the camera to Kennedy, who presents himself as an advocate for equal opportunity. The ad ends with Belafonte stating that he's voting for Kennedy. As a young junior senator from Massachusetts competing against the vastly more experienced vice president, Kennedy needed to associate himself with names and faces that the public knew and trusted. Sinatra and Belafonte helped Kennedy meet the public with an air of credibility and suave sophistication, particularly among younger and civil-rights-minded voters.

The 1964 campaign of Lyndon Johnson was the last time poverty was the centerpiece of a presidential candidate's platform. The "Great Society" was Johnson's formidable legislative suite aimed at improving living conditions for millions, and one of the most memorable ads from his campaign is entitled "Poverty." The ad features black-and-white photographs of indigent children with a male voiceover asserting that poverty is a creation of circumstance, and that these circumstances can be changed to break the cycle of destitution.[11] The musical accompaniment is haunting—a grainy recording of an acoustic guitar improvising the blues. "Poverty" is a modern political ad in every sense: it combines polemic (*sans* policy) with a soundtrack that indexes the candidate, the issue, and the voters who the ad is aimed at. The music references the South and the African-American communities whose roots are there—country blues originated in the black communities of the Mississippi Delta, even though by 1964 many from the Delta had moved to northern cities and electrified the blues. The text clearly references the ideology behind what would become known as Johnson's War on Poverty, a wide-ranging legislative suite that transformed national healthcare, housing, and education. However, the ad mentions no specific policies and is instead designed to be affectively captivating. "Poverty" also gestures toward Johnson himself, who taught

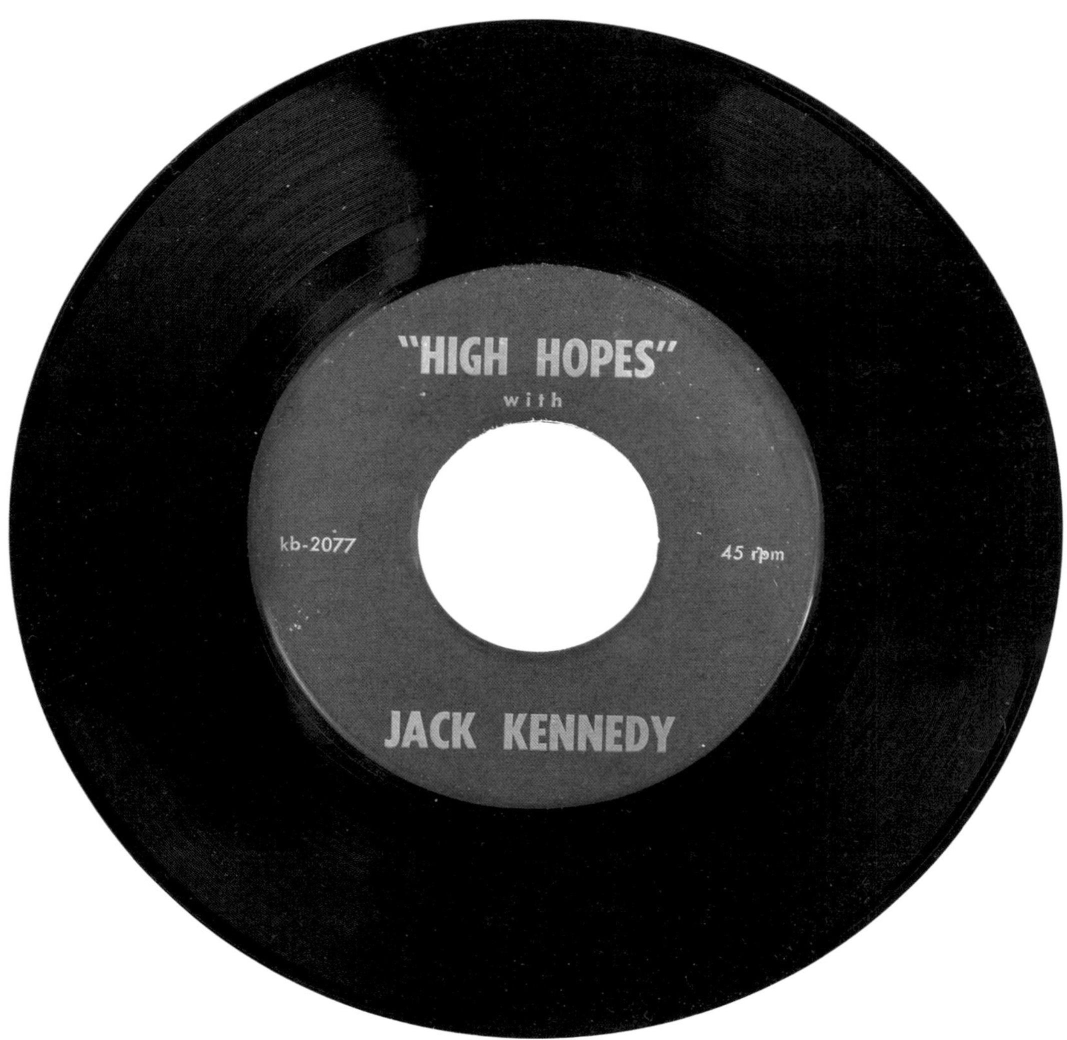

Mexican-American children in a rural school not far from his birthplace in south Texas before pursuing a political career. This particular combination of music, rhetoric, and persona has come to define campaign ads in the modern era: Ronald Reagan's "Bear" and "Morning in America," Walter Mondale's "Arms Control 5," George W. Bush's "Education Recession," and John McCain's "Spending."[12]

CONTEMPORARY CAMPAIGNS

As campaigns have grown more extravagant, theme songs have given way to campaign playlists, and rallies can now include concert-like performances. Popular legend attributes Bill Clinton's improbable triumph in the 1992 Democratic primaries to his Blues Brothers–esque saxophone performance of "Heartbreak Hotel" on *The Arsenio Hall Show*, the embodiment of baby-boomer cool. His campaign's theme song, Fleetwood Mac's "Don't Stop (Thinking about Tomorrow)," reminiscent of "Happy Days Are Here Again," captured Clinton's youthful optimism, particularly in contrast to Republican incumbent George H. W. Bush and Reform Party candidate Ross Perot. In an unusual twist, Clinton's campaign breathed life into Fleetwood Mac, and was the catalyst for a reunion tour and a Grammy-nominated live album, further

Above: A promotional copy of "High Hopes," sung by you-know-who and used in John F. Kennedy's 1960 presidential campaign.

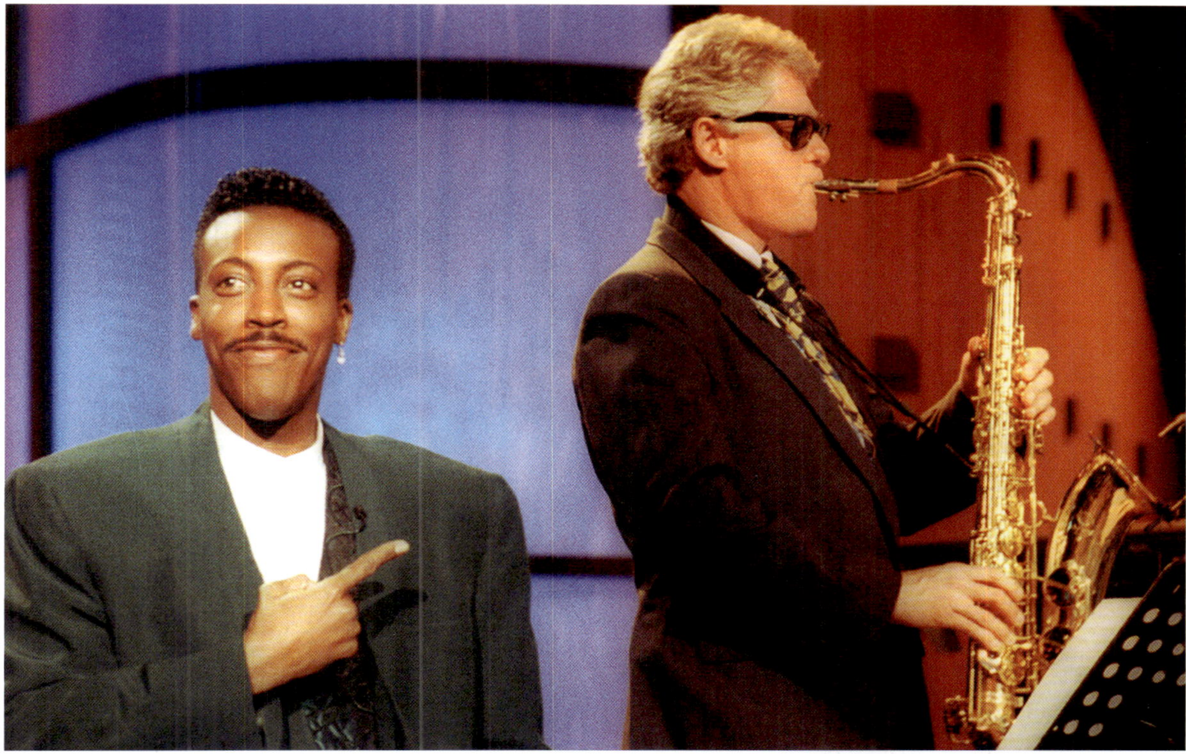

narrowing the divide between politics and pop culture. In the past two election cycles, celebrity, music, and political culture have effectively merged. Candidates now campaign and entertain as celebrities. They perform to thunderous applause like rock stars, collect Twitter followers by the millions, appear on morning and late-night shows as often as on news programs, and are pursued by a news corps that imitates the paparazzi.

Technology has also altered the sonic landscape of campaigns. With the proliferation of internet usage and the development of inexpensive digital recording, editing, and sharing software, citizens are now able to contribute to the sounds and images of politics like never before. While critics posted homemade videos of George W. Bush's gaffes, it was Barack Obama's 2008 campaign that saw tech-savvy activists creating and sharing musical tribute videos through social media platforms. Candidates communicate with the public through social media platforms like Twitter, Facebook, and YouTube, and citizens respond in kind. The most high-profile example of this was the song and video by will.i.am entitled "Yes We Can," based on Obama's concession speech after losing the 2008

New Hampshire primary. The stylishly produced black-and-white video featured numerous celebrities and notables speaking, intoning, and singing lines from the speech over Obama's voice and a hook sung by will.i.am and John Legend. The video was posted on YouTube and racked up over seventeen million views in the first month.[13] It also sparked parodies, including the slick, snarky "Yes I Can," featuring clips of John McCain talking about prolonging war in the Middle East and bombing Iran, and "No, You Can't—No Se Puede," a parody that criticizes America's disastrous wealth protection policies.[14] Both use the same visual style and music as "Yes We Can," and are constructed for an audience that recognizes the reference and revels in the satire. These types of campaign videos are not made to win over new voters, but to provide stalwarts continuously reinforced pleasure in partisanship and to sustain enthusiasm through the long campaign.

In 2016, candidates Clinton and Trump made news, positive and negative, with their campaign sounds. Both campaigns were endorsed by famous musicians,

Above: Candidate Bill Clinton performing "Heartbreak Hotel" on *The Arsenio Hall Show* on 3 June 1992.

and both were also served with cease-and-desist letters from artists who took offense to their music being used without permission. Following Obama's lead, Clinton released her official playlist just days after she launched her campaign. Its message was clear: female uplift and empowerment. Like Obama's playlists, which were overtly aimed at coalition building and bolstering a project of electoral and affective inclusion, Clinton's mix included numerous artists of color and varied genres. The mix spotlighted many female artists performing songs about fighting against long odds and succeeding. But its detractors were myriad, citing everything from the mundaneness of the mix to the fact that the oldest song was from 1999, when Clinton would have been fifty-two. These critics read the mix as contrived and pandering, a symptom of Clinton's perceived lack of authenticity.[15] In contrast, Trump's campaign playlist struck critics as not being political enough. Featuring an eclectic mix of hits from 1980s metal and classic rock to Broadway, adult contemporary, and classical music, Trump's self-curated playlist was devoid of a political message or unifying theme, save for masculine triumphalism. For his critics, this showed another dimension of his amateurism and was evidence of his lack of vision and political experience. Critic Chris Richards went so far as to label Trump's use of music as authoritarian, saying that his "[campaign songs] make everyone feel comfortable—in their indignation, in their suspicion, in their hostility."[16] But for his supporters, this was another sign of Trump's authenticity.

The ways in which music is deployed in presidential campaigns will only increase in sophistication and complexity as new technologies allow for more citizen involvement (the Bernie Sanders campaign was the recipient of several phenomenal fan-made ads) and artists assert their intellectual property rights to stop campaigns from using their music.[17] Big Data also makes marketing more effective, as information on demographics and personal habits—from red and blue neighborhoods to individuals' mobile usage and internet preferences—allows for specifically targeted ad buys. As the 2018 midterm elections loom, we should wonder what will we hear next. Will we know what music the opposition is playing, or will all of our consumption patterns reinforce partisanship to the point where our preference is to remain ignorant of both the opposing candidate's music and platform? And when will music cease to make partisan fanaticism palatable or desirable, and force us to listen to and evaluate policy, rather than playlists?

1 "God Save Great Washington," *Philadelphia Continental Journal*, 7 April 1786, cited in Benjamin S. Schoening and Eric T. Kasper, *Don't Stop Thinking about the Music: The Politics of Songs and Musicians in Presidential Campaigns* (New York: Lexington Books, 2012), p. 30.

2 This common practice was known as parody or contrafactum.

3 The lyrics are by Robert Treat Paine. See Paine, *The Works, in Verse and Prose, of the Late Robert Treat Paine, Jun. Esq.* (Boston: J. Belcher, 1812), pp. 245–247. The lyrics are also available at <potw.org/archive/potw233.html>.

4 See William T. Dargan, *Lining Out the Word: Dr. Watts Hymn Singing in the Music of Black Americans* (Berkeley: University of California Press; Chicago: Center for Black Music Research, 2006), and Charles L. Etherington, *Protestant Worship Music: Its History and Practice* (New York: Holt, Rinehart and Winston, 1962).

5 See Ron Eyerman and Andrew Jamison, *Music and Social Movements: Mobilizing Traditions in the Twentieth Century* (Cambridge: Cambridge University Press, 1998), especially p. 57ff.

6 Helen Kendrick Johnson, "The Meaning of a Song," *The North American Review*, vol. 138, no. 330 (May 1884), p. 494.

7 Benjamin S. Schoening and Eric T. Kasper, *Don't Stop Thinking about the Music*, pp. 44–45.

8 Ibid., p. 64.

9 Stuart Schimler, "Singing for the Oval Office: A History of the Political Campaign Song." Available at <presidentelect.org/art_schimler_singing.html>.

10 Benjamin S. Schoening and Eric T. Kasper, *Don't Stop Thinking about the Music*, p. 131. It is not clear why the Kennedy campaign did not seek to capitalize more explicitly on Sinatra's star power. It is possible that Sinatra's contract with Capitol Records required that he record exclusively for the label.

11 The ad can be viewed at <livingroomcandidate.org/commercials/1964/poverty>.

12 These ads can be viewed at <livingroomcandidate.org>.

13 Brian Stelter, "Finding Political News Online, the Young Pass It On," *The New York Times*, 27 March 2008.

14 See <youtu.be/KHWeUKSdHL8> and <youtu.be/gl7WwY4a9ro>.

15 See, for example, David R. Dewberry and Jonathan Millen, "Hillary Clinton's 2016 Presidential Campaign Spotify Playlist," Trax on the Trail, 25 May 2016. Available at <traxonthetrail.com/article/hillary-clinton%E2%80%99s-2016-presidential-campaign-spotify-playlist>.

16 Chris Richards, "Authoritarian Hold Music: How Donald Trump's Banal Playlist Cultivates Danger at His Rallies," *The Washington Post*, 16 March 2016. Available at <wapo.st/1VcLeDg?tid=ss_tw&utm_term=.833f3b917695>.

17 Eric T. Kasper and Benjamin S. Schoening, "The Unwelcome Use of Musical Artists and Their Songs by Political Candidates," Trax on the Trail, 18 December 2015. Available at <traxonthetrail.com/article/unwelcome-use-musical-artists-and-their-songs-presidential-candidates>.

NOBLE ROT
Elaine Ayers

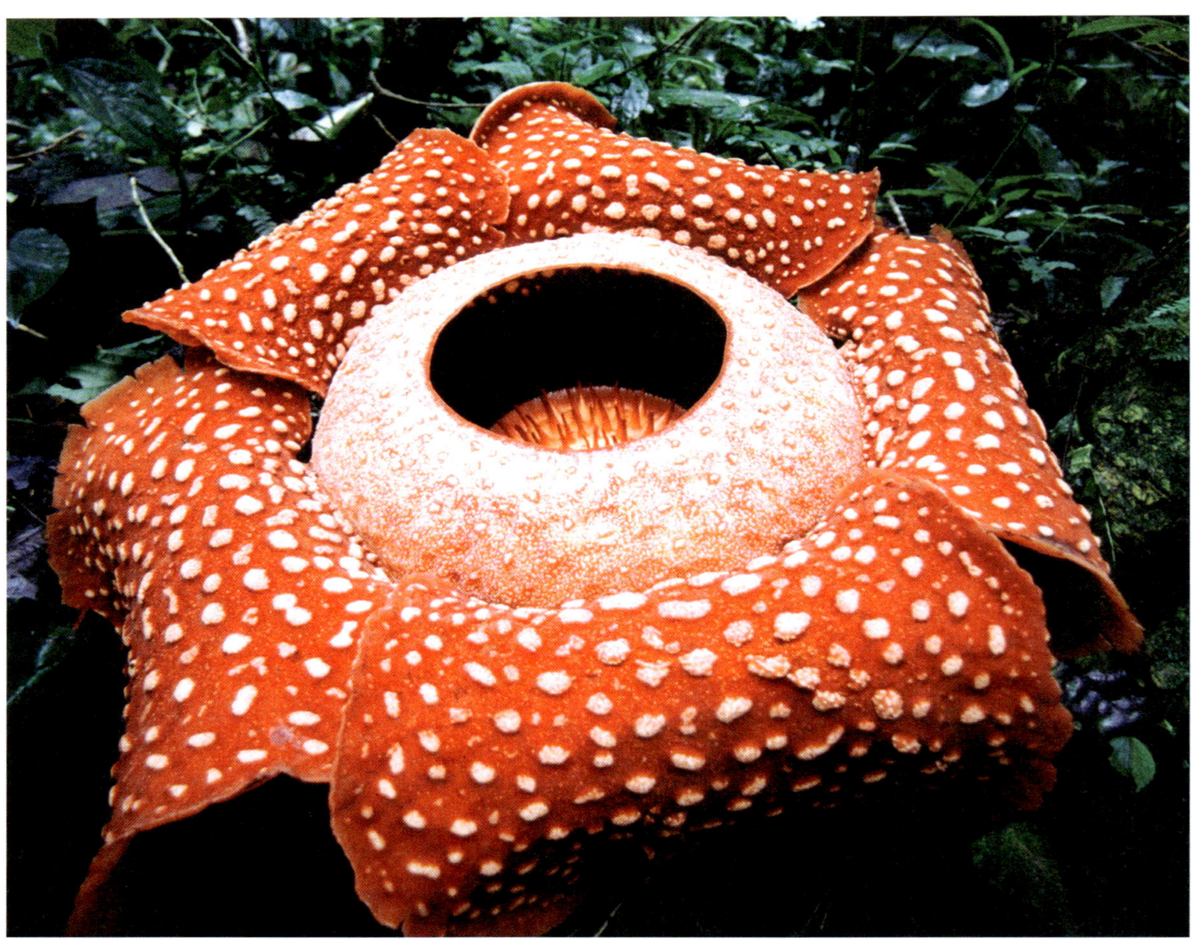

You smell *Rafflesia arnoldii* before you see it. Described variously as the scent of "decaying animal matter," "tainted beef," and "death," the fetid thickness of air hits you in waves, warning you that something is deeply wrong: that maybe you're about to stumble upon a body. Next you might see the carrion flies "always found hovering over these strange flowers," attracted by the plant's "objectionable effluvium," laying their eggs in its massive nectary and tracking out seeds on their tiny feet.[1] Finally, if you're lucky enough, you see the flower itself: a massive, five-petaled parasite growing on an unassuming vine, its dark-red body speckled with pustular protuberances, a gaping cavity revealing its sex organs to hopeful pollinators. It looks like a twisted cartoon flower, drawn too large to support its own weight. There is something disturbingly animalistic about this plant, only heightened by its corpse-like fragrance.

To be clear, this corpse flower isn't the same as the giant, phallic floral species that sparked botanical conspiracy theories in 2016 when, after lying dormant for nearly a decade, a number of its specimens bloomed in botanical gardens across the world in a seemingly coordinated attack on our senses.[2] Completely unrelated to *Amorphophallus titanum* (also known as the "giant misshapen penis" of the vegetable world), *Rafflesia arnoldii* is part of a genus most of whose species have also developed the not entirely uncommon ability to mimic the smell of

―――――――――

Above: *Rafflesia arnoldii*, the "greatest prodigy of the vegetable world."

rotting flesh to attract carrion pollinators—a kind of evolutionary olfactory symbiosis.[3] Indeed, many plants emit fragrances that mimic animal pheromones, drawing insects in with sickly sweet, musky perfumes suggesting both sexual availability and potential food sources, tricking insects into picking up their pollen to unwittingly distribute elsewhere. Some plants, like the carnivorous pitcher plants that inhabit the same Southeast Asian forests as corpse flowers, trap insects inside their cavernous mouths, slowly dissolving them in acid to extract necessary nutrients for survival.

Rafflesia arnoldii, though, is the king of flora. Exceedingly rare, and lacking most of the traits that define plant life—chlorophyll, roots, leaves—this is the largest flower in the world, and arguably the strangest. Discovered in the middle of the Sumatran rainforest in the early nineteenth century, *Rafflesia arnoldii* has defied collection, cultivation, and even, in some respects, classification, maintaining its status as one of the most unknowable creatures on earth. While chemists have recently identified the compounds that produce its undeniably corpse-like stench, *Rafflesia*'s scent seems bigger than the sum of its parts, formed as much by the flower's uncanny appearance, its fleeting rarity, and the lack of any botanical referents for describing its scent as by any combination of phenols and trimethylamines.

. . .

Enter Joseph Arnold: surgeon, botanist, explorer, and failed science fiction writer. Arnold—an overweight, bearded, surly Englishman with few friends—was no stranger to foul smells, gore, and putrefaction. At twenty-seven, he served as Surgeon-Superintendent aboard the HMS *Northampton*, an all-female convict ship that sailed for Australia in January 1815. In his months aboard the ship as it navigated the treacherous Pacific waters, Arnold kept meticulous diaries detailing his daily activities: lancing pustulent wounds, amputating gangrenous limbs, treating rampant venereal disease, mopping up bodily fluids, sometimes delivering babies. After failing to secure employment as a physician in Sydney, he decided to return to England. While temporarily docked off the coast of Java in 1815, a ship fire destroyed his natural history collections— ranging from botanical specimens to cases of insects and birds—which he had planned to sell to interested buyers at home.[4] Back in England, Arnold found

himself deeply depressed and plagued with nightmares of hooded men stalking him, knives concealed beneath their black robes. Even while studying natural history in preparation for his next trip, Arnold was haunted by what he had witnessed during his short time as surgeon aboard warships in the Napoleonic Wars; just a few years earlier, his diary listed the "purulent discharges, poultices, groans, fotor, putrid exfoliating bones, fear of h[e]morrhagy and other accompanying disagreeables," which he considered his "portion from morning till night without much hope of a diminution of them for a length of time to come."[5] The young naturalist felt stifled; he had to get out of England.

In May of 1818, Arnold trekked into the staggeringly hot rainforest outside of Padang, Western Sumatra, on the botanical expedition that would seal his fate. Dressed in a linen suit and carrying glass collection jars filled with spirits, Arnold was accompanied by Sir Thomas Stamford Raffles, administrator in the British East Indies, serving as lead; Raffles's wife, eager to make illustrations of the landscape; a local colonial officer; and dozens of Sumatran guides and porters tasked with clearing a path through the thick underbrush and carrying the team's supplies. After the group had hiked through "impenetrable forest" for a few days, one of Arnold's guides discovered what the naturalist described as "the greatest prodigy of the vegetable world": a flower so large that Arnold shook with fear, awe, and disbelief.[6] The flower measured several feet in circumference, its nectary alone able to hold fourteen pints of water, its brick-red fleshy petals "thick and covered with protuberances of a yellowish white." Arnold glanced at the "swarm of flies hovering over the mouth of the nectary," and had to hold his breath, repulsed by what he called "precisely the smell of tainted beef."[7]

The team quickly cut the flower from its host vine, packed it in a large box, and sent several porters running to bring it back to base camp. By the time they returned to camp that evening, though, Arnold "found the flower still in the box, the petals dark brown, wasted, full of Maggots & like a rotten mushroom."[8] The plant's decomposed, still-stinking body reminded

---

Opposite: Illustration of *Rafflesia patma*, a smaller relative of *arnoldii*. From the 1913 edition of Anton Kerner von Marilaun's *Pflanzenleben*.

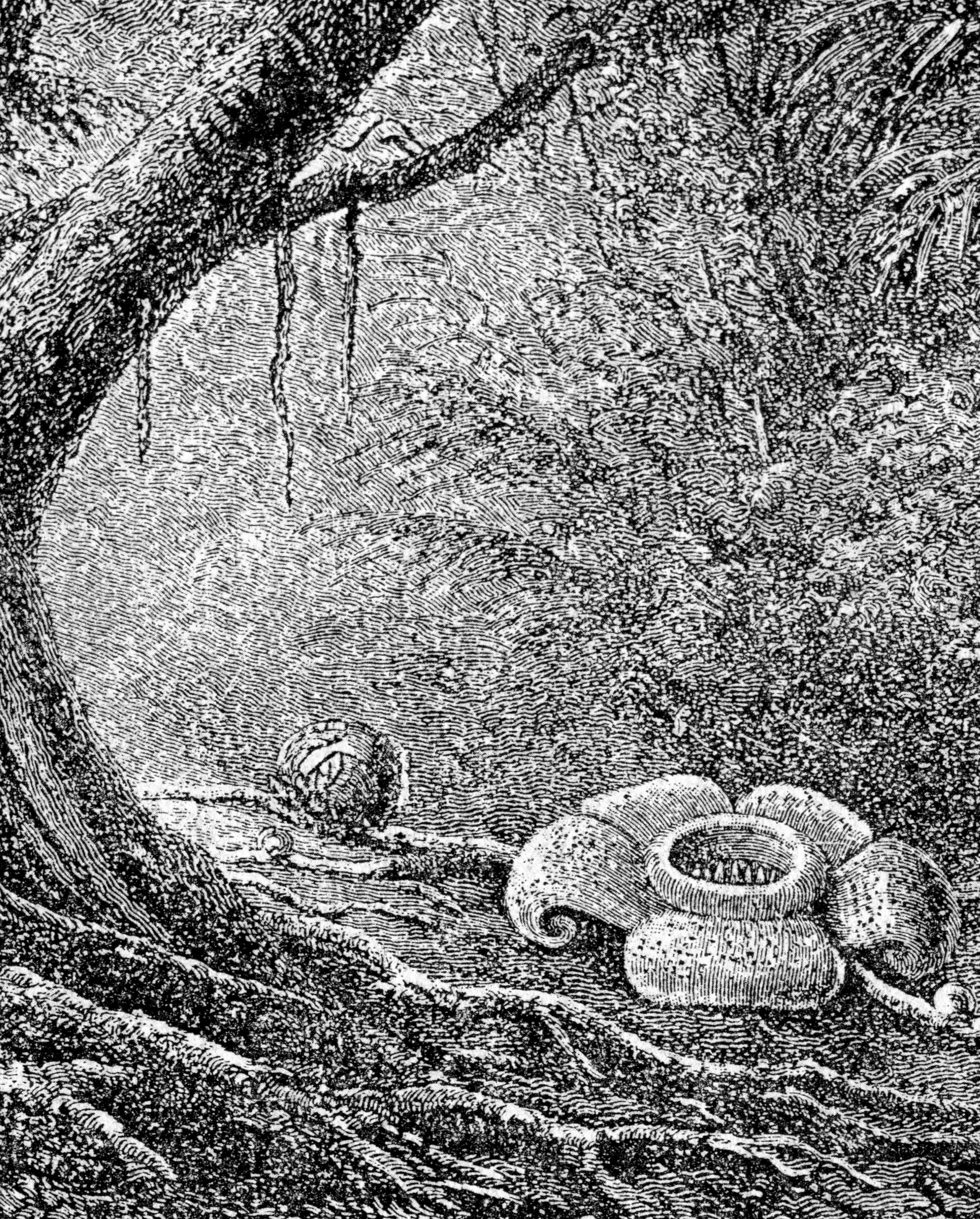

Arnold of the infected flesh he had scraped from bones while working as a ship's surgeon, a past he had tried to escape. The only recoverable part was the plant's spongy pistil (the female sex organ of the plant), which they pickled in spirits and sent back to London to be identified by Sir Joseph Banks and his librarian, Robert Brown, at the Linnean Society. By 1821, the giant flower lived on as the infamously repulsive *Rafflesia arnoldii*, a symbol of what unique horrors tropical forests might hold.[9] Illustrated, the flower had to be scaled down by more than a foot.

. . .

Arnold's first observation about the plant was that it grew best in nutrient-rich elephant shit. Fitting, perhaps, because *everything* in these Sumatran rain-forests seemed massive to the explorers; butterflies as big as birds swept past Arnold and his team, and occasional crashing sounds from the forest's interior suggested the proximity of rogue elephants—lurking tigers notwithstanding, "they alone of the animal kingdom seemed to have explored the recesses of the forest."[10] It was the luxuriant "grandeur of the vegeta-tion," though, that struck Sir Stamford Raffles most during their expedition, "the magnitude of the flowers, creepers, and trees" contrasting with the familiar stunted "pigmy vegetation" of England.[11] They tripped over rotting *Rafflesia arnoldii*, its flesh breaking down into a black, pulpy liquid, its seeds mixing with the rancid, "putrid mass" of mud, decaying organic matter, and dung.[12] The plant's magnificent, pockmarked bloom only lasted for a few days, reaching its height for only a matter of hours before decomposing, giving into the carrion larvae nesting inside of its vital organs. Even now, delaying a trip to see the flower because of an afternoon thunderstorm could mean you miss it entirely: in just a few hours, the vegetable prodigy transforms back into a pile of shit, the jungle's heat, humidity, and insect life working double-time to break down vulnerable, ripe flesh.

Joseph Arnold, for his part, fancied himself part of the Romantic tradition of tropical exploration, situating the vegetable prodigy in an environment character-ized by crashing precipices, rumbling volcanoes, and stifling heat. He attempted to record "sensory descriptions" of the landscapes he traversed; climbing a volcano in Java on an earlier voyage, Arnold noted that "it would be difficult to give such a description

of this tremendous scene as would make the reader to form an accurate idea of its terrific grandeur," never-theless recording many details, from the "vegetable mould" covering the volcano's rocks to its "very strong sulphourous smell" and the eerie absence of bird sounds from the crater's surrounding rainforest.[13] In the forest where they found *Rafflesia arnoldii*, Arnold described two-hundred-foot-high trees, whose roots, "often twisted like cables, descended like festoons almost to the water," creating "one of the most romantic scenes" he had ever witnessed.[14]

Like so many other explorers, Arnold continually agonized over how to commit the intangible sensory natural wonders he observed to paper. How, for instance, to describe smells without just comparing them to things already known? He played out his anxi-eties in an unpublished, mind-numbingly dull novel, "The Visit to the Moon: A Philosophical Romance," written from his ship desk while sailing across the Indian Ocean. In it, a young naturalist (not unlike Arnold himself) finds himself mysteriously trans-ported, during an expedition somewhere in Asia, to the barren craters of the moon. Devastatingly alone and sometimes suicidal, the naturalist struggles to communicate his terrifying lunar discoveries to his friends back on earth, unable to find words worthy of this incredible strangeness while lamenting the certain disbelief he will face if he survives his lonely journey. Although the moon presents "the most astounding discoveries and the most unheard of prodigies," the explorer fears that "this passion must necessarily be solitary": his colleagues would never believe the sights, smells, and dangers of this cold, rocky landscape.[15] Years later, Arnold echoed his protagonist's distress: "Had there been no witnesses," he wrote, "I think I should have been fearful of mentioning the dimensions of this flower."[16]

. . .

Botanists aren't quite sure where to place *Rafflesia arnoldii*, how to define its unique combination of evolu-tionary oddities. The plant's size and appearance seem to be related to its smell; most flora that emit the odor of rotting flesh tend to be oversized, and the corpse flower's fleshy texture and color undeniably appeal to carrion flies initially drawn in by its scent.[17] The plant seems to be born of its tropical environment, inextri-cable from not just its host vine but from its place in the

overwhelming and chaotic rainforest, a place of fecundity and decay.

The problem with studying *Rafflesia arnoldii*, though, is that we can't cultivate them in botanical gardens like we can with *Amorphophallus titanum*, and most other tropical plants. If you want to see the vegetable prodigy, you have to meet it on its own turf, growing in the now-endangered forests of Southeast Asia. Botanists have been able to transplant a few specimens into botanical gardens along with their hosts, but not outside of the region. Accordingly, popular culture has been rather less kind to *Rafflesia arnoldii* than to its phallic corollary. While *Amorphophallus titanum* garnered its own "live cam" so that audiences could track its three-day-long bloom cycle—minus the smell—discoveries about *Rafflesia arnoldii*'s remarkable genetic history have been run under headlines like "Giant Stinking Flower Is, Alas, from a Proper Family."[18]

Combine a few chemical compounds, and you get the smell of rotting meat; add dimethyl trisulfide, and you get a hint of cheese; benzyl alcohol, and you finish with a top note of saccharine organic matter. This is perfumery at its most basic. Corpse flower blooms, though, are so much more overwhelming than this neat potpourri of compounds. As naturalists so intimately understood, some things just can't be communicated. There are no words for the distinct smell of death, for parasitism, for such unbounded floral magnitude. Less than two weeks after discovering *Rafflesia arnoldii* growing in the forests of Western Sumatra, Joseph Arnold contracted a debilitating tropical fever. A few months later, the naturalist succumbed to his illness, dead at thirty-five. Carrion flies descended on his corpse almost immediately, attracted by the smell of his rotting flesh.

1 Eric Fitch Daglish, *The Marvels of Plant Life* (London: Thornton Butterworth, 1924).

2 Jessie Guy-Ryan, "Why Are So Many Corpse Flowers Blooming at Once?" *Atlas Obscura*, 31 July 2016. Available at <atlasobscura.com/articles/why-are-so-many-corpse-flowers-blooming-at-once>. Despite the fact that *Amorphophallus titanum* only bloom once every seven to ten years, the flowers bloomed in fifteen different botanical gardens in 2016. Between February and September, visitors flocked to view them in Adelaide, Chicago, Cornwall, Winter Park, Munich, Charleston, Kerala, New York City, Bloomington, Sarasota, Washington, DC, Denver, River Falls, Raleigh, and Hanover.

3 David Attenborough famously renamed *Amorphophallus titanum* "Titan arum" in his 1995 BBC special, *The Private Life of Plants*. Joining a centuries-long struggle to de-sex botany, Attenborough said that he felt uncomfortable repeating "giant misshapen penis" on international television, even in Latin. New species of *Rafflesia* are being consistently discovered as logging industries develop deeper into Southeast Asian rainforests. In February 2016, a team of scientists discovered, on the Philippine island of Luzon, *Rafflesia consueloae*, the smallest species of corpse flower known. Departing from its genus not just in size, *Rafflesia consueloae* emits the subtle, sweet smell of young coconuts. See John Michael M. Galindon, Perry S. Ong, and Edwino S. Fernando, "Rafflesia consueloae (Rafflesiaceae), the Smallest Among Giants; A New Species from Luzon Island, Philippines," *PhytoKeys*, vol. 61 (2016).

4 John Bastin, "The Java Journal of Dr. Joseph Arnold," *Journal of the Malaysian Branch of the Royal Asiatic Society*, vol. 46, no. 1 (1973), p. 7.

5 Entry of 29 May 1812, Joseph Arnold Journal, 1 January–31 December 1812, Mitchell Library Special Collections, C720/2, State Library of New South Wales.

6 Joseph Arnold to Dawson Turner, 9 July 1818, Joseph Arnold Collection, Linnean Society Archives, London.

7 Ibid.

8 Ibid.

9 For the full classification and description of *Rafflesia arnoldii*, along with the official announcement of Arnold's death, see Robert Brown, "An Account of a New Genus of Plants, Named Rafflesia," *Transactions of the Linnean Society of London*, vol. 13 (1821). The paper was first read before the society on 30 June 1820.

10 Sir Thomas Stamford Raffles to the Duchess of Somerset, 11 July 1818, quoted in Lady Sophia Raffles, *Memoir of the Life and Public Services of Sir Thomas Stamford Raffles*, F.R.S. (London: John Murray, 1830), p. 318.

11 Ibid.

12 Ibid., p. 317.

13 Joseph Arnold, 1 December 1815, Mitchell Library Special Collections, A1845–1847, State Library of New South Wales.

14 Joseph Arnold to Dawson Turner, 9 July 1818, Joseph Arnold Collection, Linnean Society Archives, London.

15 Joseph Arnold, "A Visit to the Moon: A Philosophical Romance" (unpublished manuscript), f. 112–113, Mitchell Library Special Collections, A1848, State Library of New South Wales.

16 Joseph Arnold to Dawson Turner, 9 July 1818, Joseph Arnold Collection, Linnean Society Archives, London.

17 For an excellent recent overview of this issue, see Jonathan Shaw, "Colossal Blossom," *Harvard Magazine*, vol. 119, no. 4 (March–April 2017).

18 Carol Kaesuk Yoon, "Giant Stinking Flower Is, Alas, From a Proper Family," *The New York Times*, 27 January 2004. Available at <nyti.ms/2jmox5W>.

CINEMATIC AIRS
Christopher Turner

In Aldous Huxley's dystopian novel, *Brave New World* (1932), the Bureau of Propaganda has invented the "feelies," which bring tactile effects to popular entertainment. By holding special knobs on their chairs, audience members could enjoy titillating experiences such as "a love scene on a bearskin rug" between "a gigantic negro and a golden-haired young brachycephalic Beta-Plus female," almost as if they were there. In 1929, Huxley had seen his first talkie, *The Jazz Singer* (1927), which he described as "the latest and most frightful creation-saving device for the production of standardized amusement." He was dismissive of the movies, believing cinemas were great factories of political distraction, where crowds soaked in "the tepid bath of nonsense. No mental effort is demanded of them, no participation; they need only sit and keep their eyes open."

In the novel, Huxley's central character attends a screening of the feely *Three Weeks in a Helicopter*, billed as: "AN ALL-SUPER-SINGING, SYNTHETIC-TALKING, COLOURED, STEREOSCOPIC FEELY WITH SYCHRONISED SCENT-ORGAN ACCOMPANIMENT." This introduction of smell into theater was not without precedent. In 1868, for a production of *The Fairy Acorn Tree*, smells were dispensed around the Alhambra Theatre in London with "vapourisers." And it is at the Alhambra where *Three Weeks in a Helicopter* is screened in the novel. Oscar Wilde, considering the staging for an 1892 production of his play *Salome*, imagined "in place of an orchestra, braziers of perfume … a new perfume for each emotion," and during MGM's *Hollywood Revue* (1928), an orange aroma was released when Charles King sang "Orange Blossom Tree."

Huxley's feely, described by one character as "first-rate," begins with an overture played on the scent-organ, to which the audience sniff and listen, transported by a "delightfully refreshing Herbal Capriccio—rippling arpeggios of thyme and lavender, of rosemary, basil, myrtle, tarragon; a series of daring modulations through the spice keys into ambergris; and a slow return through sandalwood, camphor, cedar and new-mown hay (with occasional subtle touches of discord—a whiff of kidney pudding, the faintest suspicion of pig's dung)." The film, in accordance with a culture that uses free love and sexual satisfaction as a form of social control, soon descends into pornography, and it remains unclear what role smell plays in the gymnastic gyrations that send an electric thrill through the audience. Other polysensuous extravaganzas referred to in the novel include "the famous all-howling stereoscopic feely of the gorilla's wedding" and *The Sperm Whale's Love-Life*, which made joking reference to contemporary science documentaries, a form Huxley actually admired, including his purported favorite, *The Sex Life of Lobsters*.

In 1938, Huxley emigrated to Hollywood, where, ironically given his disdain for cinema, he worked as a scriptwriter. He was tasked mainly with adapting literary classics, but also attempted, unsuccessfully, to bring *Brave New World* to the screen. In 1956, he even proposed transforming it into a three-act "musical comedy," complete with numbers like "Everybody's Happy Now" (which all sounds a bit too much like "Springtime for Hitler" in *The Producers*). Despite pitching the idea to his friend Charlie Chaplin, this bizarre scheme unfortunately also went unrealized. Notably, in his script, Huxley made the choice not to stage the feelies, deeming the representation of its multisensuous possibilities unfeasible on screen. However, in 1959, influenced by Huxley, two American films were made that used ambitious technology in the attempt to do just that, by introducing smell to cinema. The poster for one proclaimed: "FIRST They moved (1893) THEN They talked (1927) NOW They smell (1959)." The films premiered in December 1959 and January 1960, and the press dubbed their rivalry "The Battle of the Smellies."

The two films were *Behind the Great Wall*, made with the Aromarama system, conceived and developed by public relations executive Charles Weiss; and *Scent of Mystery*, which used the Smell-O-Vision process promoted by Mike Todd Jr., son of the legendary theatrical impresario and producer of the same name. By the late 1950s, television was in ascendency, and the movies sought to innovate—with 3-D, wraparound 360-degree screens, and the "smellies"—in order to

Opposite: Promotional material for *Scent of Mystery*, directed by Jack Cardiff, 1960. Courtesy Redwind Productions.

MICHAEL TODD JR.'S
SCENT OF MYSTERY
IN GLORIOUS
SMELL-O-VISION!
INCLUDING FOR THE FIRST TIME
IN ANY SOUVENIR BOOK
A HI-QUALITY LONG PLAYING RECORD.
THE HIT TUNES WITH LYRICS FROM
SCENT OF MYSTERY

see off this existential threat. Weiss showcased his technology, which used aerosol canisters to inject fragrances into the cinema's general air supply system, with a travelogue, a sweeping panorama of China featuring Buddhist temples and Mongol warriors that had already won prizes at the Venice Film Festival and the Brussels World's Fair. It was given a smell track that featured the aromas of floral processions, fireworks, and construction sites, the spicy scents of Hong Kong's street markets, and the burned resin odors of a tiger hunt.

The documentary was first shown in December 1959 at the DeMille Theater in New York, which was converted for the task at the cost of $7,500. A triggering device was connected to the projector and electronic precipitators acted as "deodorizers" to filter the air between smells. However, the *New York Post* wrote: "The great green outdoors upon one occasion came through as celery tonic." Bosley Crowther in the *New York Times* further elaborated on the film's flaws: "In between the suffusions of odors, the air in the theatre is cleared by a purifying treatment that itself leaves a sticky sweet smell, which tends to become upsetting before the film has run its full two hours. When this viewer emerged from the theatre, he happily filled his lungs with that lovely fume-laden New York ozone. It never has smelled so good."

In contrast, the more sophisticated Smell-O-Vision process, used for the comedy-mystery film *Scent of Mystery*, cost $30,000 to install and allowed smells to dissipate naturally into the air. The odors were manufactured by Professor Hans Laube, a former advertising executive from Switzerland turned "world-renowned osmologist." According to his daughter, Carmen, he thought that everything had a smell, including emotions; he once asked her to throw open the window because the room stank of ego. Laube was the inventor of a method for clearing the air in large auditoriums, and a logical extension was that he could also pipe smells in. He had shown what he called a Scentovision film, featuring several odors, as early as 1939 in the Swiss pavilion at the New York World's Fair, which was also host to Michael Todd's Hall of Music, featuring live performances by Gypsy Rose Lee. The Todds, known for their theatrical stunts and pioneering new processes, had been contemplating making a smell film for almost a decade, but it is unclear whether they first got wind of a feasible technology there. In 1943, the

New York Times reported that Scentovision "produced odors as quickly and easily as the soundtrack of a film produces sound."

There is a publicity picture of Todd Jr. and Laube sitting either side of the Smell-O-Vision master control system, or "scent energizer," which resembled a complex piece of scientific machinery. It was described in the souvenir program as a "mechanical monster": "Made of stainless steel, specially treated rubber, and glass, it looks like something out of an Atomic plant." The device, manufactured by Belock Instrument Corporation, housed a carousel of eight-inch vials each containing the highly concentrated essence of a specific scent, and had a bank of dials to regulate the concentration of odors. The 1,100-seat Todd Cinestage Theatre in Chicago, which Todd Sr. had bought and fitted with a wide, curved screen to show *Around the World in Eighty Days* (1956), was used as a laboratory for the new technology. On the back of each seat was fitted a tiny, black pipe, about three-quarters of an inch in diameter, with a spray nozzle at the tip to project smells to the viewer. A mile of pipework ran under the floor, and each nozzle was connected to the "smell brain," the huge dispensing machine that stored all the aromas to be projected. An extra track on the film carried the smell signal, which would send an electronic pulse to trigger the mechanism. A needle would then draw two centiliters of concentrate, enough to fill the auditorium, and with a faint hissing sound, right on cue, a small cloud of aroma would reach every seat in the house simultaneously.

Scent of Mystery was directed by the British director Jack Cardiff, who was known as the "Grand Master of Technicolor." He had worked as a cinematographer for Michael Powell and Emeric Pressburger on *Black Narcissus* (1947), for which he won an Oscar, and *The Red Shoes* (1948), and he had joined John Huston in an awkward tropical shoot for *The African Queen* (1951). Cardiff had just made the move to directing when Todd Sr., who had wrapped *Around the World in Eighty Days*, approached him to make an adaptation of *Don Quixote*. However, Todd died in a plane crash over New Mexico in March 1958, and the project was shelved. His son, who was keen (and now able) to emerge from his showman father's shadow, approached him to make *Scent of Mystery* instead. Cardiff was enthusiastic about shooting a $2 million "picture for the third sense." In the 1930s, he had made travelogues

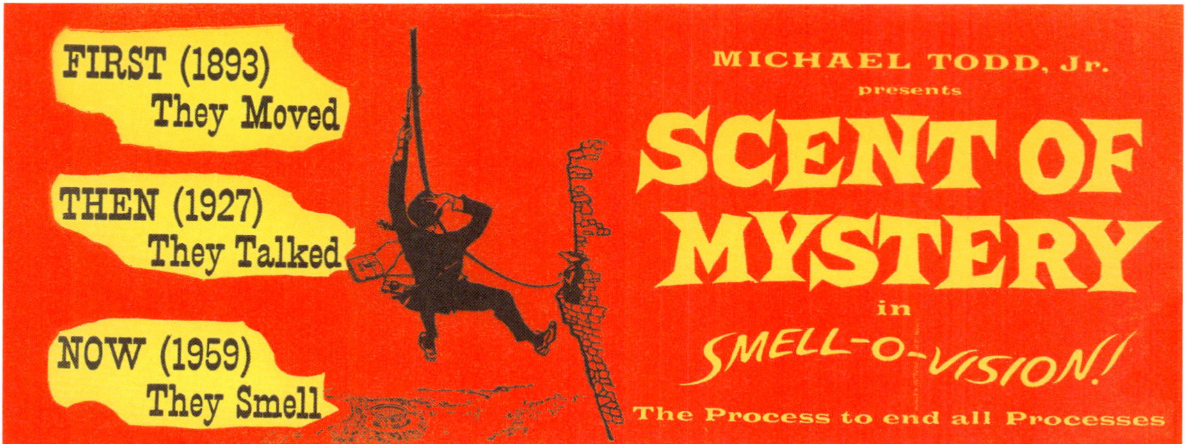

about Rome, Naples, Jerusalem, and the Bedouin in the Jordanian desert, and he decided to shoot the film entirely on location in Spain. (Todd Jr. had also first distinguished himself as the unit manager for documentary sequences about Niagara Falls and the canals of Venice.) It was shot using the special, widescreen "70mm Todd Process Camera," which gave an uncanny depth of field, adding an effect of hyperreality to the sumptuous Spanish scenery.

I had been trying to track down *Scent of Mystery* for years—it was missing from the British Film Institute archive, and all others I consulted—and I once wrote to Cardiff to ask if he had his own copies of the reels, but he was too ill to reply. (He died in 2009.) However, the film was recently reissued on DVD by Redwind Productions as *Holiday in Spain*—without the smell track, of course. It was amusing to watch it with only the illustrated list of thirty smells, printed in the program that accompanied the original screening of *Scent of Mystery*, to indicate the odors, without any clue as to when to expect them. (Helpfully, this souvenir pamphlet is reproduced with the DVD.) The dramatic point of crucial scenes was woven into the actual presence of a smell. For example, the camera lingers on bread for an unnaturally long shot, and you know that you're supposed to smell the delights of baking; or, a villain runs down a staircase to escape several rumbling casks, which crush him, and the camera pauses on his lifeless body, pickled in what you know to be the strong aroma of wine.

In 1981, John Waters released *Polyester* with an "Odorama" scratch-and-sniff card that parodied things like Smell-O-Vision. Waters's storyline featured Divine

as Francine Fishpaw, a *renifleur*—someone who is sexually gratified by odors—and the audience had to scratch the smell card when the corresponding number flashed up on screen. These included the smell of farts, socks, and roses, that were basically distinguishable in scratch and sniff only as sweet and sour. I could imagine the illustrated list of smells for *Scent of Mystery* as a similarly pungent board game, every move on which secreted an olfactory delight: "1. The faint smell of a yellow rose 2. The delectable mouth watering scent of a peach 3. The strong sharpness of wood shavings 4. Happy odor of baking bread 5. The strong pungency of a banana." There was also garlic, wine, gasoline, talcum powder, gun smoke, brandy, incense, train fumes, and even fresh air.

The film opens with a drifting, panning shot, made from a helicopter-borne camera, that follows a superimposed butterfly as it flutters into the garden of the Alhambra (appropriately the name of the cinema where *Three Weeks in a Helicopter* is screened in *Brave New World*). It alights on a flower, and the audience would have received their first smell, a rose-scented whiff of perfumed air. The second aroma would have hit them when they first encounter Peter Lorre, who plays a taxi driver and is leaning against his car devouring a ripe peach. Lorre, a fat, squat man with bulging, rolling eyes, was perhaps best known for playing a pedophile in Fritz Lang's *M* (1931). He suffered a sudden heart attack during filming in Cordoba. Local doctors diagnosed him with blocked arteries, which they alleviated

---

Above: "The process to end all processes!" Promotional material for *Scent of Mystery*.

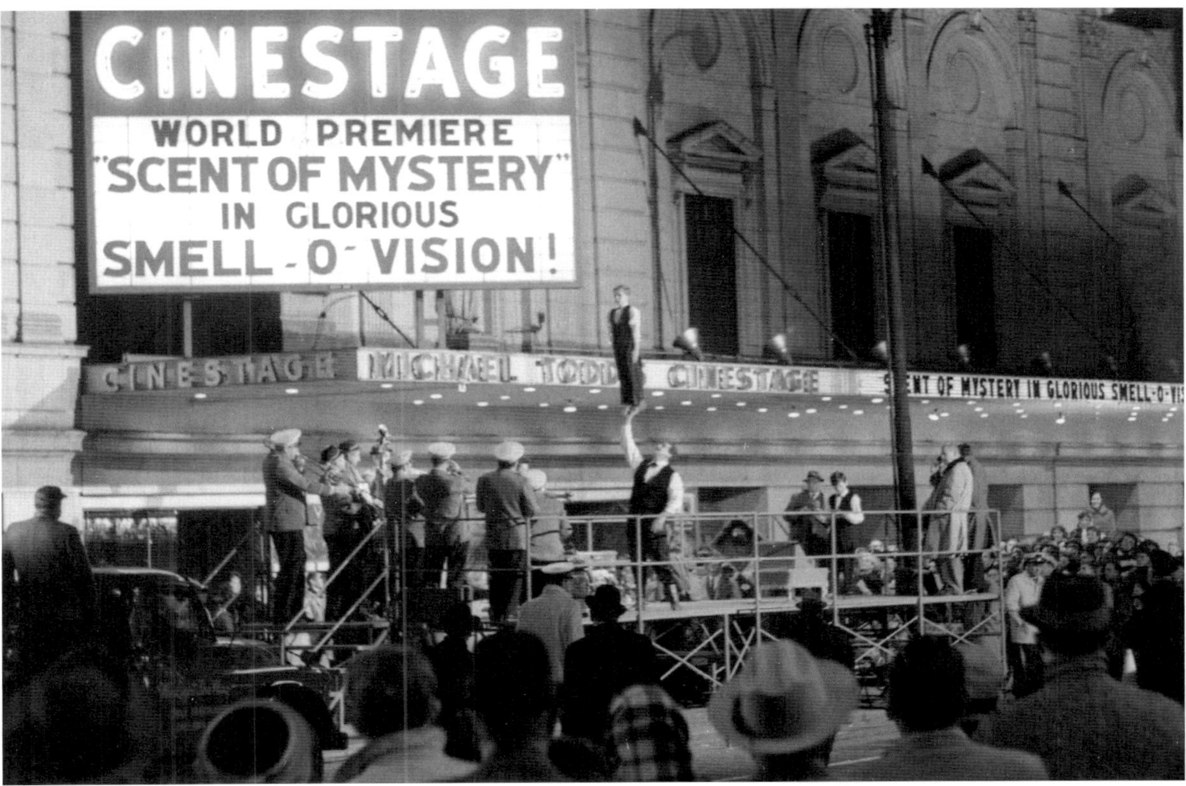

by using bloodletting, an ancient technique that seemed to work. Cardiff had to advertise for a Spanish double to cover him until he could return to the set and, even then, to do any running or other exertion.

The audience had to wait for smell No. 9, "The rare and exotic Scent of Mystery perfume," for the crucial, recurring clue to solving the murder mystery that unfolds. Our hero, Denholm Elliott (Cardiff originally cast Peter Sellers, a suggestion Todd rejected, and one can't help wishing it was him in the role), has seen a mystery woman in a large hat walking away from him and, having apparently fallen in love with her on the basis of her lingering smell, believes she is in great danger. He spends the entire movie chasing this elusive scent around Spain, shadowed by the murderer, who is identifiable from his tobacco smoke. Eventually, after sliding down a wire using his umbrella to save her from certain death, we smell No. 30, the "final wonderful and beautiful fragrance of Scent of Mystery." (One can also smell the money of the

potential marketing opportunity of the corresponding fragrance). The woman, whom we have only known by her perfume, turns around. She is played by Todd Jr.'s stepmother, Elizabeth Taylor. The movie star, who had been married three times and was recent widowed, was twenty-seven years old and at the height of her beauty and fame. "I'm married to a girl who is a few years my junior," Mike Todd had boasted. "As a matter of fact, she's a few years my junior's junior."

During filming, Cardiff asked Todd Jr. what news he had of the smells that were outlined in the script. He was shocked to discover that Todd had not yet received any samples, and suggested that they should ask for them to be sent to Spain. When Hans Laube finally sent some, well into the shoot, the director was disappointed with the results. "I took out a bottle labeled 'apricots' and inhaled excitedly," he wrote in his memoir, *Magic Hour* (1991). "It smelled of cheap eau-de-Cologne. I tried 'sea ozone.' That too smelled of eau-de-Cologne. Every sample smelled the same: a third-rate perfume, nothing at all like they were supposed to smell." The opening screening in Chicago was only a few months away, but Laube assured them

Above: Smell-O-Vision makes its debut at Chicago's Cinestage on 6 January 1960. Photo Art Shay.

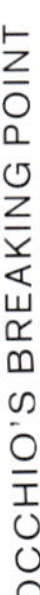

"All we

miere were
nd press,
n as they
experience
d Frank
"Glorious
to end all
he'd made a
nery worked
he only
towards the
e-Cologne."
he Warner
expensively
tion, "all
'It stinks!"
ly, as with
ema, adding
ed that the
been used
ase of the
epiphany, it

ary 1960
d the
enture,
e in the
Cardiff had
(1949), and
bringing
ertiginous
andering
der was
, which had
diff describes
ore the New
l an awful
ditioning,

fiddles with
emiere. The
cts to tubes that
t Shay.
Fisher—married
heroine of
ctory plumbing

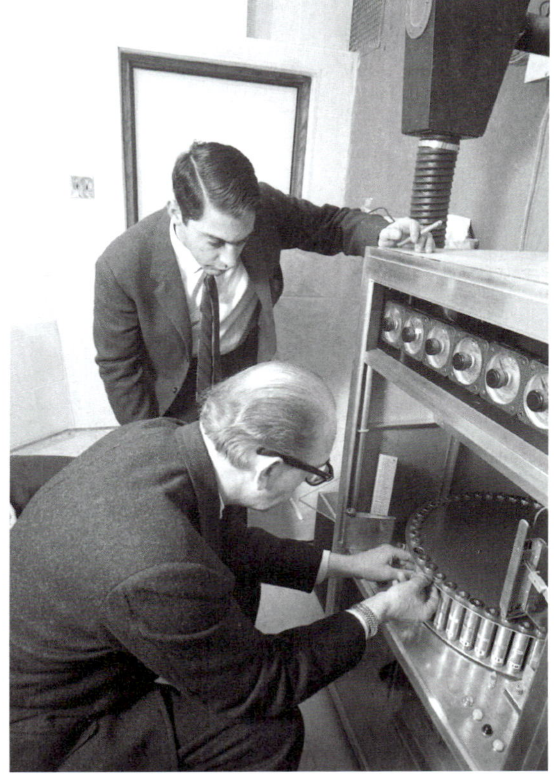

triumphantly advertising his film as 'the first smellie.'"

Cardiff later described the film as a "complete disaster," "the one film I want to erase from my memory," though he maintained that this was through no fault of his own: "It was a very interesting story with a marvelous photographic background of Spain, but the smell, for which it was made, didn't exist." *Sons and Lovers* (1960), for which he won a Golden Globe for best director and was nominated for an Academy award, came out the following year and he preferred to talk about that. In a 1986 interview, Cardiff blamed Laube for the failure, describing the professor as a "phony gentleman … a fake." The "scent energizer" was a version of the machine being operated behind the curtain at the end of *The Wizard of Oz*. "I don't know whether Michael Todd tried to sue him or not, or whether he just took it on the chin," he said.

Todd Jr., looking back on his career, dismissed the film as "just a novelty gimmick." He claimed that even if it had worked, an audience would have only been intrigued by one or two more Smell-O-Vision films. He released the film, without a smell track, as *Holiday in Spain*, but it did little business and the smellies were consigned to an afterlife in theme parks; cinemas reverted to their usual stench of stale popcorn, cigarettes, and hotdogs. For a decade, the Cinestage in Chicago was used to show adult films and, when the city bought it from Elizabeth Taylor in the 1980s, gutting it to make way for a new theater complex, the "smell brain" was still lingering in the basement. As for Laube, according to his daughter: "*Scent of Mystery* was his swan song. He lost all his money, my mom went to work, and he died about 16 years later, penniless and broken."

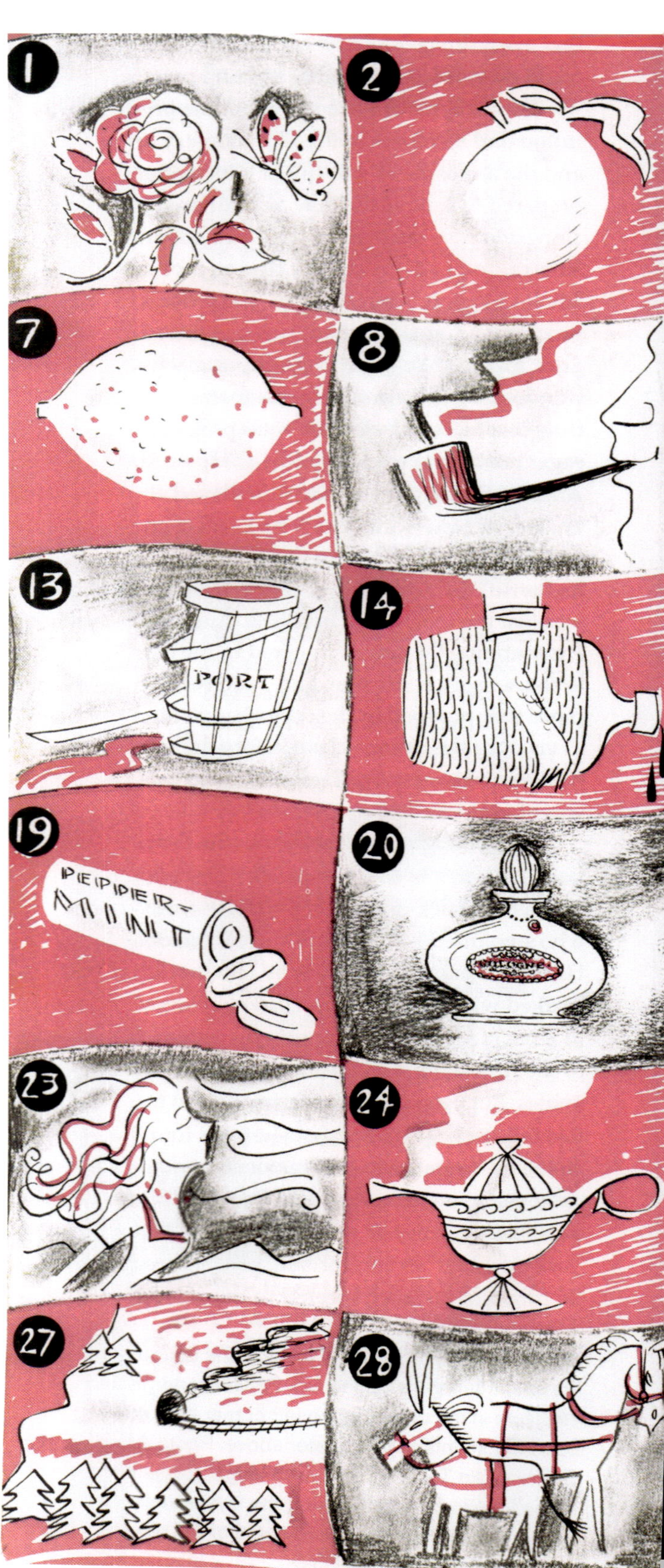

Right: Chart from brochure given out at the premiere listing the thirty scents that were pumped into the cinema for screenings of *Scent of Mystery*. Courtesy Redwind Productions.

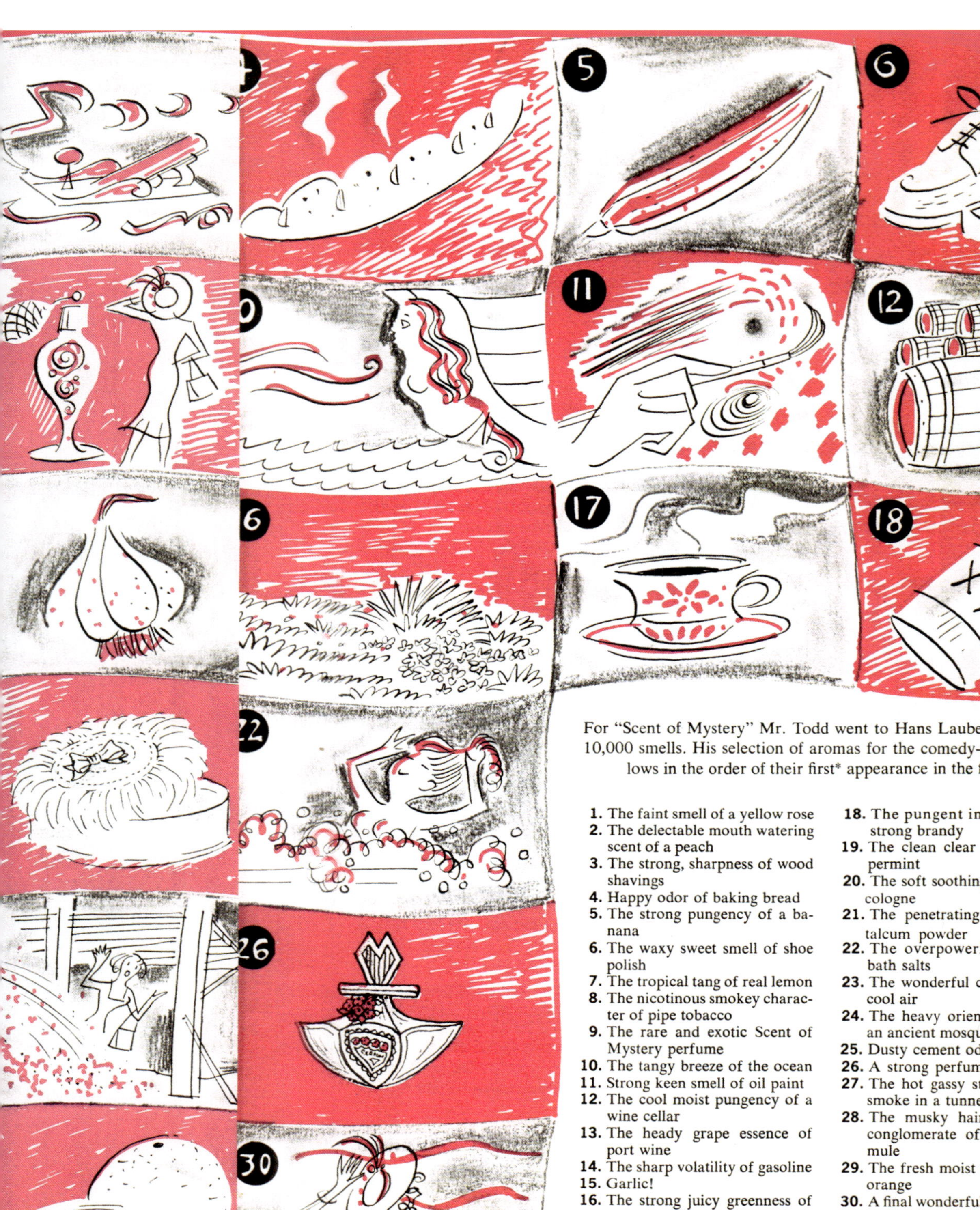

For "Scent of Mystery" Mr. Todd went to Hans Laube's library of 10,000 smells. His selection of aromas for the comedy-mystery follows in the order of their first* appearance in the film.

1. The faint smell of a yellow rose
2. The delectable mouth watering scent of a peach
3. The strong, sharpness of wood shavings
4. Happy odor of baking bread
5. The strong pungency of a banana
6. The waxy sweet smell of shoe polish
7. The tropical tang of real lemon
8. The nicotinous smokey character of pipe tobacco
9. The rare and exotic Scent of Mystery perfume
10. The tangy breeze of the ocean
11. Strong keen smell of oil paint
12. The cool moist pungency of a wine cellar
13. The heady grape essence of port wine
14. The sharp volatility of gasoline
15. Garlic!
16. The strong juicy greenness of clover and grass
17. The bracing exhilaration of steaming coffee
18. The pungent intoxication of strong brandy
19. The clean clear whiff of peppermint
20. The soft soothing fragrance of cologne
21. The penetrating sweetness of talcum powder
22. The overpowering aroma of bath salts
23. The wonderful caress of fresh cool air
24. The heavy oriental incense of an ancient mosque
25. Dusty cement odor of rubble
26. A strong perfume (cheap!)
27. The hot gassy stench of train smoke in a tunnel
28. The musky hair and leather conglomerate of a horse and mule
29. The fresh moist nose tingle of orange
30. A final wonderful and beautiful fragrance of Scent of Mystery

For the list of additional smells in the amusing cartoon "The Tale of Old Whiff" see page 33

*NOTE: *You will recognize some, which appear more than once.*

THE LUMINOSITY OF THE NOSE
D. Graham Burnett

"The Dong with a Luminous Nose" is a verse ballad of one hundred and three lines authored by the eccentric Victorian illustrator, lyricist, and polymorphous sufferer Edward Lear (1812–1888). The poem dates to the mid-1870s. The tone is madcap-moody—a griffin of twee hijinks and misshapen anguish, the sort of odd-words-in-the-mouth sing-song surrealism that gets called "nursery rhyme" or "nonsense verse." Lear and Lewis Carroll are often discussed together in this respect, as roughly contemporary progenitors of something like a veritable genre of English poetry for children that is perhaps not wholly appropriate for children (though children certainly seem to like it). Of the two authors, Lear is the more sentimentally lurid and the more inclined to write of distended or damaged body parts. All in good fun. The kind of good fun that emerges like a gleeful berserker out of a miasmatic swamp of pain and sorrow.

Paradigmatically, "The Dong with a Luminous Nose" recounts the ill-fated love of the eponymous "Dong" for a "Jumbly" girl who visits the Dong's land with others of her kind in a sieve-like vessel. Jumblies have green heads and blue hands and come from far away. The Jumbly sojourn is a whirl of joy:

While the cheerful Jumblies staid;
They danced in circlets all night long,
To the plaintive pipe of the lively Dong,
In moonlight, shine, or shade.
For day and night he was always there
By the side of the Jumbly Girl so fair …

But this idyll is soon clipped:

…the morning came of that hateful day
When the Jumblies sailed in their sieve away,
And the Dong was left on the cruel shore
Gazing—gazing for evermore, …

Within hours, hopeless pining has divested the Dong of right reason ("What little sense I once possessed / Has quite gone out of my head!"). Flushed out onto the infinite wastes of futility, the mad Dong wanders the coastal cliffs and black forests (the "great Gromboolian plain" and the "Hills of the Chankly Bore") piping plaintive dirges:

…"O somewhere, in valley or plain
Might I find my Jumbly Girl again!
For ever I'll seek by lake and shore
Till I find my Jumbly Girl once more!"

And it is here that the poem offers its immortal stroke. The gibbering Dong—exiled by desperation, haunting the nocturnal bluffs—sets to an addled stratagem: he fashions himself a large lighthouse-lantern *which he ties on his face as a prosthetic nose.* The idea is that he will use this awkward contraption as a searchlight in his doomed pursuit. The passage should be cited in its entirety:

And because by night he could not see,
He gathered the bark of the Twangum Tree
On the flowery plain that grows.
And he wove him a wondrous Nose, —
A Nose as strange as a Nose could be!
Of vast proportions and painted red,
And tied with cords to the back of his head.

Thusly accoutered, the quixotic Dong lives out his life as a ghost-glow in the hills, a nightly visitation of outcast longing, a meandering beacon of unfulfilled desire:

And all who watch at the midnight hour,
From Hall or Terrace, or lofty Tower,
Cry, as they trace the Meteor bright,
Moving along through the dreary night, —
"This is the hour when forth he goes,
The Dong with a luminous Nose!
Yonder — over the plain he goes;
He goes!
He goes;
The Dong with a luminous Nose!"

• • •

To clear the way for a proper discussion of this bizarre and affecting text, it is necessary to specify that Lear's use of the term "Dong" significantly predates the

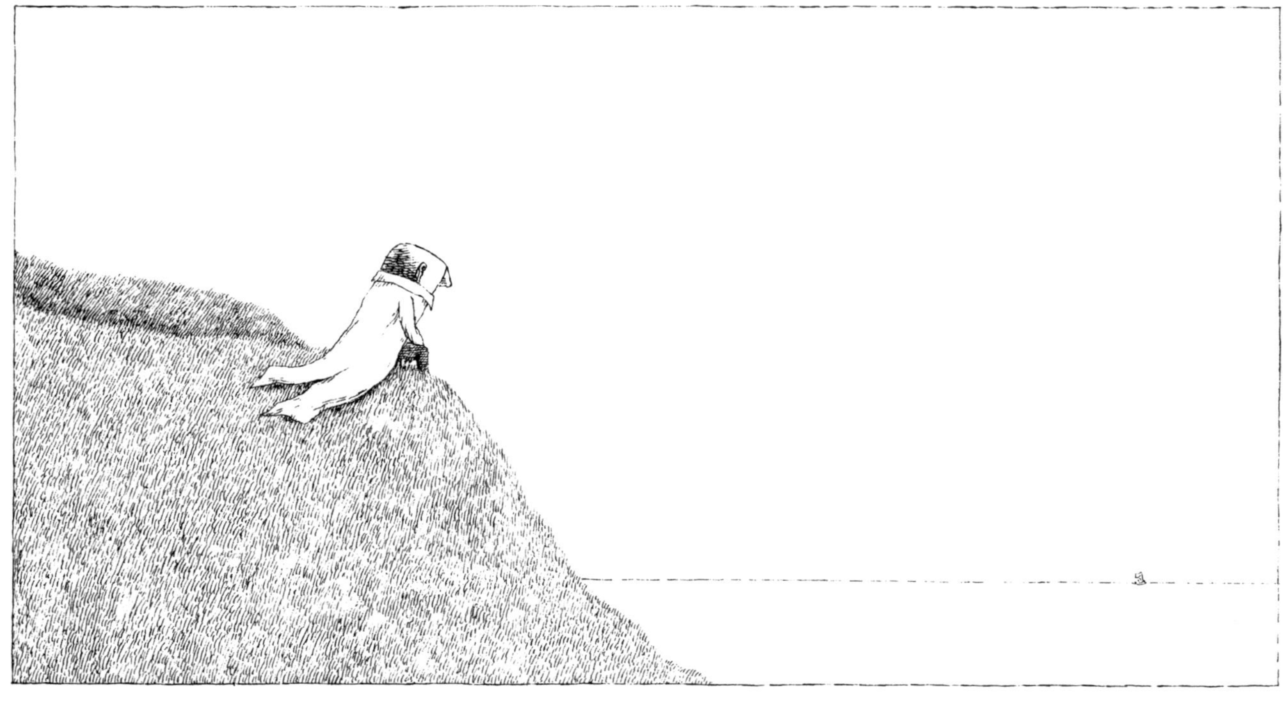

The Dong, pre-prosthesis, looks on as his Jumbly Girl
sails away.

first recorded slang usage of this word to refer to the
human penis (which dates to the interwar period). Nor
does the emergence of that bit of scurrilous argot in
the 1930s seem in any way linked to Lear's poem. In
other words, Lear neither drew on nor (as best as can
be determined) contributed to the modern cock-lexicon.
A vague air of smirk that unfortunately attaches to the
poem among contemporary readers on account of these
prurient connotations must thus be thoroughly venti-
lated if we are to access the original force and mood of
"The Dong with a Luminous Nose."

That said, commentators on the poem have been,
predictably, nearly unanimous in referencing the
phallic registers of the story. And this can hardly
be called wrong. It would be impossible entirely
to dismiss the psychological and biographical
interpretations that engage the Dong in this way.
So let us make haste both to acknowledge and then
to move past such considerations: yes, Lear had a
complicated relationship to his sexual identity, as his
biographers have documented with a scrupulousness
rivaling Lear's own detailed diaries; yes, he seems
to have been a "repressed" "homosexual" of an
identifiably tormented-Victorian variety; yes, he
experienced epileptic seizures across his life, which
seizures he appears to have believed were precipitated
by masturbation (and maybe other forms of sexual
arousal as well); yes, he wrote and illustrated a large
body of limericks, a disproportionate number of which
feature characters with large, misshapen, or bandaged
proboscises; yes, the prosthetic nature of the Dong's
nose-thing merits attention in the context of Lear's
sexual ambivalence (his own drawing of it depicts,
rather suggestively, less a nose-phallus than a kind of
nose-yoni); and finally, yes, castration anxieties are
arguably legible in the tale as a whole, particularly
when it is read against other imagery in Lear's
output—both visual and textual.

And so, in the context of these acknowledgements,
can "The Dong with a Luminous Nose" be read
as a more or less thinly veiled allegory of Lear's
abortive romantic relations with Augusta Bethell?
(Lear evidently allowed himself a dalliance with the
come-hither siren of a conventional married life.)
Yes, it would seem such a reading must be admitted.
And, going further, can the Dong be understood as a
charged figure for the lonely, ostracizing flamboyance
of non-heteronormative sexuality in one of its notable

performative accommodations to a (hostile) dominant
culture? Yes again—to some extent, presumably.

Reductive versions of the above interpretive lines
are easy to imagine. And indeed, most of them need
not be imagined, as they can actually be read in what
is now a rather large scholarly literature on Lear generally, and the Dong specifically. But we are also in
possession of a considerable number of non-reductive
treatments of the poem that inevitably cover much
of the same terrain. One thinks of Thomas Byrom's
lovely invocation of the Dong's "admirable, recreative
courage" as he confronts the futility and failure of
mondaine love—an interpretation echoed by Ina Rae
Hark, who reads the poem as a strained and painfully
self-conscious satire upon all those who cannot accommodate themselves to an existence that, in the words of
Lear, can neither be "cured" nor "cursed."[1] In a superb
essay on Lear's relationship to the Romantic tradition,
Michael O'Neill detects echoes of Shelley, Wordsworth,
and Coleridge in the fate of the Dong, as well as in the
language Lear uses to invoke his lost worlds; in the
poem's bulbous red semaphore of longing, O'Neill
senses both a barely sublated "sweaty" sensuality
together with the exquisite tenderness of a Romantic
"send-up" that "more than shivers with a frisson of the
real thing."[2] All of this feels quite correct.

But does any of this take the Dong's nose seriously
as a nose? A recent line of critical literature has turned
to Lear's work within the context of an emergent
"rhinology," and worked to recover the nose-ness
of the Dong's nose out from under nearly half a
century of Freudian, Jungian, and queer-theoretical
accretion. And so we have Hellen Giblin-Jowett
insisting directly, in her 2014 study "Smell, Smells
and Smelling in Victorian Supernatural Fiction of the
Fin de Siècle," that "despite customary interpretations
of Lear's Dong's luminous nose, *it is still possible to read
the Dong's nose as a nose*."[3] This oblique reference to the
Freudian limits of Freudian interpretation ("sometimes
a cigar is just a cigar") serves as the hinge by which
Giblin-Jowett opens onto the history of rhinoplasty, a
topic not previously dealt with in any detail in relation
to the poem—but not as irrelevant as it might seem.

This new nose literature is inextricable from a
larger interdisciplinary push toward the "history of the
senses," where a key question has for years been the
place of odor in the contested dynamics of modernism.[4]
While a concern with smell clearly plays a significant

role in the hygienic reforms of bourgeois urban culture in the second half of the nineteenth century, some scholars have of late contrasted this strain of scent-rectitude with a decadent countercurrent—one that wallowed in olfactory extremes as a form of active resistance to the odorless norms of an emergent modernity. While the Dong's nose certainly has about it more than a whiff of priapic outlawry, it must be conceded that smell-as-such has surprisingly little place in the poem.[5] To be sure, the notion of the Dong's seeking his beloved *by means of his nose* cannot but invoke scent trails and bloodhounds and the animal stirrings of olfactory desire. And yet, the poem would seem ultimately to sidestep any real engagement with smell itself. Indeed, we can go further. The poem can in fact be read as effecting a direct substitution of ocularity for olfaction, *replacing* a smelling nose with an appurtenance contrived to aid vision.[6] In this sense, "The Dong with a Luminous Nose" must be understood to participate in, and perhaps even advance, the general privileging of opticality in the domains of sense—a hegemonic philosophical and aesthetic program that only came under real critical scrutiny in the twentieth century.[7]

In a beautiful essay from 1953 entitled "Eyes and Noses," Muriel Spark quite explicitly dismissed this heavy historical torrent of eye-talk with a wave (Windows on the soul? "A fallacy; they are the windows of moods and inclinings, alarums and excursions, which act only as a magnet to more adjectives"), before electing the nose as nothing less than the probable seat of the human soul. The nose is, she declares, "our tether between spirit and substance, Heaven and Earth."[8] It is into the nose, more specifically into our nostrils, that the God of Genesis breathed the first breath of life: "The first thing that happened to Adam happened to his nose. Therefore the nose is an emblem at once of our dusty origin and our divine." Why do infants reach for noses? she asks. Because reflexively (in their angelic purity) "they doubt whether we have got souls, like themselves." By these lights, a false nose must be understood as nothing less than heresy, and Spark thereby indicts the Dong as a luciferous evasion.

Whether we would go so far or no, Spark's discussion helpfully elevates the Dong's nose-matters out of both the perfervid nightmare of *A Clockwork Orange* and the roadhouse doggerel of the man from Nantucket. At a stroke, we are reminded of the odd but undeniable philosophical seriousness of noses. This goes quite beyond the remarkable alethic mythos of Pinocchio, whose nose, after all, serves as nothing less than an *actual index of veracity*—a kind of eversion of the apodictic/epistemic organ/instrument for which Descartes searched desperately from within the black vertigo of a skeptical crisis. And beyond the bent physiognomy by which Herman Melville recast the Sperm Whale's nose-less/all-nose face into a figure for God and Satan at once. We are cast back, via the nose, to the linked problems of causality, free will, and determinism—classically epitomized within the Western tradition in the philosophical set-piece of Cleopatra's notorious nose, from which was understood to hang the Western tradition as such.[9] Nor are these metaphysical nose-problems merely antiquarian oddments. I was quite surprised to discover a recent line of work in analytic philosophy that hinges on a set of thought experiments involving dogs with luminous noses.[10] At issue? Teleology itself—the hardest question of all. The one that sits at the intersection of technical metaphysics and speculative theology.

All of which is only to suggest that a more philosophically ambitious interpretation of the Dong may not be unwarranted.

. . .

In this context, then, permit me to suggest a direction for further consideration. I wish to propose the Dong as a tragic figure for the critical limits of critical rationality. If Pinocchio can be understood as wearing the epistemic nose *par excellence* (the nose as unfailing, unflagging *truth-pointer*), the Dong's nose bodies forth the spangled delusions of all navigation by the light of reason. His is literally *the nose of no sense*. But the non-sense of this nose is by no means mere nonsense. On the contrary, it is precise. The Dong's flashing desperation-beacon offers itself as an elegantly structured allegory, figuring reason at the radiant apotheosis of its paralytic-autolytic collapse *into epistemology itself*: reason regarding reason by means of reason; the mirror held to the mirror, in (blank) reflection. Whereas Descartes's hyperbolic quest focused *la lumière naturelle* into a headlamp by which to illuminate self-evident truths, the Dong's hyperbolic quest converts his mind into its own angler-fish, fatally

---

Overleaf: The Dong in full glow.

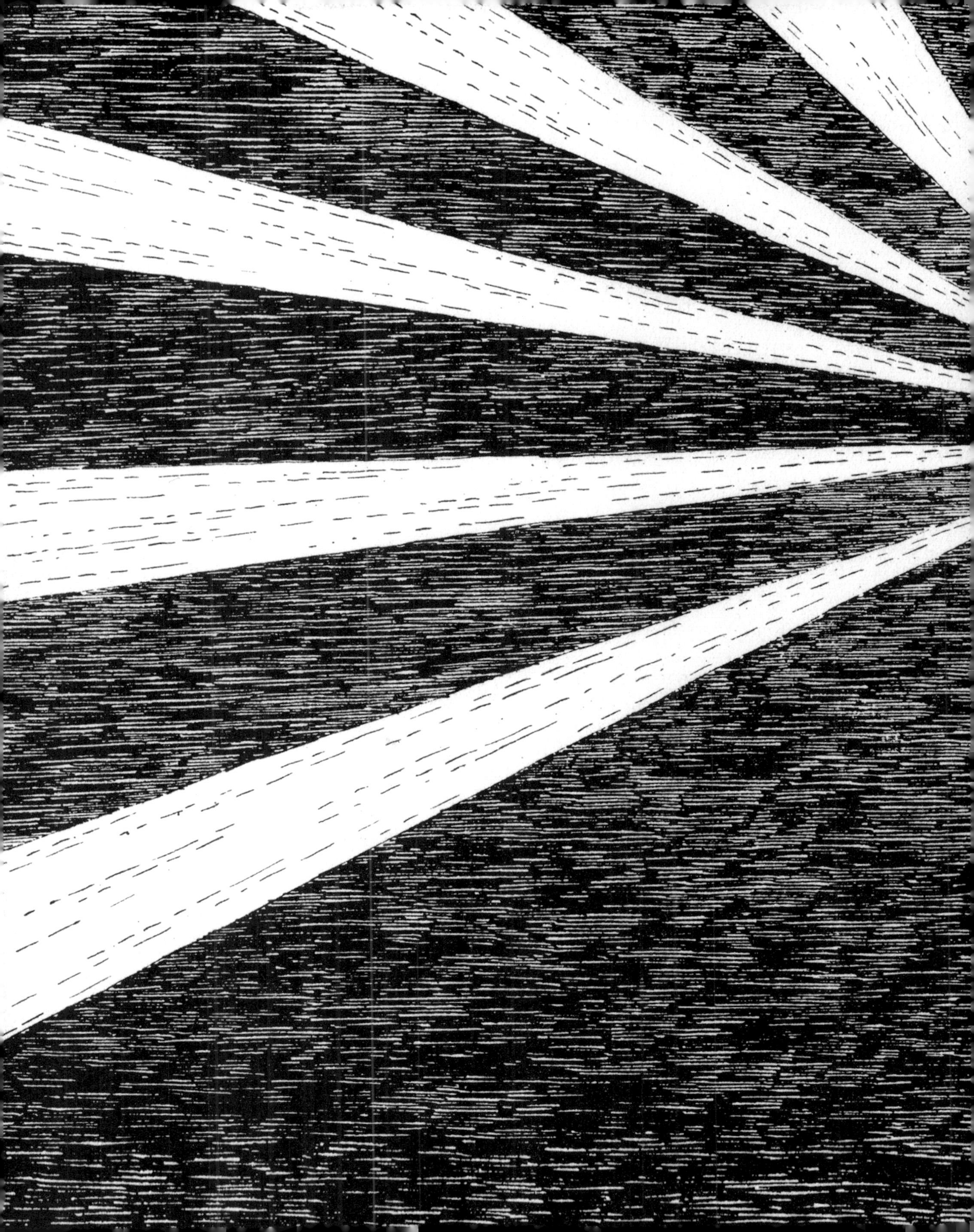

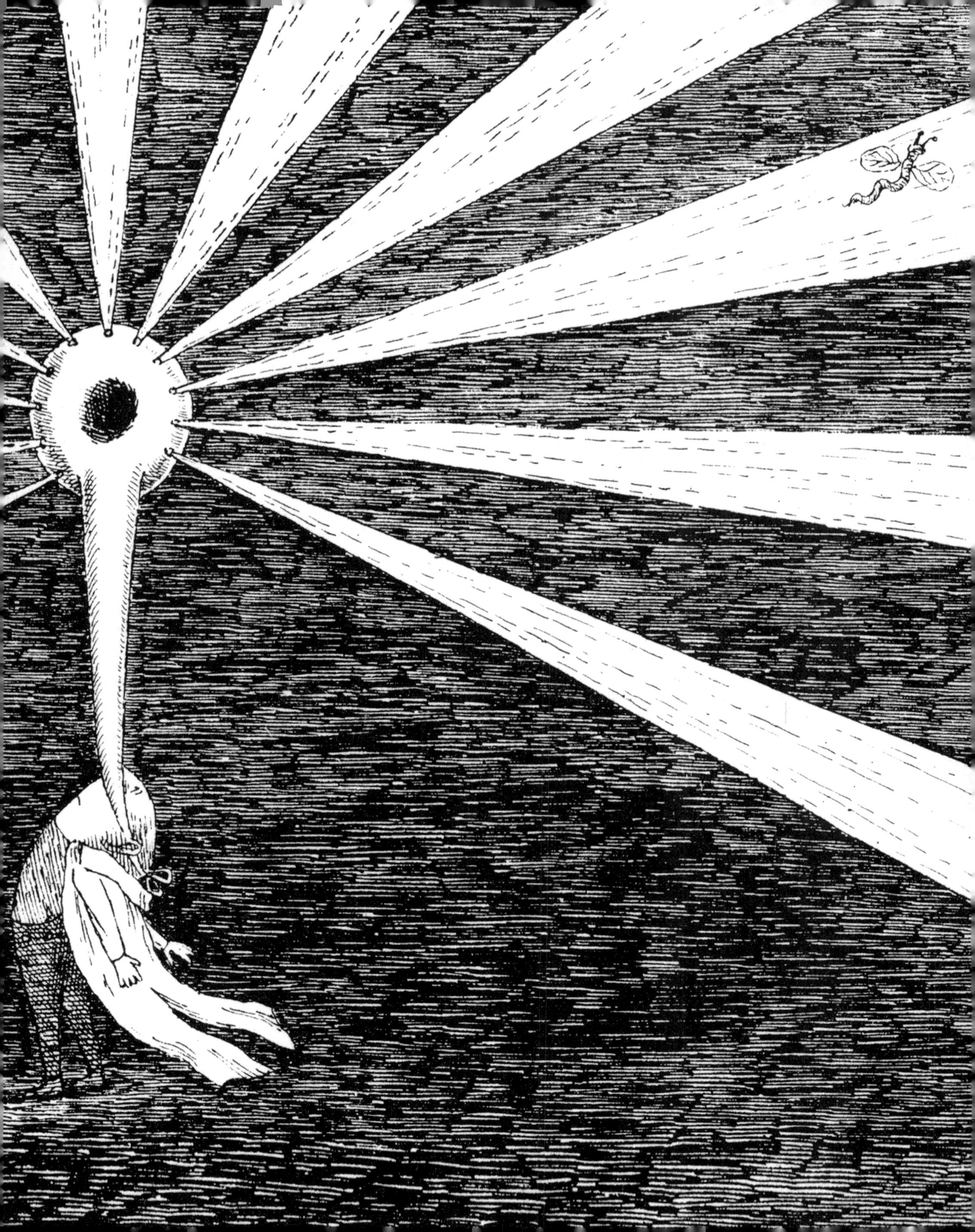

lured to the glow-worm bait at the center of its own visage. The light of reason has here been externalized, and figured as an *ignis fatuus,* equally bewitching and illusory. After all, the Dong's nose—flashing forth its disorienting rays like a laser light show; painting the looming world with streaks of dancing, incoherent luminosity—functions as a continuously blinding spectacle before his very eyes, even as it serves as a perpetual flare forever disclosing his position. Both the futility and the vanity of the involution to philosophical foundationalism would seem here to be simultaneously invoked—together with a sly nod to the notion that the narcissism of first philosophy always has its tragic origins in a displacement or compensation.

To sense the full torque of Lear's pivot on the traditional symbolic repertoire of the "light of reason," we must consider the Dong's nose in the context of two significant visual prosthetics, each of which it both signals and travesties. On the one hand, we have the whole lineage of actual head-mounted light-sources, from tongues of fire to miner's lamps.[11] For an English artist from the period, one very concrete and particular historical instance would have loomed large: the notorious head-mounted tallow candle said to have been worn by Michelangelo when he worked on his sculptures and paintings by night in solitude.[12] It is quite impossible to imagine that Lear did not hold Michelangelo's pointed pasteboard candle-cap in mind as he conceived (and depicted) the Dong's luminous accoutrement. On the other hand, we have the absolutely stereotypical head-encumbrance of every medical doctor in the nineteenth century: the "head mirror," that familiar concave reflective dish *pierced at the center* (very much like Lear's representation of the Dong's prosthetic) and used to direct light into the dark cavities of a body under investigation. Each of these devices, the head-lamp and the head-mirror, attaches to the crown of the user and extends or supplements vision: the lamp by throwing light, the mirror by reflecting it. The former, in its connection to the deep mythos of artistic representation, invokes creative power—the nocturnal demiurge that sees, and, in seeing, makes. The latter, serving as the escutcheon of medical diagnostic inquiry, invokes analytic scrutiny—the forensic gaze that will penetrate mere appearance to unveil hidden truths. Together these vision-enhancing head-devices, both the lamp

and the mirror, reify the optical aspirations of reason itself. The brilliance of Lear's patty-cake apocalypse lies in the massive leverage it brings to bear on that figural program—by means of the tiniest displacement in the fulcrum. The short move from the forehead to the nose is here nothing less than a move from insight to blindness. The Dong's is thus the nose of hysterical reason: the nose that cuts itself off to spite its face.

• • •

That might be all. But perhaps not. This juxtaposition of head-lamps and head-mirrors brings to mind the central conceit of one of the most significant works of literary criticism in the postwar period, *The Mirror and the Lamp: Romantic Theory and the Critical Tradition.* There, the American critic M. H. Abrams argued persuasively that the artistic and intellectual upheavals of the early nineteenth century were inscribed in a broad change in the dominant metaphors used to figure the mind in the canonical texts of the period: grossly speaking, out went the Platonizing image of the mind-as-mirror (which epitomized the aspirations of the mimetic paradigm itself, and with it the dream of an art that could be "true to nature"); in came the Romantic image of the mind as a shining lamp (which dramatized a new emphasis on the projective genius of the artist's vision, and with it an art of "pure expression"). The move from the mirror to the lamp was in this sense legible as a shift from a poetics of truth to one of meaning, from a readerly world of didactics to one of hermeneutics.

Abrams's central contention feels compelling and right. Right enough that one is left wondering what optical device might figure our own time—post-classical, counter-mimetic, un-Romantic, anti-hermeneutic, perfectly indifferent to didactics. Such a vehicle for our philosophical tenor would need to give us fragmentation, pixilation, vertigo, seriality, pervasiveness, flicker, hide-and-seek. If history proceeds by dialectic, we would hope for an object that can be thought of as a synthetic *Aufhebung* of mirror and lamp.

One thinks, of course, of the *disco ball,* that radiant, Dionysian planet of giddy, flashing disorientation.

And then one takes another look at Lear's depiction of the Dong's bandaged dazzle-proboscis, his flaming planetarium-prosthetic, that orbicular, ray-throwing contraption.

There is something uncanny in the conjunction.

Let me be clear: I do not wish to try to claim that Edward Lear invented the disco ball. The device, which has stimulated dance-hall swooning since the early twentieth century, has its own history. But I do wish to assert that the Dong's luminous *illinx*-beak must be understood in relation to the dominant imagery for the mind in the Western tradition, and that Lear's unsettling vision has given us an indelible figure for the cognitive euphoria-cum-derangement of modernity itself, a figure for the mind without itself, in the lonely meteor of the body. And I would like to go further. The Dong's luminous nose, I contend, is, in a very real way, still with us—hanging before our faces in every discotheque and nightclub in the world, its caterwauling rays announcing the doomed quest for both love and truth, and calling us to self-loss and abandon before the darkness.

1 Thomas Byrom, *Nonsense and Wonder* (New York: Dutton, 1977), p. 178. Edward Lear quoted in Ina Rae Hark, "Eccentricity and Victorian Angst," *Victorian Poetry*, vol. 16, no. 1/2 (Spring–Summer 1978), p. 119.

2 Michael O'Neill, "'One of the Dumms': Edward Lear and Romanticism," in *Edward Lear and the Play of Poetry*, ed. James Williams and Matthew Bevis (Oxford: Oxford University Press, 2016), p. 65.

3 Hellen Giblin-Jowett, "Smell, Smells and Smelling in Victorian Supernatural Fiction of the *Fin de Siècle*" (PhD dissertation, Newcastle University, 2014), p. 83. Italics mine.

4 For a discussion, see *The Nose Book: Representations of the Nose in Literature and the Arts*, ed. Victoria de Rijke, Lene Østermark-Johansen, and Helen Thomas (Middlesex: Middlesex University Press, 2000).

5 See Victoria de Rijke, "*Trompe-nez*: Folk, Fairy Tale and Nonsense Noses—Long, Luminous and Lecherous as Licorice," in *The Nose Book*, ed. Victoria de Rijke et al.

6 Many readers will here think of *Rudolph the Red-Nosed Reindeer*, which similarly depicts a nose that functions as an optical aid. There seems to be no genealogical links between this text (authored in 1939 in the United States) and "The Dong with a Luminous Nose," despite the striking consonances that place the two stories in sympathetic vibration.

7 The canonical discussion remains Martin Jay, *Downcast Eyes: The Denigration of Vision in Twentieth-Century French Thought* (Berkeley: University of California Press, 1993).

8 The essay originally appeared in the *Observer* on 18 January 1953. I am citing the republished version in Muriel Spark, *The Informed Air* (New York: New Directions, 2014).

9 Jimena Canales discusses the trope of Cleopatra's nose in a recent essay on causality. See Jimena Canales, "Cleopatra's Nose—and the Development of World History," in *Uncomfortable Objects*, ed. Mariana Castillo Deball (Bom Dia: Berlin, 2012).

10 The original article is Tania Lombrozo and Susan Carey, "Functional Explanation and the Function of Explanation," *Cognition*, vol. 99, no. 2 (March 2006). Also see the recent discussion in Jacob W. Dink and Lance J. Rips, "Folk Teleology and Its Implications," in *Experimental Metaphysics*, ed. David Rose (London: Bloomsbury Press, 2017), p. 227.

11 Consider, for an overview that focuses on mining lamps, Grant Wheat, "The Story of Underground Lighting," *Proceedings of the Illinois Mining Institute* (1945).

12 Giorgio Vasari, *Lives of the Artists*, trans. Mrs. Jonathan Foster, ed. Marilyn Aronberg Lavin (Mineola, NY: Dover, 2005), p. 194.

Politics stinks, they say. And at certain times more than others. Hence the need for perfumes potent enough to disguise this malodorous state of affairs. Once upon a time, it seems, perfumes would be issued long after the politician had died. For example, in the 1970s Avon brought out a fragrance line whose bottles took the form of heroic busts of George Washington, Thomas Jefferson, Abraham Lincoln, Benjamin Franklin, and Theodore Roosevelt. For its less classically inclined users, Avon also offered both Washington– and Lincoln–themed aftershaves in simpler containers. Nowadays, however, it's more prudent to pre-issue a signature scent that will cover whatever noisomeness your civic career is bound to leave in its trail. Enter Donald Trump's Empire, a fragrance he launched in 2015 just months before he began to wreak havoc with his presidential campaign. The soon-to-be candidate described the name thus: "When a man looks and feels his best he is automatically in a more powerful position. … Every man has his own empire to build. … Empire evokes this masculine drive."

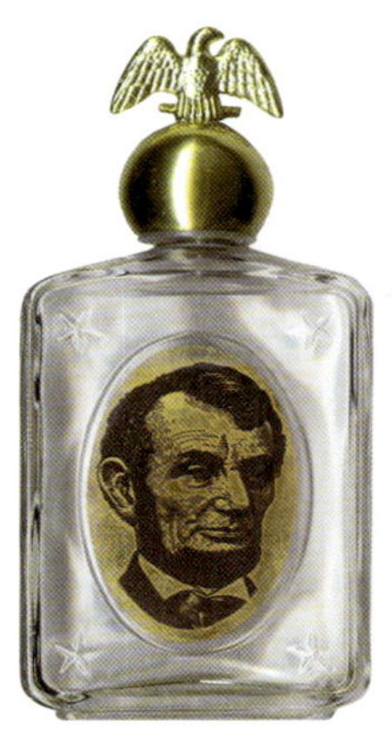
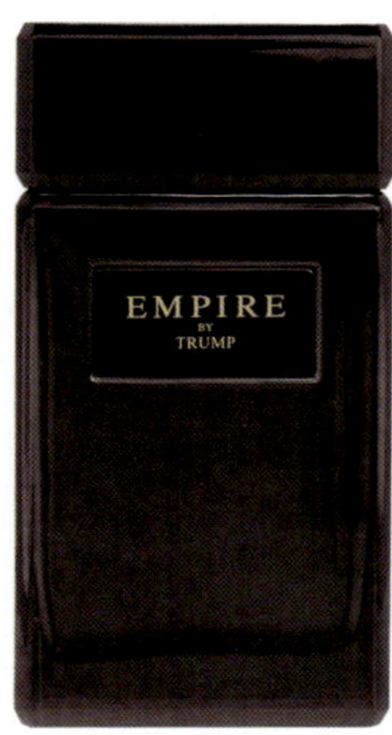

While doing this issue, we had the chance to read Zora Neale Hurston's short essay "Now Take Noses," which was published in a 1939 anthology called *Cordially Yours*. It begins: "Now take the nose for instance. Loyal and kind, from the daybreak of creation down to this present moment, it has stood before man's face and remained his best friend and adviser. … Where goes humanity there goes the faithful nose." If she is right, we apologize in advance to all our noses for where we are leading them.

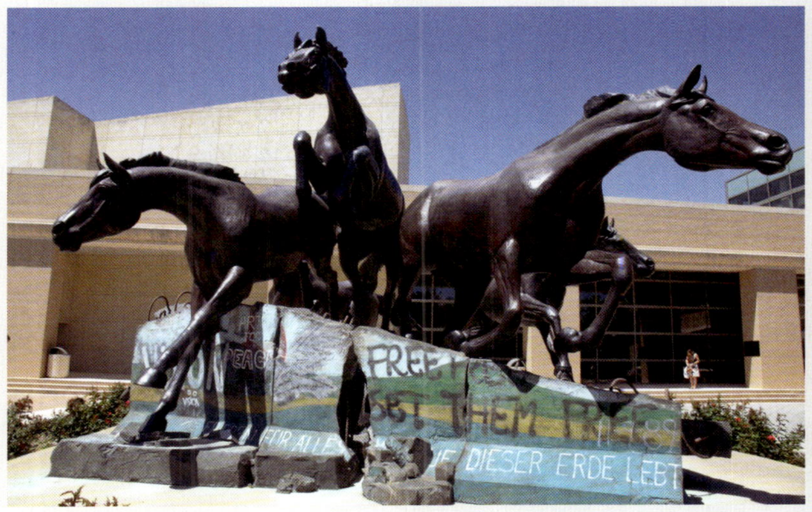

Speaking of empire, a photo of the sculpture that stands in the plaza in front of the presidential library of George H. W. Bush (see "Concrete Politics") could not be printed along with the article because the portion of the Berlin Wall incorporated into the monument is in fact only a facsimile. But we publish it here because any account of postwar German-American relations would be poorer without it. According to the sculptor, "the horses simply represent humanity and the horses represent a victory of the human spirit." Hmm. Horses, noses, humanity. Maybe some enterprising artist can concoct a *Gesamtkunstwerk* that manages to simultaneously evoke Frederic Remington, Nikolai Gogol, and Richard Bach?

While editing this issue's column on the Berlin Wall, we were, coincidentally, demolishing another wall in Berlin. This one was less of an earth-shattering event, for sure, but important nonetheless in our little world. The wall separated two rooms in our soon-to-open office and event space in Berlin, which is located close to the so-called "Red Island," the communist area of the city's Schöneberg district. Marlene Dietrich was born a couple of blocks away, and a few days ago, we saw a commemorative plaque around the corner at 155 Hauptstraße marking the building in which David Bowie lived during his Berlin years.

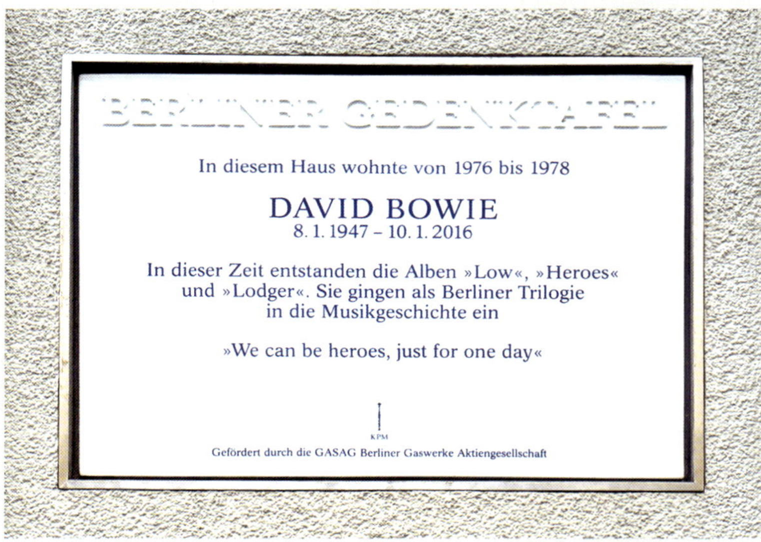

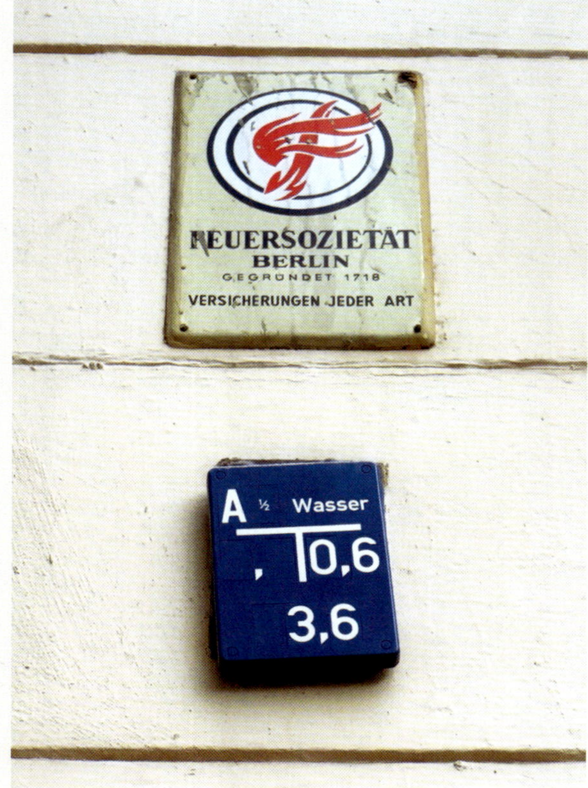

While work continues on the interior of our Berlin office, outside we discovered a different kind of plaque—one announcing that our fire insurance is provided by Feuersozietät Berlin. The sign is suggestive of the fire marks that for centuries were affixed to buildings in the United States and Britain before the advent of municipal fire departments; these marks were designed to allow each private firefighting corps to quickly identify which buildings were covered by the particular insurance company they worked for. (For more on these signs and on the history of fire insurance, see Janet Connelly's "Marks of Assurance" in issue 32.) Feuersozietät Berlin, which was founded by none other than Prussian king Friedrich Wilhelm I (father of Frederick the Great), will celebrate its three-hundredth anniversary in 2018. It was, writes William L. Evenden in *German Fire Marks*, "the first successful public law fire insurance establishment founded by a sovereign in Germany." So we are in good hands, it seems. But all this does not explain why our building's insurance company needs to be announced on its façade. Assuming that the city of Berlin will in fact dispatch its municipal fire department to put out any blazes in the building, who needs to know our insurance status? We will try to sniff out more on this burning topic for a future issue.

e-flux